Nutrition and Health Series

Adrianne Bendich, PhD, FACN, Series Editor

For further volumes:
http://www.springer.com/series/7659

Sherry A. Tanumihardjo
Editor

Carotenoids and Human Health

Humana Press

Editor
Sherry A. Tanumihardjo
Department of Nutritional Sciences
University of Wisconsin-Madison
Madison, WI, USA

ISBN 978-1-4939-5975-4 ISBN 978-1-62703-203-2 (eBook)
DOI 10.1007/978-1-62703-203-2
Springer New York Heidelberg Dordrecht London

Printed on acid-free paper

Humana Press is a brand of Springer
Springer is part of Springer Science+Business Media (www.springer.com)

Carotenoids and Human Health incorporates all areas of research interest to me from basic chemistry to whole body metabolism to public health nutrition. Chapters are written by many esteemed colleagues and friends whom I have met and worked with through the Carotenoid Research Interaction Group (CARIG), the former International Vitamin A Consultative Group (IVACG), and The HarvestPlus Biofortification program and by my colleagues and staff at the University of Wisconsin-Madison. I dedicate this book to my sons, Jeremy, Jacob, and Joel, who have endured significant amounts of time without their mom as she pursued her academic, research, and outreach endeavors to make her contributions in the world for global public health.

Sherry A. Tanumihardjo

Foreword

In 1994, a landmark study on the use of β-carotene for lung cancer prevention was published (The ATBC study) (1). It had been thought that β-carotene supplementation at a high dose would help prevent lung cancer in smokers. Much to the dismay of everyone involved in human carotenoid research, more lung cancers occurred in the β-carotene-supplemented group than in the non-supplemented group. Scientists feared that carotenoid research in humans would grind to an abrupt halt.

It did not turn out that way as this book attests. Due to research advances since 1994, we have learned a tremendous amount about carotenoid bioavailability and provitamin A carotenoid bioconversion to vitamin A. The efficiency of the bioconversion depends on many factors and varies widely depending on the particular food matrix. We can now appreciate with much more certainty the importance of provitamin A carotenoids for globally supplying vitamin A. We have also learned much more about the non-provitamin carotenoids and their links to chronic disease patterns: Cancer, eye disease, and bone disease, in particular. Carotenoids play important roles in immune function and as antioxidants, and these are two of the more likely (but not exclusive) mechanisms to explain the relationships between carotenoids and the lower prevalence of certain chronic diseases.

Owing to the growing recognition that these fascinating food components may be important in health maintenance, several chapters in this remarkable volume have been devoted to the metabolism and breakdown of carotenoids in the human body. Each and every chapter in this book has been well written by a true expert in his or her specific field. This book will be extremely useful for students and health practitioners who want to learn the most current and important research of this colorful group of photochemicals. Life would be very dull without them, indeed!

Boston, MA, USA — Robert M. Russell, MD

Reference

1. ATBC Cancer Prevention Study Group. The effect of vitamin E and β-carotene on the incidence of lung cancer and other cancers in male smokers. N Engl J Med 1994;330:1029–1035

Foreword

Series Editor Page

The great success of the Nutrition and Health Series is the result of the consistent over-riding mission of providing health professionals with texts that are essential because each includes: (1) a synthesis of the state of the science, (2) timely, in-depth reviews by the leading researchers in their respective fields, (3) extensive, up-to-date fully annotated reference lists, (4) a detailed index, (5) relevant tables and figures, (6) identification of paradigm shifts and the consequences, (7) virtually no overlap of information between chapters, but targeted, inter-chapter referrals, (8) suggestions of areas for future research and (9) balanced, data-driven answers to patient as well as health professionals' questions which are based upon the totality of evidence rather than the findings of any single study.

The Series volumes are not the outcome of a symposium. Rather, each editor has the potential to examine a chosen area with a broad perspective, both in subject matter and in the choice of chapter authors. The editor(s), whose training(s) is(are) both research and practice oriented, have the opportunity to develop a primary objective for their book, define the scope and focus, and then invite the leading authorities to be part of their initiative. The authors are encouraged to provide an overview of the field, discuss their own research and relate the research findings to potential human health consequences. Because each book is developed de novo, the chapters are coordinated so that the resulting volume imparts greater knowledge than the sum of the information contained in the individual chapters.

"Carotenoids in Human Health", edited by Sherry A. Tanumihardjo, Ph.D., clearly exemplifies the goals of the Nutrition and Health Series. Carotenoids are ubiquitous yellow, orange and red pigments found mainly in plants and are considered as major contributors to the health benefits associated with diets rich in fruits and vegetables. The major objective of this comprehensive volume is to review the growing evidence that carotenoids are bioactive molecules that can be of value to many aspects of health. The volume includes detailed data on the metabolism and food sources of carotenoids and introduces the reader to the novel plant-breeding activities, biofortification, to increase the concentration of different carotenoids in staple foods. The importance of carotenoids as a source of essential vitamin A for undernourished populations in the developing countries is a primary focus of this volume.

However, it would be highly remiss to not also review the complexities of the published clinical research with regard to supplementation with high-dose β carotene in populations at increased risk for lung cancer. Many years have passed since the ATBC study was published and two chapters in this volume (Chaps. 11 and 12) review the totality of data from relevant clinical studies so that the current and past findings can be placed in the proper perspective, especially with regard to the potential for new data to suggest that certain other carotenoids may have benefit as anti-carcinogenic agents. This up-to-date comprehensive review of the science behind the active molecules in carotenoids, as well as its value as the plant source of vitamin A, is of great importance to the nutrition community as well as for health professionals who have to answer client or patient questions about this area of clinical research.

The 20 chapters in this volume are divided into 3 sections. The first section, containing eight chapters, reviews the food sources of carotenoids and their metabolism. The first chapter reminds us that fruits and vegetables provide nearly 90 % of the carotenoid intake in the US. Of the 700 carotenoids found in nature, only about 50 are present in the human diet and have been identified in the human body. Of these, six carotenoids predominate, β-carotene, α-carotene, β-cryptoxanthin, lycopene, lutein, and zeaxanthin. Only three of the carotenoids, β-carotene, α-carotene, and β-cryptoxanthin, can be converted into retinol (vitamin A) in the body and are referred to as provitamin A carotenoids. The chapter provides references to the major international databases for carotenoid content in commonly consumed foods as well as informative tables. The second chapter, co-authored by the book's editor, describes her research into the potential of increasing the concentration of bioavailable provitamin A carotenoids as well as novel carotenoids that impart unique colors to carrots.

Carrots are a significant source of vitamin A accounting for an estimated 30 % of the dietary vitamin A in the US diet. Breeding efforts to improve food crops through biofortification have increased the nutritional value of this vegetable. The next chapter, also written by a leading investigator in the field of carotenoid metabolism, describes the last 20 years of research concerning the metabolizing enzymes and sites of their activities as well as the mechanisms of transport and absorption of the highly lipophylic carotenoids in humans. The formation of vitamin A and its carrier proteins are discussed in detail as is the storage of carotenoids and vitamin A in the liver. The seven detailed figures included in this chapter aid greatly in the understanding of the complexity of carotenoid metabolism. The importance of carotenoids in the protection of skin and eyes from UV damage is comprehensively reviewed in the next chapter that includes ten excellent figures. The antioxidant and singlet oxygen quenching reactions performed by carotenoids are well-illustrated and their biological significance is reviewed. This detailed chapter includes over 300 references and highly relevant figures and tables.

The next chapter describes the newest research on human carotenoid metabolism using stable isotopes to determine the kinetics of β-carotene and other carotenoids. Data on lycopene, lutein, and zeaxanthin as well as carotenoid mixtures are included. The following chapter describes the effects of other dietary components on carotenoid metabolism. Co-consumption of dietary lipids is an effective stimulator of carotenoid absorption. The presence of dietary fiber reduces the bioavailability of carotenoids. In light of current dietary guidelines that recommend a reduction of fat and an increase in dietary fiber intake, this chapter evaluates the impact of these dietary guidelines on carotenoid bioavailability. In addition to dietary factors affecting carotenoid absorption and metabolism, host factors also can greatly affect carotenoid bioavailability. Host factors can influence the ability to absorb, convert, and metabolize dietary carotenoids. Factors such as gender, body fat, and genetic variation play an important role in this process. The next chapter examines recent discoveries of specific carotenoid-binding proteins, as well as the existence of a diet-responsive regulatory network and the importance of genetic variation on carotenoid status. The last chapter in this section reviews the effects of gender and body composition on carotenoid status and finds that women consuming the same amount of β-carotene as age- and weight-matched men have higher serum β-carotene concentrations. Of interest, individuals with high body mass indices have lower circulating carotenoid levels and potential reasons for these differences are discussed.

The second section, with six chapters, examines the role of carotenoids in human health and begins with the importance of maternal carotenoid intake during pregnancy and lactation. This chapter emphasizes the importance of adequate carotenoid intake to assure optimal vitamin A status for the pregnant woman as well as the growing fetus; carotenoid intake is also of importance during lactation especially in developing countries where dietary sources of preformed vitamin A may not always be available. New data on the potential role of lutein in neonatal retinal function are discussed. The next chapter reviews the development of gametes, ovulation, fertilization and embryogenesis, and placental development. The importance of provitamin A carotenoids is emphasized and when there are data linking β-carotene intake specifically to outcomes, these data are discussed in detail. As mentioned above, Chaps. 11 and 12 examine the role of β-carotene in cancer risk reduction and compare its potential with that of β-cryptoxanthin (another provitamin A carotenoid) and lycopene (a non-provitamin A carotenoid) found mainly in tomatoes. The lycopene chapter contains over 200 relevant references and a comprehensive tabulation of the epidemiological studies linking diets high in lycopene-rich vegetables with reduced risk of many cancers (reminiscent of similar tables that were developed for β-carotene in the 1990s).

Three major age-related eye diseases have been associated with low lutein and zeaxanthin intakes. Lutein and zeaxanthin are found in high concentration in the macula of the retina, and this is the area of the eye that is damaged in the disease called age-related macular degeneration (AMD). Lutein and zeaxanthin are also present in the lens of the eye, which is constantly exposed to light and oxygen. Damage to the lens can result in the formation of a cataract. Retinitis pigmentosa is a disease caused by the destruction of the rod outer segments in the retina. Lutein and zeaxanthin are also present in the rods. Low intakes of foods containing lutein and zeaxanthin are associated with each of these three eye diseases and the mechanisms by which these carotenoids can protect the eye are outlined in the next chapter. The last chapter in this section examines the associations between dietary carotenoid intakes and bone health and also reviews the epidemiological data for vitamin A's effects on bone.

The last section of the volume contains six chapters that explore the global research on the importance of carotenoids in diets that may be low in many essential micronutrients including vitamin A. The first chapter in this section focuses on the public health significance of vitamin A deficiency and the importance of provitamin A carotenoids as dietary sources of vitamin A. Evidence of the efficacy of some of the major dietary interventions undertaken by the World Health Organization for increasing vitamin A status in at-risk populations and the beneficial health consequences is elaborated in the eight excellent tables and figures in this chapter. The importance of maintaining an adequate vitamin A status, especially in very young children, is clearly described in the next chapter that reviews vitamin A's role in immune function.

The final four chapters in the volume describe the newest research into increasing the sources of provitamin A carotenoids in foods, especially for populations in developing countries. Biofortification is the breeding of staple food crops to increase their micronutrient density. Successful provitamin A biofortified varieties must compete with local varieties and must be found equivalent or superior to consumers for all intended uses, including home consumption, and also must improve the vitamin A status of the targeted population. The chapter on orange sweet potato describes the many ways this important staple crop can be marketed, cooked, and preserved as it is an excellent source of provitamin A carotenoids that is well accepted by undernourished African populations. These chapters describe the agricultural, nutritional, food technology, economic, and other research efforts that have resulted in provitamin A biofortified hybrids, such as cassava, beans, sweet potatoes white potatoes and maize. In each chapter, the need to develop an understanding by consumers of the value of carotenoid rich vegetables and the involvement of governmental agencies, public and private institutions, nutrition educators, farmers, and marketers is discussed. The chapters provide a broad overview of how basic and applied sciences are contributing to the alleviation of vitamin A deficiency in underdeveloped, vitamin A-deficient populations.

The final chapter in this critically important volume is written by the editor and Dr. Harold Furr, both well-established researchers in vitamin A deficiency eradication. They remind us that eradication of vitamin A deficiency is a global effort to improve human health and prevent mortality. The chapter reviews the work of the Vitamin A Global Initiative partners that currently include the United Nations Children's Fund (UNICEF), the World Health Organization (WHO), the Canadian International Development Agency (CIDA), the United Kingdom's Department for International Development (DfID), the United States Agency for International Development (USAID), and the Micronutrient Initiative (MI). This chapter, as well as the others in this section, reiterates the importance of dietary carotenoids in the eradication of vitamin A deficiency.

"Carotenoids and Human Health" represents the newest comprehensive compilation of the status of carotenoid research as well as the status of vitamin A deficiency eradication globally. It is to the credit of Dr. Tanumihardjo and her co-authors that this volume provides an in-depth overview of the natural occurrence and biochemistry of the relevant carotenoids in the human diet and includes the latest research on the role of carotenoids and vitamin A in normal development as well as their importance in the potential prevention of certain chronic diseases. Of importance, this volume includes an in-depth review of the safety of β-carotene, related carotenoids, and vitamin A.

The logical sequence of the sections as well as the chapters within each section enhances the understanding of the latest information on the current standards of practice for clinicians, related health professionals including the physicians, dieticians, nurses, pharmacists, public health nutritionists, and others involved in the effort to reduce the adverse consequences of low vitamin A status, especially early in life. This comprehensive volume also has great value for academicians involved in the education of graduate students and post-doctoral fellows, medical students and allied health professionals who plan to interact with patients or clients with disorders that may be beneficially affected by the addition of carotenoid-containing foods or other carotenoid sources to their diets.

Cutting-edge discussions of the roles of signaling molecules, growth factors, hormones, cellular and nuclear receptors, and all of the cells directly involved in carotenoid and retinoid metabolism are included in well-organized chapters that put the molecular aspects into clinical perspective. Of great importance, the authors have provided chapters that balance the most technical information with discussions of the global importance of translational research for improving sources of dietary carotenoids and the consequent health benefits.

The volume contains over 70 detailed tables and figures that assist the reader in comprehending the complexities of the metabolism as well as the biological significance of carotenoids for human health. The over-riding goal of this volume is to provide the health professional with balanced documentation and awareness of the newest research and therapeutic approaches including an appreciation of the complexity of the relatively new field of biofortification. Hallmarks of the 20 chapters include keywords and bulleted key points at the beginning of each chapter, complete definitions of terms with the abbreviations fully defined for the reader, and consistent use of terms between chapters. There are over 1,900 up-to-date references; all chapters include a conclusion to highlight major findings. The volume also contains a highly annotated index.

This unique text provides practical, data-driven resources based upon the totality of the evidence to help the reader understand the basics, treatments, and preventive strategies that are involved in the understanding of the role carotenoids may play in healthy individuals as well as those with chronic, age-related eye diseases, cancer, immunodeficiency, or bone diseases including osteoporosis and osteoarthritis. The overarching goal of the editor is to provide fully referenced information to health professionals so they may have a balanced perspective on the value of various preventive options that are available today as well as in the foreseeable future.

In conclusion, "Carotenoids in Human Health", edited by Sherry A. Tanumihardjo, provides health professionals in many areas of research and practice with the most up-to-date, well-referenced and comprehensive volume on the current state of the science and medical uses of carotenoids with emphasis on the provitamin A carotenoids. This volume will serve the reader as the most authoritative resource in the field to date and is a very welcome addition to the Nutrition and Health Series.

Morristown, NJ, USA Adrianne Bendich, PhD, FACN

Preface

Beyond the provitamin A activity of some carotenoids and adding splashes of color to the world that we live in, carotenoids are still not considered "nutrients". Nonetheless, carotenoids are receiving increased attention as a group of phytochemicals important for optimal health. Vitamin A deficiency, particularly marginal status, continues to plague much of the world. Dietary carotenoids are a significant source of this vitamin and plant-based diets are consumed by populations most at-risk for this deficiency. Providing enhanced crops through agricultural approaches may decrease the prevalence of vitamin A deficiency if widely adopted. The over-arching goal of this book is to convince the reader that carotenoids can contribute to overall health and well-being in addition to their well-known vitamin A function.

The inspiration for *Carotenoids and Human Health* was to provide health-care and nutrition professionals and medical, graduate, and senior undergraduate students with a resource of up-to-date information on carotenoids. The different sections of the book complement each other and provide distinct areas to be used for teaching. The first section, "Carotenoid sources and metabolism", provides essential background for all readers on dietary sources of carotenoids and advanced chapters on antioxidant function, metabolism, and bioavailability that can be used in graduate-level instruction. The second section, "Carotenoids and human health", may be used by practitioners and for senior undergraduate, graduate, and medical school-level courses on the importance of carotenoids in human health and development. This section contains two chapters on pregnancy, lactation, and early life; two chapters on carotenoids and cancer; and two chapters on links of specific carotenoids to eye and bone health. Health-care and nutrition professionals will find this section most informative as they advise patients and clients. Finally, the third section, "International perspectives", is meant for courses on vitamin A and global health by emphasizing the importance of plant-based foods as sources of provitamin A carotenoids. The first two chapters are broad-based and the next three chapters are more crop-specific in an effort to show linkages between agriculture and vitamin A nutrition. The final chapter of this book provides a brief overview of methods to alleviate vitamin A deficiency and reviews some of the organizations that are dedicated to this cause.

In developing the content of this book, international representation was considered key to the success of the volume. In addition to internationally oriented researchers within the US, representations from Africa, Asia, Europe, and Mexico are among the authors. It is hoped that this book will ignite scientists, practitioners, and students to evaluate their work and endeavors in the scheme of global public health. Although carotenoids are not currently considered essential nutrients, as we move from prevention of nutrient deficiency to supporting optimal human health and prevention of disease, evidence presented in this book should compel the reader to contemplate what truly defines a nutrient.

Madison, WI, USA Sherry A. Tanumihardjo

Preface

Biography

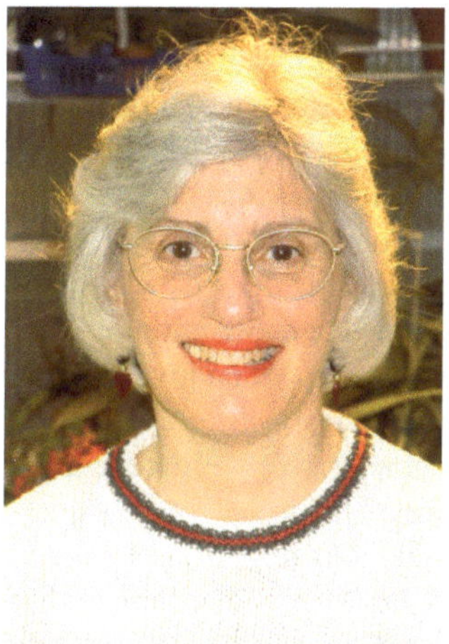

Dr. Adrianne Bendich has recently retired as Director of Medical Affairs at GlaxoSmithKline (GSK) Consumer Healthcare where she was responsible for leading the innovation and medical programs in support of many well-known brands including TUMS and Os-Cal. Dr. Bendich had primary responsibility for GSK's support for the Women's Health Initiative (WHI) intervention study. Prior to joining GSK, Dr. Bendich was at Roche Vitamins Inc. and was involved with the groundbreaking clinical studies showing that folic acid-containing multivitamins significantly reduced major classes of birth defects. Dr. Bendich has co-authored over 100 major clinical research studies in the area of preventive nutrition. Dr. Bendich is recognized as a leading authority on antioxidants, nutrition and immunity and pregnancy outcomes, vitamin safety, and the cost-effectiveness of vitamin/mineral supplementation.

Dr. Bendich, who is now President of Consultants in Consumer Healthcare LLC, is the editor of ten books including "Preventive Nutrition: The Comprehensive Guide For Health Professionals, Fourth Edition" co-edited with Dr. Richard Deckelbaum, and is the Series Editor of "Nutrition and Health" for Springer/Humana Press (http://www.springer.com/series/7659). The Series contains 40 published volumes—major new editions in 2010–2011 include Vitamin D, Second Edition edited by Dr. Michael Holick; "Dietary Components and Immune Function" edited by Dr. Ronald Ross Watson, Dr. Sherma Zibadi and Dr. Victor R. Preedy; "Bioactive Compounds and Cancer" edited by Dr. John A. Milner and Dr. Donato F. Romagnolo; "Modern Dietary Fat Intakes in Disease Promotion" edited by Dr. Fabien DeMeester, Dr. Sherma Zibadi, and Dr. Ronald Ross Watson; "Iron Deficiency and Overload" edited by Dr. Shlomo Yehuda and Dr. David Mostofsky; "Nutrition Guide for Physicians" edited by Dr. Edward Wilson, Dr. George A. Bray, Dr. Norman Temple and Dr. Mary Struble; "Nutrition and Metabolism" edited by Dr. Christos Mantzoros and "Fluid and Electrolytes in Pediatrics" edited by Leonard Feld and Dr. Frederick Kaskel. Recent volumes include: "Handbook of Drug-Nutrient Interactions" edited by Dr. Joseph Boullata and Dr. Vincent Armenti; "Probiotics in Pediatric Medicine" edited by Dr. Sonia Michail and Dr. Philip Sherman; "Handbook of Nutrition and Pregnancy" edited by Dr. Carol Lammi-Keefe, Dr. Sarah Couch and Dr. Elliot Philipson; "Nutrition and Rheumatic Disease" edited by Dr. Laura Coleman; "Nutrition and Kidney Disease" edited by Dr. Laura Byham-Grey, Dr. Jerrilynn Burrowes and Dr. Glenn Chertow; "Nutrition and Health in Developing Countries" edited by Dr. Richard Semba and Dr. Martin Bloem; "Calcium in Human Health" edited by Dr. Robert Heaney and Dr. Connie Weaver, and "Nutrition and Bone Health" edited by Dr. Michael Holick and Dr. Bess Dawson-Hughes.

Dr. Bendich served as Associate Editor for "Nutrition" the International Journal; served on the Editorial Board of the Journal of Women's Health and Gender-based Medicine, and was a member of the Board of Directors of the American College of Nutrition.

Dr. Bendich was the recipient of the Roche Research Award, is a Tribute to Women and Industry Awardee and was a recipient of the Burroughs Wellcome Visiting Professorship in Basic Medical Sciences, 2000–2001. In 2008, Dr. Bendich was given the Council for Responsible Nutrition (CRN) Apple Award in recognition of her many contributions to the scientific understanding of dietary supplements. Dr. Bendich holds academic appointments as Adjunct Professor in the Department of Preventive Medicine and Community Health at UMDNJ and has an adjunct appointment at the Institute of Nutrition, Columbia University P&S, and is an Adjunct Research Professor, Rutgers University, Newark Campus. She is listed in Who's Who in American Women.

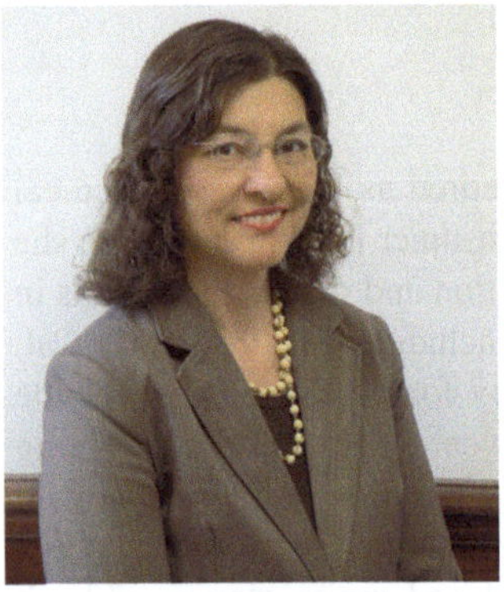

Sherry Tanumihardjo manages a progressive research and outreach team at the University of Wisconsin (UW)-Madison in the Department of Nutritional Sciences. She serves as the director of the Undergraduate Certificate in Global Health and is on the Advisory Board for the Global Health Institute at UW-Madison. She teaches both at the undergraduate and at the graduate level including international field experiences. In her research, she has almost three decades of experience with vitamin A and carotenoids. Her multidisciplinary research approach is enhanced by her broad educational background in chemistry (BS), biochemistry (MS), and nutrition (PhD). She has two main research foci including vitamin A assessment methodology and carotenoid bioavailability. Often the two overlap when investigating provitamin A carotenoids. Tanumihardjo has authored and co-authored over 100 research publications, chapters, and technical documents. Her research group works with a number of animal models (i.e., gerbils, rats, pigs, and monkeys) to answer various questions on issues related to vitamin A toxicity and deficiency and carotenoid bioavailability. Moreover, the research outcomes are often applied to the human model. In that regard, her research team has conducted studies in humans in the United States, Indonesia, South Africa, Ghana, Burkina Faso, and Zambia. She has acted as a consultant to many other studies throughout the world to assist with study design and appropriate standardization. She is a strong advocate for the promotion of nutritionally enhanced staple foods, vegetables, and fruits to enhance overall health and general well-being. This has allowed her to be an invited speaker at approximately 200 domestic and international meetings. In addition to her on-going work with nutritionally enhanced staple crops, other research efforts include the interaction of anthocyanins in purple carrots with carotenoid uptake and clearance. Further, she has developed educational materials to enhance the intake of locally grown produce in the state of Wisconsin with special emphasis on vegetables and fruits. These research and outreach efforts have been recognized as an endowed chair at UW-Madison named the Friday Chair for Vegetable Processing Research awarded to Tanumihardjo in 2009. She has chaired and co-chaired the Vitamin A and Carotenoid sessions at Experimental Biology over the years. She has served as chair of the Carotenoid Research Interaction Group (CARIG) Research Interest Section of the American Society of Nutrition (ASN) and has been on CARIG's steering committee since 2002. Her memberships to the former societies predating ASN (2005) date back to 1991 for the American Society of Nutritional Sciences and the American Society of Clinical Nutrition and to 1994 for the Society for International Nutrition Research. She has served on the Editorial Advisory Board for the *International Journal for Vitamin and Nutrition Research* since 2002, the Editorial Board for the *Journal of Nutrition* from 2005 to 2011, and for the Editorial Board for *Advances in Nutrition* since 2010. Other awards include membership on the WHO Expert Advisory Panel on Nutrition since 2012, the G. Malcolm Trout visiting scholar award lectureship at Michigan State University in 2011, the Ruth Pike Lectureship Award at Pennsylvania State University in 2007, the Alex Malaspina ILSI Future Leader Award from 2004 to 2006, and the Dannon Leadership Institute Creative Leadership training in 2001.

Acknowledgements

Although many publishers have contacted me in the past few years, I am grateful to Adrianne Bendich for her persistence at multiple Experimental Biology meetings encouraging me to consider editing this volume and in putting me in contact with Richard Hruska at Springer. A special thanks to Maureen Alexander, Developmental Editor, for her patience and making sure that all of the pieces were in place as we moved through each section of the book. Finally, I am grateful for all the work that the authors have put into their individual chapters and the encouragement of a few of them to me to see this through.

Contents

Contributors

Sara A. Arscott, PhD Department of Nutritional Sciences, University of Wisconsin-Madison, Madison, WI, USA

Raman Babu, PhD Global Maize Program, International Maize and Wheat Improvement Center, CIMMYT, Texcoco, Mexico

Neil Binkley, MD School of Medicine & Public Health, University of Wisconsin-Madison, Madison, WI, USA

William S. Blaner, PhD Department of Medicine, College of Physicians and Surgeons, Columbia University, New York, NY, USA

Megan J. Bowman, PhD Department of Horticulture, University of Wisconsin-Madision, Madison, WI, USA

Parul Christian, DrPH, MSc Department of International Health, Center for Human Nutrition, Bloomberg School of Public Health, Johns Hopkins University, Baltimore, MD, USA

Joseph Dever, PhD Department of Nutritional Sciences, University of Wisconsin-Madison, Madison, WI, USA

John W. Erdman Jr., PhD Department of Nutritional Sciences, University of Illinois at Urbana-Champaign, Urbana, IL, USA

Mieke Faber, PhD Nutritional Intervention Research Unit, Medical Research Council of South Africa, Cape Town, Western Cape Province, South Africa

Mario G. Ferruzzi, PhD Department of Food Science, Purdue University, West Lafayette, IN, USA

Department of Nutrition Science, Purdue University, West Lafayette, IN, USA

Nikki Ford, PhD Department of Nutritional Sciences, University of Texas at Austin, Austin, TX, USA

Harold C. Furr, MNS, PhD Department of Nutritional Sciences, University of Wisconsin, Madison, WI, USA

Shellen R. Goltz, PhD, RD Department of Food Science, Purdue University, West Lafayette, IN, USA

Department of Nutrition Science, Purdue University, West Lafayette, IN, USA

Xiaoming Gong, DVM, PhD Neonatology, Children's Research Institute, University of South Florida, St. Petersburg, FL, USA

Marjorie J. Haskell, BS, MPH, PhD Department of Nutrition, University of California, Davis, CA, USA

Elizabeth J. Johnson, PhD Carotenoids and Health Laboratory, Jean Mayer USDA Human Nutrition Research Center on Aging at Tufts University, Boston, MA, USA

John T. Landrum, PhD Department of Chemistry and Biochemistry, Florida International University, Miami, FL, USA

Georg Lietz, Dipl.oec.troph., PhD School of Agriculture, Food and Rural Development (AFRD), Human Nutrition Research Centre, Newcastle University, Newcastle upon Tyne, UK

Benchun Miao, PhD Nutrition and Cancer Biology Laboratory, Jean Mayer USDA Human Nutrition Research Center on aging at Tufts University, Boston, MA, USA

Raphael Mutale, BSc HarvestPlus, Department of Crop Development, c/o World Fish Centre, Lusaka, Zambia

Natalia Palacios Rojas, PhD Global Maize Program, International Maize and Wheat Improvement Center, CIMMYT, Texcoco, Mexico

Department of Agronomy, University of Wisconsin-Madison, Madison, WI, USA

Kevin Pixley, PhD Genetic Resources Program, International Maize and Wheat Improvement Center, CIMMYT, Texcoco, Mexico

Department of Agronomy, University of Wisconsin, Madison, WI

Lewis P. Rubin, MD Neonatology, Children's Research Institute, University of South Florida, St. Petersburg, FL, USA

Samantha Schmaelzle, BS Department of Nutritional Sciences, University of Wisconsin-Madison, Madison, WI, USA

Kerry Schulze, PhD Department of International Health, Center for Human Nutrition, Bloomberg School of Public Health, Johns Hopkins University, Baltimore, MD, USA

Igor O. Shmarakov, PhD Department of Medicine, College of Physicians and Surgeons, Columbia University, New York, NY, USA

Department of Biochemistry and Biotechnology, Chernivtsi National University, Chernivtsi, Ukraine

Philipp W. Simon, PhD USDA-Agricultural Research Service, Vegetable Crops Research Unit, University of Wisconsin, Madison, WI, USA

Department of Horticulture, University of Wisconsin-Madison, Madison, WI, USA

Eliab Simpungwe, PhD HarvestPlus, Zambia Country Program, c/o World Fish Centre, Lusaka, Zambia

Charles B. Stephensen, PhD Immunity and Disease Prevention Research Unit, United States Department of Agriculture, Agricultural Research Service, Western Human Nutrition Research Center, University of California, Davis, CA, USA

Rebecca Surles, PhD Global Maize Program, International Maize and Wheat Improvement Center, CIMMYT, Texcoco, Mexico

Guangwen Tang, PhD Carotenoids and Health Laboratory, Jean Mayer USDA Human Nutrition Research Center on Aging, Friedman School of Nutrition Science and Policy, Tufts University, Boston, MA, USA

Sherry A. Tanumihardjo, MS, PhD Department of Nutritional Sciences, University of Wisconsin-Madison, Madison, WI, USA

Paul van Jaarsveld Nutritional Intervention Research Unit, Medical Research Council of South Africa, Caper Town, Western Cape Province, South Africa

Rohini Vishwanathan, PhD Carotenoids and Health Laboratory, Jean Mayer USDA Human Nutrition Center on Aging at Tufts University, Boston, MA, USA

Xiang-Dong Wang, MD, PhD Nutrition and Cancer Biology Laboratory, Jean Mayer USDA Human Nutrition Research Center on Aging at Tufts University, Boston, MA, USA

Jason J. Yuen, MS Department of Medicine, College of Physicians and Surgeons, Columbia University, New York, NY, USA

Section I
Carotenoid Sources and Metabolism

Chapter 1
Food Sources of Carotenoids

Sara A. Arscott

Key Points

- Carotenoids are a class of ubiquitous yellow, orange, and red pigments found in nature and regarded as major contributors to the purported health benefits of a diet rich in fruits and vegetables. They are an important source of vitamin A in many diets and may protect from development of degenerative diseases such as macular degeneration, cancer, and heart disease.
- Carotenoids vary greatly among foods; and their concentration is influenced by many factors, including genetics, climate, maturity, cultivation practices, and processing and storage methods.
- Quantification of carotenoids in foods is complicated by their inherent variability and instability. Nonetheless, several databases list the representative carotenoid content of foods to use to better understand dietary carotenoid intake of individuals and populations.
- This chapter serves as an overview of food sources of carotenoids, sources of variation in food carotenoids, and the effects of food processing and preparation on carotenoid stability.

Keywords Content • Food • Fruits • Sources • Variability • Vegetables

Introduction

A large number of epidemiological studies have linked diets rich in fruits and vegetables with reduced risk of cancer and other chronic diseases [1–6]. Carotenoids are one class of phytochemicals that contribute to their status as "functional foods" and are regarded as a major contributor to their purported health benefits. Carotenoids are a diverse and widespread group of fat-soluble, yellow, orange, and red pigments synthesized exclusively in bacteria, fungi, and higher plants, and which serve as the sole source for animals. They are especially abundant in yellow-orange and in dark green leafy vegetables. In humans, the most well-known function of some carotenoids (the provitamin A carotenoids) is enzymatic conversion in the body to vitamin A. Vitamin A is essential for growth, reproduction, and immune function. Vitamin A nutrition remains a challenge in many parts of the developing world where deficiency leads to high disease and mortality rates, especially in children. Carotenoids may

S.A. Arscott Ph.D. (✉)
Department of Nutritional Sciences, University of Wisconsin-Madison, 1415 Linden Dr, Madison, WI 53706, USA
e-mail: arscott@nutrisci.wisc.edu

S.A. Tanumihardjo (ed.), *Carotenoids and Human Health*, Nutrition and Health,
DOI 10.1007/978-1-62703-203-2_1,

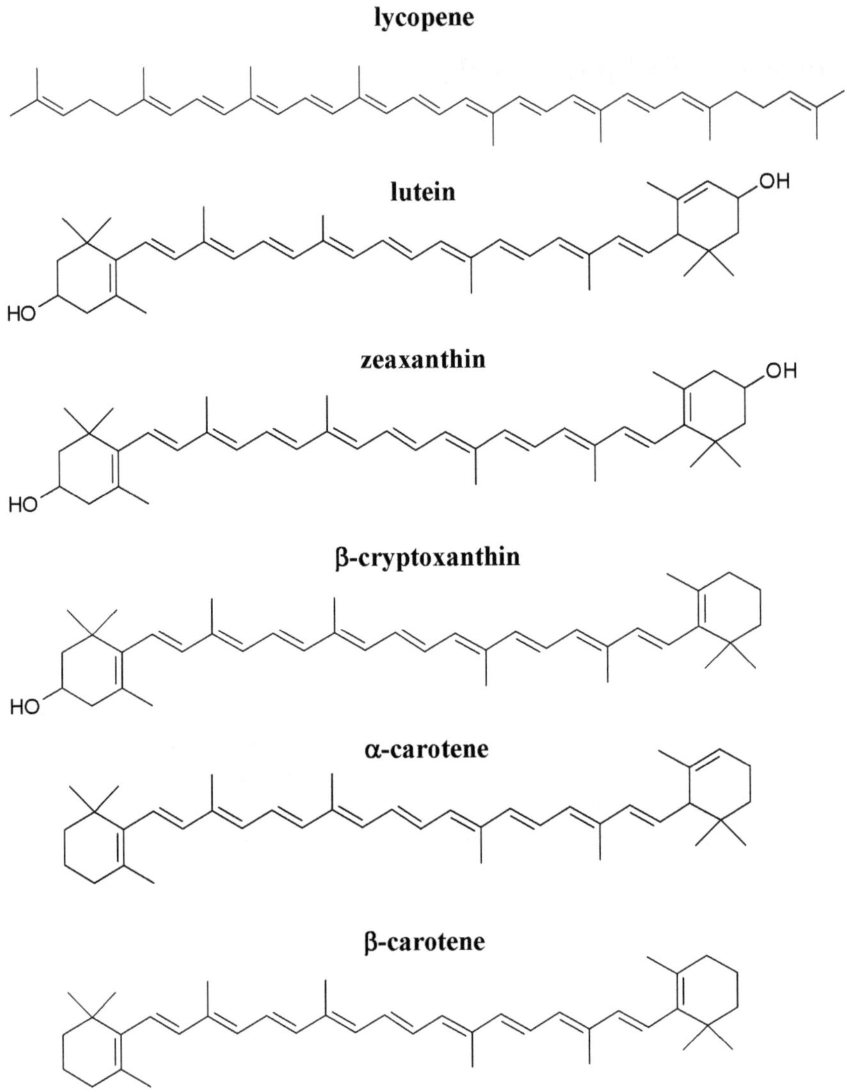

Fig. 1.1 Structures of carotenoids commonly found in foods

also play an important role in photoprotection in the eye [7, 8], enhancing immune function [9, 10], and prevention of chronic disease [11–14]. Information on individual- and population-level carotenoid intake relies on accurate knowledge about amounts in foods. For these reasons, the sources and content of carotenoids in food are of major interest to researchers, nutritionists, food processors, manufacturers, and consumers.

Over 700 carotenoids have been characterized in nature [15]. They are secondary plant compounds synthesized and localized in cellular plastids. Their major roles in plants are as accessory light harvesting pigments in chloroplasts of photosynthetic tissues, absorbing light mostly in the blue-green wavelength range, and in chromoplasts of non-photosynthetic tissues such as fruits, flowers, and roots. They also serve to mediate photoprotection through quenching the excess energy of chlorophyll or singlet oxygen and as an attractant to pollinators as in flowers.

Structurally, carotenoids are a related family of C_{40} isoprenoid polyene compounds, the majority of which are composed of eight isoprenoid units, like β-carotene (Figure 1.1). Hydrocarbons, such as α- and β-carotene, found in carrots, are referred to as carotenes and oxygenated derivatives, such as lutein and β-cryptoxanthin, found predominantly in corn and tangerines, respectively, are referred to as xanthophylls. The most characteristic feature of carotenoids is their conjugated double-bond chain that forms a chromophore responsible for the characteristic colors ranging from colorless (phytoene), to yellow (lutein), orange (β-carotene), and red (lycopene). This structure allows carotenoids to act in the energy transfer reactions of photosynthesis and as antioxidants.

Several tables and databases of the carotenoid content of foods have been compiled to aid in classifying certain carotenoids of interest and quantification of intake [16–20]. Analytical methods of carotenoid analysis have improved greatly in the last couple of decades and the use of high-performance liquid chromatography (HPLC) has facilitated more accurate separation and quantification of the wide array of different carotenoid pigments often present in a single food. However, inherent difficulties exist in accurately quantifying food carotenoids.

The carotenoid content of foods is highly variable and is affected by a number of factors including genotype (variety or cultivar), season, geography, cultivation variation, stage of maturity at harvest, and postharvest storage conditions. Thus, identifying absolute carotenoid content of a type of fruit, vegetable, or other food is not possible and should more reasonably be considered as a range of values. Additionally, processing of foods can lead to quantitative as well as qualitative changes because carotenoids are susceptible to isomerization and oxidation. Also, food processing and cooking can disrupt the matrix of a food which can have an impact on bioavailability and should be considered when evaluating intake. Lastly, while the analytical method itself is subject to several sources of error [21], the main problem with carotenoid analysis lies in their inherent instability. In spite of the challenges, databases serve as references for general ranges of the principle carotenoids found in foods: β-carotene, α-carotene, β-cryptoxanthin, lycopene, lutein, and zeaxanthin. Some databases have also served as sources for estimating individual- and population-level carotenoid intake [18, 22–25] and the analytical effort behind the databases has helped to elucidate not only the levels but also the nature, distribution, and variability of food carotenoids.

This chapter serves as an overview of food sources of carotenoids, sources of variation in food carotenoids, and the effects of food processing and preparation on carotenoid stability.

Food Sources of Carotenoids

Fruits and vegetables provide nearly 90 % of the carotenoid intake in the USA [25]. Of the hundreds of carotenoids found in nature, upwards of 50 are present in the human diet and have been identified in the human body [26]. Of these, 6 carotenoids predominate, β-carotene, α-carotene, β-cryptoxanthin, lycopene, lutein, and zeaxanthin. Most nutrition research has focused on these carotenoids and they have been extensively studied for their potential effects and association to several disease processes [11–14]. Three of these carotenoids, β-carotene, α-carotene, and β-cryptoxanthin, can be converted to retinol (vitamin A) in the body and are referred to as provitamin A carotenoids. Quantification of these carotenoids in foods facilitates an understanding of fruit and vegetable sources of vitamin A. In the past, carotenoid quantification was focused on total vitamin A activity. With the recognition of beneficial effects of carotenoids on human health, independent of their vitamin A activity, accurate quantification of individual carotenoids has become paramount.

While this chapter is focused on the six predominant carotenoids, improvements in analytical techniques have led to more specific and detailed information on carotenoids such as phytoene in tomatoes [27], violaxanthin in mangoes [20], and lactucaxanthin in lettuce [28]. The health implications of these carotenoids are not yet known.

In 1998, the United States Department of Agriculture (USDA) collaborated with the Nutrition Coordinating Center (NCC) at the University of Minnesota to release the USDA–NCC Carotenoid

Database for the US Foods as an update to the original 1993 USDA-National Cancer Institute (NCI) Carotenoid Database [19]. The database lists 215 foods and can be accessed online at http://www.nal.usda.gov/fnic/foodcomp/Data/car98/car98.html. It was originally developed from a review of published articles reporting food carotenoid values. Better analytical methods based on HPLC and more references in the literature allowed the 1998 release to improve upon the original database by including a greater variety of fruits and vegetables and a number of other sources of carotenoids in the US diet including eggs, butter, margarine, corn meal, and mixed dishes. Additionally, different forms of a particular food such as raw, cooked, canned, and frozen were separated unlike the earlier version which aggregated them.

The USDA–NCC database is the most comprehensive documentation of carotenoid content of a wide range of US foods to date, and was incorporated into the USDA National Nutrient Database for Standard Reference [29]. Table 1.1 presents selected foods from that database. The database lists the food content of β-carotene, α-carotene, β-cryptoxanthin, lycopene, and lutein plus zeaxanthin as μg per 100 g fresh weight. Lutein and zeaxanthin, both oxygenated xanthophylls, are not always separated by some analytical techniques and often grouped together. Confidence codes associated with each carotenoid value were established as a summary of five quality indices (analytic method, quality control, number of samples, sample handling, and sampling plan). A confidence code of "A" means that the user can have considerable confidence in the value; "B" indicates some problems existed regarding the data that the values were based on, and "C" represents the lowest confidence based on limited quantity or quality of data. While a "C" rating is analytically acceptable, the value lacks the carotenoid variability inherent in food and may not be representative of available foods. Only 2 % of individual carotenoid values were assigned an "A," 14 % "B," and 84 % "C." This suggests that as of 1999, there existed a considerable dearth of robust data on food carotenoids in the USA. As analytical techniques continue to improve and a wider variety of foods analyzed, it will be important to update databases such as the USDA–NCC database to reflect the range of carotenoid levels in foods.

Several reviews and databases on international food carotenoids have been published. A review, published in 2009 on food sources of carotenoids, intake, stability, and bioavailability, provides a table of 68 foods, mostly of plant origin, and their range of the six primary carotenoids [30]. The table includes data sourced from 27 published articles between the years 2000 and 2007, referencing foods from many different countries. A European carotenoid database developed from a number of studies was reported in 2001 by O'Neill and others [18] and was used to determine comparative intakes of carotenoids across five countries. Heinonen and others [31] reported the carotenoid composition of Finnish foods. Hart and Scott [32] analyzed the carotenoid content of commonly consumed fruits and vegetables in the UK. West and Poortvliet [16] compiled international food carotenoid data with special emphasis on developing countries using the same expert data system as the USDA–NCC Carotenoid database, but with relaxed inclusion criteria due to lower availability of sensitive analytical tools in many developing countries. An Austrian Carotenoid Database was developed in 2000 to assess the average carotenoid values of commonly eaten vegetables from different areas of Austria [33]. Carotenoid content of commonly consumed foods in Denmark [34], Korea [35], and Indonesia [36, 37] has been published.

Recently, Rodriguez-Amaya and others [20] published an update to the Brazilian food carotenoid database and critically reviewed factors affecting carotenoid composition. The database is a combination of analytical work with that of other laboratories. Important in their process was the optimization and continual assessment of methodology for different foods. Different food matrices require different methods to assure complete release of carotenoids from the matrix as well as limit degradation and isomerization. The data for many of the foods span years of harvest, varietal differences, regional variation, maturity, temperature, farming practices, and raw versus processed foods, and clearly demonstrate carotenoid variation.

In spite of carotenoid variation, several generalizations can be made regarding content and profiles in many fruits and vegetables. β-Carotene is the most widely distributed carotenoid in foods [38] and

Table 1.1 Content of major carotenoids in selected foods (μg/100 g)[a]

Food	α-Carotene	β-Carotene	β-Cryptoxanthin	Lutein+Zeaxanthin	Lycopene
	Mean[b]				
	Range[c]				
Apricots	0	6,640	0	0	65
		1,520–19,270			
Asparagus, raw	12	493	–	–	–
	0–17	317–581			
Avocado, raw	28	53	36	–	–
	28–28	52–53	22–50		
Banana, raw	5	21	0–70	0	0
	0–15				
Beans, green, raw	68	377	0	640	0
	44–90	252–510		590–690	
Beet greens, raw	5	3,405	–	–	–
	0–14	2,181–5,028			
Broccoli, raw	1	779	0	2,445	0
	0–2	398–2,330		2,060–2,830	
Brussels sprouts, raw	6	450	0	1,590	
	0–11	340–530			
Cabbage, raw	0	65	0	310	0
		58–80			
Carrot, raw	4,649	8,836	–	–	–
	2,600–9,710	3,577–14,700			
Collards, raw	238	3,323	80	–	–
		2,284–5,400			
Corn, sweet, yellow, canned, whole kernels, drained	33	30	0	884	
		8–44		520–1,197	0
Egg, whole, raw, fresh	0	0	0	55	–
Grapefruit, raw, pink and red	5	603	12	13	1,462
	0–14	248–2,343	0–30	0–20	160–3,362
Kale, raw	0	9,226	0	39,550	0
		4,720–14,600			
Lettuce, cos or romaine, raw	0	1,272	0	2,635	0
		1,200–1,345			
Lettuce, iceberg, raw	2	192	0	352	0
	0–4	114–330			
Mango, raw	17	445	11	–	–
		395–495			
Melon, cantaloupe, raw	27	1,595	0	40	0
	9–61	1,377–1,847			
Nectarine, raw	0	101	59	–	–
		100–103			
Okra, raw	28	432	–	–	–
Orange, raw	16	51	122	187	–
	14–20	40–59			
Orange juice, raw	2	4	15	36	–
	1–3	3–5	14–16	28–44	
Papaya, raw	0	276	761	75	0
		62–910	517–1,264		

(continued)

Table 1.1 (continued)

Food	α-Carotene	β-Carotene	β-Cryptoxanthin	Lutein + Zeaxanthin	Lycopene
Peach, raw	1	97	24	57	0
	0–3	76–112	12–30	10–80	
Peas, geen, raw	19	485	–	–	–
	16–26	340–557			
Pepper, sweet, green,	22	198			
raw	0–34	81–276	–	–	–
Pepper, sweet, red,	59	2,379	2,205	–	–
raw		1,940–2,978			
Pumpkin, canned, no	4,795	6,940	0	0	0
salt	2,170–7,420	3,060–10,820			
Spinach	0	5,597	0	11,938	
		3,970–8,900		9,500–15,940	0
Squash, summer, crookneck and straight, raw	0	90		290	0
Squash, summer, zucchini, with skin, raw	0	410	0	2,125	0
Squash, winter, acorn, raw	0	220	0	38	0
Squash, winter,	834	4,226	–	–	–
butternut, raw	732–935	1,360–8,378			
Sweet potato, raw	0	9,180	–	–	–
		5,029–16,000			
Tangerine, raw	14	71	485	243	0
		68–73			
Tomato, red, ripe, raw	112	393	0	130	3,025
	0–223	115–700			879–4,200
Watermelon, raw	0	295	103	17	4,868
		287–310	0–310		

[a]Source: USDA–NCC Carotenoid Database for the US Foods—1998. The data for the US foods were obtained from many sources and may represent different growing years, growing areas, cultivars, processing techniques, lengths and conditions of storage, and possibly different methods of analysis

[b]Weighted means of the carotenoid values from each reference/study based on sampling plan ratings; 0, value is a true analytical zero value (<detection limit); –, unreported value (does not necessarily mean a zero value)

[c]Minimum and maximum values

is valued as the most potent provitamin A carotenoid because in the human body β-carotene is broken down by β-carotene monooxygenase in the mucosa of the small intestine, into two retinal molecules, which are reduced to vitamin A (retinol). β-Carotene is primarily found in dark orange fruits and vegetables such as mango, apricot, cantaloupe, carrots, red peppers, sweet potatoes, and pumpkins, and green vegetables such as broccoli, kale, and chard. Table 1.2 lists daily per capita supply of primary carotenoids from fruits and vegetables to the US population and the carotenoids identified and quantified in those foods. α-Carotene often accompanies β-carotene, but at much lower concentrations. It is present in high amounts in carrots and some varieties of squash and pumpkins. In the US diet, carrots are the greatest source of α-carotene, and this carotenoid in human plasma uniquely indicates high carrot consumption [39–41]. Both α-carotene and β-cryptoxanthin can also supply vitamin A, but because only half of each molecule has the necessary unsubstituted β-ionone ring, they theoretically have only 50 % the activity of β-carotene.

Table 1.2 Daily per capita supply of primary carotenoids from fruits and vegetables to the US population and carotenoids identified and quantified in those foods. Foods selected based on high per capita supply of primary carotenoids[a]

Food	α-Carotene	β-Carotene	β-Cryptoxanthin	Lutein + Zeaxanthin	Lycopene	Source
	Per capita availability[b,c], μg/day Carotenoids identified and quantified in food[d]					
Broccoli	0.11	82.6	0.00	259.4	0.00	
	All-*trans* β-carotene, **all-*trans* lutein**, all-*trans* lutein epoxide 9-*cis* lutein 9′-*cis* lutein, 13-*cis* lutein, 13′-*cis* lutein, all-*trans* zeaxanthin, 9-*cis* zeaxanthin, all-*trans* neoxanthin, 9-*cis* neoxanthin, all-*trans* violaxanthin					[47, 113]
Carrot	590.8	1122.9	–	–	–	
	α-carotene, **all-*trans* β-carotene**, 9-*cis* β-carotene, 13-*cis* β-carotene, γ-carotene, ζ-carotene, β-zeacarotene, lutein, lycopene					[59, 114, 118, 127]
Corn	10.5	9.5	0.00	280.9	0.00	
	α-carotene, β-carotene, β-cryptoxanthin, **all-*trans* lutein**, 9-*cis* lutein, 9′-*cis* lutein, 13-*cis* lutein, 13′-*cis* lutein, **all-*trans* zeaxanthin**, and 9-*cis* zeaxanthin					[47, 61]
Grapefruit, red or pink	0.4	49.2	1.0	1.1	119.3	
	α-carotene, **β-carotene**, β-cryptoxanthin, *cis*-β-cryptoxanthin, lutein, zeaxanthin, **lycopene**, phytoene, phytofluene, ζ-carotene					[115, 116, 121]
Kale	0.00	25.8	0.00	110.7	0.00	
	β-carotene, **all-*trans* lutein**, all-*trans* lutein epoxide, 9-*cis* lutein, 9′-*cis* lutein, 13-*cis* lutein, 13′-*cis* lutein, all-*trans* zeaxanthin, 9-*cis* zeaxanthin, violaxanthin, neoxanthin					[47, 63, 88]
Lettuce, cos or romaine	0.00	173.8	0.00	360.0	0.00	
	β-carotene, **all-*trans* lutein**, 9-*cis* lutein, 9′-*cis* lutein, 13-*cis* lutein, 13′-*cis* lutein, all-*trans* zeaxanthin, 9-*cis* zeaxanthin,					[47, 119]
Cantaloupe	3.1	184.7	0.00	4.6	0.00	
	α-carotene, **β-carotene**, lutein, β-cryptoxanthin					[121, 122]
Orange	12.5	39.7	95.0	145.7	–	
	α-carotene, β-carotene, α-cryptoxanthin, **β-cryptoxanthin**, **all-*trans* lutein**, **all-*trans* zeaxanthin**, ***cis*-violaxanthin**, luteoxanthin, neochrome, mutatoxanthin, β-citaurin, phytoene, phytofluene					[47, 65, 115, 116, 121]
Pumpkin	243.5	352.4	0.00	0.00	0.00	
	Antheraxanthin, **α-carotene**, **all-*trans* β-carotene**, lutein, zeaxanthin, violaxanthin, ζ-carotene					[20, 123–125, 127]

(continued)

Table 1.2 (continued)

Food	α-Carotene	β-Carotene	β-Cryptoxanthin	Lutein + Zeaxanthin	Lycopene	Source
Spinach	0.00	176.1	0.00	375.7	0.00	
	All-*trans* β-carotene, **all-*trans* lutein**, 9-*cis* lutein, 9′-*cis* lutein, 13-*cis* lutein, all-*trans* lutein epoxide, neolutein, all-*trans* zeaxan thin, 9-*cis* zeaxanthin, all-*trans* neoxanthin, 9-*cis* neoxanthin, all-*trans* violaxanthin					[47, 113, 118]
Sweet potato	0.00	600.2	–	–	–	
	All-*trans* β-carotene, 13-*cis* β-carotene, β-cryptoxanthin, ipomoeaxanthin					[126–128]
Tangerine	0.7	3.5	23.8	11.9	0.00	
	α-carotene, β-carotene, α-cryptoxanthin, **β-cryptoxanthin**, **lutein**, **zeaxanthin**, lycopene, zeinoxanthin, violaxanthin, ***cis*-violaxanthin**, luteoxanthin, neochrome, mutatoxanthin, antheraxanthin, β-citaurin, phytoene, phytofluene					[65, 115–117, 122]
Tomato	123.5	433.4	0.00	143.4	3335.8	
	β-carotene, lutein, **lycopene**, γ-carotene, neurosporene, ζ-carotene, phytoene, phytofluene					[27, 104, 120]
Watermelon, red	0.00	56.15	19.60	3.24	926.50	
	β-carotene, lutein, β-cryptoxanthin, **all-*trans* lycopene,** *cis*-lycopene, neoxanthin, phytofluene					[56, 122, 129]

[a] Adapted from Kopsell and Kopsell, 2006 [130]

[b] Per capita availability of primary carotenoids calculated from USDA/ERS Food Availability (per capita) Data System 2009 multiplied by carotenoid content reported in USDA–NCC Carotenoid Database for the US Foods—1998. Food availability data reflects fresh fruit or vegetable availability data, represents food disappearance into the marketing system, and includes substantial quantities of nonedible food portions and food lost to human use through waste, trimming, cooking, and spoilage in the home and marketing system. Data typically overestimate amounts of food and nutrients people actually ingest.

[c] A zero value is a true analytical zero value (<detection limit), while an unreported carotenoid value ("–") does not necessarily mean a zero value. See text and Table 1.1 footnotes for more information regarding the USDA–NCC Carotenoid Database for the US Foods 1998.

[d] Carotenoids in bold text identify those reported in highest concentration

β-Cryptoxanthin is the principle carotenoid in many tropical orange-fleshed fruits and is found in high concentrations in tangerines, oranges, and certain mangos and papayas. In colder climates, β-cryptoxanthin is found at lower concentrations in fruits such as peaches, nectarines, and red peppers. Epidemiological studies suggest that β-cryptoxanthin may play a role in protection from inflammatory diseases such as arthritis [42], angina pectoris [43], and osteoporosis [44] (see Chap. 14).

Major sources of lutein include green vegetables such as broccoli, brussels sprouts, peas, string beans, and leaves. Dietary intake and plasma concentrations of both lutein and zeaxanthin, the yellow pigments found in the macula of the human retina, have an inverse relationship with the risk of macular degeneration [45, 46]. Lutein and zeaxanthin are structural isomers and are not provitamin A carotenoids. Lutein, a dihydroxy derivative of α-carotene, is normally present in plant tissues at much higher concentrations than zeaxanthin, a dihydroxy derivative of β-carotene, and the ratio of these two carotenoids can vary [47]. The major role of lutein in photosynthesis is proposed as the reason for its abundance over zeaxanthin in many green plant tissues [48]. Some varieties of corn are an exception to this, where zeaxanthin is the major pigment [38, 47]. Zeaxanthin is also found in high amounts in egg yolks, dark leafy greens, certain yellow-orange fruits, and vegetables such as squash, oranges, and orange peppers, Japanese persimmons, and Chinese wolfberries (*Lycium barbarum*) [7, 49].

Lycopene, an unsaturated acyclic hydrocarbon carotenoid with an open hydrocarbon chain, is the principle red pigment found primarily in tomatoes and tomato products, watermelon, and pink grapefruit. Due to lack of the β-ionone ring, lycopene has no vitamin A activity, and typically occurs naturally as the all-*trans* form. Lycopene is the most potent *in vitro* antioxidant of all carotenoids found in appreciable amounts in humans [50]. A meta-analysis of 11 case–control studies and 10 cohort studies showed that high tomato consumption modestly reduced the relative risk of prostate cancer in men [51]. While lycopene is proposed to be the phytochemical responsible for this benefit, the mechanistic actions of whole tomato, lycopene, and other tomato carotenoids have been implicated.

Variation of carotenoid composition

The carotenoids in leafy and non-leafy green vegetables are found in the chloroplasts and the hydroxycarotenoids are unesterified. The principle carotenoids, lutein, β-carotene, violaxanthin, and neoxanthin, exist in relatively consistent proportions, although the absolute concentrations vary considerably [20]. In contrast, in ripe fruit, the carotenoids are located in the chromoplasts, the xanthophylls are mostly esterified with fatty acids, and the carotenoid composition and proportion are much more variable and complex. In root crop vegetables, like carrots and sweet potatoes, carotenes predominate, whereas in typical yellow maize, the xanthophylls predominate. Carotenoids dissolved in the oily droplets of orange or yellow fruits or sweet potatoes are more accessible for absorption in the gut [52], likely due to greater solubility, as compared to the carotenoids sequestered in crystalline form, as in carrots, or complexed to proteins, as in the chloroplasts of leafy green vegetables. These factors are important when considering bioavailability and for researchers concerned with carotenoid and vitamin A intake.

Variety, genotype, season, stage of maturity, geographic location, climate, and growing conditions affect the carotenoid composition in a given food. Significant genetic variation exists within species of fruits and vegetables. The lycopene content of 49 hydroponically grown and environmentally controlled tomato accessions varied up to ninefold higher than the reported average content [53] of 30 mg/kg [19, 54]. Eighteen cultivars of tomatoes had a range of lycopene content from 43 to 120 mg/kg [55]. Total carotenoid concentration of 27 watermelon cultivars varied from 37 to 122 mg/kg [56]. Lutein content ranged from 150 to 337 μg/g dry weight in six varieties of greenhouse-grown lettuce [57] and from 10 to 22 μg/g fresh weight in four varieties of hydroponically grown lettuce [28]. Differences among cultivars have been noted for acerola [20], banana [58], carrot [59, 60], corn [61], guava [20], kale [62–67], mango, melon, orange [65], papaya [58], peach, pepper [66, 67], pumpkins, and squashes [20, 58].

Seasonal and geographic effects on the carotenoid content of fruits and vegetables have also been widely studied. In general, elevated temperature and greater exposure to sunlight may increase carotenogenesis in fruits, but may also promote photodegradation [20]. The lycopene content of ripe tomatoes harvested at six different times of year varied from 7,061 μg/100 g in mid-summer (July) to 11,969 μg/100 g in March; however, no definite seasonal trend or correlation with solar radiation or temperature was found for total carotenoids [68]. This study demonstrated the negative effects hot temperatures may have on lycopene accumulation in tomatoes. In agreement, Toor and others [69] found 31 % lower lycopene content of greenhouse-grown tomatoes in the summer months. However, Zanfini and others [70] found lower carotenoid content in winter-grown greenhouse tomatoes than in summer. Aherne and others [71] tested four different tomato types in two geographic regions (Ireland and Spain) and concluded that geographic location had a more pronounced effect on carotenoid content than variety. However, effects of geographic location may be primarily due to differences in environmental conditions. In three different tomato varieties grown in three different locations, lycopene content was different only in the salad tomato grown in different regions [70]. The regions had comparable climatic conditions in terms of temperature and UV radiation.

Carotenoid profiles of Hass avocados grown in different regions of southern California were similar, with moderate variation in amounts of different carotenoids [72]. The greatest variation was observed over different months of harvest, with increases of over tenfold for β-carotene, violaxanthin, 9′-*cis*-neoxanthin, and lutein-5,6-epoxide, and up to 26-fold for α-carotene and neoxanthin in fruits from one region between January and September. Potatoes showed an effect of year of harvest on total carotenoids [73]. Thirty-two to 56 % lower levels in 1 year may have been due to higher levels of solar radiation coupled with drought conditions.

Leafy vegetables grown in open fields were found to have lower carotenoid levels in the summer than in the winter [31, 74]. However, marketed, minimally processed endive and New Zealand spinach grown under plastic roofs were found to have significantly higher carotenoid content in the summer than in the winter [75]. Plastic roofs may have either protected the carotenoids from photodegradation in the summer or led to lower carotenoid accumulation in the winter.

Maturation or ripening of fruits is usually accompanied by enhanced carotenogenesis [76, 77]. This process typically proceeds through degradation of chloroplasts and their photosynthetic structures, along with the disappearance of chlorophyll and the characteristic chloroplast carotenoids, β-carotene, lutein, and violaxanthin. The up-regulation of enzymes in the carotenogenic pathway results in the massive *de novo* synthesis of carotenoids that accumulate in developing chromoplasts, namely, carotenes, cryptoxanthin, zeaxanthin, and violaxanthin [78, 79]. Patterns and extent of pigment accumulation during maturation are related to the expression of the corresponding biosynthetic genes.

Lycopene, β-carotene, and total carotenoid levels were highest at full ripeness of greenhouse-grown cherry tomatoes [79]. Increased levels of carotenoids with increasing ripeness have been noted for mango [68, 80, 81], guava [82], papaya [83], and pepper cultivars (*Capsicum* species) [67, 84–87]. However, as indicated earlier, not all carotenoids necessarily increase during ripening. Howard and others [67] found that β-cryptoxanthin, β-carotene, α-carotene, and zeaxanthin all increased during ripening of seven different pepper varieties, while lutein was reduced to non-detectable in all varieties except the yellow bell pepper. Similarly, lutein content decreased during ripening in two pink-fleshed varieties of guava [82]. This phenomenon occurs during ripening in fruits as chloroplast carotenoids such as lutein gradually disappear as a consequence of chloroplast degeneration into chromoplasts.

In leafy vegetables, the ripening pattern and carotenoid accumulation are not well-defined. In four different Indonesian leafy vegetables, the mature leaves had 24 % greater total provitamin A carotenoids than young leaves [36]. Mature kale leaves from conventional farms contained significantly higher levels of β-carotene and lutein than the young leaves; violaxanthin had an unusually high concentration in the young leaves; and neoxanthin had nearly the same concentration in young and old leaves [88]. In contrast, kale from an organic farm had similar concentrations of carotenoids in both young and old leaves. Content of total carotenoids in field-grown baby spinach harvested at three different growth stages over three different growing periods tended to increase at the later stages and also increased during 5 or 9 days of storage at 10 °C [89]. In agreement, Azevedo-Meleiro and others [75] found that the carotenoid concentrations in the mature leaves of endive and lettuce were two to four times greater than those in young leaves. In contrast, they found that the younger leaves of New Zealand spinach had slightly higher carotenoid levels than the mature leaves. The growth habit of the different plants may explain the difference, where lettuce and endive are headed, with dark green older, outer leaves, and lighter green younger, inner leaves. The spinach leaves are distributed along a stem with younger leaves slightly greener than older leaves.

Cultivation practices can also affect carotenoid content. A comparison of hydroponically and conventionally grown lettuce found 10–30 % lower carotenoid content in hydroponically cultivated lettuce [28]. Organically farmed mandarin orange juice contained about 40 % more total carotenoids than conventionally grown mandarin juice [90] and organically grown kale contained higher concentrations of all carotenoids than kale grown conventionally on a neighboring farm [91]. In contrast, however, juice from conventionally grown red grapefruit had significantly higher lycopene concentrations, which were inversely proportional to ascorbic acid concentrations [92]. Kale, grown hydroponically with increasing rates of NO_3-nitrogen (N) treatment and a static ratio of NO_3-N:NH_4-N, showed no increase in carotenoid content on a fresh weight (FW) basis, but both lutein and β-carotene increased linearly when calculated on a dry weight (DW) basis [93]. The form of nitrogen also mattered, with increases in carotenoid pigment in kale expressed either on an FW or a DW basis when NO_3-N increased from 0 to 100 % of the ratio of NO_3-N:NH_4-N. The authors concluded that N management should be considered when designing crop programs to maximize carotenoids. These examples illustrate that food crop inputs and production practices have influence on carotenoid concentration; however, while one particular practice may favorably influence carotenoid accumulation, the concentration of other nutrients and phytochemicals may vary and must be assessed if the desire is to maximize the overall nutritional density of a certain food.

The above examples of carotenoid variability are by no means exhaustive. There are many variables that affect pigment accumulation in plants and while it may be possible to make generalizations about the influence of one variable, the reality is that numerous variables exert their influence during growth, maturation, and ripening. Carotenoid synthesis and accumulation in plants may be determined by many factors, but just as important to the food manufacturer and consumer are the influences on carotenoid stability after harvest. Not only industrial-scale food processing, cooking, and storage can have a marked effect on content, but also form of carotenoid acids, heat treatment, and exposure to light and oxygen can promote degradation and isomerization of the all-*trans*-carotenoids to the *cis*-isomers. Slicing or juicing of fruits can release organic acids that can promote isomerization; however, thermal processing has the strongest influence on this process.

Thermal and mechanic processing of fruits and vegetables has the potential to improve the bioavailability of carotenoids due to the disruption of the matrix of the cellular structures [94, 95]; however, they can also cause significant loss of carotenoids [96] and introduce *cis–trans* isomerization [97]. All carotenoids can undergo *cis–trans* isomerization and while the *trans* form is the usual configuration in nature, both forms can be found in fruits and vegetables [47]. Heat treatment, exposure to light and oxygen, and organic acid release through slicing and juicing can promote isomerization. *Cis–trans* isomers differ in their intestinal absorption in humans; therefore, processes that increase isomerization may adversely affect bioavailability and the resulting vitamin A value of foods. Thus, in order to maximize carotenoid bioavailability, a balance must be sought during processing to disrupt the matrix, but not result in excessive losses from heat and oxidation.

Most research on degradation and isomerization during processing and cooking has focused on β-carotene and lycopene and while some generalizations may be brought forward, the extent of changes in content or isomeric profile ultimately depends on the food matrix, temperature, duration, oxygen exposure, and severity of processing. Significant degradation of β-carotene is seen with deep-frying [96], dehydration [97], and extrusion [98]. Degradative products tend to be *cis*-isomers and epoxides and are also promoted by contact with acids, light, and heat. Dehydration techniques have an impact on losses. Sun-dried spinach (10 h) had greater β-carotene losses (43 %) than oven-dried (10 h at 65 °C) [97]. Freeze-drying carrots preserves β-carotene levels significantly compared with other drying methods [98] and lutein [99] and β-carotene appear to be fairly stable during mild to moderate heat processing [97, 99–103].

The effects of processing on tomato lycopene content and isomerization have been extensively studied and reviewed [104, 105]. More than 80 % of dietary lycopene is consumed from processed tomato products [104] and is present almost exclusively in the all-*trans* form. Lycopene appears to be much more resistant to isomerization and degradation [97, 99, 106], retaining its all-*trans* form during thermal processing of tomatoes while β-carotene and lutein experienced extensive isomerization [107].

Many aspects of food preparation impact carotenoid stability. In addition to those already mentioned, storage condition, packaging, freezing, lipid composition, additional antioxidant constituents, specific food matrices, contact with food acids, surface area, porosity, and enzymatic oxidation during slicing, peeling, pulping, or juicing can all contribute to variability in food carotenoid levels.

Considerations of variety, season, stage of maturity, growing practices, storage, and processing are important not only for growers, food processors, and consumers but also for researchers trying to understand carotenoid and provitamin A intake in populations for the purpose of epidemiological studies. Seasonal variations in dietary intake and serum concentrations of carotenoids of different populations have been observed [31, 108–112]. Coupled with the variability in carotenoid content of foods, the classification and stratification of carotenoid and food intake patterns in populations become more complicated and may affect the association with disease risk.

References

1. Dauchet L, Amouyel P, Hercberg S, Dallongeville J. Fruit and vegetable consumption and risk of coronary heart disease: a meta-analysis of cohort studies. J Nutr. 2006;136:2588–93.
2. Hung HC, Joshipura KJ, Jiang R, Hu FB, Hunter D, Smith-Warner SA, Colditz GA, Rosner B, Spiegelman D, Willett WC. Fruit and vegetable intake and risk of major chronic disease. J Natl Cancer Inst. 2004;96:1577–84.
3. Riboli E, Norat T. Epidemiological evidence of the protective effects of fruit and vegetables on cancer risk. Am J Clin Nutr. 2003;78:559S–69.
4. Lee JE, Männistö S, Spiegelman D, Hunter DJ, Bernstein L, van den Brandt PA, Buring JE, Cho E, English DR, Flood A, Freudenheim JL, Giles GG, Giovannucci E, Håkansson N, Horn-Ross PL, Jacobs EJ, Leitzmann MF, Marshall JR, McCullough ML, Miller AB, Rohan TE, Ross JA, Schatzkin A, Schouten LJ, Virtamo J, Wolk A, Zhang SM, Smith-Warner SA. Intakes of fruit, vegetables, and carotenoids and renal cell cancer risk: a pooled analysis of 13 prospective studies. Cancer Epidemiol Biomarkers Prev. 2009;18:1730–9.
5. Zhang CX, Ho SC, Chen YM, Fu JH, Cheng SZ, Lin FY. Greater vegetable and fruit intake is associated with a lower risk of breast cancer among Chinese women. Int J Cancer. 2009;125:181–8.
6. Mente A, de Koning L, Shannon H, Anand S. A systematic review of the evidence supporting a causal link between dietary factors and coronary heart disease. Arch Intern Med. 2009;169:659–69.
7. Sommerburg O, Keunen JEE, Bird AC, van Kujik FJGM. Fruits and vegetables that are sources for lutein and zeaxanthin: the macular pigment in human eyes. Br J Ophthalmol. 1998;82:907–10.
8. Johnson EJ, Hammond BR, Yeum KJ, Qin J, Wang XD, Castaneda C, Snodderly DM, Russell RM. Relation among serum and tissue concentrations of lutein and zeaxanthin and macular pigment density. Am J Clin Nutr. 2000;71:1555–62.
9. Garcia AL, Rühl R, Herz U, Koebnick C, Schweigert FJ, Worm M. Retinoid- and carotenoid-enriched diets influence the ontogenesis of the immune system in mice. Immunology. 2003;110:180–7.
10. Hughes DA. Effects of carotenoids on human immune function. Proc Nutr Soc. 1999;58:713–8.
11. Tang L, Jin T, Zeng X, Wang JS. Lycopene inhibits the growth of human androgen-independent prostate cancer cells in vitro and in BALB/c nude mice. J Nutr. 2005;135:287–90.

12. Seifried HE, McDonald SS, Anderson DE, Greenwald P, Milner JA. The antioxidant conundrum in cancer. Cancer Res. 2003;63:4295–8.
13. Finley JW. Proposed criteria for assessing the efficacy of cancer reduction by plant foods enriched in carotenoids, glucosinolates, polyphenols and selenocompounds. Ann Bot. 2005;95:1075–96.
14. Granado F, Olmedilla B, Blanco I. Nutritional and clinical relevance of lutein in human health. Br J Nutr. 2003;90:487–502.
15. Britton G, Liaaen-Jenson S, Pfander H, editors. Carotenoids handbook. Basel, Switzerland: Birkhauser; 2004.
16. West CE, Poortvliet EJ. The carotenoid content of foods with special reference to developing countries. The Netherlands: Department of Human Nutrition, Wageningen Agricultural University; 1993.
17. Mangels AR, Holden JM, Beecher GR, Forman MR, Lanza E. Carotenoid content of fruits and vegetables: an evaluation of analytic data. J Am Diet Assoc. 1993;93:284–96.
18. O'Neill ME, Carroll Y, Corridan B, Olmedilla B, et al. A European carotenoid database to assess carotenoid intakes and its use in a five-country comparative study. Br J Nutr. 2001;85:499–507.
19. Holden JM, Eldridge AL, Beecher GR, Buzzard IM, Bhagwat S, Davis CS, Douglass LW, Gebhardt S, Haytowitz D, Schakel S. Carotenoid content of U.S. Foods: an update of the database. J Food Compost Anal. 1999;12: 169–96.
20. Rodriguez-Amaya DB, Kimura M, Godoy HT, Amaya-Farfan J. Updated Brazilian database on food carotenoids: factors affecting carotenoid composition. J Food Compost Anal. 2008;21:445–63.
21. Rodriguez-Amaya DB. Food carotenoids: analysis, composition, and alterations during storage and processing of foods. Forum Nutr. 2003;56:35–7.
22. Chug-Ahuja JK, Holden LM, Forman MR, Mangels AR, Beecher GR, Lanza E. The development and application of a carotenoid database for fruits, vegetalbes, and selected multicomponent foods. J Am Diet Assoc. 1993;93: 318–23.
23. Forman MR, Lanza E, Yong LC, Holden JM, Graubard BI, Beecher GR, Melitz M, Brown ED, Smith JC. The correlation between two dietary assessments of carotenoid intake and plasma carotenoid concentrations: application of a carotenoid food-composition database. Am J Clin Nutr. 1993;58:519–24.
24. Michaud DS, Giovannucci EL, Ascherio A, Rimm EB, Forman MR, Sampson L, Willett WC. Associations of plasma carotenoid concentrations and dietary intake of specific carotenoids in samples of two prospective cohort studies using a new carotenoid database. Cancer Epidemiol Biomarkers Prev. 1998;7:283–90.
25. USDA ERS Food Availability (Per Capita) Data System; Nutrient Availability. Available from: http://www.ers.usda.gov/data-products/food-availability-(per-capita)-data-system.aspx. Accessed July 2011.
26. Khachik F, Spangler CJ, Smith Jr JC, Canfield LM, Steck A, Pfander H. Identification, quantification, and relative concentrations of carotenoids and their metabolites in human milk and serum. Anal Chem. 1997;69:1873–81.
27. Khachik F, Carvalho L, Bernstein PS, Muir GJ, Zhao DY, Katz NB. Chemistry, distribution, and metabolism of tomato carotenoids and their impact on human health. Exp Biol Med. 2002;227:845–51.
28. Kimura M, Rodriguez-Amaya DR. Carotenoid composition of hydroponic leafy vegetables. J Agric Food Chem. 2003;51:2603–7.
29. USDA National Nutrient Database for Standard Reference, Release 21. Composition of Foods Raw, Processed, Prepared. 2008. Available from: http://www.nal.usda.gov/fnic/foodcomp/search/. Accessed July 2011.
30. Maiani G, Castón MJ, Catasta G, Toti E, Cambrodón IG, Bysted A, Granado-Lorencio F, Olmedilla-Alonso B, Knuthsen P, Valoti M, Böhm V, Mayer Miebach E, Behsnilian D, Schlemmer U. Carotenoids: actual knowledge on food sources, intakes, stability and bioavailability and their protective role in humans. Mol Nutr Food Res. 2009;53:S194–218.
31. Heinonen MI, Ollilainen V, Linkola EK, Varo PT, Koivistoinen PE. Carotenoids in Finnish foods: vegetables, fruits, and berries. J Agric Food Chem. 1989;37:655–9.
32. Hart DJ, Scott KJ. Development and evaluation of an HPLC method for the analysis of carotenoids in foods, and the measurement of the carotenoid content of vegetables and fruits commonly consumed in the UK. Food Chem. 1995;54:101–11.
33. Murkovic M, Gams K, Draxl S, Pfannhauser W. Development of an Austrian carotenoid database. J Food Compost Anal. 2000;13:435–40.
34. Leth T, Jakobsen J, Andersen NL. The intake of carotenoids in Denmark. Eur J Lipid Sci Technol. 2000;102: 128–32.
35. Kim Y-N, Giraud DW, Driskell JA. Tocopherol and carotenoid content of selected Korean fruits and vegetables. J Food Compost Anal. 2007;20:458–65.
36. Hulshof PLM, Chao-Xu, van de Bovenkamp P, Muhilal, West CE. Application of a validated method for the determination of provitamin A carotenoids in Indonesian foods of different maturity and origin. J Agric Food Chem. 1997;45:1174–1179.
37. Setiawan B, Sulaeman A, Giraud DW, Driskell JA. Carotenoid content of selected Indonesian fruits. J Food Compost Anal. 2001;14:169–76.

38. Rodriguez-Amaya DB. A guide to carotenoid analysis in foods. Washington, D.C.: ILSI Press; 2001.
39. Campbell DR, Gross MD, Martini MC, Grandits GA, Slavin JL, Potter JD. Plasma carotenoids as biomarkers of vegetables and fruit intake. Cancer Epidemiol Biomarkers Prev. 1994;3:493–500.
40. Yang Z, Zhang Z, Penniston KL, Binkley N, Tanumihardjo SA. Serum carotenoid concentrations in postmenopausal women from the United States with and without osteoporosis. Int J Vitam Nutr Res. 2008;78:105–11.
41. Tanumihardjo SA, Horvitz MA, Porter-Dosti M, Simon PW. Serum α- and β-carotene concentrations qualitatively respond to sustained carrot feeding. Exp Biol Med. 2009;234:1250–6.
42. Pattison DJ, Symmons DP, Lunt M, Welch A, Bingham SA, Day NE, Silman AJ. Dietary beta-cryptoxanthin and inflammatory polyarthritis: results from a population-based prospective study. Am J Clin Nutr. 2005;82:451–5.
43. Ford ES, Giles WH. Serum vitamins, carotenoids, and angina pectoris: findings from the National Health and Nutrition Examination Survey III. Ann Epidemiol. 2000;10:106–16.
44. Sugiura M, Nakamura M, Ogawa K, Ikoma Y, Ando F, Shimokata H, Yano M. Dietary patterns of antioxidant vitamin and carotenoid intake associated with bone mineral density: findings from post-menopausal Japanese female subjects. Osteoporos Int. 2011;22:143–52.
45. Moeller SM, Parekh N, Tinker L, Ritenbaugh C, Blodi B, Wallace RB, Mares JA, CAREDS Research Study Group. Associations between intermediate age-related macular degeneration and lutein and zeaxanthin in the Carotenoids in Age-related Eye Disease Study (CAREDS): ancillary study of the Women's Health Initiative. Arch Ophthalmol. 2006;124:1151–62.
46. Whitehead AJ, Mares JA, Danis RP. Macular pigment: a review of current knowledge. Arch Ophthalmol. 2006;124:1038–45.
47. Humphries JM, Khachik F. Distribution of lutein, zeaxanthin, and related geometrical isomers in fruit, vegetables, wheat, and pasta products. J Agric Food Chem. 2003;51:1322–7.
48. Mathis P, Schenck CC. The functions of carotenoids in photosynthesis. In: Britton G, Goodwin TW, editors. Carotenoid chemistry and biochemistry. Oxford: Pergamon Press; 1982. p. 339–482.
49. Weller P, Breithaupt DE. Identification and quantification of zeaxanthin esters in plants using liquid chromatography-mass spectrometry. J Agric Food Chem. 2003;51:7044–9.
50. Di Mascio P, Kaiser S, Sies H. Lycopene as the most efficient biological carotenoid singlet oxygen quencher. Arch Biochem Biophys. 1989;274:532–8.
51. Etminan M, Takkouche B, Caamaño-Isorna F. The role of tomato products and lycopene in the prevention of prostate cancer: a meta-analysis of observational studies. Cancer Epidemiol Biomarkers Prev. 2004;13:340–5.
52. de Pee S, West CE, Permaesih D, Martuti S, Muhilal, Hautvast JG. Orange fruit is more effective than are dark green, leafy vegetables in increasing serum concentrations of retinol and β-carotene in schoolchildren in Indonesia. Am J Clin Nutr. 1998;68:1058–67.
53. Adalid AM, Roselló S, Nuez F. Evaluation and selection of tomato accessions (*Solanum section Lycopersicon*) for content of lycopene, β-carotene and ascorbic acid. J Food Compos Anal. 2010;23:613–8.
54. Kuti JO, Konuru HB. Effects of genotype and cultivation environment on lycopene content in red-ripe tomatoes. J Agric Food Chem. 2005;85:2021–6.
55. Lenucci MS, Cadinu D, Taurino M, Piro G, Dalessandro G. Antioxidant composition in cherry and high-pigment tomato cultivars. J Agric Food Chem. 2006;54:2606–13.
56. Perkin-Veazie P, Collins JK, Davis AR, Roberts W. Carotenoid content of 50 watermelon cultivars. J Agric Food Chem. 2006;54:2593–7.
57. Nicolle C, Carnat A, Fraisse D, Lamaison J, Rock E, Michel H, Amouroux P, Remesy C. Characterisation and variation of antioxidant micronutrients in lettuce (*Lactuca sativa folium*). J Sci Food Agric. 2004;84:2061–9.
58. Wall MM. Ascorbic acid, vitamin A, and mineral composition of banana (*Musa* sp.) and papaya (*Carica papaya*) cultivars grown in Hawaii. J Food Compost Anal. 2006;19:434–45.
59. Nicolle C, Simon G, Rock E, Amouroux P, Remesy C. Genetic variability influences carotenoid, vitamin, phenolic, and mineral content in white, yellow, purple, orange, and dark-orange carrot cultivars. J Amer Soc Hort Sci. 2004;129:523–9.
60. Arscott SA, Tanumihardjo SA. Carrots of many colors provide basic nutrition and bioavailable phytochemicals acting as a functional food. Compr Rev Food Sci Food Saf. 2010;9:223–39.
61. Kurilich AC, Juvik JA. Quantification of carotenoid and tocopherol antioxidants in *Zea mays*. J Agric Food Chem. 1999;47:1948–55.
62. Kurilich AC, Tsau GJ, Brown A, Howard L, Klein BP, Jeffrey EH, Kushad M, Wallig MA, Juvik JA. Carotene, tocopherol, and ascorbate contents in subspecies of *Brassica oleracea*. J Agric Food Chem. 1999;47:1576–81.
63. Kopsell DA, Kopsell DE, Lefsrud MG, Curran-Celentano J, Dukach LE. Variation in lutein, beta-carotene, and chlorophyll concentrations among Brassica oleracea cultigens and seasons. HortScience. 2004;39:361–4.
64. Mercadante AZ, Rodriguez-Amaya DB. Effects of ripening, cultivar differences, and processing on the carotenoid composition of mango. J Agric Food Chem. 1998;46:128–30.

65. Dhuique-Mayer C, Fanciullino A-L, Dubois C, Ollitrault P. Effect of genotype and environment on citrus juice carotenoid content. J Agric Food Chem. 2009;57:9160–8.
66. Simonne AH, Simonne EH, Eitenmiller RR, Mills HA, Green NR. Ascorbic acid and provitamin A contents in unusually colored bell peppers (*Capsicum annuum* L.). J Food Compost Anal. 1997;10:299–311.
67. Howard LR, Talcott ST, Brenes CH, Villalon B. Changes in phytochemical and antioxidant activity of selected pepper cultivars (*Capsicum* species) as influenced by maturity. J Agric Food Chem. 2000;48:1713–20.
68. Raffo A, La Malfa G, Fogliano V, Maiani G, Quaglia G. Seasonal variation in antioxidant components of cherry tomatoes (*Lycopersicon esculentum* cv. Naomi F1). J Food Compos Anal. 2006;19:11019.
69. Toor RK, Savage GP, Lister CE. Seasonal variations in the antioxidant composition of greenhouse grown tomatoes. J Food Compost Anal. 2006;19:1–10.
70. Zanfini A, Dreassi E, La Rosa C, D'Addario C, Corti P. Quantitative variations of the main carotenoids in Italian tomatoes in relation to geographic location, harvest time, varieties, and ripening stage. Ital J Food Sci. 2007;19:181–90.
71. Aherne SA, Jiwan MA, Daly T, O'Brien NM. Geographical location has greater impact on carotenoid content and bioaccessibility from tomatoes than variety. Plant Foods Hum Nutr. 2009;64:250–6.
72. Lu QY, Zhang Y, Wang Y, Wang D, Lee RP, Gao K, Byrns R, Heber D. California Hass Avocado: profiling of carotenoids, tocopherol, fatty acid, and fat content during maturation and from different growing areas. J Agric Food Chem. 2009;57:10408–13.
73. Griffiths DW, Dale MFB, Morris WL, Ramsay G. Effects of season and postharvest storage on the carotenoid content of *Solanum phureja* potato tubers. J Agric Food Chem. 2007;55:379–85.
74. Ramos DMR, Rodriguez-Amaya DB. Determination of the vitamin A value of common Brazilian leafy vegetables. J Micronut Anal. 1987;3:147–55.
75. de Azevedo-Meleiro CH, Rodriguez-Amaya DB. Carotenoid of endive and New Zealand spinach as affected by maturity, season and minimal processing. J Food Compost Anal. 2005;18:845–55.
76. Rodriguez-Amaya DB. Nature and distribution of carotenoids in foods. In: Charalambous G, editor. Shelf-life studies of foods and beverages. Chemical, biological, physical, and nutritional aspects. Amsterdam: Elsevier Science Publishers; 1993. p. 547–89.
77. Rodriguez-Amaya DB, Porcu OM, Azevedo-Meleiro CH. Variation in the carotenoid composition of fruits and vegetables along the food chain. In: Desjardins Y, editor. Conference: Proceedings of the 1st international symposium on human health effects of fruits and vegetables FAVHEALTH 2005, Quebec City, Canada, 17–20 August 2005, Acta Horticulturae. 2007. p. 387–94.
78. Roca M, Hornero-Méndez D, Gandul-Rojas B, Mínguez-Mosquera MI. Stay-green phenotype slows the carotenogenic process in *Capsicum annuum* (L.) fruits. J Agric Food Chem. 2006;54:8782–7.
79. Raffo A, Leonardi C, Fogliano V, Ambrosino P, Salucci M, Gennaro L, Buglianesi R, Giuffrida F, Quaglia G. Nutritional value of cherry tomatoes (*Lycopersicon esculentum* Cv. Naomi F1) harvested at different ripening stages. J Agric Food Chem. 2002;50:6550–6.
80. Vázquez-Caicedo AL, Sruamsiri P, Carle R, Neidhart S. Accumulation of all-*trans*-β-carotene and its 9-*cis* and 13-*cis* stereoisomers during postharvest ripening of nine Thai mango cultivars. J Agric Food Chem. 2005;53:4827–35.
81. Ornelas-Paz JD, Failla ML, Yahia EM, Gardea-Bejar A. Impact of the stage of ripening and dietary fat on in vitro bioaccessibility of β-carotene in "Ataulfo" Mango. J Agric Food Chem. 2008;56:1511–6.
82. González IA, Osorio C, Meléndez-Martínez AJ, González-Miret ML, Heredia FJ. Application of tristimulus colorimetry to evaluate colour changes during ripening of Colombian guava (*Psidium guajava* L.) varieties with different carotenoid pattern. Int J Food Sci Technol. 2011;46:840–8.
83. Schweiggert RM, Steingass CB, Mora E, Esquivel P, Carle R. Carotenogenesis and physico-chemical characterictics during maturation of red fleshed papaya fruit (*Carica papaya* L.). Food Res Int. 2011;44:1373–80.
84. Davies BH, Matthews S, Kirk JTO. The natures and biosynthesis of the carotenoids of different colour varieties of *Capsicum annuum*. Phytochemistry. 1970;9:797–805.
85. Minguez-Mosquera MI, Horneo-Mendez D. Comparative study of the effects of paprika processing on the carotenoids in peppers (*Capsicum annuum*) of the Bola and Agridulce varieties. J Agric Food Chem. 1994;42:1555–60.
86. Markus F, Daood HG, Kapitany J, Biacs PA. Change in the carotenoid and antioxidant content of spice red pepper (paprika) as a function of ripening and some technological factors. J Agric Food Chem. 1999;47:100–7.
87. Hornero-Mendez D, de Guevera RGL, Minguez-Mosquera MI. Carotenoid biosynthesis changes in five red pepper (*Capsicum annuum* L.) cultivars during ripening. Cultivar selection for breeding. J Agric Food Chem. 2000;48:3857–64.
88. de Azevedo CH, Rodriguez-Amaya DB. Carotenoid composition of kale as influenced by maturity, season, and minimal processing. J Sci Food Agric. 2005;85:591–7.

89. Bergquist SA, Gertsson UE, Olsson ME. Influence of growth stage and postharvest storage on ascorbic acid and carotenoid contant and visual quality of baby spinach (*Spinacia oleracea* L.). J Sci Food Agric. 2006;86: 346–55.
90. Beltrán-González F, Pérez-López AJ, López-Nicolás JM. Effects of agricultural practices on instrumental colour, mineral content, carotenoid composition, and sensory quality of mandarin orange juice, cv. Hernandina. J Sci Food Agric. 2008;88:1731–8.
91. Mercadante AZ, Rodriguez-Amaya DB. Carotenoid composition of a leafy vegetable in relation to some agricultural variables. J Agric Food Sci. 1991;39:1094–7.
92. Lester G. Organic vs conventionally grown Rio Red whole grapefruit and juice: comparison of production inputs, market quality, consumer acceptance, and human health-bioactive compounds. J Agric Food Chem. 2007;55:4474–80.
93. Kopsell DA, Kopsell DE, Curran-Celentano J. Carotenoid pigments in kale are influenced by nitrogen concentration and form. J Sci Food Agric. 2007;87:900–7.
94. Erdman Jr JW, Bierer TL, Gugger ET. Absorption and transport of carotenoids. Ann NY Acad Sci. 1993;691:76–85.
95. Castenmiller JJM, West CE, Linssen JPH, van het Hof KH, Voragen AGJ. The food matrix of spinach is a limiting factor in determining the bioavailability of β-carotene and to a lesser extent of lutein in humans. J Nutr. 1999;129:349–55.
96. Sulaeman A, Keeler L, Taylor SL, Giraud DW, Driskell JA. Carotenoid content, physicochemical, and sensory qualities of deep-fried carrot chips as affected by dehydration/rehydration, antioxidant, and fermentation. J Agric Food Chem. 2001;49:3253–61.
97. Yadav SK, Sehgal S. Effect of home processing on ascorbic acid and β-carotene content of spinach (*Spinacia oleracia*) and amaranth (*Amaranthus tricolor*) leaves. Plant Foods Hum Nutr. 1995;47:125–31.
98. Desobry SA, Netto FM, Labuza TP. Preservation of β-carotene from carrots. Crit Rev Food Sci Nutr. 1998;38:381–96.
99. Khachik F, Goli MB, Beecher GR, Holden J, Lusby WR, Tenorio MD, Barrera MR. Effect of food preparation on qualitative and quantitative distribution of major carotenoid constituents of tomatoes and several green vegetables. J Agric Food Chem. 1992;40:390–8.
100. Khachik F, Beecher GR, Whittaker NF. Separation, identification, and quantification of the major carotenoid and chlorophyll constituents in extracts of several green vegetables by liquid chromatography. J Agric Food Chem. 1986;34:603–16.
101. Khachik F, Beecher GR. Separation and identification of carotenoids and carotenol fatty acid esters in some squash products by liquid chromatography. 1. Quantification of carotenoids and related esters by HPLC. J Agric Food Chem. 1988;36:929–37.
102. Lessin W, Catigani G, Schwartz SJ. Quantification of *cis-trans* isomers of provitamin A carotenoids in fresh and processed fruits and vegetables. J Agric Food Chem. 1997;45:3728–32.
103. Mosha TC, Pace RD, Adeyeye S, Laswai HS, Mtebe K. Effect of traditional processing practices on the content of total carotenoid, β-carotene, α-carotene, and vitamin A activity of selected Tanzanian vegetables. Plant Foods Hum Nutr. 1997;50:189–201.
104. Shi J. Lycopene in tomatoes: chemical and physical properties affected by food processing. Crit Rev Biotechnol. 2000;20:293–334.
105. Boileau AC, Erdman Jr JW. Impact of food processing on content and bioavailability of carotenoids. In: Krinsky NI, Mayne ST, Sies H, editors. Carotenoids and health. New York: Marcel Dekker, Inc; 2004. p. 209–28.
106. Nguyen ML, Schwartz SJ. Lycopene stability during food processing. Proc Soc Exp Biol Med. 1998;218:101–5.
107. Nguyen M, Francis D, Schwartz S. Thermal isomerization susceptibility of carotenoids in different tomato varieties. J Sci Food Agric. 2001;81:910–7.
108. Olmedilla B, Granado F, Blanco I, Rojas-Hidalgo E. Seasonal and sex-related variations in six serum carotenoids, retinol, and α-tocopherol. Am J Clin Nutr. 1994;60:106–10.
109. Granado-Lorencio F, Olmedilla-Alonso B, Herrero-Barbudo C, Blanco-Navarro I. Pérez-Sacristán. Seasonal variation of serum α- and β-cryptoxanthin and 25-OH-vitamin D_3 in women with osteoporosis. Osteoporosis Int. 2008;19:717–20.
110. Rautalahti M, Albanes D, Haukka J, Roos E, Virtamo J. Seasonal variation of serum levels of β-carotene and α-tocopherol. In: Waldron KW, Johnson IT, Fenwich GR, editors. Food and cancer prevention: chemical and biological aspects. Cambridge, UK: The Royal Society of Chemistry; 1993. p. 146.
111. Ito Y, Ochiai J, Sasaki R, Suzuki S, Kusuhara Y, Morimitsu Y, Otani M, Aoki K. Serum concentrations of carotenoids, retinol, and alpha-tocopherol in healthy persons determined by high-performance liquid chromatography. Clin Chim Acta. 1990;24:131–44.
112. Ziegler RG, Wilcox III HB, Mason TJ, Bill JS, Virgo PW. Seasonal variation in intake of carotenoids and vegetables and fruits among white men in New Jersey. Am J Clin Nutr. 1987;45:107–14.

113. Larsen E, Christensen LP. Simple saponification method for the quantitative determination of carotenoids in green vegetables. J Agric Food Chem. 2005;53:6598–602.
114. Simon PW, Wolff ZY. Carotenes in typical and dark orange carrots. J Agric Food Chem. 1987;35:1017–22.
115. Agocs A, Nagy V, Szabo Z, Mark L, Ohmacht R, Deli J. Comparative study of the carotenoid composition of the peel and the pulp of different citrus species. Innov Food Sci Emerg Technol. 2007;8:390–4.
116. Xu C, Fraser PD, Wang W, Bramley PM. Differences in the carotenoid content of ordinary citrus and lycopene-accumulating mutants. J Agric Food Chem. 2006;54:5474–81.
117. Navarro P, Pérez-López AJ, Mercader MT, Carbonell-Barrachina AA, Gabaldon JA. Antioxidant activity, color, carotenoids composition, minerals, vitamin C, and sensory quality of organic and conventional mandarin juice, cv. Orogrande. Food Sci Technol Int. 2011;17:241–8.
118. Kopas-Lane LM, Warthesen JJ. Carotenoid photostability in raw spinach and carrots during cold storage. J Food Sci. 1995;60:773–6.
119. Mou B. Genetic variation of beta-carotene and lutein contents in lettuce. J Amer Soc Hort Sci. 2005;130:870–6.
120. Tonucci LH, Holden JM, Beecher GR, Khachik F, Davis CS, Mulokozi G. Carotenoid content of thermally processed tomato-based food products. J Agric Food Chem. 1995;43:579–86.
121. Isabelle M, Lee BL, Lim MT, Koh W, Huang D, Ong CN. Antioxidant activity and profiles of common fruits in Singapore. Food Chem. 2010;123:77–84.
122. Fleshman MK, Lester GE, Riedl KM, Kopec RE, Narayanasamy S, Curley Jr RW, Schwartz SJ, Harrison EH. Carotene and novel apocarotenoid concentrations in orange-fleshed *Cucumis melo* melons: determinations of β-carotene bioaccessibility and bioavailability. J Agric Food Chem. 2011;59:4448–54.
123. Breithaupt DE, Bamedi A. Carotenoid esters in vegetables and fruits: a screening with emphasis on β-cryptoxanthin esters. J Agric Food Chem. 2001;49:2064–70.
124. Provesi JG, Dias CO, Amante ER. Changes in carotenoids during processing and storage of pumpkin puree. Food Chem. 2011;128:195–202.
125. Kurz C, Carle R, Schieber A. HPLC-DAD-MS^n characterization of carotenoids from apricots and pumpkins for the evaluation of fruit product authenticity. Food Chem. 2008;110:522–30.
126. Kimura M, Kobori CN, Rodriguez-Amaya DB, Nestel P. Screening and HPLC methods for carotenoids in sweet-potato, cassava and maize for plant breeding trials. Food Chem. 2007;100:1734–46.
127. Khachik F, Beecher GR. Application of a C-45-β-carotene as an internal standard for quantification of carotenoids in yellow/orange vegetables by liquid chromatography. J Agric Food Chem. 1987;35:732–8.
128. Ishiguro K, Yoshinaga M, Kai Y, Maoka T, Yoshimoto M. Composition, content, and antioxidative activity of the carotenoids in yellow-fleshed sweetpotato (*Ipomoea batatas* L.). Breed Sci. 2010;60:324–9.
129. Chandrika UG, Fernando KSSP, Ranaweera KKDS. Carotenoid content and *in vitro* bioaccessibility of lycopene from guava (*Psidium guajava*) and watermelon (*Citrullus lanatus*) by high performance liquid chromatography diode array detection. Int J Food Sci Nutr. 2009;60:558–66.
130. Kopsell DA, Kopsell DE. Accumulation and bioavailability of dietary carotenoids in vegetable crops. Trends in Plant Science. 2006;11:499–507.

Chapter 2
Carrots of Various Colors

Samantha Schmaelzle and Sherry A. Tanumihardjo

Key Points

- Orange carrots are one of the most widely consumed vegetables and are a significant source of provitamin A carotenoids in the US diet. Breeding efforts to increase the nutritional value of carrots through biofortification have been on the rise.
- Through biofortification, carrots of multiple hues have been bred. The different pigments in the carrots are phytochemical components shown to have potential health benefits beyond providing vitamin A. For example, purple carrots are purple because of anthocyanins, which act as antioxidants, and red carrots are red because of lycopene, which may aid in heart disease prevention. Purple–white, purple–yellow, purple–orange, purple–red, purple–orange–red (POR), red–orange, and orange–yellow have successfully been bred.
- From previous research on solid colored carrots, carrots such as the POR variety will have anthocyanins, β-carotene, and lycopene, respectively, because of their different color components.
- Plant breeders should be encouraged to develop these carrots to provide sources of vitamin A precursors and other phytochemicals.
- Consuming these whole vegetables could have a greater reduction in disease risk than individual compounds, but further research is needed. The consumption of these carrots could provide not only vitamin A but also other functional compounds that have disease-fighting properties and enhance the well-being of humans.

Keywords α-Carotene • α-Retinol • Anthocyanins • Biofortification • Rainbow carrots

Introduction

Carrots are one of the most popular vegetables in the USA and fresh-market carrot consumption has been increasing over the past few decades [1]. Since the introduction of "cut and peel" carrots into the market place, which are also commonly called baby carrots, carrot consumption has increased by 50% in the USA. Carrots are a significant source of vitamin A in the form of α- and β-carotene

S. Schmaelzle, B.S. • S.A. Tanumihardjo, M.S., Ph.D. (✉)
Department of Nutritional Sciences, University of Wisconsin-Madison, 1415 Linden Dr, Madison, WI 53706, USA
e-mail: sherry@nutrisci.wisc.edu

S.A. Tanumihardjo (ed.), *Carotenoids and Human Health*, Nutrition and Health,
DOI 10.1007/978-1-62703-203-2_2, © Springer Science+Business Media New York 2013

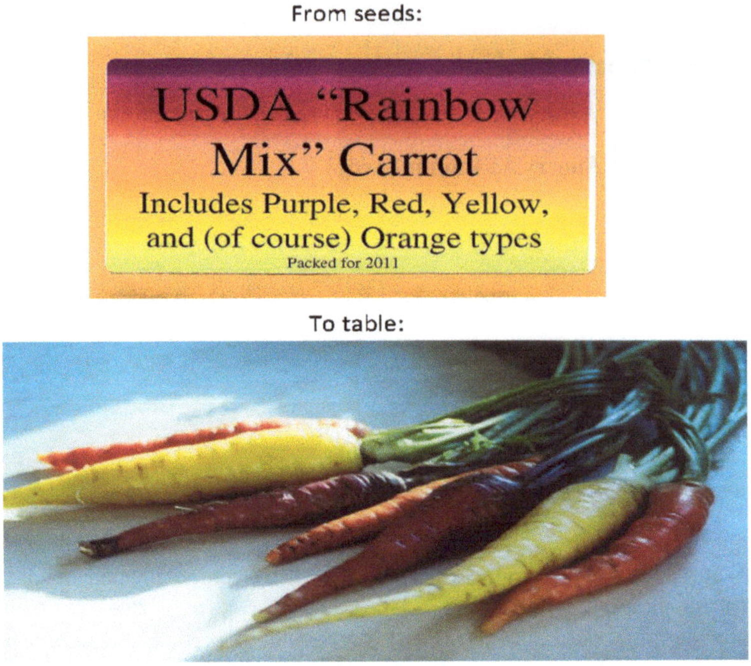
From seeds:
USDA "Rainbow Mix" Carrot
Includes Purple, Red, Yellow, and (of course) Orange types
Packed for 2011
To table:

Fig. 2.1 For over a decade, "rainbow" carrot seeds have been distributed to community and youth gardeners in Wisconsin and at various outreach efforts around the world. The harvested carrots are then used as demonstration tools to emphasize color variety among vegetables and their health benefits

accounting for an estimated 30% of the dietary vitamin A in the US diet [2]. Breeding efforts to improve food crops through biofortification (discussed extensively in Chap. 17) have increased the nutritional value of this vegetable [3, 4]. For carrots, biofortification has included increasing the provitamin A content (i.e., α- and β-carotene) as well as other bioactive compounds such as lutein, lycopene, and anthocyanins. These horticultural approaches for improving the nutritional quality and visual appeal of our food supply provide a sustainable, inexpensive complement to medical and social programs for preventing human disease [3].

Different colors of fruits and vegetables are due to pigmented disease-fighting phytochemicals, which is one reason the 2010 Dietary Guidelines recommend choosing a variety of fruits and vegetables [5]. Different colors of carrots (i.e., purple, red, white, yellow, and orange; Fig. 2.1) have been around for hundreds of years; however, orange carrots have been the predominant carrot available on the US grocery shelves. Colored carrots have a wide variation of pigments that have different biological benefits when consumed, such as providing vitamin A and decreased chronic disease risks [6]. Because carrots are so widely accepted and consumed among people especially in the USA, increasing the nutrient content could have exponential health benefits. Carrot breeders have developed new lines of novelty carrots that have multiple colors (and therefore, multiple phytochemicals) available in one carrot. For example, the POR carrot has a purple cortex with an orange and red core due to the presence of anthocyanins, α- and β-carotene, and lycopene, respectively [7].

Carotenoids are present in fruits and vegetables that have yellow, orange, and red pigmentation. Carotenoids protect chlorophyll from photooxidation and are accessory, light-harvesting pigments and photoreceptors [3]. Some carotenoids have provitamin A activity, meaning that they can be converted to vitamin A in the body. Other carotenoids support vision (see Chap. 13) and have antioxidant activity (see Chap. 4) in the body. Vitamin A obtained from the diet in fruits and vegetables is often recommended rather than from preformed sources (i.e., retinyl acetate or retinyl palmitate) because of the potential for hypervitaminosis A with supplements and fortified foods [8–10]. When consumed as plant provitamin A carotenoids, the body has more control over how much provitamin A is converted to retinol [11].

Flavonoids are a large group (~4,000 identified) of polyphenolic compounds that are expressed in plants, largely in fruits and vegetables [12]. Isoflavones, flavones, and anthocyanins are a few categories of flavonoids based on their chemical structure and function [13]. Anthocyanins in purple carrot include cyanidin-3-(2″-xylose-6-glucose-galactoside), cyanidin-3-(2″-xylose-galactoside), cyanidin-3-(2″-xylose-6′-sinapoyl-glucose-galactoside), cyanidin-3-(2″-xylose-6′-(4 coumuroyl) glucose-galactoside), and the major one, cyanidin-3-(2″-xylose-6′-feruloyl-glucose-galactoside) [14]. Flavonoids have dietary benefits such as antiallergy, anti-inflammatory, antitumor, and antioxidant characteristics [12]. Evidence exists that certain flavonoids can prevent platelet aggregation [13]. Indeed, dietary intake of flavonoids is quite high compared to other dietary antioxidants, such as vitamins C and E [12].

This chapter outlines why these "rainbow" carrots are important for human consumption, explains the carotenoids and/or phytochemicals in each of the colored carrots, and suggests the health benefit of incorporating multiple pigments into new types.

Types of Carrots, Their Phytochemicals, and Health Benefits

Solid colored carrots have been studied for nutritive benefits and color components to the point that they have been considered a "functional food" [15]. The pigments found in plants play important roles in plant metabolism and visual attraction in nature [3]. The pigments in carrots serve an important role in promoting health because they have been associated with reduced risk of atherosclerosis, cancer, and inflammation [16]. In general, phytochemicals have mechanisms of action in the body including antioxidant effects, modulation of detoxifying enzymes, stimulation of the immune system, modulation of hormone metabolism, and antibacterial and antiviral effects. Fruits and vegetables that are brightly colored—yellow, orange, red, green, blue, and purple—generally contain high amounts of phytochemicals and nutrients. Phytochemicals present in different types of carrots include not only the carotenoids but also flavonoids, such as red or blue anthocyanins.

Orange carrots. Orange carrots predominantly contain α- and β-carotene, both of which are orange pigments. These readily available carrots in the USA are high in vitamin A, which is essential for healthy eyes, cell growth, and reproduction. β-Carotene usually receives most attention and α-carotene, another provitamin A carotenoid in carrots, is often overlooked. The human body converts β-carotene directly to vitamin A, which is also important in strengthening the immune system by keeping the skin, lungs, and intestinal track in order (see Chap. 16). α- and β-Carotene are also antioxidants, which are important to fight against heart disease and trap free radicals. α-Carotene may be more powerful than β-carotene in inhibiting processes that may lead to tumor growth (see Chap. 11). α-Carotene is centrally cleaved in the intestinal brush border and reduced to α-retinol and retinol [17]. Biofortification of orange carrots has resulted in carrots with very high levels of α- and β-carotene [4, 14].

Yellow carrots. Yellow carrots contain predominantly the xanthophyll lutein, which is important for healthy eyes and in the fight against macular degeneration (see Chap. 13). Lutein may also prevent lung and other cancers and reduce the risk of atherosclerosis. A human study determined that yellow carrot lutein was 65% as bioavailable as that from a lutein in oil supplement [18].

Red carrots. The rich red pigment in red carrots is lycopene, which is a pigment also found in red tomatoes and pink watermelon. Lycopene is associated with a reduced risk of serum lipid oxidation, heart disease prevention, and a wide variety of cancers (see Chap. 12). Lycopene from red-pigmented carrots is about 40% as bioavailable as that from tomato paste [19]. For consumers who do not like tomatoes, having another food source of lycopene that is widely accepted would be a great option.

Purple and black carrots. Purple carrots get their pigmentation from phytochemicals called anthocyanins that act as powerful antioxidants to sequester harmful free radicals in the body [15, 20]. Sometimes the pigments are so dark that the carrots are called "black." Anthocyanins may prevent heart disease by acting as anti-inflammatory agents and reducing lipid oxidation [15]. Purple carrots were one of the first types to be consumed by humans in the Middle East [21]. Grassman et al. [22] evaluated different colored carrots and their antioxidant capacity. Solid colored purple carrots contained the most phenolic compounds and therefore may lead to higher antioxidant capacity in the human body.

White carrots. Although white carrots lack pigment, they are still a great source of dietary fiber. In comparative studies, white carrots are generally used as a control because they lack the pigmented phytochemicals that colored carrots hold [20].

Rainbow carrots. Efforts to breed carrots of several colors have been on the rise. Purple–white, purple–yellow, purple–orange, purple–red, POR, red–orange, and orange–yellow have successfully been bred. Because multicolored carrots are fairly new types, limited research and information are available on their phytochemical content and effects in animal or human models. From previous research on solid colored carrots, carrots such as the POR variety will have anthocyanins, β-carotene, and lycopene, respectively, because of their different color components. Rainbow carrot seeds have been distributed to community and youth gardeners to build awareness and to use the harvested carrots to demonstrate the diversity of pigments in vegetables (Fig. 2.1).

In Vitro Research

Sun et al. [20] determined the phytochemical profile and antioxidant capacity of seven colored carrots: purple–yellow, purple–orange, red, dark orange, orange, yellow, and white. Anthocyanins were the major phytochemical in purple–yellow and purple–orange carrots, and chlorogenic acid was a major compound in all carrots. Carotenoids did not contribute substantially to total antioxidant capacity, but correlated with it. Purple–yellow carrots had the highest antioxidant capacity, followed by purple–orange carrots, and the other carrots did not differ from each other. These results demonstrate that purple carrots have high antioxidant capacity and content, and therefore human consumption of these carrots may be beneficial.

Animal Research

Animal research is often performed to look at tissue storage and bioefficacy of the provitamin A carotenoids to make vitamin A. Studies of this sort are either not possible with humans due to the invasiveness of looking at tissue distribution or require isotopic tracers, which are expensive. Although not all animals are good models for carotenoid metabolic studies, Mongolian gerbils are useful and have been extensively used for provitamin A carotenoid studies including carrots [7, 14, 23].

Two animal studies used biofortified high β-carotene orange carrots and purple carrots to assess the bioavailability of the β-carotene in Mongolian gerbils [14]. In the first study, gerbils received a diet containing powdered orange, purple, white alone, or white carrot with a β-carotene supplement. In the second study, high-β-carotene orange, orange, purple, or white carrot powder diets were fed. After 21 days of feeding, the effects of carrot type or supplement on serum and liver β-carotene, α-carotene, and vitamin A concentrations were analyzed.

Liver stores of β-carotene and vitamin A did not differ between orange and purple carrot diets, when equal amounts of β-carotene from each of the diets were consumed [14]. Therefore, the anthocyanins from the purple carrot did not interfere with the bioavailability of β-carotene. Second, both the orange and the purple carrot diet resulted in higher liver vitamin A concentrations compared with the supplement, demonstrating that carotenoids from whole foods fed throughout the day are more consistently converted to vitamin A than single supplement doses. Finally, high-β-carotene carrots resulted in more than twofold higher β-carotene and 10% higher vitamin A liver stores compared with typical orange carrots [14]. These results suggest that high-β-carotene carrots may be an alternative source of vitamin A to typical carrots in areas of vitamin A deficiency. This was the first study to show that biofortified high-β-carotene orange carrots increase the vitamin A concentration in liver when compared with typical orange carrots in gerbils.

In another animal study, Mills et al. [7] measured the antioxidant potential and vitamin A bioefficacy of four biofortified carrot varieties—purple/orange, POR, orange/red, and orange. Each type of carrot was fed to Mongolian gerbils ($n = 11$/group, 6 groups) for 4 weeks. After treatment, antioxidant capacity, carotenoid, and retinol concentrations were analyzed in the liver and serum. Liver antioxidant capacity and vitamin A stores from the four colored carrot-fed gerbils were significantly higher than the white carrot-fed negative control group. Antioxidant capacity was also higher than the vitamin A-supplemented positive control group [7], suggesting that the bioactive compounds in the colored carrots enhanced liver antioxidant capacity.

Indeed, the antioxidant capacity of serum did not differ among the treatment groups, but was greater in the liver extracts from gerbils fed colored carrots compared with gerbils fed white carrots [7]. Antioxidant feeding interventions have mixed results, either showing little or no effect on antioxidant capacity in serum. This study may have been too short to see a serum antioxidant effect and serum is likely not a sensitive indicator of what is occurring at the tissue level.

Bioavailability competition between lycopene and β-carotene in the orange/red carrot variety may occur. In previous research, orange/red carrots fed to humans [19] and gerbils [23] showed lower bioavailability of lycopene than when fed tomato paste, which does not contain as much β-carotene as the red carrot. Intake of the orange and orange/red carrots yielded similar vitamin A bioefficacies in the gerbils [23]; and therefore, lycopene bioavailability may be more negatively affected than β-carotene bioefficacy when the two carotenoids interact.

The enhancement of liver antioxidant capacity observed in gerbils consuming biofortified carrots was likely due to the combined bioactivities of multiple compounds rather than the individual activities of carotenoids, anthocyanins, or phenolic acids, illustrating the synergistic benefit associated with intake of whole foods.

Human Studies with Various Colored Carrots

Unlike animal studies where absolute bioefficacy can be measured directly from liver stores of vitamin A, human bioavailability studies with various solid colored carrots have examined relative bioavailability using serum concentration changes over time with chronic feeding. Several human studies have shown varying bioavailabilities of specific phytochemicals from different colored carrots.

Two studies showed that lycopene and β-carotene are bioavailable from red carrots in humans [19]. The first study fed muffins made from red carrots at 5 mg lycopene/day compared with white carrots as a negative control for a period of 11 days. The second study determined the effect of carrot fiber on lycopene bioavailability by feeding tomato paste muffins with or without white carrots. Lycopene and β-carotene were bioavailable from red carrot, but lycopene absorption was negatively affected by carrot fiber. Combined results from both studies suggested that lycopene in red carrot is 44% as bioavailable as that from tomato paste and a serum plateau occurred at ≥20 mg lycopene/day [19].

Anthocyanins from purple carrots are bioavailable and can be absorbed intact as shown by a feeding study [24]. Varying amounts (250–500 g) of raw or cooked purple carrots were fed to human subjects. The four different anthocyanins observed were found intact in plasma by 30 min and peaked at 2 h after consumption. Cooking of the carrots increased the recovery of some anthocyanins. The reduced recovery of anthocyanins from the larger amount of carrots fed suggested saturation of absorption mechanisms.

Lutein bioavailability from yellow carrot was examined in humans by feeding 1.7 mg lutein/day from yellow carrots or a lutein supplement dissolved in oil, and white carrots as a negative control [18]. The subjects were fed carrot smoothies, muffins, and soup for breakfast and lunch for 7 days. The lutein from yellow carrots significantly increased serum concentrations and was found to be 65% as bioavailable as the lutein supplement. The yellow carrot treatment also maintained serum β-carotene concentrations, whereas the lutein treatment did not. Bioavailability of crystalline lutein, which is the form found in most supplements, is highly variable between and within subjects [25]. While yellow carrots are not a concentrated source of lutein compared to other vegetables such as green leaves, they may serve as an alternative bioavailable source of lutein especially considering the popularity of carrots in the US diet.

All of this research demonstrated that the compounds in these carrots had high bioavailability. However, a study with two different orange carrots did not show a difference in α- and β-carotene uptake and clearance in the serum between the two types [4]. Subjects received all three treatments of white, orange, or dark orange carrot muffins for 11 days with a 10-day washout period between treatments. The lack of difference between the orange and dark orange carrots may have been due to the prolonged time that the subjects were on a low carotenoid diet causing more bioconversion to vitamin A. Other tissues may have shown differences but were not accessible as in the animal studies with a similar design [14].

Arscott et al. [26] determined that anthocyanins in purple–orange carrots do not influence the bioavailability of β-carotene in young women. Using three treatment groups (i.e., purple/orange, orange, and white carrot smoothies) Arscott conducted a 3×3 crossover, acute feeding trial with five female subjects. Subjects were fed a carrot-containing breakfast after a carotenoid and anthocyanin washout period and blood samples were taken periodically for the next week. Both the orange and purple–orange carrot β-carotene peaks were elevated, but not different, suggesting that anthocyanins had no effect on β-carotene concentrations in serum. No effect of treatment was found for plasma antioxidant activity, which is a similar outcome as the animal study [7]. The design of this study is valuable, but a higher number of subjects and acute studies combined with chronic feedings might show a greater effect of the different compounds interacting with one another.

Conclusion

Further research with multicolored carrots and humans must be done to determine the interactions of beneficial compounds because they may compete with each other for release or uptake from the carrot. This research could lead to more varieties of carrots on grocery shelves and into the hands of consumers. The development of new and more potent sources of provitamin A carotenoids in horticultural crops, including carrots, and improvement of production shelf-life and consumer acceptance of these crops can make an important contribution to improving human health [3]. Increasing vegetable consumption, including carrots, was associated with modest weight loss in obese individuals [27]. In taste evaluation, the carrots of various colors were well-received and liked by consumers, especially when they were not blindfolded [28]. With this information, plant breeders should be encouraged to develop these carrots to provide sources of both vitamin A precursors and phytochemicals. Consuming these whole foods has an equal or greater reduction in disease risk than individual compounds [29].

As described in the multicolored carrot research, consuming fruits and vegetables that contain multiple bioactive compounds may have a more synergistic benefit than simply taking supplements or individual compounds. The consumption of these carrots could provide not only vitamin A but also other functional compounds that have disease-fighting properties and could enhance the well-being of humans.

References

1. USDA Economic Research Service. Factors affecting carrot consumption in the United States. In: Lucier G, Lin BH, editors. 2007. Available from: http://www.ers.usda.gov/Publications/VGS/2007/03Mar/VGS31901/. Accessed Oct 2011.
2. Simon PW. Breeding carrot, cucumber, onion and garlic for improved quality and nutritional value. Hortic Bras. 1992;11:171–3.
3. Simon PW. Plant pigments for color and nutrition. Hortic Sci. 1997;32:12–3.
4. Tanumihardjo SA, Horvitz MA, Porter Dosti M, Simon PW. Serum α- and β-carotene concentrations qualitatively respond to sustained carrot feeding. Exp Biol Med. 2009;234:1250–6.
5. United States Department of Health and Human Services, U.S.D.A., and United States Dietary Guidelines Committee. Report of the Dietary Guidelines Advisory Committee on the Dietary Guidelines for Americans, 2010. 2010.
6. Krebs-Smith SM, Kantor LS. Choose a variety of fruits and vegetables daily: understanding the complexities. J Nutr. 2001;131:487S–501.
7. Mills JP, Simon PW, Tanumihardjo SA. Biofortified carrot intake enhances liver antioxidant capacity and vitamin A status in Mongolian gerbils. J Nutr. 2008;138:1692–8.
8. Penniston KL, Tanumihardjo SA. Vitamin A in dietary supplements and fortified foods: too much of a good thing? J Am Diet Assoc. 2003;103:1185–7.
9. Penniston KL, Tanumihardjo SA. The acute and chronic toxic effects of vitamin A. Am J Clin Nutr. 2006;83:191–201.
10. Ribaya-Mercado JD, Solomons NW, Medrano Y, Bulux J, Dolnikowski GG, Russell RM, Wallace CB. Use of the deuterated-retinol-dilution technique to monitor the vitamin A status of Nicaraguan schoolchildren 1 y after initiation of the Nicaraguan national program of sugar fortification with vitamin A. Am J Clin Nutr. 2004;80:1291–8.
11. Tanumihardjo SA. Food-based approaches for ensuring adequate vitamin A nutrition. Compr Rev Food Sci Food Saf. 2008;7:373–81.
12. Buhler DR, Miranda C. Antioxidant activities of flavonoids. Oregon State University. 2000. http://lpi.oregonstate.edu/f-w00/flavonoid.html. Accessed 21 Oct 2011.
13. Marzocchella L, Fantini M, Benevenuto M, Masuelli L, Tresoldi I, Modesti A, Bei R. Dietary flavonoids: molecular mechanisms of action as anti-inflammatory agents. Recent Pat Inflamm Allergy Drug Discov. 2011;5(3):200–20.
14. Porter Dosti M, Mills JP, Simon PW, Tanumihardjo SA. Bioavailability of β-carotene (βC) from purple carrots is the same as typical orange carrots while high-βC carrots increase βC stores in Mongolian gerbils (*Meriones unguiculatus*). Br J Nutr. 2006;96:258–67.
15. Arscott SA, Tanumihardjo SA. Carrots of many colors provide basic nutrition and bioavailable phytochemicals acting as a functional food. Compr Rev Food Sci Food Saf. 2010;9:223–39.
16. Simon PW, Tanumihardjo SA, Clevidence BA, Novotny JA. Role of color and pigments in breeding, genetics, and nutritional improvement of carrots. In: Culver CA, Wrolstad RE, editors. Color quality of fresh and processed foods, ACS Symposium Series 983. Washington, DC: ACS Books; 2008. p. 151–66.
17. Tanumihardjo SA, Howe JA. Twice the amount of α-carotene isolated from carrots is as effective as β-carotene in maintaining the vitamin A status of Mongolian gerbils. J Nutr. 2005;135:2622–6.
18. Molldrem KL, Li J, Simon PW, Tanumihardjo SA. Lutein and β-carotene from lutein-containing yellow carrots are bioavailable in humans. Am J Clin Nutr. 2004;80:131–6.
19. Horovitz MA, Simon PW, Tanumihardjo SA. Lycopene and β-carotene are bioavailable from lycopene 'red' carrots in humans. Eur J Clin Nutr. 2004;58:803–11.
20. Sun T, Simon PW, Tanumihardjo SA. Antioxidant phytochemicals and antioxidant capacity of biofortified carrots (*Daucus carota L.*) of various colors. J Agric Food Chem. 2009;57:4142–7.
21. Simon PW. Domestication, historical development, and modern breeding of carrot. Plant Breed Rev. 2000;19:157–90.

22. Grassmann J, Schnitzler WH, Habegger R. Evaluation of different colored carrot cultivars on antioxidant capacity based on their carotenoid and phenolic contents. Int J Food Sci Nutr. 2007;58:603–11.
23. Mills JP, Simon PW, Tanumihardjo SA. β-Carotene from red carrot maintains vitamin A status, but lycopene bioavailability is lower relative to tomato paste in Mongolian gerbils. J Nutr. 2007;137:1395–400.
24. Kurilich AC, Clevidence BA, Britz SK, Simon PW, Novotny JA. Plasma and urine responses are lower for acylated vs nonacylated anthocyanins from raw and cooked purple carrots. J Agric Food Chem. 2005;53:6537–42.
25. Tanumihardjo SA, Li J, Porter Dosti M. Lutein absorption is facilitated with cosupplementation of ascorbic acid in young adults. J Am Diet Assoc. 2005;105:114–8.
26. Arscott SA, Simon PW, Tanumihardjo SA. Anthocyanins in purple-orange (*Daucus carota L*) do not influence the bioavailability of β-carotene in young women. J Agric Food Chem. 2010;58:2877–81.
27. Tanumihardjo SA, Valentine AR, Zhang Z, Whigham LD, Lai HJ, Atkinson RL. Strategies to increase vegetable or reduce energy and fat intake induce weight loss in adults. Exp Biol Med. 2009;234:542–52.
28. Surles RL, Weng N, Simon PW, Tanumihardjo SA. Carotenoid profiles and consumer sensory evaluation of specialty carrots (*Daucus carota*) of various colors. J Agric Food Chem. 2004;52:3417–21.
29. Buijsse B, Feskens EJ, Kwape L, Kok FJ, Kromhout D. Both α- and β-carotene, but not tocopherols and vitamin C, are inversely related to 15-year cardiovascular mortality in Dutch elderly men. J Nutr. 2008;138:344–50.

Chapter 3
Carotenoid Metabolism and Enzymology

Igor O. Shmarakov*, Jason J. Yuen*, and William S. Blaner

Key Points

- Carotenoids are plant-derived lipophilic compounds with a common chemical structure of eight isoprenoid units. The major carotenoids that are present in human tissues are primarily the polyunsaturated hydrocarbon carotenes β-carotene and lycopene and the oxygen-containing xanthophylls β-cryptoxanthin, lutein, and zeaxanthin. These carotenoids function in the body as retinoid (vitamin A) precursors and antioxidants.
- Carotenoid lipophilicity determines the specific features of carotenoid metabolic processing, and its relationship with and great dependence on lipid metabolism. This includes intestinal absorption of carotenoids from mixed micelles, facilitated uptake of carotenoids into cells mediated by the members of class B scavenger receptor protein family, lipoprotein transportation in the circulation, and oxygenase-mediated cleavage of carotenoids to form retinoids or apocarotenals.
- Dietary-derived carotenoids are transported in the postprandial circulation in chylomicrons and in the fasting circulation distributed among VLDL, LDL, and HDL. β-Carotene and lycopene are predominantly found in VLDL and LDL, whereas lutein and zeaxanthin are distributed equally between LDL and HDL.
- The presence of the polyunsaturated double bonds in the chemical structure of carotenoids underlies their ability to undergo nonenzymatic isomerization, singlet oxygen quenching, and electron transfer during oxidation/reduction reactions. These polyunsaturated double bonds are also sites of specific enzymatic cleavage, which is mediated by members of the nonheme iron-containing oxygenase family, specifically by BCMO1 (β-carotene-15,15′-monooxygenase, EC 1.14.99.36) and BCMO2 (β-carotene-9′,10′-monooxygenase, EC 1.14.99.n2).

---

* Shmarakov and Yuen contributed equally to this work.

I.O. Shmarakov, Ph.D.
Department of Medicine, College of Physicians and Surgeons, Columbia University, 630 W. 168th Street, New York, NY 10032, USA

Department of Biochemistry and Biotechnology, Chernivtsi National University, 2 Kotsyubynskyi Street, Chernivtsi, 58000, Ukraine

J.J. Yuen, M.S. • W.S. Blaner, Ph.D. (✉)
Department of Medicine, College of Physicians and Surgeons, Columbia University, 630 W. 168th Street, New York, NY 10032, USA
e-mail: wsb2@columbia.edu

S.A. Tanumihardjo (ed.), *Carotenoids and Human Health*, Nutrition and Health,
DOI 10.1007/978-1-62703-203-2_3, © Springer Science+Business Media New York 2013

- BCMO1 is a cytosolic protein, characterized as a carotenoid central cleavage enzyme, and is solely responsible for retinoid (vitamin A and its metabolites) formation from carotenoid precursors. BCMO2 is a mitochondrial protein, which catalyzes asymmetric cleavage of carotenoids, regulating carotene and xanthophyll degradation, and formation of apocarotenoid derivatives.

Keywords Beta-carotene • Lycopene • Retinoid • Lipoprotein • SR-BI • CD36

Abbreviations

ABC	ATP-binding cassette
ACO	apocarotenoid-15,15′-oxygenase
Apo	apolipoprotein
BCMO1	β-carotene-15,15′-monooxygenase
BCMO2	β-carotene-9′,10′-monooxygenase
CD36	cluster of differentiation 36
CR	chylomicron remnant
CRBP-II	cellular retinol binding protein type II
EZ	ezetimibe
HDL	high-density lipoprotein
HSC	hepatic stellate cell
ISX	intestine specific homeobox
LDL	low-density lipoprotein
LPL	lipoprotein lipase
LRAT	lecithin-retinol acyltransferase
MEF2	myocyte enhancer factor 2
NPC1L1	Niemann-Pick C1-like 1
PPAR	peroxisome proliferator-activated receptor
PPRE	peroxisome proliferator response element
RAR	retinoic acid receptor
RPE65	retinal pigment epithelium-specific protein 65 kDa
RXR	retinoid X receptor
SR-BI	scavenger receptor class B type I
T_3	triiodothyronine
TR	thyroid hormone receptor
TRE	thyroid hormone response element
UCP1	uncoupling protein 1
VLDL	very low density lipoprotein

Introduction

Dietary intake of carotenoids has been associated with reduced risks of various cancers [1], cardiovascular diseases, metabolic syndrome and obesity [2, 3], as well as cataract formation [4] and macular degeneration [5]. These beneficial health effects of dietary carotenoids have made the study of their bioavailability, absorption and metabolism an area of considerable interest, since humans cannot synthesize these molecules *de novo* and must obtain them from the diet. The proposed biological actions of carotenoids are numerous, and include their involvement in gene regulation [6], as well as their protective roles as antioxidants [7]. Despite all the nutritive properties of carotenoids, the molecular mechanisms underlying their metabolism remain to be fully established. In this chapter, we discuss the metabolic processes of carotenoid absorption and transport across the intestinal mucosa, including the numerous transformations involved in their metabolism. Much of the research attention focused on carotenoids is centered on their metabolic fate as retinoid (vitamin A) precursors. The bioconversion of provitamin A carotenoids to retinoids is therefore covered at length in this chapter.

Bioavailability and Dietary Factors

Of all the known carotenoids that exist in nature, humans ingest no less than 40 that are common in fruits and vegetables [8]. The carotenoids found in human plasma are limited, however, and are largely represented by the polyunsaturated hydrocarbons β-carotene, α-carotene, and lycopene, and the lipophilic xanthophylls β-cryptoxanthin, lutein, and zeaxanthin [8, 9]. Other xanthophylls and their metabolites, such as phytofluene and phytoene, have also been detected in low concentrations in human blood [9]. The rest of the dietary carotenoids, despite their relative abundance in green leafy vegetables, are generally absent in human tissues; neoxanthin, for example, which is ubiquitously present in higher plants, has never been reported to be detected in human blood [8]. It has been speculated that neoxanthin and other xanthophylls may be poorly absorbed in the intestine due to their polar carbonyl groups [8]. The molecular properties of lipophilicity and non-polarity may therefore determine the bioavailability of carotenoids, and the higher bioavailability of carotenes may be due to how readily accessible they are for uptake by enterocytes in the intestinal lumen. Indeed, more lipophilic carotenoids are more likely to accumulate in circulation. A diet study, in which healthy subjects ingested one serving per day of spinach for a week, showed significant increases in plasma levels of lutein and β-carotene, while the more polar neoxanthin and violaxanthin remained below quantifiable levels [10]. *In vitro* studies with differentiated Caco-2 cells, a human intestinal cell line, have also shown lipophilicity of carotenoids to be positively associated with their uptake [11, 12]. Together, these results suggest that the bioavailability of carotenoids is at least in part determined by their structural properties, which may determine their solubility in the mixed luminal components of bile salts, biliary phospholipids, and dietary lipids.

The initial step in the digestion of carotenoids involves their release from the food matrix, which begins in the stomach and continues into the duodenum. The carotenoids are then solubilized in lipid droplets and transferred to mixed micelles along with other dietary lipids. In many cases, these critical steps of micellization, in which carotenoids are transferred from the food matrix to micelles, constitute the bottleneck in the absorption process, especially when the carotenoids are embedded in the fibrous cell walls of fruits and vegetables. This is evidenced by the very low recovery of ingested carotenoids in the aqueous phase of the duodenal contents; as a result of which, only a small fraction is available for intestinal uptake [13]. The food matrix is therefore a major determinant of carotenoid bioavailability, and its physical disruption by means of heat or mechanical processing improves absorption [14–19]. Thus, the overall bioaccessibility of carotenoids is determined by the efficiency at which carotenoids are transferred from the food matrix to micelles [8, 20]. As expected, the hydrocarbon carotenes have been observed to be more sensitive to luminal conditions [21], underscoring the influence of lipophilicity on their transfer to micelles. The presence of dietary fat in the intestinal chyme is therefore important, and has the greatest impact of all the dietary factors that influence carotenoid absorption [22]. It has long been understood that co-ingestion of fat is required for the absorption of carotenoids from a meal, and studies have demonstrated markedly enhanced carotenoid absorption with increasing amounts of dietary lipids [23, 24]. In addition to the amount, the structural composition of the co-ingested lipids also affects postprandial levels of carotenoids; long-chain fatty acyl groups, for example, are significantly more effective than medium-chain fatty acyl groups at enhancing absorption of β-carotene [25]. Failla and colleagues explored comprehensively the effects of amount and structure of triglycerides on carotenoid absorption, and found that while the addition of triglycerides increased the *in vitro* micellization of hydrocarbon carotenes, it did not affect that of the more polar xanthophylls. Moreover, the bioaccessibility of the carotenes was influenced by the chain length, but not by the degree of unsaturation, of the fatty acyl groups [22].

Much remains to be understood about the processing of carotenoids in the intestinal lumen, which is made ever more complicated by the myriad of interactions among dietary components. In addition to the effects of dietary fat, the amount and quality of dietary fiber also influence, often decrease, the bioavailability of carotenoids [26]. Other factors involve carotenoid–carotenoid interactions [27–31]. It has been reported that oral administration of a combined dose of β-carotene and lutein to human subjects resulted in reduced plasma levels of both carotenoids, as compared to their levels when ingested separately [31, 32]. *In vitro* studies have also evidenced competition between lycopene and β-carotene for absorption, each mutually inhibiting transit of the other through a Caco-2 cell monolayer [29]. To the contrary, however, another study carried out in human subjects showed that β-carotene consumption could improve lycopene absorption [30], while lycopene had no effect on β-carotene absorption [31]. These observed carotenoid–carotenoid interactions may be dependent on the specific carotenoid concentrations employed in the studies and further investigations will be needed to systematically resolve these inconsistencies.

Absorption into the Intestinal Mucosa

After incorporation into micelles, carotenoids are taken up by enterocytes at the apical mucosal surface of the brush border membrane [33]. The linear association observed between the lipophilicity of carotenoids and uptake from mixed micelles suggests a process of passive diffusion across the plasma membrane of epithelial cells [11, 34, 35]. In further support of this classical view on intestinal lipid absorption, *in vitro* experiments with Caco-2 cells have also demonstrated enhanced carotenoid uptake when the cells displayed compromised membrane integrity [11, 12]. Intestinal absorption and tissue accumulation are known to vary across animal species [12, 36, 37]. Furthermore, inter-individual variability in intestinal absorption and plasma accumulation has been observed in human subjects given pharmacological doses of β-carotene [38]. These physiological disparities cannot be explained by an unregulated passive diffusion process across the intestinal epithelium, and instead suggest some level of selectivity in a facilitated uptake process. In fact, Caco-2 cells exhibit isomer specificity, preferring the uptake of all-*trans*-β-carotene over the *cis*-conformations [29]. Additionally, kinetic studies have provided evidence for a saturable, receptor-mediated mechanism that is also time- and concentration-dependent [29].

At present, there is general consensus that class B scavenger receptors expressed on the membrane brush border play a role in facilitating the transport of β-carotene, lycopene, and lutein [39–42]. Scavenger receptor class B type 1 (SR-BI) is a member of the ATP-binding cassette (ABC) transporter superfamily, which mediates the selective uptake of cholesterol and cholesterol esters, and has an important role in reverse cholesterol transport [43, 44]. Cluster of differentiation 36 (CD36) is another member of the class B scavenger receptor family, and is known to mediate the transport of fatty acids into cells [45–47]. Both SR-BI and CD36 are expressed in the human intestinal epithelium [48, 49], where they can facilitate the uptake of β-carotene as well as cholesterol; transient transfection of COS-7 cells, a model cell line for recombinant protein expression, with either SR-BI or CD36 conferred on the cells the ability to absorb membrane-soluble lipids, including β-carotene, with similar efficiency [39]. The involvement of both of these receptors in cholesterol uptake suggests that carotenoids may be absorbed into the intestinal epithelium via the same mechanisms involved in cholesterol transport. This hypothesis is supported by the observation that consumption of plant sterols decreased both cholesterol absorption and carotenoid bioavailability in humans [50]. Dietary carotenoids also reduce cholesterol absorption in rats [51]. The differences in distribution, however, of SR-BI and CD36 along the length of the human small intestine suggest different functional roles for these homologous receptors. SR-BI is expressed throughout the small intestine, while CD36 is not expressed in the duodenum [49]. These expression profiles suggest that CD36 is likely to be the major facilitator of dietary lipid uptake in the jejunum and the ileum, where the absorption of monoacylglycerols and free fatty acids takes place [52], while SR-BI may be responsible for mediating the uptake of the more hydrophobic lipid molecules in the duodenum [39], where carotenoids are thought to be mainly absorbed. Indeed, *in vivo* experiments have shown the absorption of β-carotene to be significantly impaired in *Sr-bI* knockout (*Sr-bI*$^{-/-}$) mice, although this difference was observed only in mice fed a high-fat, high-cholesterol diet [39]. Interestingly, when fed a basal diet, β-carotene absorption was equally low in *Sr-bI*$^{-/-}$ and wild-type mice [39]. These data indicate that while SR-BI plays a role in the uptake of β-carotene in the small intestine, its efficiency as a carotenoid transporter is dependent on the presence of other dietary lipids. This observation is consistent with diet studies that showed increased postprandial levels of carotenoids with higher fat intake [24, 53]. Conversely, transgenic mice overexpressing *Sr-bI* in the intestine showed a 10-fold increase in plasma lycopene levels after 30 days of dietary supplementation [42]. *In vitro* experiments have also associated SR-BI with the uptake of lycopene [42] and lutein [40], as well as β-carotene [41] in Caco-2 cells. These findings convincingly establish a role for SR-BI in the intestinal uptake of carotenoids.

Much less is known about CD36 and its role in carotenoid uptake in the intestine. CD36 recognizes a number of ligands including cholesterol and free fatty acids, and it plays a critical role in the intestinal uptake of very long chain fatty acids [54, 55], but its involvement in carotenoid uptake has yet to be systematically studied. While the ability of CD36 to facilitate the uptake of β-carotene has been demonstrated in transfected COS-7 cells [39], the inhibition of CD36 with anti-CD36 antibodies did not affect β-carotene transport in Caco-2 cells [41]. These results suggest that while CD36 can facilitate the absorption of carotenoids, it probably does not contribute significantly to total carotenoid absorption in the intestine. Consistent with this view, the pattern of CD36's distribution along the intestine is instead more suggestive of an important role in fatty acid transport [49, 55, 56]. Further studies will be needed to determine the extent of CD36's contribution to carotenoid uptake in the intestine.

While all the data point to SR-BI as the major carotenoid transporter in the intestine, there are suggestions that other apical membrane receptors may be involved. Since SR-BI is highly expressed in the duodenum where it is known to facilitate the transport of many lipophilic molecules, including various cholesterol esters, phospholipids, and triglycerides [57–59], the impairment of carotenoid uptake in its absence may not be very surprising. Through its hydrophobic transmembrane domain, SR-BI mediates the bidirectional flux of free cholesterol and cholesterol esters down a concentration gradient [60–62]. Likewise, the SR-BI-mediated transport of carotenoids may be a facilitated-diffusion process that requires no energy expenditure [20]. Such a model may be supported by the linear rates of uptake observed in studies of Caco-2 cells, in response to physiological doses of carotenoids [40], but it probably does not account for all regulation that occurs at the level of uptake by the enterocyte. Importantly, antibodies raised against SR-BI receptors did not fully inhibit carotenoid uptake in Caco-2 cells [41, 42]. Treatment of the cells with ezetimibe (EZ), a known inhibitor of cholesterol transport, further inhibited β-carotene uptake in an additive fashion, implying different targets of inhibition [41]. The mechanism by which EZ inhibits cholesterol transport is not fully understood, but EZ has been reported to target Niemann-Pick C1-like 1 (NPC1L1) [63], which has been associated with the intestinal absorption of cholesterol [64, 65]. NPC1L1 is also highly expressed on the intestinal epithelium, making it a candidate receptor for carotenoids. The *in vitro* inhibition of NPC1L1, however, does not impair lycopene uptake by Caco-2 cells [42]. Collectively, these experiments suggest that there may be other brush border membrane receptors involved, or other mechanisms in place, that contribute to the facilitated absorption of carotenoids into the intestinal epithelium.

Processing and Efflux from the Enterocyte

Within the intestinal mucosa, provitamin A carotenoids are either cleaved to form retinal or incorporated intact into chylomicrons. In the human intestine, where the majority of carotenoid cleavage takes place [66], 55–75 % of the absorbed β-carotene is enzymatically converted into retinaldehyde, which is further reduced to retinol by retinaldehyde reductase and converted to retinyl ester by lecithin-retinol acyltransferase (LRAT, EC 2.3.1.135), with the aid of cellular retinol binding protein type II (CRBP-II) [67]. β-Carotene is therefore a major dietary source of vitamin A for humans [68]. The retinyl esters formed are then incorporated into chylomicrons along with intact carotenoids for secretion and transport in the circulation, via the lymphatic system. Chylomicrons are the major lipoprotein particles secreted by enterocytes in the postprandial state, and they are essential for the transport of all dietary fat and fat-soluble nutrients in the blood [69, 70]. These processes are summarized in Fig. 3.1.

The basolateral secretion of carotenoids into the lymph is dependent on the assembly and secretion of apolipoprotein B (apoB)-containing chylomicrons, which is induced by the presence of lipid micelles on the apical surface of intestinal cells and mediated by apolipoprotein A-IV (apoA-IV) [69, 71–73]. As such, the transfer of carotenoids across the intestinal mucosa is dependent on the presence of dietary lipids, which regulates the assembly of chylomicrons that serve as their transport vehicles in the plasma. The extent of carotenoid incorporation into chylomicrons may be determined by the

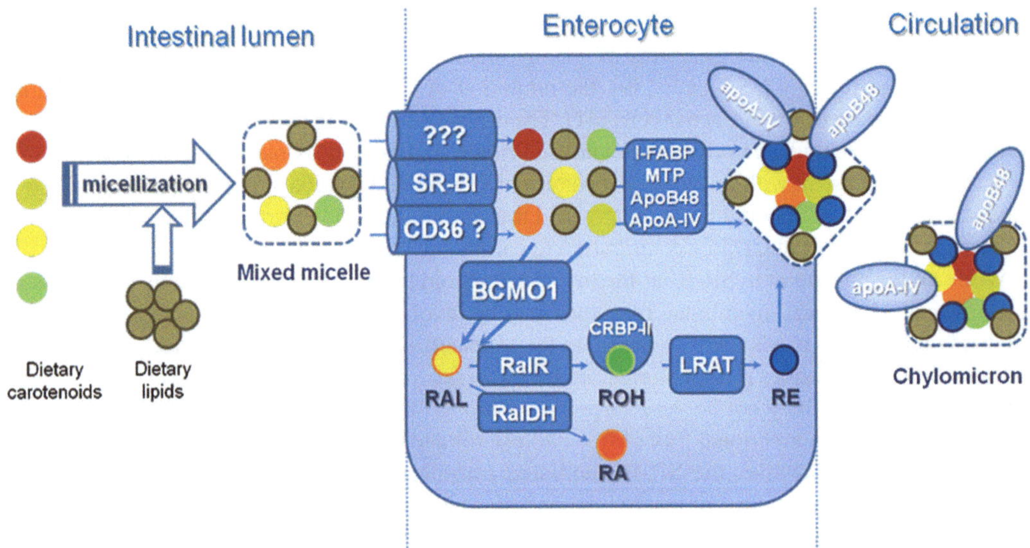

Fig. 3.1 Absorption and metabolism of carotenoids in the intestine. Within the lumen of the intestine, carotenoids (predominantly β-carotene, lycopene, β-cryptoxanthin, lutein, and zeaxanthin) are released from the food matrix, solubilized in lipid droplets and transferred to mixed micelles along with other dietary lipids. After incorporation into micelles, carotenoids are delivered to the apical mucosal surface of the brush border membrane, where they are taken up by the enterocyte via a receptor-mediated mechanism that involves scavenger receptor class B type 1 (SR-BI). It also has been proposed that CD36 and possibly other unidentified apical membrane receptors may facilitate carotenoid uptake into the enterocyte. Inside the enterocyte, proretinoid carotenoids (β-carotene and β-cryptoxanthin) may be acted upon by BCMO1 to form retinaldehyde (RAL), which can then be reduced to retinol (ROH) by retinal reductases (RalR) or oxidized to retinoic acid (RA) by retinal dehydrogenases (RalDH). Retinol bound to cellular retinol binding protein type II (CRBP-II) is esterified by lecithin-retinol acyltransferase (LRAT) to form retinyl ester, which is packaged into apolipoprotein B (apoB)-containing chylomicrons along with intact carotenoids and other dietary fats for secretion and transport in the circulation [39–42, 67]

structural properties of the different carotenoid species [29]. In parallel with evidence for isomer discrimination at the level of cellular uptake, During et al. found that, within Caco-2 cells, all-*trans*-β-carotene was preferentially incorporated into chylomicrons over the *cis*-isomers [29]. These investigators reported linear rates of secretion, as well as uptake, in response to increasing initial concentrations of β-carotene administered, up to 6 μM and saturating at 10 μM [29]. The greater variability observed for the basolateral secretion, versus cellular uptake, of the different carotenoids tested, further points to the involvement of intracellular mechanisms [29], possibly in the selective transport of carotenoids through the secretory pathway, as has been observed in the preferential packaging of nascent, instead of preformed, triglycerides into chylomicrons [74].

Very little is known about the molecular mechanisms for carotenoid discrimination and transport within the enterocyte. Likewise, any intracellular processing remains largely unknown, and evidence for it is limited to inferences from the detection of carotenoid metabolites in the postprandial plasma. All-*trans*-β-carotene, for example, has been reported to accumulate in the plasma of human subjects who ingested only 9-*cis*-β-carotene. This observation suggests the occurrence of isomerization during the absorption process [75]. *In vitro* experiments, however, have failed to show accumulation of all-*trans*-β-carotene in the basolateral medium when Caco-2 cell monolayers were incubated with 9-*cis*-β-carotene [29]. More recently, it has been reported that lycopene is isomerized in intestinal cells [76] from the more prevalent dietary form, the all-*trans* configuration, to the potentially more biologically active *cis*-isomers in human subjects [76, 77].

There may also be further regulation that takes place after uptake into the brush border membrane. Carotenoids taken up by the intestinal epithelia may be selectively excreted back into the intestinal lumen, perhaps in a process similar to that described for the excretion of phytosterols by ABC transporters [8, 78]. The expression of ABC transporters in the enterocyte is known to be induced by plant sterols as a means to selectively transport non-cholesterol sterols back into the intestinal lumen [79, 80]. Plant sterols decrease serum levels of both cholesterol and carotenoids [81], and this reduction, at least in cholesterol levels, is due to lower intestinal absorption [82]. So, it is possible that the ABC transporters involved in the transport of sterols are also responsible for the reduced absorption of cholesterol and carotenoids. But there is no definitive evidence for the resecretion of carotenoids from the enterocyte back into the intestinal lumen. The detection, however, of carotenoids in human bile [83] may be taken to suggest this possibility, since these same ABC transporters are known to play a role in the biliary secretion of cholesterol.

On the whole, the molecular mechanisms underlying the cellular translocation and metabolism of intact carotenoids in the human intestine remain unknown. The bulk of our current knowledge on the subject is instead focused on the well-characterized enzymatic conversion of provitamin A carotenoids to retinoids.

Transport and Metabolism in the Circulation

Chylomicrons secreted into the basolateral side of the intestinal epithelia are drained into the mesenteric lymphatic vessels and carried to the venous blood via the thoracic duct [84]. By way of the intestinal lymphatics, lipid transport circumvents first-pass hepatic metabolism, and the carotenoids and retinyl ester associated with chylomicrons are available for uptake by extrahepatic tissues. In the circulation, chylomicrons are quickly metabolized to chylomicron remnants (CRs) in a process characterized by the loss of triglyceride content, through hydrolysis catalyzed by lipoprotein lipase (LPL), and the subsequent acquisition of apolipoprotein E (apoE), which signals hepatic clearance. During this transit period, retinyl ester is also hydrolyzed, following significant hydrolysis of triglyceride, and retinol can be taken up by peripheral tissues. Retinyl ester is a substrate for LPL, and its hydrolysis in the postprandial plasma contributes significantly to extra-hepatic stores of retinol; 25 % of chylomicron retinyl ester is hydrolyzed for peripheral uptake [85, 86]. Plasma response of different carotenoids has

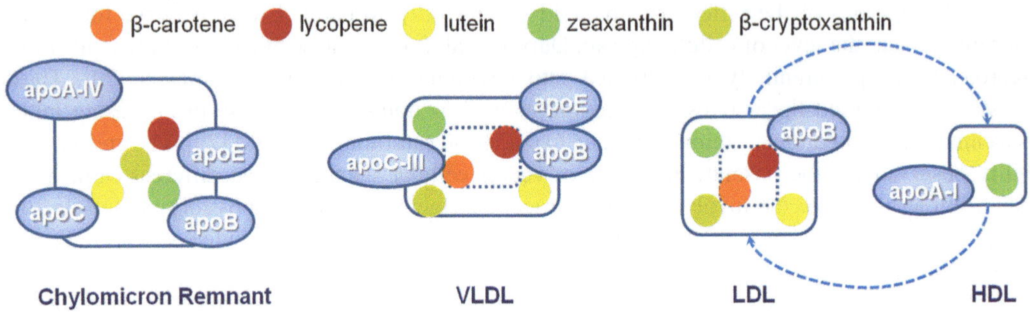

Fig. 3.2 Carotenoid distribution among different lipoprotein classes. Carotenoids are transported in the circulation as components of lipoproteins. In the fasting state, the majority (55 %) of plasma carotenoid is transported on low-density lipoproteins (LDL); approximately 33 % is associated with high-density lipoprotein (HDL), with the remainder associated with very low-density lipoprotein (VLDL). β-Carotene and lycopene are associated predominantly with LDL and VLDL, while lutein and zeaxanthin are distributed equally between LDL and HDL. The xanthophylls are carried close to the particle's surface where they are more likely to be transferred between lipoproteins (especially between LDL and HDL), whereas the lipophilic carotenes occupy the inner core and have less contact with other lipoproteins, thus preventing exchange [91–93]

been observed to differ in the postprandial state. Work by Novotny et al., following the plasma concentrations of [^{13}C]lutein and [^{13}C]β-carotene after ingestion of kale isotopically labeled with ^{13}C and served to human volunteers with 30 g of oil, established that lutein is first detected between 3 and 6 h, and β-carotene between 4 and 6 h, after dose consumption [87]. Interestingly, the time of peak plasma lutein concentrations in these subjects ranged between 10 and 36 h, whereas β-carotene exhibited a double peak in plasma, with the first peak occurring between 8 and 10 h and the second occurring between 24 and 36 h [85]. Comparative studies of carotenoid absorption carried out in preruminant calves by Bierer et al. established for this species that lutein peaked earlier in serum (12 h after dosing) than did the less polar lycopene, α-carotene, and β-carotene (16, 24, and 24 h, respectively) [88]. It should be noted that, for both the human and preruminant calf studies, intestine-derived chylomicrons were not separated from liver-derived lipoproteins; thus, the reported times to peak plasma concentrations likely reflect both intestinal uptake and resecretion from the liver. Before newly absorbed carotenoids can be cleared from the circulation, the CRs must be made small enough by triglyceride hydrolysis to enter the perisinusoidal space in the liver where absorption occurs [89]. Here, the binding of apoE on the surface of the CR to hepatic low-density lipoprotein (LDL) receptors is critical for the endocytosis of the remnant particle into hepatocytes [90].

Within the liver, carotenoids can be accumulated or secreted back into the circulation as a component of very low density lipoprotein (VLDL). In the fasting state, 10–19 % of plasma carotenoids is transported on VLDL; the majority (55 %) is found in LDL, and around 33 % is associated with high-density lipoproteins (HDL). β-Carotene and lycopene are predominantly found in LDL and VLDL, while lutein and zeaxanthin are distributed equally between LDL and HDL [91, 92]. This difference in distribution is consistent with the observation that lipoprotein transfer of carotenoids occurs mainly with xanthophylls [93], which may be accounted for by the hydrophobicity of the molecules; the polar xanthophylls are localized to the surface of the particle where they are more likely to be transferred between lipoproteins, while the lipophilic carotenes occupy the inner core of lipoproteins where they are physically shielded from this effect (see Fig. 3.2) [92]. Because the majority of carotenoids circulating in the blood is carried within the core of VLDL and LDL particles [94], tissues expressing high levels of LDL receptors, such as the liver and adrenal glands, will accumulate high levels of these carotenoids. Cellular uptake of carotenoids may also depend on whether the tissue expresses other cell surface receptors. SR-BI and CD36 have been implicated in the tissue uptake of carotenoids; for example, the selective uptake of xanthophylls in the cells of the retina involves SR-BI [95], and CD36 has been reported to play an important role in facilitating the uptake of lycopene and lutein by adipose tissue [96].

Given that carotenoids follow the same metabolic pathways as dietary lipids in the enterocyte and in the circulation, the proteins involved in the processes of absorption and transport will also indirectly affect plasma carotenoid levels. This notion is supported by findings of altered plasma carotenoid concentrations in human subjects with genetic polymorphisms of genes involved in lipid metabolism, including apoB and apoA-IV [97]. Recent studies on the variability of plasma carotenoid concentrations in human populations have also shown that the observed differences can at least in part be explained by multiple genetic variations in genes involved in lipoprotein metabolism and lipid transfer [98, 99].

Tissue Uptake and Accumulation

Tissues are able to selectively take up carotenoids from the circulation, depending on expression of membrane receptors, SR-BI and/or CD36, as well as LDL receptors and possibly other unidentified cell surface proteins. Within tissues, carotenoids can be utilized either for retinoid production or as antioxidants. In the case of adipose tissue, where much of the body's carotenoid accumulates, they can also be released back into the circulation. β-Carotene, lycopene, and lutein are carotenoids that are predominantly found in adipose tissue, and they are thought to be taken up by adipocytes via CD36 in a facilitated-uptake process [96]. Carotenoid levels in adipose tissue are site-specific, and most carotenoids accumulate in higher concentrations in the adipose tissue of the abdomen than in the other major adipose depots of the body, the buttocks and thighs [100]. Abdominal adipose carotenoids have been found to be significantly correlated with serum levels and dietary intake, and it has been proposed that these levels may be used as a reliable indicator of carotenoid status [100].

The liver is another organ with a large capacity for carotenoid accumulation. Carotenoids arrive at the liver in lipoprotein remnant particles, which are taken up via endocytosis into hepatocytes, where they can accumulate. Once dissociated from lipoprotein remnants, carotenoids can be transferred to hepatic stellate cells (HSCs) in a process that has yet to be elucidated. Several studies performed in animal models suggest that HSCs can also accumulate β-carotene [101, 102], albeit at lower levels than in hepatocytes; the accumulation of β-carotene and lycopene, for example, has been shown in GRX cells, an *in vitro* model of murine HSCs [100]. HSCs have also been demonstrated to accumulate all-*trans*-lycopene in their lipid droplets, where they have been observed to isomerize to *cis*-conformations [103].

In the eyes, high concentrations of the xanthophylls lutein and zeaxanthin are found in the retinal pigment epithelium of the neural retina. Often referred to as macular pigments, the levels of these xanthophylls in the macula of the retina correlate with dietary intake [28], and their accumulation may be explained in part by the preferential uptake of zeaxanthin, as opposed to β-carotene, in a process that appears to be entirely dependent on SR-BI [95]. On the other hand, genetic variations in CD36 have been associated with altered plasma and retina concentrations of lutein [104]. The presence of specific pathways for the transfer of lutein and zeaxanthin from the blood into the retina is proposed to involve specific xanthophyll-binding proteins [105]; the Pi isoform of glutathione S-transferase has a high affinity for zeaxanthin [106], and a lutein-binding protein has been identified as a member of a protein family collectively referred to as steroidogenic acute regulatory protein [107, 108].

Carotenoids can also accumulate in high levels in human skin. Measurements using Raman microscopy have revealed a non-homogeneous distribution of carotenoids across the epidermis, with pronounced peak levels at the skin surface [109]. This distribution is proposed to occur because carotenoids are transported via sweat glands to the surface of the skin, where they can then penetrate into the epidermis. The process is not unlike the topical application of carotenoids, the source of which, in this case, is originally the serum. Indeed, carotenoid concentrations in the skin have been observed to be positively correlated with serum levels [110]. As such, the concentration of carotenoids in the epidermis is higher in areas of the body with higher density of sweat glands, such as the palms, the soles, and the forehead [109]. Carotenoids may protect the skin from UV-induced photooxidative damage by acting as antioxidants or UV-absorbing pigments [109, 110]. In human skin, topically applied β-carotene can be converted to retinyl ester, which may also play a protective role against acute UV exposure and its cytotoxic effects [111, 112].

Intracellular Metabolism

Dietary carotenoids can be converted into a number of biologically active products owing to their unique chemical structure, which consists of eight isoprenoid units and the associated polyunsaturated double bonds. These structural characteristics underlie the capacity of carotenoids for isomerization, singlet oxygen quenching, and electron transfer during oxidation/reduction reactions (see Fig. 3.3) [92, 113, 114]. Some of these reactions can be mediated by specific enzymes that catalyze oxidative cleavage of specific double bonds. In contrast to specific enzymatic cleavage, carotenoids can also be modified to a number of compounds by nonenzymatic chemical transformations, due to the high reactivity of their conjugated double bonds [115]. These products can be formed in tissues through reaction with reactive oxygen species, which are generated in normal physiological processes, and can be further modified and eliminated from the body. Carotenoid oxidation products formed *in vitro* have been extensively studied, especially as compounds formed in oxidative conditions where carotenoids act as antioxidants [116, 117]. Because of the presence of several potential "sites of reaction," carotenoid enzymatic processing has been a subject of debate for decades, and we are still far from having a definitive metabolic picture. Whenever a carotenoid metabolite is identified in

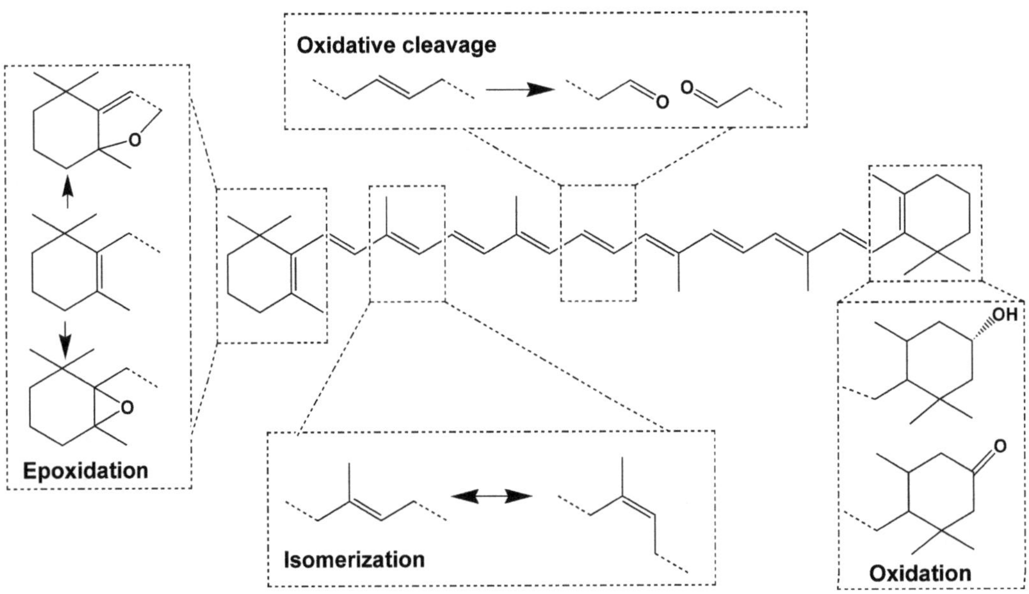

Fig. 3.3 Potential sites within the β-carotene molecule which can undergo enzymatic cleavage, oxidation, epoxidation, and isomerization. The unique chemical structure of eight isoprenoid units with their associated polyunsaturated double bonds underlies the capacity of carotenoids for enzymatic cleavage, oxidation, epoxidation, and isomerization [92, 115, 116, 129]

a tissue, the question is invariably raised as to whether it is a product of specific enzymatic activity or simply a by-product of nonspecific reactions. Because of this, it is often unclear which of the numerous carotenoid derivatives may truly be metabolically significant.

β-Carotene conversion to retinoid was the first carotenoid metabolic transformation to be systematically studied in animal tissues, owing to the biological significance of retinoids [68]. Although the *in vivo* enzymatic reaction was first described in 1930 by Moore [118], β-carotene oxygenase activity was only demonstrated in 1965 when two groups of investigators, Goodman and Huang [119] and Olson and Hayaishi [120], independently showed that rat small intestine homogenates can enzymatically cleave β-carotene at the central 15,15′-carbon double bond to yield two molecules of vitamin A aldehyde (retinal/retinaldehyde). At around the same time, an alternative metabolic pathway for eccentric cleavage was proposed [121]. The initial debate around central versus eccentric cleavage of β-carotene *in vivo* was not settled until the enzymes responsible for these pathways were cloned and characterized [122]. Now termed BCMO1 (β-carotene-15,15′-monooxygenase, EC 1.14.99.36) and BCMO2 (β-carotene-9′,10′-monooxygenase, EC 1.14.99.n2), these enzymes belong to the carotenoid oxygenase family and catalyze central and eccentric β-carotene cleavage, respectively [122]. The human genome encodes at least three members of this protein family, which share about 40 % amino acid sequence identity [123]. The third member of this family is retinoid isomerohydrolase RPE65, which catalyzes the isomerization of all-*trans*-retinyl ester to 11-*cis*-retinol in the retina, a critical step in the visual cycle essential for normal vision [124–126].

An additional pathway for carotenoid metabolism in mammals is characterized by the oxidation of a secondary hydroxyl group, which may or may not involve the migration of the double bond in a β-ring to form an ε-ring [127, 128]. Such reactions have been proposed to be mediated by NAD-dependent dehydrogenases in the liver [129]. The specific enzymes responsible for these oxidation reactions have not been identified, nor have the biological activities of the resulting ketocarotenoids been established, even though these compounds have been detected in physiologically significant levels in human plasma [130]. As pointed out by Nagao, these carotenoid derivatives may have biological activities related to the α, β-unsaturated carbonyl group present in a number of these compounds [8], which has been associated with the suppression of free radical generation and cancer cell proliferation [131].

Carotenoid Cleavage Enzymes and Their Metabolic Roles

Carotenoid Central Cleavage and BCMO1

The sole pathway for carotenoid (mainly β-carotene) conversion to retinoids is the central cleavage reaction, which is catalyzed by the cytosolic enzyme β-carotene 15,15′-monooxygenase (BCMO1 EC 1.14.99.36, systematic name β-carotene:oxygen 15,15′-oxidoreductase (bond-cleaving)). There is no consensus in the literature regarding a standard nomenclature for the central cleavage enzyme, and several acronyms are in use: CMO1, BCO1, BCDO1, BCDO, and BCMO. For many years, the enzyme was termed β-carotene 15,15′-dioxygenase (EC 1.13.11.21 and EC 1.18.3.1) because of an early biochemical characterization that incorrectly implicated a dioxygenase reaction mechanism [119, 120]. It was subsequently demonstrated—using a partially purified chicken intestine BCMO1 preparation, isomerically pure β-carotene as substrate and $^{17}O_2$ and $H_2{}^{18}O$ as oxygen sources—that the enzymatic cleavage of the central carbon 15,15′-double bond in β-carotene actually involves a monooxygenase-type mechanism [132]. Thus, the enzyme has been renamed β-carotene 15,15′-monooxygenase (EC 1.14.99.36) to reflect the correct reaction mechanism. This enzymatic reaction, which yields two retinaldehyde molecules, proceeds in three stages: epoxidation of the 15,15′-double bond, hydration of the double bond leading to ring opening, and oxidative cleavage of

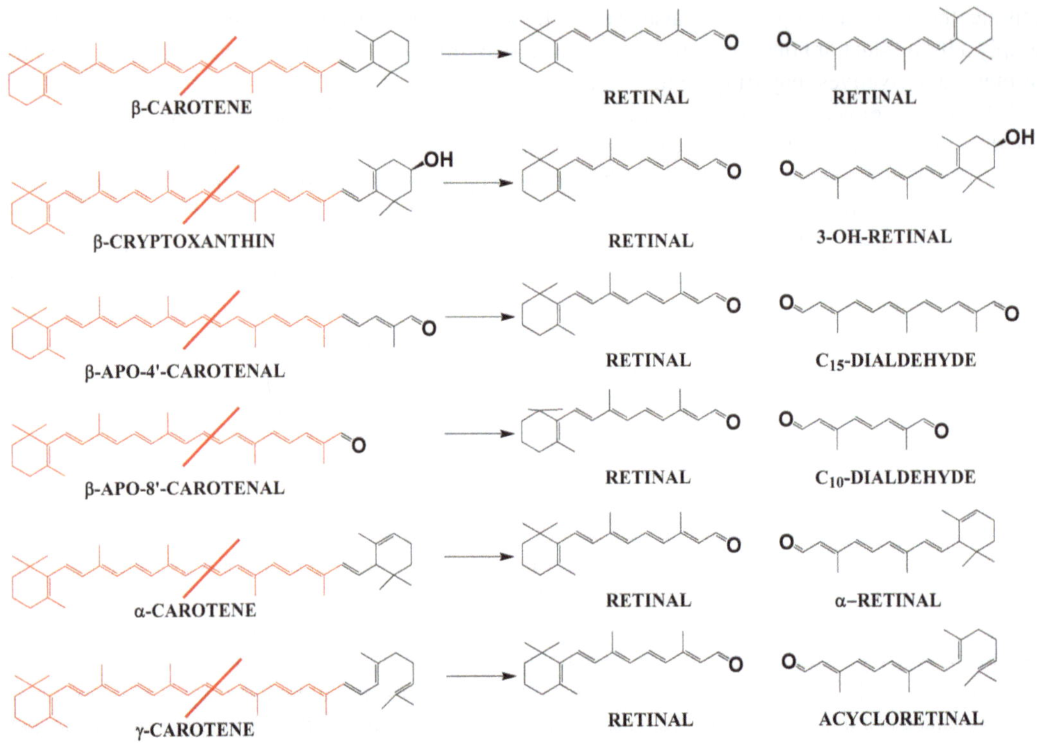

Fig. 3.4 Substrate specificity of BCMO1 reported in the literature. Recombinant BCMO1 is reported in the literature to catalyze cleavage of β-carotene, β-cryptoxanthin, β-apo-4′-carotenal, β-apo-8′-carotenal, α-carotene, and γ-carotene, but not β-apo-12′-carotenal, lutein, zeaxanthin, or lycopene. At least one half-site of an unsubstituted β-ionone ring in a substrate with a molecular mass greater than C_{30} is required to allow for cleavage of the central carbon 15,15′-double bond [143–145]

the diol formed [132, 133]. During the reaction, a substrate carbocation intermediate is formed, which is stabilized by cation-π interactions with the two aromatic residues in the substrate-binding cleft of BCMO1 [134]. Two oxygen atoms from two different sources are used, molecular oxygen and water; one retinaldehyde incorporates an oxygen atom from dioxygen, and the other retinaldehyde receives an oxygen from water [132].

In humans, the *Bcmo1* gene is located on chromosome 16. The gene sequence is evolutionarily conserved throughout the animal kingdom [122]. Molecular cloning and characterization of BCMO1 has been reported for the homologous enzyme from various species, including fruit flies [135], chickens [136], mice [137–139], bovines [140], and zebrafish [141]. The first attempt to characterize human BCMO1 was made by Yan et al. [142], but complete molecular cloning and characterization of the human enzyme was done in 2002 by Lindqvist and Andersson [143]. Amino acid comparison of human BCMO1 with the homologous enzymes from mice, rats, chickens, zebra fish, and fruit flies showed sequence identity of 85 %, 84 %, 67 %, 56 %, and 22 %, respectively [123].

Recombinant human BCMO1 is a hydrophilic protein of 547 amino acids with a predicted molecular weight of 62,637 Da. The active BCMO1 enzyme is an oligomer with Fe^{2+} ions as metal ligands in the active site [143]. It catalyzes the cleavage of β-carotene with the highest activity, followed by β-cryptoxanthin, β-apo-4′-carotenal, β-apo-8′-carotenal, α-carotene, and γ-carotene. It does not, however, catalyze the cleavage of β-apo-12′-carotenal, lutein, zeaxanthin, or lycopene, suggesting that at least one half-site of an unsubstituted β-ionone ring in a substrate with a molecular mass greater than C_{30} is required for cleavage of the central carbon 15,15′-double bond (see Fig. 3.4) [143–145].

Cleavage of the most common dietary carotenoid, β-carotene, results in two molecules of retinaldehyde, which can be further converted to retinol or retinoic acid by retinaldehyde reductases or retinaldehyde dehydrogenases, respectively [146].

BCMO1 belongs to the nonheme iron-containing oxygenase family. Although the BCMO1 crystal structure has not been resolved, information is available regarding other members of its protein family, including native bovine RPE65 [125] and apocarotenoid-15,15′-oxygenase (ACO) from *Synechocystis* PCC 6803 [147]. Based on the solved crystal structures of these proteins, all iron (II)-dependent oxygenases, including BCMO1, are predicted to share a common seven-bladed β-propeller structural motif, with Fe^{2+} coordinated in a near-perfect octahedral arrangement by four histidines [147]. Sequence alignments within the carotenoid cleavage oxygenase family clearly show that the most highly conserved regions are within the β strands that form the propeller, strongly suggesting that all members of the family have the same β-propeller motif and may therefore be modeled along the lines of the structures of RPE65 and ACO [125, 133]. A large hydrophobic tunnel permeating the protein molecule leads from the surface to the active site defined by the position of iron. The shape of this tunnel appears to determine substrate specificity of the carotenoid cleavage oxygenases [133]. Based on this information, it seems likely that the crystal structure for BCMO1 will soon be resolved.

Using RNA blotting and immunostaining techniques, Lindqvist and Anderson showed that the human *Bcmo1* gene is highly expressed in the mucosa of the digestive tract and the parenchymal cells of the liver [148]. These tissues are most commonly used as sources for purifying or studying the native enzyme, and its physiological role in these tissues has been well-established. In addition to the small intestine and liver, human BCMO1 is also present at high levels in non-digestive tissues, including kidneys (proximal and distal convoluted tubules) and, to a lesser extent, steroidogenic tissues such as testes (Leydig and Sertoli cells) and ovaries (granulose cells and theca interna), as well as prostate (epithelium and stroma), skeletal muscle (muscle fibers), skin (epidermis) [148], and eyes (retinal and ciliary body pigment epithelia) [142, 148]. A similar expression pattern of *Bcmo1* is observed in mice, where expression of the enzyme is detected in small intestine, liver, testes, kidneys, retina, and skin [136, 137, 139]. Further insight into liver BCMO1 distribution has been provided by experiments performed on mice, which revealed that *Bcmo1* is predominantly expressed in hepatic stellate cells [102].

Regulation of BCMO1 Activity

BCMO1 activity is subject to transcriptional regulation, mainly by tissue-specific negative feedback mechanisms [66], In addition, enzymatic activity may vary due to genetic variation among different species [149] and within the human population [150–152]. One of the major factors that affect intestinal *Bcmo1* expression is dietary retinoids. Several studies have shown that intestinal β-carotene cleavage activity was enhanced by retinoid deficiency, and reduced by high levels of supplementary retinoids in the diet [153, 154]. BCMO1 activity in the intestine of rats was observed to be decreased by up to 79 %, 88 %, and 67 % after oral administration of retinyl acetate, all-*trans*-retinoic acid, and 9-*cis*-retinoic acid, respectively. Conversely, retinoid deficiency was observed to upregulate *Bcmo1* gene expression, which was then suppressed by all-*trans*-retinoic acid or 9-*cis*-retinoic acid. Similar effects were observed when β-carotene and apo-8′-carotenal were orally administered; BCMO1 activity in the rat intestine was decreased by up to 79 % and 56 %, respectively [153]. Furthermore, apo-12′-carotenal and the retinoic acid receptor alpha (RARα) antagonist, Ro 41-5253, significantly increased intestinal BCMO1 activity by 55 % and 94 %, respectively [154]. *Bcmo1* gene expression in the lungs and testes was also suppressed by all-*trans*-retinoic acid or 9-*cis*-retinoic acid in retinoid-deficient rats. In the liver, however, *Bcmo1* gene expression was only decreased by all-*trans*-retinoic

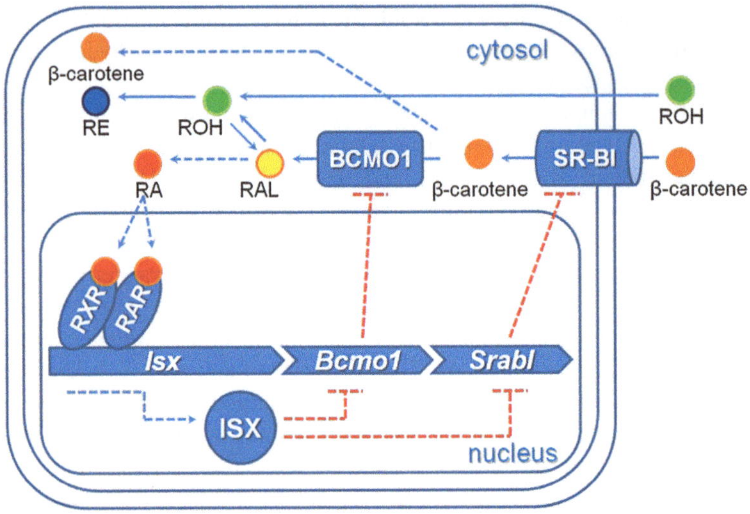

Fig. 3.5 Negative feedback regulation of β-carotene absorption and metabolism in the intestine. Sufficient intake of retinoids and/or proretinoid carotenoids from the diet leads to the formation of retinoic acid in the enterocyte. Retinoic acid, acting via retinoic acid receptors, induces expression of intestinal transcription factor (ISX), which represses expression of both SR-B1 and BCMO1, decreasing further β-carotene absorption and central cleavage [155, 156]

acid and not 9-*cis*-retinoic acid, and renal expression was not affected by treatment with either retinoid. Together, these data suggest that *Bcmo1* gene expression in some tissues may be downregulated by retinoic acid, thus affecting β-carotene conversion to retinaldehyde [153].

Seino et al. were the first to establish a role for intestine specific homeobox (ISX) transcription factor in the regulation of retinoid metabolism [155]. These investigators showed that retinoid-deficiency decreased *Isx* expression and increased *Bcmo1* expression in the duodenum and the jejunum of wild-type mice. In *Isx*-deficient ($Isx^{LacZ/LacZ}$) mice, however, retinoid-deficiency did not increase *Bcmo1* expression in the duodenum and the jejunum. These results suggest that ISX participates in retinoid metabolism by regulating *Bcmo1* expression in the proximal intestine. Furthermore, Lobo et al. showed, using both mouse models and human cell lines, that in addition to *Bcmo1* expression, lipid absorption by SR-BI in the intestine was also subject to control by retinoid signaling [156]. Retinoic acid signaling was shown to induce expression of the intestinal transcription factor ISX, which in turn suppressed expression of both SR-BI and BCMO1 [156]. The increase in intestinal SR-BI expression and systemic β-carotene accumulation in *Bcmo1*-knockout ($Bcmo1^{-/-}$) mice were prevented by dietary retinoids, via induction of ISX expression. These elegant studies reveal a diet-responsive regulatory network that controls β-carotene absorption and retinoid production by negative feedback regulation (see Fig. 3.5).

Tissues other than the intestine also have complex regulatory mechanisms for regulating *Bcmo1* expression, one of which is summarized in Fig. 3.6. Analysis of the human *Bcmo1* gene promoter has demonstrated that the gene contains a peroxisome proliferator response element (PPRE), to which binds peroxisome proliferator-activated receptor (PPAR)γ [157]. PPARγ is essential but not sufficient for the induction of human *Bcmo1* gene expression, which is dependent on the cooperation between PPARγ and the transcription factor myocyte enhancer factor 2 (MEF2) isoforms [158]. Interestingly, the same regulatory pattern exists for CRBP-II, the molecular partner of BCMO1 in the intestine. *Crbp-II* gene expression is regulated through PPAR/RXR heterodimers bound to nuclear receptor response elements present in the *Crbp-II* gene promoter [159].

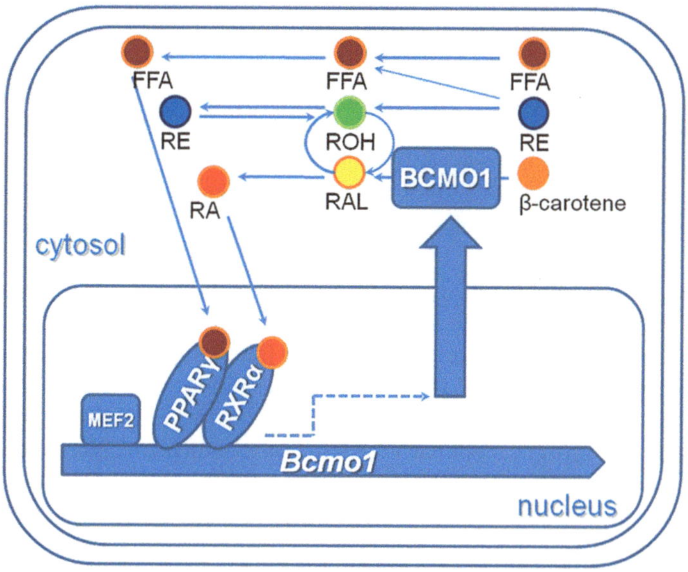

Fig. 3.6 Proposed mechanism for regulating human *Bcmo1* gene expression in liver and peripheral tissues. The human *Bcmo1* gene promoter contains a peroxisome proliferator response element (PPRE), and peroxisome proliferator-activated factor (PPAR)γ dimerized with retinoid X receptor (RXR) binds to this site. The natural ligands for these receptors, free fatty acids (FFA) for PPARs and 9-*cis*-retinoic acid (RA) for RXRs, can activate *Bcmo1* expression. Activation of human *Bcmo1* gene expression is further dependent on cooperation between PPARγ and myocyte enhancer factor 2 (MEF2) isoforms [157, 158]

The observation of enhanced *Bcmo1* expression in Caco-2 cells by triiodothyronine (T_3), which is inhibited by actinomycin D, led Yamaguchi and Suruga [160] to the conclusion that the expression of the *Bcmo1* gene might be regulated by T_3 at the transcriptional level. However, these researchers were unable to make a clear assessment of whether the observed upregulation was directly a result of thyroid hormone receptor (TR) binding to thyroid hormone response elements (TREs) or due to enhanced PPARγ transcriptional activity induced by T_3 treatment of human intestinal cells. Nevertheless, these findings suggest that T_3 might contribute to regulating β-carotene conversion to retinoid in the human small intestine [160]. Similar transcriptional dynamics were observed in experiments performed on rats [161]. Studying the influence of alcohol administration, which results in the decrease of hepatic retinoid levels, these investigators detected increased mRNA levels of *Bcmo1*, *Bcmo2*, *Pparγ*, *Pparα*, and *Trβ*, and the corresponding increases in the protein levels of BCMO2, PPARγ, and PPARα. These findings support the idea that BCMO1 is transcriptionally regulated by PPARγ in a process that may involve TRβ.

Several animal studies have shown that *Bcmo1* expression can be regulated by other carotenoids. For instance, lycopene intake downregulates *Bcmo1* expression in the adrenal glands and kidneys of rats [162]. Decreases in expression of *Pparγ* and its target gene *Fabp3* in the adrenal glands and kidneys were observed to parallel expression levels for *Bcmo1*. A mechanism for how lycopene and its metabolites influence *Bcmo1* expression has not been clarified, but at least two lycopene metabolites, 10′-apolycopen-10′-oic acid and 14′-apolycopen-14′-oic acid, did not have an effect on *Bcmo1* expression in mice [163]. Lutein was observed to inhibit β-carotene cleavage enzyme activity in rat enterocytes [164]. Flavonoids such as luteolin, quercetin, and rhamnetin, which have a catechol structure in their B-ring, are remarkably efficient at inhibiting BCMO1 activity in a noncompetitive manner [165, 166]. This may be important for BCMO1 in the intestine, where it may be exposed to these flavonoids.

Physiological Roles of BCMO1

The metabolic function of BCMO1 as the central cleavage enzyme is now well-characterized; its activity constitutes the sole pathway for the biosynthesis of retinoids from carotenoid precursors, which contributes significantly towards satisfying retinoid needs in the human body. In times of dietary insufficiency, a steady level of retinoids can be maintained in peripheral tissues by local central cleavage of carotenoids, especially in tissues that are sensitive to retinoid levels, such as epithelial tissues and the steroidogenic cells [140, 148].

Experiments with genetically modified animals have shown broad physiological roles for BCMO1 in extra-intestinal tissues. In addition to impairment in β-carotene metabolism, which results in its accumulation in large quantities in tissues [102, 146, 167], BCMO1 deficiency alters the metabolism of other carotenoids. *Bcmo1*$^{-/-}$ mice fed lycopene showed significant differences in tissue accumulation as compared to wild-type mice; lycopene concentrations were decreased in liver, spleen, and thymus, and increased in prostate, seminal vesicles, testes, and brain. Moreover, alterations were observed in the distribution of lycopene isomers; in *Bcmo1*$^{-/-}$ mice, the percent of *cis*-isomers were significantly increased in all the tissues examined, with the exception of testes [168].

BCMO1-deficiency has been independently associated with altered lipid homeostasis. Even when maintained on a retinoid-sufficient chow diet, *Bcmo1*$^{-/-}$ mice developed fatty liver and displayed elevated serum levels of unesterified fatty acids, suggesting a regulatory role for BCMO1 in lipid metabolism that is independent of retinoid status. This mutant mouse model was also more susceptible to high-fat diet-induced impairments in fatty acid metabolism [102, 167].

BCMO1 is proposed to influence adipocyte physiology by contributing directly to retinoic acid production in an adipose-specific manner [169, 170]. *Bcmo1*$^{-/-}$ mice have elevated expression of PPARγ-regulated marker genes that are associated with adipogenesis in visceral adipose tissues [167]. In mature mouse adipocytes, β-carotene, but not all-*trans*-retinol, is metabolized to retinoic acid, and its signaling via RARs decreases the expression of PPARγ and CCAAT/enhancer-binding protein α, which are key lipogenic transcription factors. This is proposed to reduce the lipid content of mature adipocytes. Oral administration of β-carotene, but not all-*trans*-retinol, was reported to induce retinoid signaling and decrease PPARγ expression in white adipose tissue of retinoid-deficient mice [171]. Similarly, retinaldehyde directly derived from β-carotene cleavage has also been implicated in the regulation of adipocyte physiology; by binding to PPARγ and RXRs, retinaldehyde is proposed to antagonize their activities [172]. Because β-carotene is a critical physiological precursor for retinoid production in adipose tissue, provitamin A carotenoids may act as dietary regulators of body fat reserves. Amengual et al. [173] have recently proposed that β-carotene intake may have different consequences on body adiposity in subjects carrying different *Bcmo1* functional gene variants and proposed the involvement of β-carotene and *Bcmo1* in human obesity [173]. However, this notion is contradicted by studies involving ferrets, which showed that chronic supplementation with β-carotene resulted in hypertrophy of white adipocytes and a general increase in body weight. Moreover, these animals had decreased amounts of brown-like multilocular adipocytes in the retroperitoneal depot and decreased UCP1 content in different fat depots, which suggests a lower thermogenic capacity [174]. Most importantly, the idea that provitamin A carotenoids may be dietary regulators of body fat reserves is strongly contradicted by human trials of β-carotene as a cancer chemopreventative. These studies failed to show any correlation between dietary carotenoid intake and body mass index in large human cohorts, even after many years of supplementation with high doses of β-carotene [175–178].

Interestingly, an additional potential function for BCMO1 has been proposed recently based on microarray analysis of cadmium-exposed *Caenorhabditis elegans* and Hepa 1–6 murine hepatoma cells. These studies suggest that *Bcmo1* may act as an early cadmium-responsive gene that is highly inducible by cadmium. Because BCMO1 is highly conserved across many species, the transcriptional response to cadmium may also be conserved [179].

Carotenoid Eccentric Cleavage and BCMO2

In 2001, Kiefer et al. cloned and characterized a second carotenoid-cleaving enzyme termed β-carotene 9′,10′-monooxygenase (EC 1.14.99.n2, BCMO2, also known as CMO2, BCO2, BCDO2), which catalyzes asymmetric cleavage of carotenoids [180]. BCMO2 requires Fe^{2+} as an essential cofactor for reaction, yielding one molecule of β-apo-10′-carotenal and one molecule of β-ionone when β-carotene is used as substrate. The BCMO2 protein shares about 40 % amino acid sequence identity with BCMO1 and is expressed in many of the same tissues. Immunohistochemical analysis of BCMO2 expression revealed that the eccentric cleavage enzyme is expressed in cell types that also express BCMO1, including epithelial cells in the mucosa of the small intestine and the stomach, parenchymal cells in the liver, Leydig and Sertoli cells in testes, kidney tubules, adrenal glands, exocrine pancreas, and retinal pigment epithelia and ciliary body epithelia in the eyes [181]. BCMO2 is uniquely expressed in cardiac and skeletal muscle cells, prostate and endometrial connective tissue, and endocrine pancreas [181].

Recently, Amengual and coworkers showed that BCMO2 is a mitochondrial carotenoid oxygenase with broad substrate specificity, accepting a wider variety of substrates compared to BCMO1 [182]. BCMO2 catalyzes the conversion of both carotenes and xanthophylls. Investigation of vertebrate BCMO2 substrate recognition demonstrated that both the central polyene chain backbone and the ionone-ring structures are important in substrate specificity [182]. Hu et al., using recombinant ferret BCMO2 as a model for carotenoid metabolism, demonstrated that the enzyme catalyzes the eccentric cleavage of both all-*trans*-β-carotene and the 5-*cis*- and 13-*cis*-isomers of lycopene at the 9′,10′-double bond but not all-*trans*-lycopene [183]. The enzyme can interact with both the β- and 3-OH-ionone rings of carotenoids, removing both ionone rings from the substrate by oxidative cleavage at positions C9,C10 or C9′,C10′, resulting in the formation of a set of products, including 3-OH-β-ionone, 3-OH-α-ionone, β-ionone, 3-OH-α-apo-10′-carotenal, 3-OH-β-apo-10′-carotenal, β-apo-10′-carotenal, and C_{14}-dialdehyde rosafluene (see Fig. 3.7) [182, 184]. Enzyme kinetic analysis indicated that zeaxanthin and lutein are preferentially cleaved by BCMO2 over β-cryptoxanthin and that BCMO2 cleavage activity is higher towards lycopene *cis*-isomers compared to β-carotene [182–184].

The physiological importance of eccentric cleavage and the metabolic function of BCMO2 are still unclear. Until the molecular cloning of BCMO1 and BCMO2, it had been proposed that, in addition to the central cleavage pathway, eccentric cleavage of carotenoids could give rise to retinoid formation from β-carotene. According to this proposed pathway, β-carotene could be cleaved randomly at any position along its isoprenoid backbone to form β-apocarotenals of different chain lengths. By analyzing retinoic acid formation from β-apocarotenals, a mechanism similar to β-oxidation of fatty acids was proposed by Wang et al. [185]. More recent studies, however, performed on genetically modified animals showed that *Bcmo2*-deficiency neither influences retinoid tissue stores nor impairs retinoid metabolism [182]. Only the absence of BCMO1 alters tissue retinoid stores, which implies that BCMO1 is the sole enzyme responsible for retinoid formation from carotenoids [102, 146, 167, 182].

Several *in vivo* observations of *Bcmo2*-deficient animals revealed altered carotenoid metabolism, suggesting an important role for BCMO2 in carotene and xanthophyll degradation. These studies also confirm broad carotenoid substrate specificity for BCMO2. Inhibition of BCMO2 activity in a tissue-specific manner caused no adverse developmental or health consequences and did not affect serum and liver retinoid levels. Mutations resulting in a loss of BCMO2 function, however, cause excessive carotenoid accumulation in chicken skin [186], bovine adipose tissue and milk [187, 188], and a yellow fat phenotype in sheep [189]. *Bcmo2*-deficient mice display altered carotenoid homeostasis, and carotenoids accumulate excessively in several tissues, including blood, heart, liver, and adipose [182, 190]. In hepatic mitochondria obtained from *Bcmo2*-deficient mice, the accumulated carotenoids are proposed to induce key markers of mitochondrial dysfunction, including manganese

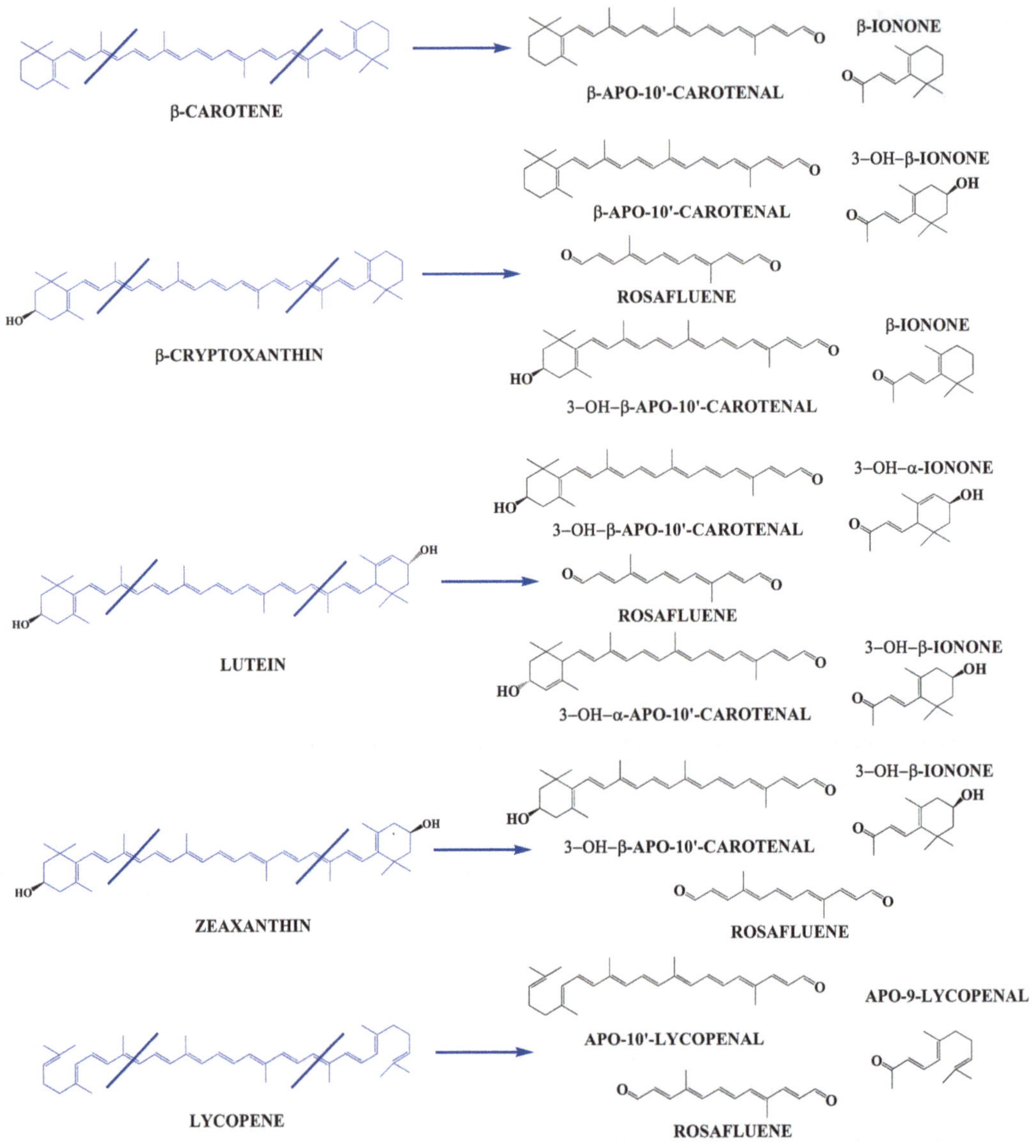

Fig. 3.7 Substrate specificity of BCMO2 reported in the literature. Recombinant BCMO2 is reported to have a relatively broad specificity for catalyzing oxidative cleavage of carotenoid substrates which possess both a polyene backbone and ionone-ring structures. Cleavage occurs at positions C9,C10 and C9′,C10′ [182–184]

superoxide dismutase, and reduce rates of ADP-dependent respiration. This impairment was associated with an induction of phospho-MAP kinase and phospho-AKT, markers of cell signaling pathways related to oxidative stress and disease. Administration of carotenoids to HepG2 cells, a human hepatoma cell line, depolarized mitochondrial membranes and resulted in the production of reactive oxygen species [182]. These studies underscore the importance of regulated carotenoid eccentric cleavage in extra-intestinal tissues for the channeling of carotenoid substrates towards the formation of desirable compounds with predictable biological properties, in order to prevent potential damaging effects arising from autooxidation [116, 191, 192]. Products of autooxidation formed from free radical attack on carotenoids may be more toxic prooxidants than the original free radicals. As a cause of oxidative stress induction [116], carotenoid oxidation products may lead to oxidative damage of different cellular components [117, 192], resulting in high cytotoxicity [116, 193]. Regulated formation of carotenoid metabolites may also be beneficial for cell survival. Apo-10′-lycopenoic acid treatment of human bronchial epithelial cells was associated with the induction of phase II detoxifying/antioxidant enzymes [194]. BCMO2 is predominantly located in mitochondria, where reactive oxygen species are produced in large quantities.

There is growing research interest into whether carotenoid eccentric cleavage products formed by BCMO2 activity may act as biologically active mediators in transcription regulation, and whether these are significant for regulating other metabolic pathways [163, 195, 196]. Several methodological approaches have been employed in an attempt to prove the hypothesis that apocarotenoid signaling involves nuclear receptors, including RARs, RXRs, and PPARs; however, β-apo-8′-carotenoic acid, β-apo-14′-carotenoic acid, β-cyclocitral, β-cyclogernanic acid, β-ionone, β-ionylideneacetaldehyde, β-ionylideneacetic acid and β-apo-13-carotenone, have no significant transactivational activity for the RARs when compared with all-*trans*-retinoic acid. This suggests that the potential biological effects of these apocarotenoids are mediated by mechanisms that are independent of RARs [197]. Studies with COS-1 cells, devoted to the investigation of different β-apocarotenoids on RXRα signaling showed that among the compounds tested, β-*apo*-13-carotenone can antagonize the activation of RXRα by 9-*cis*-retinoic acid, at concentrations as low as 1 nM. Molecular modeling studies revealed that β-*apo*-13-carotenone undergoes molecular interactions as an antagonist of RXRα, suggesting a possible function of β-apocarotenones in RXRα signaling [198]. The ability of eccentric cleavage products to repress PPAR and RXR activation and the biological responses induced by their respective agonists have been demonstrated *in vitro* and *in vivo* for β-*apo*-14′-carotenal (apo14), but not for other structurally related apocarotenals. However, these observed effects involved apo14 concentrations as high as 10 μM, which cannot be achieved through normal dietary intake of β-carotene [196]. *Apo*-10′-lycopenoic acid, used in micromolar concentrations (3–10 μM), transactivates the retinoic acid receptor β (RARβ) promoter *in vitro*. Although induction of RARβ expression was achieved *in vitro*, *in vivo* serum concentrations of this compound during its supplementation were not reported to exceed 20 nM [199].

These findings raise a question about the relative importance of these compounds *in vivo*, as the reported concentrations for β-carotene and lycopene in human serum under conditions of dietary supplementation are not higher than 0.7 and 1.3 μM, respectively [200, 201], and tissue concentrations for the most abundant carotenoids are found to be within the ng/g range [202]. In humans, the predominant lycopenals in the blood, *apo*-8′- and *apo*-12′-lycopenals, are observed in picomolar concentrations [201]. Although *in vitro* experiments employing human recombinant BCMO2 expression in *Escherichia coli* showed that BCMO2 can catalyze the formation of β-*apo*-10′-carotenal from β-carotene [203], only ^{14}C-β-*apo*-8′-carotenal can be detected in vivo in human plasma after dose consumption of isotopically labeled β-carotene [204]. In both *Bcmo1*-deficient and wild-type mice, *apo*-10′-carotenal and *apo*-12′-carotenal were the only β-apocarotenals detected in the serum and liver [102], and β-*apo*-10′-carotenol was identified as the major β-carotene cleavage product in white adipose tissue of *Bcmo1*$^{-/-}$ mice [173]. In rats, lycopene is cleaved *in vivo* at different positions to produce *apo*-12′-lycopenal, and other unidentified metabolites, in addition to *apo*-8′-lycopenal in liver [205].

Little is known about *Bcmo2* gene regulation. In contrast to *Bcmo1*, *Bcmo2* expression is minimally affected by retinoid status, as reported by Luvizotto et al. [161]. *Bcmo2* expression is highly correlated with *Ppar* expression, suggesting potential involvement of *Ppar*s in the regulation of *Bcmo2* expression. Studies have shown increases in *Bcmo2* mRNA expression in *Bcmo1*-deficient animals [102, 168], suggesting the possible existence of a coordinated regulatory process that regulates expression levels of both carotene monooxygenases. The observed elevation in *Bcmo2* expression is related to increased tissue concentrations of β-carotene and/or increased levels of apo-10′- or apo-12′-carotenals formed by BCMO2 [102]. All-*trans*-lycopene supplementation in ferrets upregulated *Bcmo2* expression in lung tissue. In rats, however, lycopene intake did not affect *Bcmo2* gene expression in the adrenal glands or in most other tissues, but *Bcmo2* expression was reduced in the kidneys, lungs, and mucosal cells [162]. In mice, treatment with an equimolar amount of 14′-apolycopen-14′-oic acid upregulated *Bcmo2* expression, whereas all-*trans*-lycopene downregulated the expression of the enzyme [163].

Conclusions and Future Directions

Carotenoids have been a subject of considerable research for many decades. Much of this research has focused on the abilities of carotenoids to serve as retinoid precursors and antioxidants. The last decade has been especially fruitful for gaining understanding of carotenoid metabolism and actions; during this period, the studies of carotenoid metabolism and actions have undergone a *"second birth."* The molecular cloning and characterization of *Bcmo1* and *Bcmo2* have resolved the longstanding controversy over whether retinoid formation involves solely central carotenoid cleavage or both central and asymmetric cleavage of carotenoids. The identification of how ISX acts in a negative feedback loop to influence *Bcmo1* expression in response to dietary retinoid availability has greatly extended our understanding of carotenoid absorption and metabolism. Similarly, the identification of cell surface transporters, which facilitate carotenoid uptake into enterocytes and other cells within the body, has advanced our understanding of carotenoid metabolism.

Yet a great number of questions regarding carotenoid metabolism and actions still remain to be answered. One of the major questions that needs to be resolved concerns whether carotenoid metabolites, formed enzymatically, or carotenoid derivatives formed nonenzymatically, have specific physiologically important actions within the body. Do apocarotenoids formed through BCMO2 action have specific physiological roles in the body? Do some of these act through nuclear hormone receptors? How do nonenzymatically formed carotenoid derivatives influence cellular and tissue actions? Another area in need of further research centers on carotenoid processing in intestinal cells following absorption from the diet. What processes are important for assuring carotenoid incorporation into nascent chylomicrons? How are these similar to or different from those of other dietary lipids? What processes and/or factors are important for facilitating cellular carotenoid uptake, metabolism and accumulation within the body after absorption?

There is also need for the validation of new animal models, especially induced mouse mutants, for use in studying carotenoid metabolism. Are these mouse models the appropriate ones for use in extrapolating human carotenoid metabolism? This is an important research need given the growing controversy in data obtained using different animal models, which limits their practical implementation and application to humans.

Overall, our understanding of carotenoid metabolism and actions has grown remarkably in the last decade. Many older questions and controversies have been resolved. However, many new and important questions regarding carotenoid metabolism and actions have also arisen from recent work. Undoubtedly, the next decade will see many of these questions resolved by new research.

Acknowledgments The work described in this chapter that was carried out in the authors' laboratory was supported by grants R01 DK068437, R01 DK079221, and RC2 AA019413 from the National Institutes of Health.

References

1. Chatterjee M, Janarthan M. Biological activity of carotenoids: its implications in cancer risk and prevention. Curr Pharm Biotechnol. 2012;13(1):180–90.
2. Riccioni G, D'Orazio N, Speranza L, et al. Carotenoids and asymptomatic carotid atherosclerosis. J Biol Regul Homeost Agents. 2010;24(4):447–52.
3. Villaca Chaves G, Goncalves de Souza G, Cardoso de Matos A, et al. Serum retinol and beta-carotene levels and risk factors for cardiovascular disease in morbid obesity. Int J Vitam Nutr Res. 2010;80(3):159–67.
4. Wegner A, Khoramnia R. Cataract is a self-defence reaction to protect the retina from oxidative damage. Med Hypotheses. 2011;76(5):741–4.
5. Zhou H, Zhao X, Johnson EJ, et al. Serum carotenoids and risk of age-related macular degeneration in a Chinese population sample. Invest Ophthalmol Vis Sci. 2011;52(7):4338–44.
6. Stahl W, Ale-Agha N, Polidori MC. Non-antioxidant properties of carotenoids. Biol Chem. 2002;383(3–4):553–8.
7. Stahl W, Sies H. Bioactivity and protective effects of natural carotenoids. Biochim Biophys Acta. 2005;1740(2):101–7.
8. Nagao A. Absorption and metabolism of dietary carotenoids. Biofactors. 2011;37(2):83–7.
9. Bendich A, Olson JA. Biological actions of carotenoids. FASEB J. 1989;3(8):1927–32.
10. Asai A, Yonekura L, Nagao A. Low bioavailability of dietary epoxyxanthophylls in humans. Br J Nutr. 2008;100(2):273–7.
11. Sugawara T, Kushiro M, Zhang H, Nara E, Ono H, Nagao A. Lysophosphatidylcholine enhances carotenoid uptake from mixed micelles by Caco-2 human intestinal cells. J Nutr. 2001;131(11):2921–7.
12. Baskaran V, Sugawara T, Nagao A. Phospholipids affect the intestinal absorption of carotenoids in mice. Lipids. 2003;38(7):705–11.
13. Tyssandier V, Reboul E, Dumas JF, et al. Processing of vegetable-borne carotenoids in the human stomach and duodenum. Am J Physiol Gastrointest Liver Physiol. 2003;284(6):G913–23.
14. Rock CL, Lovalvo JL, Emenhiser C, Ruffin MT, Flatt SW, Schwartz SJ. Bioavailability of beta-carotene is lower in raw than in processed carrots and spinach in women. J Nutr. 1998;128(5):913–6.
15. Gartner C, Stahl W, Sies H. Lycopene is more bioavailable from tomato paste than from fresh tomatoes. Am J Clin Nutr. 1997;66(1):116–22.
16. Stahl W, Sies H. Uptake of lycopene and its geometrical isomers is greater from heat-processed than from unprocessed tomato juice in humans. J Nutr. 1992;122(11):2161–6.
17. van het Hof KH, de Boer BC, Tijburg LB, et al. Carotenoid bioavailability in humans from tomatoes processed in different ways determined from the carotenoid response in the triglyceride-rich lipoprotein fraction of plasma after a single consumption and in plasma after four days of consumption. J Nutr. 2000;130(5):1189–96.
18. van Het Hof KH, West CE, Weststrate JA, Hautvast JG. Dietary factors that affect the bioavailability of carotenoids. J Nutr. 2000;130(3):503–6.
19. Rich GT, Bailey AL, Faulks RM, Parker ML, Wickham MS, Fillery-Travis A. Solubilization of carotenoids from carrot juice and spinach in lipid phases: I. Modeling the gastric lumen. Lipids. 2003;38(9):933–45.
20. Yonekura L, Nagao A. Intestinal absorption of dietary carotenoids. Mol Nutr Food Res. 2007;51(1):107–15.
21. Blanquet-Diot S, Soufi M, Rambeau M, Rock E, Alric M. Digestive stability of xanthophylls exceeds that of carotenes as studied in a dynamic *in vitro* gastrointestinal system. J Nutr. 2009;139(5):876–83.
22. Huo T, Ferruzzi MG, Schwartz SJ, Failla ML. Impact of fatty acyl composition and quantity of triglycerides on bioaccessibility of dietary carotenoids. J Agric Food Chem. 2007;55(22):8950–7.
23. Roodenburg AJ, Leenen R, van het Hof KH, Weststrate JA, Tijburg LB. Amount of fat in the diet affects bioavailability of lutein esters but not of alpha-carotene, beta-carotene, and vitamin E in humans. Am J Clin Nutr. 2000;71(5):1187–93.
24. Unlu NZ, Bohn T, Clinton SK, Schwartz SJ. Carotenoid absorption from salad and salsa by humans is enhanced by the addition of avocado or avocado oil. J Nutr. 2005;135(3):431–6.
25. Borel P, Tyssandier V, Mekki N, et al. Chylomicron beta-carotene and retinyl palmitate responses are dramatically diminished when men ingest beta-carotene with medium-chain rather than long-chain triglycerides. J Nutr. 1998;128(8):1361–7.
26. O'Connell O, Ryan L, O'Sullivan L, Aherne-Bruce SA, O'Brien NM. Carotenoid micellarization varies greatly between individual and mixed vegetables with or without the addition of fat or fiber. Int J Vitam Nutr Res. 2008;78(4–5):238–46.
27. van den Berg H. Carotenoid interactions. Nutr Rev. 1999;57(1):1–10.
28. Wang Y, Illingworth DR, Connor SL, Barton Duell P, Connor WE. Competitive inhibition of carotenoid transport and tissue concentrations by high dose supplements of lutein, zeaxanthin and beta-carotene. Eur J Nutr. 2010;49(6):327–36.

29. During A, Hussain MM, Morel DW, Harrison EH. Carotenoid uptake and secretion by CaCo-2 cells: beta-carotene isomer selectivity and carotenoid interactions. J Lipid Res. 2002;43(7):1086–95.
30. Johnson EJ, Qin J, Krinsky NI, Russell RM. Beta-carotene isomers in human serum, breast milk and buccal mucosa cells after continuous oral doses of all-trans and 9-cis beta-carotene. J Nutr. 1997;127(10):1993–9.
31. van den Berg H, van Vliet T. Effect of simultaneous, single oral doses of beta-carotene with lutein or lycopene on the beta-carotene and retinyl ester responses in the triacylglycerol-rich lipoprotein fraction of men. Am J Clin Nutr. 1998;68(1):82–9.
32. Kostic D, White WS, Olson JA. Intestinal absorption, serum clearance, and interactions between lutein and beta-carotene when administered to human adults in separate or combined oral doses. Am J Clin Nutr. 1995;62(3):604–10.
33. Harrison EH. Mechanisms of digestion and absorption of dietary vitamin A. Annu Rev Nutr. 2005;25:87–103.
34. Scita G, Aponte GW, Wolf G. Uptake and cleavage of beta-carotene by cultures of rat small intestinal cells and human lung fibroblasts. Methods Enzymol. 1993;214:21–32.
35. Hollander D, Ruble Jr PE. beta-carotene intestinal absorption: bile, fatty acid, pH, and flow rate effects on transport. Am J Physiol. 1978;235(6):E686–91.
36. Slifka KA, Bowen PE, Stacewicz-Sapuntzakis M, Crissey SD. A survey of serum and dietary carotenoids in captive wild animals. J Nutr. 1999;129(2):380–90.
37. Asai A, Terasaki M, Nagao A. An epoxide-furanoid rearrangement of spinach neoxanthin occurs in the gastrointestinal tract of mice and *in vitro*: formation and cytostatic activity of neochrome stereoisomers. J Nutr. 2004;134(9):2237–43.
38. Borel P, Grolier P, Mekki N, et al. Low and high responders to pharmacological doses of beta-carotene: proportion in the population, mechanisms involved and consequences on beta-carotene metabolism. J Lipid Res. 1998;39(11):2250–60.
39. van Bennekum A, Werder M, Thuahnai ST, et al. Class B scavenger receptor-mediated intestinal absorption of dietary beta-carotene and cholesterol. Biochemistry. 2005;44(11):4517–25.
40. Reboul E, Abou L, Mikail C, et al. Lutein transport by Caco-2 TC-7 cells occurs partly by a facilitated process involving the scavenger receptor class B type I (SR-BI). Biochem J. 2005;387(Pt 2):455–61.
41. During A, Dawson HD, Harrison EH. Carotenoid transport is decreased and expression of the lipid transporters SR-BI, NPC1L1, and ABCA1 is downregulated in Caco-2 cells treated with ezetimibe. J Nutr. 2005;135(10):2305–12.
42. Moussa M, Landrier JF, Reboul E, et al. Lycopene absorption in human intestinal cells and in mice involves scavenger receptor class B type I but not Niemann-Pick C1-like 1. J Nutr. 2008;138(8):1432–6.
43. Rigotti A, Miettinen HE, Krieger M. The role of the high-density lipoprotein receptor SR-BI in the lipid metabolism of endocrine and other tissues. Endocr Rev. 2003;24(3):357–87.
44. Yancey PG, Kawashiri MA, Moore R, et al. *In vivo* modulation of HDL phospholipid has opposing effects on SR-BI- and ABCA1-mediated cholesterol efflux. J Lipid Res. 2004;45(2):337–46.
45. Hajri T, Han XX, Bonen A, Abumrad NA. Defective fatty acid uptake modulates insulin responsiveness and metabolic responses to diet in CD36-null mice. J Clin Invest. 2002;109(10):1381–9.
46. Febbraio M, Abumrad NA, Hajjar DP, et al. A null mutation in murine CD36 reveals an important role in fatty acid and lipoprotein metabolism. J Biol Chem. 1999;274(27):19055–62.
47. Coburn CT, Knapp Jr FF, Febbraio M, Beets AL, Silverstein RL, Abumrad NA. Defective uptake and utilization of long chain fatty acids in muscle and adipose tissues of CD36 knockout mice. J Biol Chem. 2000;275(42):32523–9.
48. Werder M, Han CH, Wehrli E, Bimmler D, Schulthess G, Hauser H. Role of scavenger receptors SR-BI and CD36 in selective sterol uptake in the small intestine. Biochemistry. 2001;40(38):11643–50.
49. Lobo MV, Huerta L, Ruiz-Velasco N, et al. Localization of the lipid receptors CD36 and CLA-1/SR-BI in the human gastrointestinal tract: towards the identification of receptors mediating the intestinal absorption of dietary lipids. J Histochem Cytochem. 2001;49(10):1253–60.
50. Richelle M, Enslen M, Hager C, et al. Both free and esterified plant sterols reduce cholesterol absorption and the bioavailability of beta-carotene and alpha-tocopherol in normocholesterolemic humans. Am J Clin Nutr. 2004;80(1):171–7.
51. Nicolle C, Cardinault N, Aprikian O, et al. Effect of carrot intake on cholesterol metabolism and on antioxidant status in cholesterol-fed rat. Eur J Nutr. 2003;42(5):254–61.
52. Hajri T, Abumrad NA. Fatty acid transport across membranes: relevance to nutrition and metabolic pathology. Annu Rev Nutr. 2002;22:383–415.
53. Brown MJ, Ferruzzi MG, Nguyen ML, et al. Carotenoid bioavailability is higher from salads ingested with full-fat than with fat-reduced salad dressings as measured with electrochemical detection. Am J Clin Nutr. 2004;80(2):396–403.
54. Drover VA, Nguyen DV, Bastie CC, et al. CD36 mediates both cellular uptake of very long chain fatty acids and their intestinal absorption in mice. J Biol Chem. 2008;283(19):13108–15.

55. Drover VA, Ajmal M, Nassir F, et al. CD36 deficiency impairs intestinal lipid secretion and clearance of chylomicrons from the blood. J Clin Invest. 2005;115(5):1290–7.
56. Nassir F, Wilson B, Han X, Gross RW, Abumrad NA. CD36 is important for fatty acid and cholesterol uptake by the proximal but not distal intestine. J Biol Chem. 2007;282(27):19493–501.
57. Thuahnai ST, Lund-Katz S, Williams DL, Phillips MC. Scavenger receptor class B, type I-mediated uptake of various lipids into cells. Influence of the nature of the donor particle interaction with the receptor. J Biol Chem. 2001;276(47):43801–8.
58. Urban S, Zieseniss S, Werder M, Hauser H, Budzinski R, Engelmann B. Scavenger receptor BI transfers major lipoprotein-associated phospholipids into the cells. J Biol Chem. 2000;275(43):33409–15.
59. Hauser H, Dyer JH, Nandy A, et al. Identification of a receptor mediating absorption of dietary cholesterol in the intestine. Biochemistry. 1998;37(51):17843–50.
60. Yancey PG, Bortnick AE, Kellner-Weibel G, de la Llera-Moya M, Phillips MC, Rothblat GH. Importance of different pathways of cellular cholesterol efflux. Arterioscler Thromb Vasc Biol. 2003;23(5):712–9.
61. Thuahnai ST, Lund-Katz S, Dhanasekaran P, et al. Scavenger receptor class B type I-mediated cholesteryl ester-selective uptake and efflux of unesterified cholesterol. Influence of high density lipoprotein size and structure. J Biol Chem. 2004;279(13):12448–55.
62. Connelly MA, de la Llera-Moya M, Monzo P, et al. Analysis of chimeric receptors shows that multiple distinct functional activities of scavenger receptor, class B, type I (SR-BI), are localized to the extracellular receptor domain. Biochemistry. 2001;40(17):5249–59.
63. Garcia-Calvo M, Lisnock J, Bull HG, et al. The target of ezetimibe is Niemann-Pick C1-Like 1 (NPC1L1). Proc Natl Acad Sci USA. 2005;102(23):8132–7.
64. Davis Jr HR, Zhu LJ, Hoos LM, et al. Niemann-Pick C1 Like 1 (NPC1L1) is the intestinal phytosterol and cholesterol transporter and a key modulator of whole-body cholesterol homeostasis. J Biol Chem. 2004;279(32):33586–92.
65. Sane AT, Sinnett D, Delvin E, et al. Localization and role of NPC1L1 in cholesterol absorption in human intestine. J Lipid Res. 2006;47(10):2112–20.
66. Lietz G, Lange J, Rimbach G. Molecular and dietary regulation of beta, beta-carotene 15,15′-monooxygenase 1 (BCMO1). Arch Biochem Biophys. 2010;502(1):8–16.
67. Herr FM, Wardlaw SA, Kakkad B, Albrecht A, Quick TC, Ong DE. Intestinal vitamin A metabolism: coordinate distribution of enzymes and CRBP(II). J Lipid Res. 1993;34(9):1545–54.
68. Grune T, Lietz G, Palou A, et al. Beta-carotene is an important vitamin A source for humans. J Nutr. 2010;140(12):2268S–85.
69. Hussain MM. A proposed model for the assembly of chylomicrons. Atherosclerosis. 2000;148(1):1–15.
70. Iqbal J, Hussain MM. Intestinal lipid absorption. Am J Physiol Endocrinol Metab. 2009;296(6):E1183–94.
71. Lu S, Yao Y, Meng S, Cheng X, Black DD. Overexpression of apolipoprotein A-IV enhances lipid transport in newborn swine intestinal epithelial cells. J Biol Chem. 2002;277(35):31929–37.
72. Lu S, Yao Y, Cheng X, et al. Overexpression of apolipoprotein A-IV enhances lipid secretion in IPEC-1 cells by increasing chylomicron size. J Biol Chem. 2006;281(6):3473–83.
73. Carriere V, Vidal R, Lazou K, et al. HNF-4-dependent induction of apolipoprotein A-IV gene transcription by an apical supply of lipid micelles in intestinal cells. J Biol Chem. 2005;280(7):5406–13.
74. Mansbach 2nd CM, Parthasarathy S. A re examination of the fate of glyceride-glycerol in neutral lipid absorption and transport. J Lipid Res. 1982;23(7):1009–19.
75. You CS, Parker RS, Goodman KJ, Swanson JE, Corso TN. Evidence of cis-trans isomerization of 9-cis-beta-carotene during absorption in humans. Am J Clin Nutr. 1996;64(2):177–83.
76. Richelle M, Sanchez B, Tavazzi I, Lambelet P, Bortlik K, Williamson G. Lycopene isomerisation takes place within enterocytes during absorption in human subjects. Br J Nutr. 2010;103(12):1800–7.
77. Ross AB, Vuong LT, Ruckle J, et al. Lycopene bioavailability and metabolism in humans: an accelerator mass spectrometry study. Am J Clin Nutr. 2011;93(6):1263–73.
78. Lu K, Lee MH, Patel SB. Dietary cholesterol absorption; more than just bile. Trends Endocrinol Metab. 2001;12(7):314–20.
79. Plat J, Nichols JA, Mensink RP. Plant sterols and stanols: effects on mixed micellar composition and LXR (target gene) activation. J Lipid Res. 2005;46(11):2468–76.
80. Berge KE, Tian H, Graf GA, et al. Accumulation of dietary cholesterol in sitosterolemia caused by mutations in adjacent ABC transporters. Science. 2000;290(5497):1771–5.
81. Plat J, Kerckhoffs DA, Mensink RP. Therapeutic potential of plant sterols and stanols. Curr Opin Lipidol. 2000;11(6):571–6.
82. Plat J, Mensink RP. Effects of diets enriched with two different plant stanol ester mixtures on plasma ubiquinol-10 and fat-soluble antioxidant concentrations. Metabolism. 2001;50(5):520–9.
83. Leo MA, Ahmed S, Aleynik SI, Siegel JH, Kasmin F, Lieber CS. Carotenoids and tocopherols in various hepatobiliary conditions. J Hepatol. 1995;23(5):550–6.

84. O'Driscoll CM. Anatomy and physiology of lymphatics. In: Charman WN, Stella VJ, editors. Lymphatic transport of drugs. Boca Raton, FL: CRC Press, Inc; 1992. p. 1–35.
85. van Bennekum AM, Kako Y, Weinstock PH, et al. Lipoprotein lipase expression level influences tissue clearance of chylomicron retinyl ester. J Lipid Res. 1999;40(3):565–74.
86. Blaner WS, Obunike JC, Kurlandsky SB, et al. Lipoprotein lipase hydrolysis of retinyl ester. Possible implications for retinoid uptake by cells. J Biol Chem. 1994;269(24):16559–65.
87. Novotny JA, Kurilich AC, Britz SJ, Clevidence BA. Plasma appearance of labeled beta-carotene, lutein, and retinol in humans after consumption of isotopically labeled kale. J Lipid Res. 2005;46(9):1896–903.
88. Bierer TL, Merchen NR, Erdman Jr JW. Comparative absorption and transport of five common carotenoids in preruminant calves. J Nutr. 1995;125(6):1569–77.
89. Wisse E, De Zanger RB, Charels K, Van Der Smissen P, McCuskey RS. The liver sieve: considerations concerning the structure and function of endothelial fenestrae, the sinusoidal wall and the space of Disse. Hepatology. 1985;5(4):683–92.
90. Cooper AD. Hepatic uptake of chylomicron remnants. J Lipid Res. 1997;38(11):2173–92.
91. Clevidence BA, Bieri JG. Association of carotenoids with human plasma lipoproteins. Methods Enzymol. 1993;214:33–46.
92. Krinsky NI, Johnson EJ. Carotenoid actions and their relation to health and disease. Mol Aspects Med. 2005;26(6):459–516.
93. Tyssandier V, Choubert G, Grolier P, Borel P. Carotenoids, mostly the xanthophylls, exchange between plasma lipoproteins. Int J Vitam Nutr Res. 2002;72(5):300–8.
94. Ziouzenkova O, Winklhofer-Roob BM, Puhl H, Roob JM, Esterbauer H. Lack of correlation between the alpha-tocopherol content of plasma and LDL, but high correlations for gamma-tocopherol and carotenoids. J Lipid Res. 1996;37(9):1936–46.
95. During A, Doraiswamy S, Harrison EH. Xanthophylls are preferentially taken up compared with beta-carotene by retinal cells via a SRBI-dependent mechanism. J Lipid Res. 2008;49(8):1715–24.
96. Moussa M, Gouranton E, Gleize B, et al. CD36 is involved in lycopene and lutein uptake by adipocytes and adipose tissue cultures. Mol Nutr Food Res. 2011;55(4):578–84.
97. Borel P, Moussa M, Reboul E, et al. Human plasma levels of vitamin E and carotenoids are associated with genetic polymorphisms in genes involved in lipid metabolism. J Nutr. 2007;137(12):2653–9.
98. Borel P, Moussa M, Reboul E, et al. Human fasting plasma concentrations of vitamin E and carotenoids, and their association with genetic variants in apo C-III, cholesteryl ester transfer protein, hepatic lipase, intestinal fatty acid binding protein and microsomal triacylglycerol transfer protein. Br J Nutr. 2009;101(5):680–7.
99. Lietz G, Hesketh J. A network approach to micronutrient genetics: interactions with lipid metabolism. Curr Opin Lipidol. 2009;20(2):112–20.
100. Chung HY, Ferreira AL, Epstein S, Paiva SA, Castaneda-Sceppa C, Johnson EJ. Site-specific concentrations of carotenoids in adipose tissue: relations with dietary and serum carotenoid concentrations in healthy adults. Am J Clin Nutr. 2009;90(3):533–9.
101. Lakshman MR, Asher KA, Attlesey MG, Satchithanandam S, Mychkovsky I, Coutlakis PJ. Absorption, storage, and distribution of beta-carotene in normal and beta-carotene-fed rats: roles of parenchymal and stellate cells. J Lipid Res. 1989;30(10):1545–50.
102. Shmarakov I, Fleshman MK, D'Ambrosio DN, et al. Hepatic stellate cells are an important cellular site for beta-carotene conversion to retinoid. Arch Biochem Biophys. 2010;504(1):3–10.
103. Teodoro AJ, Perrone D, Martucci RB, Borojevic R. Lycopene isomerisation and storage in an *in vitro* model of murine hepatic stellate cells. Eur J Nutr. 2009;48(5):261–8.
104. Borel P, de Edelenyi FS, Vincent-Baudry S, et al. Genetic variants in BCMO1 and CD36 are associated with plasma lutein concentrations and macular pigment optical density in humans. Ann Med. 2011;43(1):47–59.
105. Li B, Vachali P, Bernstein PS. Human ocular carotenoid-binding proteins. Photochem Photobiol Sci. 2010;9(11):1418–25.
106. Bhosale P, Larson AJ, Frederick JM, Southwick K, Thulin CD, Bernstein PS. Identification and characterization of a Pi isoform of glutathione S-transferase (GSTP1) as a zeaxanthin-binding protein in the macula of the human eye. J Biol Chem. 2004;279(47):49447–54.
107. Li B, Vachali P, Frederick JM, Bernstein PS. Identification of StARD3 as a lutein-binding protein in the macula of the primate retina. Biochemistry. 2011;50(13):2541–9.
108. Bhosale P, Li B, Sharifzadeh M, et al. Purification and partial characterization of a lutein-binding protein from human retina. Biochemistry. 2009;48(22):4798–807.
109. Lademann J, Meinke MC, Sterry W, Darvin ME. Carotenoids in human skin. Exp Dermatol. 2011;20(5):377–82.
110. Terao J, Minami Y, Bando N. Singlet molecular oxygen-quenching activity of carotenoids: relevance to protection of the skin from photoaging. J Clin Biochem Nutr. 2011;48(1):57–62.
111. Antille C, Tran C, Sorg O, Saurat JH. Topical beta-carotene is converted to retinyl esters in human skin ex vivo and mouse skin *in vivo*. Exp Dermatol. 2004;13(9):558–61.

112. Lademann J, Schanzer S, Meinke M, Sterry W, Darvin ME. Interaction between carotenoids and free radicals in human skin. Skin Pharmacol Physiol. 2011;24(5):238–44.
113. Krinsky NI. The antioxidant and biological properties of the carotenoids. Ann N Y Acad Sci. 1998;854:443–7.
114. Britton G. Structure and properties of carotenoids in relation to function. FASEB J. 1995;9(15):1551–8.
115. Nagao A. Oxidative conversion of carotenoids to retinoids and other products. J Nutr. 2004;134(1):237S–40.
116. Siems W, Salerno C, Crifo C, Sommerburg O, Wiswedel I. Beta-carotene degradation products—formation, toxicity and prevention of toxicity. Forum Nutr. 2009;61:75–86.
117. Sommerburg O, Karius N, Siems W, et al. Proteasomal degradation of beta-carotene metabolite-modified proteins. Biofactors. 2009;35(5):449–59.
118. Moore T. Vitamin A and carotene: the absence of the liver oil vitamin A from carotene. VI. The conversion of carotene to vitamin A *in vivo*. Biochem J. 1930;24(3):692–702.
119. Goodman DS, Huang HS. Biosynthesis of vitamin A with rat intestinal enzymes. Science. 1965;149:879–80.
120. Olson JA, Hayaishi O. The enzymatic cleavage of beta-carotene into vitamin A by soluble enzymes of rat liver and intestine. Proc Natl Acad Sci USA. 1965;54(5):1364–70.
121. Glover J. The conversion of beta-carotene into vitamin A. Vitam Horm. 1960;18:371–86.
122. Wyss A. Carotene oxygenases: a new family of double bond cleavage enzymes. J Nutr. 2004;134(1):246S–50.
123. von Lintig J. Colors with functions: elucidating the biochemical and molecular basis of carotenoid metabolism. Annu Rev Nutr. 2010;30:35–56.
124. Cai X, Conley SM, Naash MI. RPE65: role in the visual cycle, human retinal disease, and gene therapy. Ophthalmic Genet. 2009;30(2):57–62.
125. Kiser PD, Golczak M, Lodowski DT, Chance MR, Palczewski K. Crystal structure of native RPE65, the retinoid isomerase of the visual cycle. Proc Natl Acad Sci USA. 2009;106(41):17325–30.
126. Moiseyev G, Takahashi Y, Chen Y, et al. RPE65 is an iron(II)-dependent isomerohydrolase in the retinoid visual cycle. J Biol Chem. 2006;281(5):2835–40.
127. Khachik F, Beecher GR, Goli MB, Lusby WR, Smith Jr JC. Separation and identification of carotenoids and their oxidation products in the extracts of human plasma. Anal Chem. 1992;64(18):2111–22.
128. Etoh H, Utsunomiya Y, Komori A, Murakami Y, Oshima S, Inakuma T. Carotenoids in human blood plasma after ingesting paprika juice. Biosci Biotechnol Biochem. 2000;64(5):1096–8.
129. Yonekura L, Kobayashi M, Terasaki M, Nagao A. Keto-carotenoids are the major metabolites of dietary lutein and fucoxanthin in mouse tissues. J Nutr. 2010;140(10):1824–31.
130. Khachik F, de Moura FF, Chew EY, et al. The effect of lutein and zeaxanthin supplementation on metabolites of these carotenoids in the serum of persons aged 60 or older. Invest Ophthalmol Vis Sci. 2006;47(12):5234–42.
131. Murakami A, Takahashi D, Kinoshita T, et al. Zerumbone, a Southeast Asian ginger sesquiterpene, markedly suppresses free radical generation, proinflammatory protein production, and cancer cell proliferation accompanied by apoptosis: the alpha, beta-unsaturated carbonyl group is a prerequisite. Carcinogenesis. 2002;23(5):795–802.
132. Leuenberger MG, Engeloch-Jarret C, Woggon W-D. The reaction mechanism of the enzyme catalyzed central cleavage of β-carotene to retinal. Angew Chem Int Ed. 2001;40(14):2613–7.
133. Kloer DP, Schulz GE. Structural and biological aspects of carotenoid cleavage. Cell Mol Life Sci. 2006;63(19–20):2291–303.
134. Poliakov E, Gentleman S, Chander P, et al. Biochemical evidence for the tyrosine involvement in cationic intermediate stabilization in mouse beta-carotene 15, 15′-monooxygenase. BMC Biochem. 2009;10:31.
135. von Lintig J, Vogt K. Filling the gap in vitamin A research. Molecular identification of an enzyme cleaving beta-carotene to retinal. J Biol Chem. 2000;275(16):11915–20.
136. Wyss A, Wirtz G, Woggon W, et al. Cloning and expression of beta, beta-carotene 15,15′-dioxygenase. Biochem Biophys Res Commun. 2000;271(2):334–6.
137. Paik J, During A, Harrison EH, Mendelsohn CL, Lai K, Blaner WS. Expression and characterization of a murine enzyme able to cleave beta-carotene. The formation of retinoids. J Biol Chem. 2001;276(34):32160–8.
138. Wyss A, Wirtz GM, Woggon WD, et al. Expression pattern and localization of beta, beta-carotene 15,15′-dioxygenase in different tissues. Biochem J. 2001;354(Pt 3):521–9.
139. Redmond TM, Gentleman S, Duncan T, et al. Identification, expression, and substrate specificity of a mammalian beta-carotene 15,15′-dioxygenase. J Biol Chem. 2001;276(9):6560–5.
140. Morales A, Rosas A, Gonzalez A, et al. Cloning of the bovine beta-carotene-15,15′-oxygenase and expression in gonadal tissues. Int J Vitam Nutr Res. 2006;76(1):9–17.
141. Lampert JM, Holzschuh J, Hessel S, Driever W, Vogt K, von Lintig J. Provitamin A conversion to retinal via the beta, beta-carotene-15,15′-oxygenase (bcox) is essential for pattern formation and differentiation during zebrafish embryogenesis. Development. 2003;130(10):2173–86.
142. Yan W, Jang GF, Haeseleer F, et al. Cloning and characterization of a human beta, beta-carotene-15,15′-dioxygenase that is highly expressed in the retinal pigment epithelium. Genomics. 2001;72(2):193–202.
143. Lindqvist A, Andersson S. Biochemical properties of purified recombinant human beta-carotene 15,15′-monooxygenase. J Biol Chem. 2002;277(26):23942–8.

144. Kim YS, Oh DK. Substrate specificity of a recombinant chicken beta-carotene 15,15′-monooxygenase that converts beta-carotene into retinal. Biotechnol Lett. 2009;31(3):403–8.
145. Kim YS, Park CS, Oh DK. Hydrophobicity of residue 108 specifically affects the affinity of human beta-carotene 15,15′-monooxygenase for substrates with two ionone rings. Biotechnol Lett. 2010;32(6):847–53.
146. Fierce Y, de Morais Vieira M, Piantedosi R, Wyss A, Blaner WS, Paik J. *In vitro* and *in vivo* characterization of retinoid synthesis from beta-carotene. Arch Biochem Biophys. 2008;472(2):126–38.
147. Kloer DP, Ruch S, Al-Babili S, Beyer P, Schulz GE. The structure of a retinal-forming carotenoid oxygenase. Science. 2005;308(5719):267–9.
148. Lindqvist A, Andersson S. Cell type-specific expression of beta-carotene 15,15′-mono-oxygenase in human tissues. J Histochem Cytochem. 2004;52(4):491–9.
149. von Lintig J, Hessel S, Isken A, et al. Towards a better understanding of carotenoid metabolism in animals. Biochim Biophys Acta. 2005;1740(2):122–31.
150. Lindqvist A, Sharvill J, Sharvill DE, Andersson S. Loss-of-function mutation in carotenoid 15,15′-monooxygenase identified in a patient with hypercarotenemia and hypovitaminosis A. J Nutr. 2007;137(11):2346–50.
151. Ferrucci L, Perry JR, Matteini A, et al. Common variation in the beta-carotene 15,15′-monooxygenase 1 gene affects circulating levels of carotenoids: a genome-wide association study. Am J Hum Genet. 2009;84(2):123–33.
152. Leung WC, Hessel S, Meplan C, et al. Two common single nucleotide polymorphisms in the gene encoding beta-carotene 15,15′-monoxygenase alter beta-carotene metabolism in female volunteers. FASEB J. 2009;23(4):1041–53.
153. Takitani K, Zhu CL, Inoue A, Tamai H. Molecular cloning of the rat beta-carotene 15,15′-monooxygenase gene and its regulation by retinoic acid. Eur J Nutr. 2006;45(6):320–6.
154. Bachmann H, Desbarats A, Pattison P, et al. Feedback regulation of beta, beta-carotene 15,15′-monooxygenase by retinoic acid in rats and chickens. J Nutr. 2002;132(12):3616–22.
155. Seino Y, Miki T, Kiyonari H, et al. Isx participates in the maintenance of vitamin A metabolism by regulation of beta-carotene 15,15′-monooxygenase (Bcmo1) expression. J Biol Chem. 2008;283(8):4905–11.
156. Lobo GP, Hessel S, Eichinger A, et al. ISX is a retinoic acid-sensitive gatekeeper that controls intestinal beta, beta-carotene absorption and vitamin A production. FASEB J. 2010;24(6):1656–66.
157. Boulanger A, McLemore P, Copeland NG, et al. Identification of beta-carotene 15, 15′-monooxygenase as a peroxisome proliferator-activated receptor target gene. FASEB J. 2003;17(10):1304–6.
158. Gong X, Tsai SW, Yan B, Rubin LP. Cooperation between MEF2 and PPARgamma in human intestinal beta, beta-carotene 15,15′-monooxygenase gene expression. BMC Mol Biol. 2006;7:7.
159. Takase S, Suruga K, Goda T. Regulation of vitamin A metabolism-related gene expression. Br J Nutr. 2000;84 Suppl 2:S217–21.
160. Yamaguchi N, Suruga K. Triiodothyronine stimulates CMO1 gene expression in human intestinal Caco-2 BBe cells. Life Sci. 2008;82(13–14):789–96.
161. Luvizotto RA, Nascimento AF, Veeramachaneni S, Liu C, Wang XD. Chronic alcohol intake upregulates hepatic expression of carotenoid cleavage enzymes and PPAR in rats. J Nutr. 2010;140(10):1808–14.
162. Zaripheh S, Nara TY, Nakamura MT, Erdman Jr JW. Dietary lycopene downregulates carotenoid 15,15′-monooxygenase and PPAR-gamma in selected rat tissues. J Nutr. 2006;136(4):932–8.
163. Reynaud E, Aydemir G, Ruhl R, Dangles O, Caris-Veyrat C. Organic synthesis of new putative lycopene metabolites and preliminary investigation of their cell-signaling effects. J Agric Food Chem. 2011;59(4):1457–63.
164. van Vliet T, van Schaik F, Schreurs WH, van den Berg H. *In vitro* measurement of beta-carotene cleavage activity: methodological considerations and the effect of other carotenoids on beta-carotene cleavage. Int J Vitam Nutr Res. 1996;66(1):77–85.
165. Nagao A, Maeda M, Lim BP, Kobayashi H, Terao J. Inhibition of beta-carotene-15,15′-dioxygenase activity by dietary flavonoids. J Nutr Biochem. 2000;11(6):348–55.
166. Bando N, Muraki N, Murota K, Terao J, Yamanishi R. Ingested quercetin but not rutin increases accumulation of hepatic beta-carotene in BALB/c mice. Mol Nutr Food Res. 2010;54 Suppl 2:S261–7.
167. Hessel S, Eichinger A, Isken A, et al. CMO1 deficiency abolishes vitamin A production from beta-carotene and alters lipid metabolism in mice. J Biol Chem. 2007;282(46):33553–61.
168. Lindshield BL, King JL, Wyss A, et al. Lycopene biodistribution is altered in 15,15′-carotenoid monooxygenase knockout mice. J Nutr. 2008;138(12):2367–71.
169. Tourniaire F, Gouranton E, von Lintig J, et al. beta-Carotene conversion products and their effects on adipose tissue. Gene Nutr. 2009;4(3):179–87.
170. Reichert B, Yasmeen R, Jeyakumar SM, et al. Concerted action of aldehyde dehydrogenases influences depot-specific fat formation. Mol Endocrinol. 2011;25(5):799–809.
171. Lobo GP, Amengual J, Palczewski G, Babino D, von Lintig J. Carotenoid-oxygenases: key players for carotenoid function and homeostasis in mammalian biology. Biochim Biophys Acta. 2012;1821(1):78–87.
172. Ziouzenkova O, Orasanu G, Sharlach M, et al. Retinaldehyde represses adipogenesis and diet-induced obesity. Nat Med. 2007;13(6):695–702.

173. Amengual J, Gouranton E, van Helden YG, Hessel S, Ribot J, et al. Beta-carotene reduces body adiposity of mice via BCMO1. PLoS One. 2011;6(6):e20644.
174. Sanchez J, Fuster A, Oliver P, Palou A, Pico C. Effects of beta-carotene supplementation on adipose tissue thermogenic capacity in ferrets (*Mustela putorius furo*). Br J Nutr. 2009;102(11):1686–94.
175. Olmedilla B, Granado F, Southon S, et al. A European multicentre, placebo-controlled supplementation study with alpha-tocopherol, carotene-rich palm oil, lutein or lycopene: analysis of serum responses. Clin Sci (Lond). 2002;102(4):447–56.
176. The effect of vitamin E and beta carotene on the incidence of lung cancer and other cancers in male smokers. The Alpha-Tocopherol, Beta Carotene Cancer Prevention Study Group. N Engl J Med. 1994;330(15):1029–35.
177. Omenn GS, Goodman GE, Thornquist MD, et al. Risk factors for lung cancer and for intervention effects in CARET, the Beta-Carotene and Retinol Efficacy Trial. J Natl Cancer Inst. 1996;88(21):1550–9.
178. Kamangar F, Qiao YL, Yu B, et al. Lung cancer chemoprevention: a randomized, double-blind trial in Linxian, China. Cancer Epidemiol Biomarkers Prev. 2006;15(8):1562–4.
179. Cui Y, Freedman JH. Cadmium induces retinoic acid signaling by regulating retinoic acid metabolic gene expression. J Biol Chem. 2009;284(37):24925–32.
180. Kiefer C, Hessel S, Lampert JM, et al. Identification and characterization of a mammalian enzyme catalyzing the asymmetric oxidative cleavage of provitamin A. J Biol Chem. 2001;276(17):14110–6.
181. Lindqvist A, He YG, Andersson S. Cell type-specific expression of beta-carotene 9′,10′-monooxygenase in human tissues. J Histochem Cytochem. 2005;53(11):1403–12.
182. Amengual J, Lobo GP, Golczak M, et al. A mitochondrial enzyme degrades carotenoids and protects against oxidative stress. FASEB J. 2011;25(3):948–59.
183. Hu KQ, Liu C, Ernst H, Krinsky NI, Russell RM, Wang XD. The biochemical characterization of ferret carotene-9′,10′-monooxygenase catalyzing cleavage of carotenoids *in vitro* and *in vivo*. J Biol Chem. 2006; 281(28):19327–38.
184. Mein JR, Dolnikowski GG, Ernst H, Russell RM, Wang XD. Enzymatic formation of apo-carotenoids from the xanthophyll carotenoids lutein, zeaxanthin and beta-cryptoxanthin by ferret carotene-9′,10′-monooxygenase. Arch Biochem Biophys. 2011;506(1):109–21.
185. Wang XD, Russell RM, Liu C, Stickel F, Smith DE, Krinsky NI. Beta-oxidation in rabbit liver *in vitro* and in the perfused ferret liver contributes to retinoic acid biosynthesis from beta-apocarotenoic acids. J Biol Chem. 1996;271(43):26490–8.
186. Eriksson J, Larson G, Gunnarsson U, et al. Identification of the yellow skin gene reveals a hybrid origin of the domestic chicken. PLoS Genet. 2008;4(2):e1000010.
187. Tian R, Pitchford WS, Morris CA, Cullen NG, Bottema CD. Genetic variation in the beta, beta-carotene-9′, 10′-dioxygenase gene and association with fat colour in bovine adipose tissue and milk. Anim Genet. 2010;41(3):253–9.
188. Berry SD, Davis SR, Beattie EM, et al. Mutation in bovine beta-carotene oxygenase 2 affects milk color. Genetics. 2009;182(3):923–6.
189. Vage DI, Boman IA. A nonsense mutation in the beta-carotene oxygenase 2 (BCO2) gene is tightly associated with accumulation of carotenoids in adipose tissue in sheep (*Ovis aries*). BMC Genet. 2010;11:10.
190. Ford NA, Clinton SK, von Lintig J, Wyss A, Erdman Jr JW. Loss of carotene-9′,10′-monooxygenase expression increases serum and tissue lycopene concentrations in lycopene-fed mice. J Nutr. 2010;140(12):2134–8.
191. Siems W, Wiswedel I, Salerno C, et al. Beta-carotene breakdown products may impair mitochondrial functions–potential side effects of high-dose beta-carotene supplementation. J Nutr Biochem. 2005;16(7):385–97.
192. van Helden YG, Keijer J, Knaapen AM, et al. Beta-carotene metabolites enhance inflammation-induced oxidative DNA damage in lung epithelial cells. Free Radic Biol Med. 2009;46(2):299–304.
193. Alija AJ, Bresgen N, Sommerburg O, Siems W, Eckl PM. Cytotoxic and genotoxic effects of beta-carotene breakdown products on primary rat hepatocytes. Carcinogenesis. 2004;25(5):827–31.
194. Lian F, Wang XD. Enzymatic metabolites of lycopene induce Nrf2-mediated expression of phase II detoxifying/antioxidant enzymes in human bronchial epithelial cells. Int J Cancer. 2008;123(6):1262–8.
195. Linnewiel K, Ernst H, Caris-Veyrat C, et al. Structure activity relationship of carotenoid derivatives in activation of the electrophile/antioxidant response element transcription system. Free Radic Biol Med. 2009;47(5):659–67.
196. Ziouzenkova O, Orasanu G, Sukhova G, et al. Asymmetric cleavage of beta-carotene yields a transcriptional repressor of retinoid X receptor and peroxisome proliferator-activated receptor responses. Mol Endocrinol. 2007;21(1):77–88.
197. Marsh RS, Yan Y, Reed VM, Hruszkewycz D, Curley RW, Harrison EH. β-Apocarotenoids do not significantly activate retinoic acid receptors α or β. Exp Biol Med (Maywood). 2010;235(3):342–8.
198. Eroglu A, Hruszkewycz DP, Curley Jr RW, Harrison EH. The eccentric cleavage product of beta-carotene, beta-apo-13-carotenone, functions as an antagonist of RXRalpha. Arch Biochem Biophys. 2010;504(1):11–6.
199. Lian F, Smith DE, Ernst H, Russell RM, Wang XD. Apo-10′-lycopenoic acid inhibits lung cancer cell growth *in vitro*, and suppresses lung tumorigenesis in the A/J mouse model *in vivo*. Carcinogenesis. 2007; 28(7):1567–74.

200. Edwards AJ, Vinyard BT, Wiley ER, et al. Consumption of watermelon juice increases plasma concentrations of lycopene and beta-carotene in humans. J Nutr. 2003;133(4):1043–50.
201. Kopec RE, Riedl KM, Harrison EH, et al. Identification and quantification of apo-lycopenals in fruits, vegetables, and human plasma. J Agric Food Chem. 2010;58(6):3290–6.
202. Khachik F, Carvalho L, Bernstein PS, Muir GJ, Zhao DY, Katz NB. Chemistry, distribution, and metabolism of tomato carotenoids and their impact on human health. Exp Biol Med (Maywood). 2002;227(10):845–51.
203. Kim YS, Yeom SJ, Oh DK. Production of beta-apo-10′-carotenal from beta-carotene by human beta-carotene-9′,10′-oxygenase expressed in E. coli. Biotechnol Lett. 2011;33(6):1195–200.
204. Ho CC, de Moura FF, Kim SH, Clifford AJ. Excentral cleavage of beta-carotene *in vivo* in a healthy man. Am J Clin Nutr. 2007;85(3):770–7.
205. Gajic M, Zaripheh S, Sun F, Erdman Jr JW. Apo-8′-lycopenal and apo-12′-lycopenal are metabolic products of lycopene in rat liver. J Nutr. 2006;136(6):1552–7.

Chapter 4
Reactive Oxygen and Nitrogen Species in Biological Systems: Reactions and Regulation by Carotenoids

John T. Landrum

Key Points

- ROS/RNS originate primarily from oxygen reduction processes, differ markedly in reactivity and lifetimes, and are essential high fidelity sensors of the redox status in cells.
- High levels of ROS/RNS can trigger positive feedback mechanisms and overwhelm antioxidant capacity leading to oxidative stress and apoptosis.
- Carotenoids function as antioxidants but react principally with only the most reactive radicals.
- Carotenoid cation radicals are long-lived, their formation disrupts radical oxidative mechanisms and are readily reduced by ascorbate, glutathione, and tocopherol.
- Carotenoids in the skin and retina are protective against the light-induced action of singlet oxygen.
- Evidence supports the argument that carotenoid cleavage products serve a role in cell signaling and regulation.

Keywords Carotenoids • Apo-carotenals • Reactive oxygen species (ROS) • Reactive nitrogen species (RNS) • Oxidative stress • Singlet oxygen

Introduction

The principal components of living cells are electron-rich and contain abundant carbon in reduced oxidation states. The formal oxidation state of carbon in CO_2 produced in respiration is 4+ contrasting with 0 in glucose and 1− in alkenes. From a thermodynamic perspective, the success of living systems, composed primarily of low-valent carbon but immersed in an atmosphere high in oxygen, is truly remarkable. The unique triplet electronic ground-state of molecular oxygen confers on it a kinetic inertness toward reaction with most organic molecules that potentiates management of oxygen as an electron sink. Reactive oxygen species (ROS) are the practical consequence of the adoption of oxygen as the terminal electron acceptor in aerobic metabolism. Generation of reactive nitrogen species (RNS), including ${}^{\bullet}NO$, is also principally the result of reactions involving reduced

J.T. Landrum, Ph.D. (✉)
Department of Chemistry and Biochemistry, Florida International University, 11200 SW 8th St, Miami, FL 33199, USA
e-mail: landrumj@fiu.edu

S.A. Tanumihardjo (ed.), *Carotenoids and Human Health*, Nutrition and Health,
DOI 10.1007/978-1-62703-203-2_4, © Springer Science+Business Media New York 2013

oxygen species [1]. Although many ROS are clearly toxic, organisms have developed a range of protective mechanisms to manage the destructive consequences of ROS that are produced by reduction of molecular O_2 [2–4].

An evolutionary adaptation is the recruitment of ROS as high fidelity sensors of the redox status of cells and as signaling molecules [1, 2, 5]. Specialization of enzyme systems and mechanisms to control the production of ROS/RNS at specific times and locations enable regulation of intra- and intercellular processes [6]. The production of energy within mitochondria, the metabolism and detoxification of lipophilic substances in peroxisomes, the generation of oxygen and nitrogen radicals as signaling molecules, and the production of ROS during the immune response of leukocytes, all involve the reduction of molecular oxygen and ROS generation, such as H_2O_2 and O_2^-. Reduced oxygen is activated to participate in further reactions capable of promoting oxidation of biological components. The major site of oxygen reduction within a eukaryotic cell is the mitochondrion; however, other organelles are also implicated in ROS production. Cytosolic oxidases are associated with the endoplasmic reticulum, peroxisomes, lysosomes, and chloroplasts, which are sites of ROS generation in animals and plants [7, 8]. In the liver, 20 % of oxygen consumption occurs in peroxisomes, which function in lipid metabolism [9]. Management of ROS occurs by an effective series of strategies: containment, interception, diversion, and deactivation. Localization of ROS production within mitochondria and peroxisomes isolates them and protects sensitive reactive cellular components and structures (e.g., DNA, proteins, lipids, and carbohydrates) from oxidation and participation in radical reactions [10–14]. Many ROS are too polar or short-lived to diffuse across lipid membranes. Interception and diversion of the oxidizing potential of ROS by glutathione and similarly poised biological redox couples buffer the potential within cells and provides a defense against wayward ROS [15].

A host of proteins and enzymes are efficient at further reducing activated forms of oxygen and compete with the destructive unregulated oxidative consequences of ROS. They shuttle the oxidizing potential of ROS away from sensitive structures and cellular components by diverting them to catabolize cellular waste and toxins [16]. Several enzyme systems utilize the oxidizing potential of reactive, low-valent oxygen intermediates to carry out metabolic processes. These enzymes enable direct reaction, or deactivation of primary and secondary ROS, including H_2O_2, O_2^-, $^1O_2$, and peroxylipids, as well as RNS, including nitric oxide, peroxynitrite, and nitrogen dioxide [17]. This deactivation of ROS is accomplished by the action of antioxidants and enzyme systems that accumulate at effective concentrations within the cell and its specific cellular compartments where ROS levels are highest. Many are rapidly synthesized in response to the actions of ROS [18–20].

Chronic inflammatory events and/or exposure to mitogens can upset the balance between production and neutralization of ROS. ROS can trigger cytokine release, production of matrix metallooxygenases, and chemotactic attraction of leukocytes resulting in increased intra- and extracellular release of ROS. Chemotactic attraction of macrophages that release ROS can accelerate such imbalances [21–25]. Repeated oxidative stress can lead to functional and/or structural damage to organelles, cells, and tissues, and can produce pathogenic conditions associated with many diseases (Table 4.1). ROS detection is almost impossible in experimental settings, posing special challenges. Identifying specific ROS and generation sites within the subcellular spaces requires detection of products and/or use of suitable indicators [26]. Direct detection of specific ROS and their actions is possible in certain well-controlled systems and recently developed methods provide new approaches [26–29].

Oxidative stress is assessed by secondary measurements of different biochemical events and products (e.g., peroxidation of lipids; malondialdehyde generation [30, 31]; protein degradation [8]; "nicked," cleaved, or oxidized DNA [32]; and the lipid oxidation associated cellular responses of cytokine production [33]). These diverse measures assess different events and processes that neither conform to a single definition of oxidative stress nor definitively diagnose the causative events that triggered their production. We are invariably forced to assemble the circumstantial evidence from a multitude of indirect measurements. Despite these limitations, during the past decade work has progressed, particularly in assessing the dynamics of the interplay of ROS and transcription.

Table 4.1 Diseases and degenerative processes that are ROS-linked [34–41]

Atherosclerosis
Alzheimer's disease
Neurodegenerative diseases
Cardiac disease
Chronic obstructive pulmonary disease
Ischemic–reperfusion injury
Crohn's disease
Age-related macular degeneration
Cataract
Rheumatoid arthritis
Osteoporosis
Osteolytic implant failure
Diabetes
Autoimmune diseases
Cancers
Skin
Lung
Prostate
Ovarian
Colon
Hepatic

Essential Functions of Reactive Oxygen Species and Reactive Nitrogen Species

ROS/RNS serve many essential functions *in vivo* (Table 4.2) [5, 9, 42, 43].

The body of evidence demonstrating that many ROS act as signal transducers is compelling [72]. The natural interplay resulting from the generation and deactivation of ROS (as well as ROS-generated signal molecules, e.g., prostaglandins, interleukins), is a delicately balanced system essential to normal cellular function [73]. Generation of oxygen radicals is involved in the mechanism of vascular smooth muscle to sense the partial pressure of O_2 and regulate vasoconstriction and paradoxically also dilation [42]. Hydrogen peroxide is a signal molecule involved in activation of chemotaxis of neutrophils and macrophages, an action essential for the immune response to bacterial infection [21, 69, 70]. However, generation of ROS by white blood cells sets the stage for the possibility that unregulated ROS production will result in oxidative stress and/or an inflammatory response that can disrupt the homeostatic redox balance in extracellular spaces.

Generation of high levels of ROS can trigger feedback mechanisms, overwhelm antioxidant capacity, and result in persistent, excessive ROS production causing subcellular, cellular, and tissue damage [73]. These actions of ROS are widely implicated in the pathogenesis of a diverse number of diseases (Table 4.1). Chronic ROS exposure is associated with damage of the normally impermeable inner mitochondrial membranes and can pose a risk to the entire cellular apparatus by enabling normally contained ROS to diffuse into the surrounding cytosol through the porous outer membrane [37, 74]. Extensive research has implicated dysfunction of mitochondria in the pathogenesis of cardiac, neurological, and other diseases [37, 75, 76]. Cyclooxygenases (COX) reduce levels of reactive and pro-oxidative hydroperoxides, including fatty acid hydroperoxides, diverting their ability to participate in unregulated free radical chain reactions. COX are also important for the conversion of arachadonic acid into prostaglandins, including PGH-2, a potent vasoconstrictor. However, prostaglandins are able to upregulate transcription of ROS generating enzymes [77, 78]. ROS-stimulated PGH-2 production is linked to Alzheimer pathogenesis [71, 77, 79].

Table 4.2 Essential actions of oxygen and nitrogen free radicals

Plants
Metabolism [44]
Immune response [45–48]
Growth and development [49]
Cell growth [50]
Control of plant form [51]
Seed germination [48, 52]
Modulation of gene expression [5]
Animals
Immune response [53, 54]
Vasodilation [55–57]
Growth and development
Bone and cartilage maintenance (osteoclasts, osteoblasts)[58–62]
Milk properties and function [63–65]
Necrotizing enterocolitis [66]
Embryonic development [67]
Modulation of gene expression [8]
Cell differentiation [8]
Differentiation [68]
Macrophage chemotaxis [21, 69, 70]
Detoxification of xenobiotics [71]

In 1989, Halliwell and Gutteridge defined antioxidants as, "any substance that when present at low concentrations compared with that of an oxidizable substrate, significantly delays or inhibits oxidation of that substrate" [80]. Many of the important biological antioxidants work synergistically in networks [17]. *In vivo* and *in vitro* studies provide support that carotenoids, tocopherols, ascorbate, phytopolyphenols, and glutathione are antioxidants that function as a combined redox buffering system within the cell [81–83]. These components provide antioxidant protection in lipophilic membrane environments, the aqueous cytosol, and extracellular compartments [17]. The ability of antioxidants to equilibrate at aqueous/lipid (cytosolic/membrane) interfaces is a critical feature for efficient antioxidant protection of cellular components [81, 84, 85]. The large number of antioxidants together with the antioxidant enzyme creates a natural but complex redundancy within the biological systems, which can mask the antioxidant role of single components [86]. The leakage of ROS past the antioxidant defenses within a cell creates oxidative stress through the undesirable oxidative reactions that degrade lipids, proteins, DNA, and carbohydrates often leading to additional ROS generation via the activation of pro-inflammatory transcription factors such as nuclear factor κB (NF-κB), activated protein-1, peroxisome-proliferator receptors, and the induction of COX and P450 enzymes [18, 72]. Hydroxylation, oxidation, and nitration that result from ROS alter the solubility and the reactivity of small molecules and can influence the tertiary structure of proteins and/or their ability to interact with each other.

Carotenoids are Demonstrated *In Vivo* Antioxidants

Carotenoids function as antioxidants in many living systems [87–89]. Their proposed role and that of their metabolites in maintaining the optimal function of numerous biochemical processes is supported by epidemiological evidence, *in vitro* experiments, cell culture studies, and genetic knockout models [90–98]. The intensely colored, electron-rich, and lipophilic carotenoids are poly-isoprenoid derived compounds synthesized in plants, bacteria, fungi, and algae. They cannot be synthesized by higher animals but are often modified by oxidation or reduction of the terminal end groups [99]. Carotenoids are essential to photosynthesis and have been recruited by higher animals for many functions [100, 101]. Dietary carotenoids are well-known for their ability to produce coloration, most notably in birds and also in arthropods (insects, arachnids, and crustaceans), reptiles, and amphibians [102–107]. Producing the evidence needed to unambiguously conclude that dietary carotenoids are critically important antioxidants has been challenging because antioxidant function is largely redundant. The multi-layered antioxidant mechanisms present within biological systems protect against catastrophic dysfunction when a single component is restricted. The natural, water-soluble reducing agents, glutathione and ascorbate, are present *in vivo* at levels of 1–10 mM and react directly with many ROS [108]. Vitamin E, a lipid-soluble component, is transported *in vivo* by lipoproteins, and is an effective antioxidant present at levels of ~30 μmol L^{-1} in human serum [109, 110]. Antioxidant enzymes are upregulated in response to increased ROS generation thereby ameliorating any diminished efficiency of small molecule antioxidants [18, 19].

In the photosynthetic apparatus of higher plants, carotenoids protect the photosynthetic antenna proteins from damage by ROS and their secondary products, particularly, $^1O_2$ and O_2^{1-} [111–113]. In a photic environment, chloroplasts in plants may generate 20 times more ROS than the mitochondria and pose a formidable risk of oxidative stress to the cell, primarily in the form of singlet oxygen [44]. In humans, the antioxidant action of carotenoids has also been unambiguously demonstrated in the skin, where singlet oxygen is photochemically generated [114]. In other tissues, the complex interplay of carotenoids with other antioxidants and oxidant/antioxidant regulatory processes remains an imposing task to fully elucidate [114–123].

Carotenoids may possibly act *in vivo* as pro-oxidants [124–127]. Concern was raised that high level supplemental β-carotene may have acted via pro-oxidant pathways to increase lung cancer rates in smokers in the ABTC and CARET studies [128–130]. An interpretation of this observation involving the action of carotenoid oxidation products as transcription regulators has emerged in recent years [131–135]. Although the potential pro-oxidant activity of carotenoids is often considered to be a recent revelation, Trevor Goodwin insightfully discussed this possibility as well as the antioxidant function in his comprehensive monograph on carotenoids in 1954 [136]. Following the initial addition of a free radical to a carotenoid (4.1), a carotenoid carbon radical is produced that has the capability to participate in the fully allowed propagation steps of a free radical chain reaction. These steps include the addition of ground-state molecular dioxygen generating a carotenoid peroxyradical (4.2). Abstraction of hydrogen from an alkyl group or lipid produces a carotenoid hydroperoxide capable of promoting oxidation of other biomolecules, (4.3) and (4.4). The carotenoid hydroperoxide generated in (4.3) can decompose by homolytic peroxide bond cleavage to generate two new radicals, (4.4). The hydroxyl radical generated in (4.4) will react rapidly and indiscriminantly at a diffusion-limited rate with the first alkyl group it encounters (4.5). A lipid hydroperoxide is formed in an analogous sequence (4.6) [124]. Once a lipid radical is generated, the propagating chain reaction (4.7), can continue consuming lipids regenerating new radicals, producing an equivalent of lipid peroxide during each cycle, and geometrically increasing the oxidative stress until the process is dampened by antioxidant interception of the radical intermediates.

$$\text{Car} + \text{R}^{\bullet} \rightarrow \text{R} - \text{Car}^{\bullet} \quad \text{Addition of Radical} \quad \text{R} = \text{alkyl, HOO, and OH} \tag{4.1}$$

$$\text{R} - \text{Car}^{\bullet} + \text{O}_2 \rightarrow \text{R} - \text{Car} - \text{OO}^{\bullet} \quad \text{Addition of Oxygen} \tag{4.2}$$

$$\text{R} - \text{Car} - \text{OO}^{\bullet} + \text{R} - \text{H} \rightarrow \text{R}^{\bullet} + \text{R} - \text{Car} - \text{OOH} \quad \text{H} - \text{Abstraction} \tag{4.3}$$

$$\text{R} - \text{Car} - \text{OOH} \rightarrow \text{R} - \text{Car} - \text{O}^{\bullet} + \text{HO}^{\bullet} \quad \text{Homolysis} \tag{4.4}$$

$$\text{HO}^{\bullet} + \text{R} - \text{H} \rightarrow \text{R}^{\bullet} + \text{H}_2\text{O} \quad k \sim 1 \times 10^9 \text{M}^{-1}\text{s}^{-1} \quad \text{H} - \text{Abstraction} \tag{4.5}$$

$$\text{R} - \text{Car} - \text{O}^{\bullet} + \text{L} - \text{H} \rightarrow \text{R} - \text{Car} - \text{OH} + \text{L}^{\bullet} \quad \text{H} - \text{Abstraction} \quad (\text{L} = \text{lipid}) \tag{4.6}$$

$$\text{L}^{\bullet} + \text{O}_2 \rightarrow \text{LOO}^{\bullet} + \text{LH} \rightarrow \text{LOOH} + \text{L}^{\bullet} \quad \text{Lipid Peroxyl Radical} \tag{4.7}$$

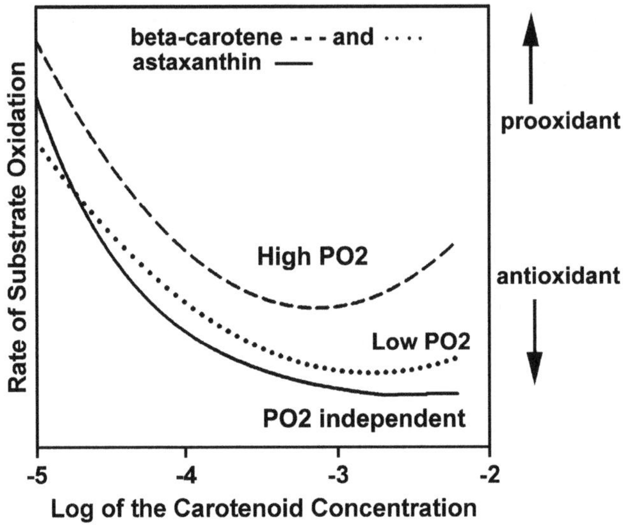

Fig. 4.1 The rate of oxidation of lipid and consumption of oxygen are dependent on carotenoid identity, concentration, and oxygen partial pressure (PO_2). For astaxanthin, the rate of oxidation decreases as the carotenoid concentration increases. Because the astaxanthin radical is slow to react with oxygen it cannot participate as a pro-oxidant at high concentrations (*solid line*). β-Carotene is also an effective antioxidant at low concentrations of oxygen and the rate of oxidation decreases with increasing concentration of β-carotene (*dotted line*). At high partial pressures of oxygen (ca. 1 atm.) β-carotene behaves as an antioxidant at low concentrations (ca. $<10^{-4}$ M) but becomes a pro-oxidant when concentrations exceed 10^{-3} M, (*dashed line*)

In vitro models of free radical oxidation of β-carotene demonstrate that the dependence of the rate of oxygen consumption in this chain reaction is a function of the β-carotene concentration and produces a “U”-shaped curve. Significant catalytic, pro-oxidant activity will occur when the oxygen partial pressure and β-carotene levels are high (Fig. 4.1) [124, 126].

When the concentrations of β-carotene and oxygen are sufficiently high, the rate of the pro-oxidant free radical chain reaction accelerates. Comparison of a number of carotenoids demonstrates that they are not all equally prone to act as pro-oxidants. The presence of oxygen substituents on the ionone ring, such as those found in astaxanthin, stabilize the intermediate carotenoid carbon-centered radical and reduce its reactivity toward molecular oxygen. This disrupts the pro-oxidant mechanism by enabling Car$^{\bullet}$ to react more rapidly with reductants regenerating the carotenoid than its reaction with O_2 [126]. Zeaxanthin, a dihydroxy carotenoid, is actively accumulated in the human macula and is widely accepted to function as an antioxidant [137–139]. Significantly, it too lacks the ability to participate in pro-oxidant behavior [126]. By contrast, the carotenoids, lycopene and β-carotene, which lack oxygen substituents exhibit both pro-oxidant and antioxidant abilities *in vitro* [126]. Pro-oxidant activity for β-carotene (as measured by malondialdehyde generation) in rat liver microsomes occurred at 760 mmHg of O_2 but not at the normal partial pressure of 150 mmHg [140]. There appears to be little evidence that sustainable, pro-oxidant free radical chain reactions involving carotenoids occur at the low partial pressures of O_2 and the low concentrations of carotenoids found *in vivo*. A substantial and growing body of evidence indicates that carotenoid-derived oxidation products (especially *apo*-carotenoid cleavage products [141, 142]) participate in cell signaling, triggering transcription of both pro-oxidant and antioxidant metabolic processes [18, 131, 134, 143].

The Identity and Sources of ROS/RNS Generated *In Vivo*

Although molecular dioxygen must be abundant within cells for the efficient generation of energy by aerobic metabolism, the concentration of free O_2 is controlled and is at very low levels within cells, organelles, and the intracellular spaces. In mammals, oxygen is principally bound to myoglobin and hemoglobin, and free dioxygen levels are limited by strong equilibrium binding constants with these proteins. Intracellular free oxygen partial pressures have been measured and values are around 40 mmHg (ca. 3.7×10^{-4} M) [144–146]. Within the guinea pig retina, a rapidly respiring aerobic tissue, the partial pressure of oxygen at the position of the retinal pigment epithelium and outer segments is 50 mmHg, dropping further in the inner retinal layers [146]. Low oxygen tensions combined with the high activation energy of O_2 with singlet-state biomolecules protects the sensitive cellular components from spontaneously oxidizing in respiration.

Generation of Singlet Oxygen

The high-energy, singlet excited state of molecular oxygen [formed either by photosensitization (4.8) and (4.9) or chemical reactions (4.10)–(4.12)] and the various partially reduced states of oxygen (e.g., O_2^{1-}, H_2O_2, $HO^{\bullet}$) are either directly or indirectly the oxidants responsible for the indiscriminant and damaging reactions associated with oxidative stress. *In vivo* singlet oxygen is also chemically produced by myeloperoxidase and chloroperoxidases via the generation of hypochlorite [147].

$$\text{Sens} \xrightarrow{h\nu} \text{Sens}^* \tag{4.8}$$

$$\text{Sens}^* + {}^3O_2 \rightarrow \text{Sens} + {}^1O_2 \quad k \cong 10^9\,\text{M}^{-1}\text{s}^{-1} \quad \text{Photosensitization} \tag{4.9}$$

$$^{\bullet}OH + O_2^{1-} \rightarrow {}^1O_2 + OH^{1-} \tag{4.10}$$

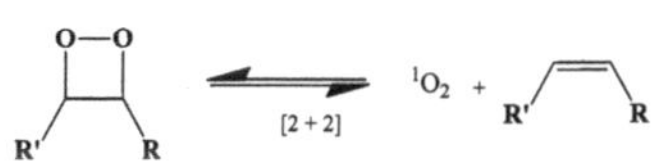

Decomposition of 1,2-endoperoxides (4.11)

$$H_2O_2 + OCl^- \rightarrow {}^1O_2 + H_2O + Cl^- \tag{4.12}$$

The potential for reaction of the activated intermediates formed from oxygen within biological systems is significant but varies with the nature of the intermediate/ROS. Singlet oxygen is able to react with biomolecules by several mechanisms [113, 148]. The most important of these lead to lipid peroxides by the addition to the double bonds of unsaturated fatty acids (Scheme 4.1a), or aldehydes, and ketones (Scheme 4.1c, d).

The unique environmental stress resulting from light and oxygen sets the stage for $^1O_2$ generation (4.9). These conditions are characteristic of leaves in plants, as well as the skin and eyes of animals. Unique adaptations protect these tissues from the photochemically initiated damage associated with singlet oxygen. The xanthophylls present within the light harvesting proteins of the chloroplast, the macular xanthophylls present within the inner retinal layers of primates including humans, and carotenes accumulated in the deep layers of the dermis function in exactly this manner [87, 111, 114, 137, 138, 149, 150].

Generation of Reactive Forms of Oxygen by Reduction

The reduction of molecular oxygen by the sequential transfer of electrons during oxidative metabolism produces the intermediate, low-valent oxygen species, superoxide, and peroxide, leading to the

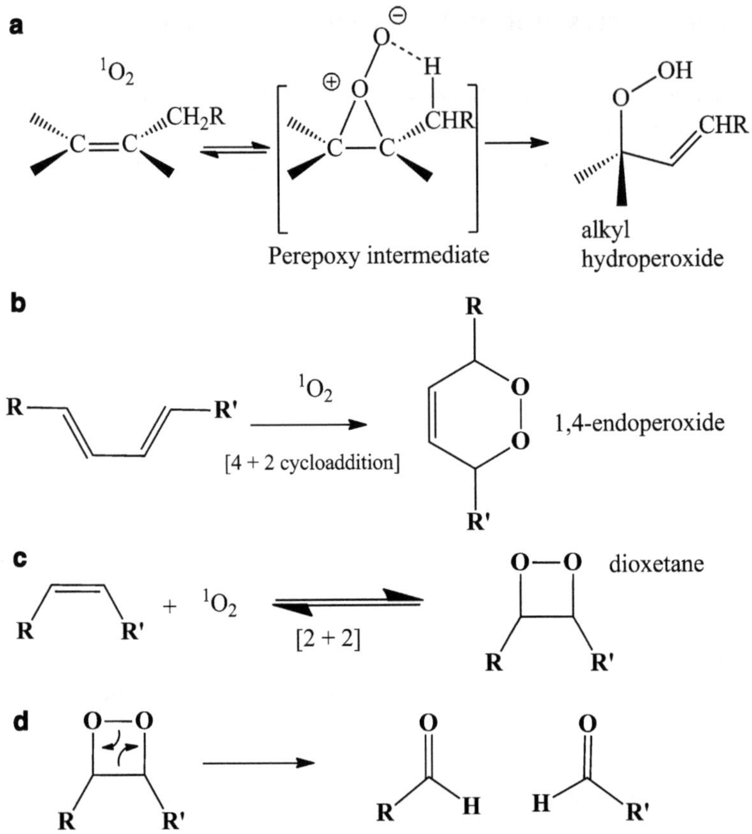

Scheme 4.1 Reactions of singlet oxygen

formation of hydroxyl radicals. Reduction of oxygen occurs extensively within mitochondria by reaction with NADPH oxidase and also within the cytosol with xanthine oxidase (4.13) [12, 151–153].

$$^3O_2 \xrightarrow{e^-\text{(NADPH Oxidase)}} O_2^{\bullet-} \tag{4.13}$$

Superoxide undergoes dismutation, a thermodynamically favorable ($K_{eq}=4\times10^{20}$ at pH=7) self-oxidation-reduction to generate hydrogen peroxide and oxygen. The reaction rate for the dismutation reaction in the absence of catalyst is slow, (4.14) [154].

$$2O_2^{\bullet-} + 2H_2O \rightleftharpoons O_2 + HO_2^- + OH^- \quad k \le 0.3\,M^{-1}s^{-1} \text{ Dismutation of Superoxide} \tag{4.14}$$

Because superoxide is a weak base, its protonation can produce small amounts of neutral, hydrogen dioxide, (4.15) [154]. As indicated by the pK_a, the equilibrium at physiological pH lies heavily toward the superoxide ion with $\frac{[O_2^-]}{[HO_2]} \cong \frac{320}{1}$.

$$O_2^{\bullet-} + H^+ \rightleftharpoons HO_2^{\bullet} \quad pKa_{HO_2^{\bullet}} = 4.7 \tag{4.15}$$

Bimolecular dismutation of superoxide and its neutral conjugate acid, $HO_2^{\bullet}$, is rapid (4.16), [154], and would be a major reaction process of superoxide if the enzyme, superoxide dismutase (SOD), was not abundant. Formation of hydrogen dioxide is not significant to the transport of superoxide as a neutral component across membranes.

$$O_2^{\bullet -} + HO_2^{\bullet} \rightleftharpoons O_2 + HO_2^{-} \quad k = 1\times10^{8}\,M^{-1}s^{-1} \tag{4.16}$$

The importance of controlling superoxide *in vivo* is demonstrated by the ubiquitous presence of SOD, which catalyzes the dismutation of superoxide anions at a diffusion limited rate, (4.17).

$$2O_2^{\bullet -} + 2H^{+} \xrightarrow{SOD} H_2O_2 + O_2 \quad k = \sim 10^{10}\,M^{-1}s^{-1} \tag{4.17}$$

In addition to producing hydrogen peroxide, superoxide reacts rapidly with either free Fe^{3+} reducing it to Fe^{2+}, (4.18a), or free Cu^{2+} to form Cu^{1+}, (4.18b). The oxygen product formed by the superoxide reduction of transition metal ions can be singlet oxygen [154].

$$O_2^{\bullet -} + Fe^{3+} \rightarrow Fe^{2+} + {}^{1}O_2 \quad k = 10^{6}\,M^{-1}s^{-1} \tag{4.18a}$$

$$O_2^{\bullet -} + Cu^{2+} \rightarrow Cu^{1+} + {}^{1}O_2 \tag{4.18b}$$

The monohydrogen peroxide as produced in (4.16) is a fairly strong base and will fully protonate immediately upon generation *in vivo* (4.19).

$$HO_2^{1-} + H^{+} \rightleftharpoons H_2O_2 \quad pKa_{H_2O_2} = 11.96 \quad \text{Protonation of Monohydrogen Peroxide} \tag{4.19}$$

Cupric or ferric ions acting as a Lewis acid can catalyze the dismutation of superoxide by a mechanism that may involve direct coordination of one molecule of superoxide, which is then activated for reduction by a second superoxide molecule (4.20a) and (4.20b) [154].

$$2O_2^{\bullet -} + 2H_2O \xrightarrow{Fe^{3+}} O_2 + H_2O_2 + 2OH^{-} \tag{4.20a}$$

$$2O_2^{\bullet -} + 2H_2O \xrightarrow{Cu^{2+}} O_2 + H_2O_2 + 2OH^{-} \tag{4.20b}$$

The hydrogen peroxide formed by dismutation of superoxide is able to participate in an Fe^{2+}-catalyzed disproportionation that generates singlet oxygen (4.21) [154]. Catalase functions by a similar stoichiometry to (4.21). Homolysis of the peroxide bond, (4.22), is able to generate hydroxyl radicals, but it is a relatively slow reaction in the absence of a catalyst.

$$2H_2O_2 \xrightarrow{Fe^{2+}\text{ or Catalase}} 2H_2O + O_2 \tag{4.21}$$

$$H_2O_2 \rightarrow 2HO^{\bullet} \quad \text{Homolysis of the peroxide bond} \tag{4.22}$$

In the presence of cuprous or ferrous ions, the Fenton reaction can generate hydroxyl radicals (4.23a) and (4.23b).

$$H_2O_2 + Cu^{1+} \rightarrow Cu^{2+} + OH^{-} + HO^{\bullet} \quad \text{Copper Catalyzed Fenton Reaction} \tag{4.23a}$$

$$H_2O_2 + Fe^{2+} \rightarrow Fe^{3+} + OH^{-} + HO^{\bullet} \quad k = 10^{3} - 10^{6}\,M^{-1}s^{-1} \quad \text{Iron Catalyzed Fenton Reaction} \tag{4.23b}$$

Cuprous ion has a larger rate constant than ferrous ion for catalytic decomposition of H_2O_2 to form hydroxyl radical. Generally, both free iron and copper ion concentrations are low under physiological conditions. For iron this is thought to be ~10^{-9} M [155–158]. Hypohalous acid is generated in peroxisomes within macrophages by myeloperoxidase (4.24) [159, 160]. Highly reactive hydroxyl radical is principally generated *in vivo* as a consequence of hydrogen peroxide and hypohalous acid via the Fenton reaction (4.23a) and (4.23b) and (4.25) [161]. The levels of iron and copper ions rise as a result of excessive proteolytic degradation of metalloproteins during oxidative stress [162]. Catalase intercepts hydrogen peroxide reducing hydroxyl radical production and the subsequent oxidative stress. Knockout mice lacking catalase develop normally but are sensitive to oxidative stress in specific tissues due to an inability to deactivate hydrogen peroxide [163]. Hydroxyl radical and singlet oxygen are formed rapidly during respiratory burst in phagocytosis by neutrophils and macrophages by reaction of superoxide with hypochlorous acid (4.25) [162]. Antibacterial activity has been attributed to hypothiocyanous acid formed in a reaction similar to (4.24) from thiocyanate anion, which is present in significant levels (mM) in saliva and may be a source of hydroxyl radicals [162].

$$H_2O_2 + Cl^- \rightarrow HOCl + H_2O \quad \text{Myeloperoxidase in macrophages} \tag{4.24}$$

$$O_2^{\bullet-} + HOCl \rightleftharpoons {}^1O_2 + Cl^- + HO^{\bullet} \quad k \sim 8\times10^6 \tag{4.25}$$

A primary reaction of hydroxyl radical is the initiation of peroxidation by abstraction of hydrogen, (4.26), forming an alkyl radical. The pro-oxidative chain propagation reaction steps, (4.27a) and (4.27b), result in the formation alkyl peroxides. Rates of hydroxyl reactions are diffusion-limited, $k \sim 10^9$–10^{10} [164].

$$R-H + HO^{\bullet} \rightarrow R^{\bullet} + H_2O \quad \text{Initiation} \tag{4.26}$$

$$R^{\bullet} + O_2 \rightarrow RO_2^{\bullet} \quad \text{Propagation 1} \tag{4.27a}$$

$$RO_2^{\bullet} + R-H \rightarrow RO_2H + R^{\bullet} \quad \text{Propagation 2} \tag{4.27b}$$

The often-mentioned Haber-Weiss reaction is not a significant source of hydroxyl radical *in vivo*. This reaction involves an electron transfer from superoxide to hydrogen peroxide, (4.28), and is too sluggish to compete with the rapid reaction of superoxide through other pathways [162, 165].

$$O_2^{\bullet-} + H_2O_2 \rightleftharpoons O_2 + HO^- + HO^{\bullet} \quad \text{slow, insignificant physiologically} \quad k \sim 0.41\ \text{mol}^{-1}\text{s}^{-1} \tag{4.28}$$

Although important and informative, this series of reactions of oxygen species fails to place these actors clearly on their stage, in play with a supporting cast and script, i.e., within cells and organelles at critical and specific times during cellular processes. The identities of participating enzymes, their localization within (or outside of) the cell, and the timing of the events associated with ROS generation (and deactivation) are fundamental to understanding the need for specific antioxidants and the importance of the physicochemical properties that underlie their ability to provide protection. Different ROS vary in their sites of generation, reactivity, and polarity, which necessitate cellular control mechanisms that include different antioxidants.

Generation of Reactive Forms of Nitrogen

Nitric oxide is an important signal molecule in smooth muscle as well as other physiological processes. It is formed by the oxidation of the L-arginine guanidium group [166]. Many RNS are formed as a consequence of reactions between oxygen radicals, particularly superoxide, with nitric oxide. Peroxynitrite is produced by a diffusion-controlled reaction of superoxide and nitric oxide (4.29) [108]. Few cellular reactions can compete for superoxide in the presence of nitric oxide. Peroxynitrite participates in several important reactions that lead to the production of additional RNS and free radicals. The rapid reaction of peroxynitrite with carbon dioxide at physiological levels (ca. 1 mM) produces the unstable nitrosoperoxocarboxylate anion (I), which readily decomposes to carbonate anion radical and nitrogen dioxide (4.30) [35]. The production of hydroxyl radical requires a disfavored protonation of peroxynitrite ion followed by (relatively slow) homolysis (4.31) and (4.32). The carbonate anion radical and nitrogen dioxide are both involved in the steps of protein nitration.

$$^{\bullet}NO + O_2^{\bullet-} \rightarrow ONOO^{1-} \quad k = 6.9 \times 10^9\,M^{-1}s^{-1} \quad \text{Formation of Peroxynitrite} \tag{4.29}$$

$$ONOO^{1-} + CO_2 \rightarrow [ONOO-CO_2^-, I] \rightarrow {}^{\bullet}CO_3^- + {}^{\bullet}NO_2 \quad k = 5.8 \times 10^4\,M^{-1}s^{-1} \tag{4.30}$$

The peroxynitrite anion is a weak base and its conjugate acid, hydrogen peroxynitrite has a pK_a of 5.9. Hence, at physiological pH the ratio of the peroxynitrite anion to its conjugate acid is near 20:1. Peroxynitrite exists predominantly as the *cis*-isomer; the conjugate acids of the isomers exhibit different pK_a values, with the *trans* form being weaker. Its pK_a is about 8; therefore, its protonated form will dominate by 10:1 at physiological pH [164]. Homolysis of hydrogen peroxynitrite, (4.32), leads to generation of hydroxyl radical and nitrogen dioxide, but it is slow and a small contributor to hydroxyl radical production [167].

$$ONOO^{1-} + H^+ \rightarrow HOONO \quad pKa_{HOONO} = 5.9 \tag{4.31}$$

$$HOONO \rightarrow HO^{\bullet} + {}^{\bullet}NO_2 \quad \text{Homolysis of Peroxynitrite O} - \text{O bond} \tag{4.32}$$

Singlet oxygen is formed by nitrogen dioxide directly accepting an electron from superoxide, (4.33), or a reaction of superoxide and $^{\bullet}NO_2$ forming peroxynitrate, (4.34), which decomposes to nitrite anion and singlet oxygen (4.35).

$$O_2^{\bullet-} + {}^{\bullet}NO_2 \rightarrow NO_2^- + {}^1O_2 \tag{4.33}$$

$$O_2^{\bullet-} + {}^{\bullet}NO_2 \rightarrow O_2NOO^{1-} \quad \text{Formation of Peroxynitrate} \tag{4.34}$$

$$O_2NOO^{1-} \rightarrow NO_2^- + {}^1O_2 \quad \text{Peroxynitrate decomposition} \tag{4.35}$$

Instead of direct decomposition, the intermediate nitrosoperoxocarboxylate anion, I, (see (4.30)) can rearrange as shown in (4.36). The rearrangement product, II, is a potent nitrating agent similar in its reactivity to acyl nitrates (4.37) [168]. Nitrogen dioxide produced by peroxynitrite decomposition can abstract H from tyrosine OH as shown in (4.38).

$$[ONOO-CO_2^-, I] \xrightarrow{\text{rearrangement}} [O_2NO-CO_2^-, II] \tag{4.36}$$

$$R-H + [O_2NO-CO_2^-\ II] \rightarrow R-NO_2 + HCO_3^{1-} \tag{4.37}$$

$$^{\bullet}NO_2 + AR-OH \rightarrow AR-O^{\bullet} + HONO \quad \text{Hydrogen Abstraction} \tag{4.38}$$

The specific oxidants that are produced in natural systems vary markedly among tissues owing to differences in the physical, chemical, and physiological stresses present. Skin and eyes are exposed to high levels of light and oxygen that can lead to the efficient and direct photogeneration of singlet oxygen. By contrast, lung tissue is exposed to high concentrations of oxygen (as well as numerous environmental oxidants, such as components in smoke), but in the absence of light, oxidative stress is initiated by mechanisms that do not include photosensitization of O_2 [169]. The consequence is that the proportions of the specific ROS will vary and the subcellular sites of generation will also be different. Mitochondrial dysfunction and presence of macrophages are notable sources of ROS and oxidative stress [37, 74, 170]. The natural presence of resident or "fixed" macrophages (i.e., neutrophils) that serve "house-keeping" functions within tissues, phagocytosing bacteria, debris, and necrotic tissue, provide a mechanism for chemical generation of singlet oxygen (4.10)–(4.12), (4.18a), (4.18b), (4.21), and (4.25), superoxide (4.13), peroxide, alkyl peroxides (4.16), (4.17), and (4.20), and peroxynitrite (4.29). Importantly, neutrophil-generated radicals will be released within the intercellular space.

Table 4.3 Estimates of half-lives for prominent reactive oxygen species

Reactive oxygen species	Half-life	Diffusion distance
Hydroxyl radical [34, 172]	1×10^{-9} s	40–50 Å [34], 93 Å [172]
Alkoxyl radical ($RO^{\bullet}$) [34]	1×10^{-6} s	
Singlet oxygen ($^1O_2$) [34]	1×10^{-6} s	
Peroxynitrite ($ONOO^{1-}$)	0.05–1 s	
Nitric oxide ($NO^{\bullet}$) [35, 173]	0.002–10 s	~1 mm
Nitrogen dioxide ($^{\bullet}NO_2$) [174]	10 μs	
Carbonate anion radical ($CO_3^{\bullet-}$) [175]	1,500 ms	
Peroxyl radical ($ROO^{\bullet}$) [34]	~7 s	
Alkyl and hydroperoxides (ROOH) [176]	~4 min	
Superoxide (O_2^{1-}) [177]	Seconds–minutes	
Seminquinone radical anion ($Q^{1-\bullet}$) [34, 178, 179]	Days, 50–200 μs [178]	0.6 μm
Carotenoid cation radical ($Car^{+\bullet}$) [180]	~200 s	
β-Carotene cation radical (β-$Car^{+\bullet}$) [181]	1.4–14 min.	

The existence of cellular processes shared by different cell types and tissues argue that common antioxidant mechanisms must also be important. The universal presence of SOD, at concentrations of 10^{-6} to 10^{-7} M, existentially supports this line of reasoning [108]. Understanding the fundamental character of each ROS, its mechanisms of generation, and reactions can provide insight into the genesis of oxidative stress in dissimilar tissues and when common or unique mechanisms may be operative. Among the important distinguishing properties of oxidant species is their reactive half-lives, which provides both a measure of their reactivity and an estimate of the distance they can diffuse from their point of generation prior to reaction. The polarity of a ROS and its site of generation combined with the half-life provide limits that define which cellular components and structures will be imperiled by its production [171, 172]. Table 4.3 summarizes estimates for prominent ROS half-lives and some diffusion distances.

Identifying the mechanism(s) of ROS formation and their interaction with antioxidants that are physiologically abundant provide the basis to distinguish which are significant to specific organelles, cell types, or tissues. *In vitro* data that demonstrate an antioxidant can mechanistically react or deactivate a specific oxidant do not establish its significance to the physiological well-being of an organism and it may be hard to do so convincingly even with controlled clinical studies. Many species are effective as antioxidants *in vitro* but simply may not be properly localized, present insufficiently high concentrations, or be too rapidly depleted to play a meaningful role *in vivo*. Depletion of an antioxidant or knockout of antioxidant enzyme systems are not generally possible to observe in humans (except when they occur as spontaneous genetic defects).

Properties of Individual ROS

Singlet Oxygen

As described earlier, molecular dioxygen is sensitized by interaction with the triplet excited states of chromophores generated by the absorption of visible or UV light (4.8) and (4.9). The steps of this process are illustrated by Scheme 4.2, showing the role carotenoids may play in quenching.

Examples of some typical photosensitizers include natural heme, chlorophylls, riboflavin, tryptophan, components of lipofuscin [182–184], bilirubin, and other conjugated chromophores, all of which absorb light in the blue to UV [97, 113, 148, 185]. (For a comprehensive review of biological sensitizers of oxygen see [185].)

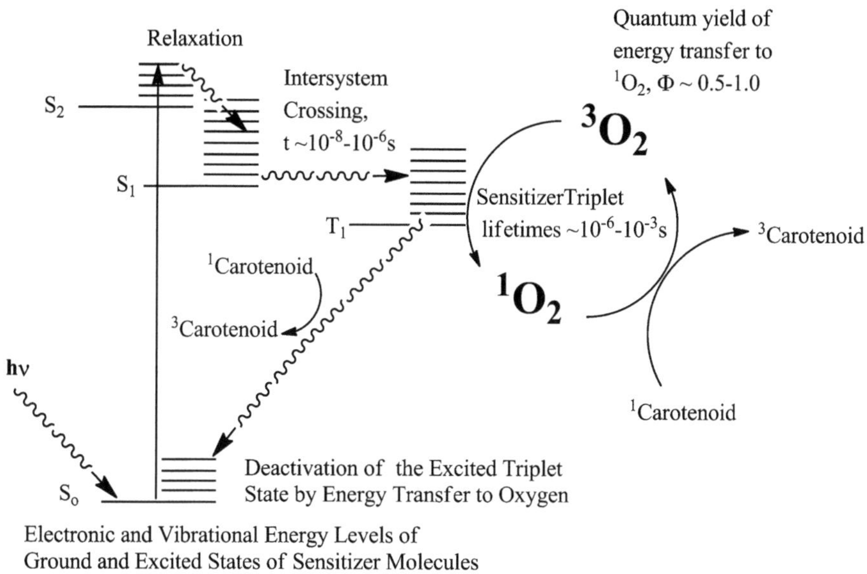

Scheme 4.2

Ground-state oxygen would react exothermically with virtually all biological molecules but the high activation energy required for initiation slows these reactions to nearly imperceptible rates. Oxygen exists in a triplet ground-state having two unpaired electrons, whereas biological molecules exist in a singlet ground-state with no unpaired electrons. Reactions that produce a net change in the spin-state of the system are quantum mechanically forbidden [186]. Singlet oxygen is generated in many biological systems by the action of light and this process is the most widely recognized source of this reactive, excited state, $^1O_2$ ($^1\Delta_g$), which is an activated form that behaves chemically as an electrophile but is *not* a free radical. $^1O_2$ can also be produced by chemical reactions including oxidation of superoxide and decomposition of peroxynitrite and peroxynitrate, see (4.10)–(4.12), (4.18a), (4.18b), (4.21), (4.25), (4.33), and (4.35) [187–191]. The reaction between O_2^- and H_2O_2, often referred to as the Haber-Weiss reaction (4.28), has been advocated as a source of $^1O_2$ but the rate of this process is too slow to be competitive relative to alternative reactions of O_2^{1-} and H_2O_2 *in vivo* [165]. Singlet oxygen may be a major component among the toxic species generated by chemical steps in phagocytosis [187]. Reactions of $^1O_2$ with singlet-state organic alkenes, particularly unsaturated lipids such as arachidonic acid, are rapid and fully spin-allowed. The energy difference between the ground-state and singlet excited state of oxygen is 94 kJ mol^{-1} (22.4 kcal mol^{-1}) [113].

Light having wavelengths shorter than 1,276 nm (near IR) provides sufficient energy to produce singlet oxygen from its ground-state but direct absorption of light by the oxygen triplet ground-state to produce $^1O_2$ does not occur efficiently. The difference in the ground and excited spin-states makes the process spin-forbidden. The combination of the added potential energy in the singlet oxygen moiety and the energy associated with the C–O bond formation confers on $^1O_2$ the ability to behave in a pernicious fashion within the cell. Carbon–oxygen bond energies are around 90 kcal mol^{-1}. It is significant that light in the visible or even near UV lacks sufficient energy to fully break covalent chemical bonds, which have bond energies of 80–100 kcal mol^{-1}. Rates of singlet oxygen reactions with unsaturated fatty acids range from 1,000 to 30,000 times faster than those with ground-state triplet oxygen [148, 192].

Triplet excited state sensitizers activate oxygen by direct transfer of energy, (4.9), producing $^1O_2$ by a rapid, efficient, and fully spin-allowed process. Heme proteins, as well as other photosensitizers, are distributed widely in membranes and the aqueous compartment of the cell. Free heme, produced by the degradation of myoglobin and hemoglobin, can be an important sensitizer and source of singlet oxygen. Rarely, genetic defects such as that which causes *erythropoietic protoporphyria* can result in accumulation of large quantities of free heme within the dermis leading to the generation of pathological levels of $^1O_2$ and an extreme sensitivity to light [116, 119]. As already noted, chemical generation of singlet oxygen is also an important process. Reaction C in Scheme 4.1 is a reversible process *in vitro* and thermal decomposition of synthetic dioxetanes is a convenient method used to study the efficiency of singlet oxygen quenchers or the reactions of singlet oxygen *in vitro* [148]. Biochemical generation of $^1O_2$ is dependent on processes that are associated with high O_2^- levels and formation of peroxynitrite. These conditions are most commonly encountered in mitochondria, peroxisomes, and macrophages.

The question of whether direct enzymatic action generates appreciable quantities of singlet oxygen remains incompletely answered. A recent report describes electron paramagnetic resonance (EPR) evidence using spin-traps for singlet oxygen that $^1O_2$ is generated during the p450 hydroxylation in rat liver microsomes [193]. Kerver et al. reported evidence of singlet oxygen generation in rat liver and small intestine mitochondria and concluded that a non-enzymatic dismutation reaction, see (4.20a), was the most probable source [194].

Superoxide, Peroxide, Hydroxyl Radical, and Peroxynitrite

Superoxide ($t_{1/2}$ ~ Seconds–Minutes)

Superoxide is generated directly and efficiently *in vivo* by a 1 e^- reduction of molecular oxygen and is a free radical. In neutrophils, superoxide is generated by NADPH oxidase and is concentrated within phagosomes (4.13). Xanthine oxidase is an abundant enzyme present within blood where its role in the production of superoxide has been associated with ischemia/reperfusion injury [195, 196]. Secondary ROS that form from superoxide include singlet oxygen, H_2O_2, peroxynitrite, hypohalites (HOX, X = Cl, Br, SCN), and hydroxyl radical [5, 26, 40, 113, 148, 167, 197]. These secondary ROS, in combination with superoxide, give rise to the effective toxic reactions responsible for bacterial cell death during respiratory burst following phagocytosis [21, 198, 199].

Mitochondrial Versus Cytosolic Superoxide

Estimates indicate that as much as 5 % of all oxygen molecules entering the terminal step of mitochondrial electron transport are released as superoxide ions [11, 200]. The rate of superoxide generation increases at elevated oxygen concentrations; however, in certain types of smooth muscle, hypoxia may also induce greater production of superoxide and ROS [152]. Production of superoxide occurs normally in many tissues, e.g., smooth muscle, cornea epithelium. Xanthine oxidase, a superoxide generator associated with tissues where oxidative stress is involved in pathogenesis [63, 201], is found in the cytosol and incorporated into milk fat as a source of superoxide and peroxide. Cytosolic xanthine oxidase activation may precede mitochondrial dysfunction [202, 203]. Loss of integrity in the mitochondrial outer membrane caused by cytosolic ROS may be equally or more important than mitochondrial ROS generation to the dysfunction of mitochondria. There is some dispute of whether mitochondria are the principal source of ROS within the cell [7, 204].

In reperfusion of cardiac tissue following ischemia, mitochondrial dysfunction and reduction of O_2 by complex I is accepted as a major component of ROS production [170]. Oxidation of the purine base, guanosine, within mitochondria, producing 8-hydroxyguanosine, occurs at a rate 10,000 times greater than within the nucleus where oxidative phosphorylation does not occur [205]. Reaction between molecular oxygen and complex I (NADH dehydrogenase and its associated iron-sulfur cluster, N2), has been argued to be the source of superoxide [76, 206, 207] but recent research suggests that hydrogen peroxide is the likely product formed by reaction of O_2 with complex I and that superoxide is a product of other enzyme systems [153]. A recent review discusses the role of different sites of superoxide production [12]. A significant concern in the production of superoxide by the mitochondrial enzyme system is the topological question of whether superoxide is released on the inner side of the mitochondrial membrane or on the outer side and into the cytosol [14]. The nuclear transcription factor NrF2, which activates the nuclear transcription of phase II antioxidants via the antioxidant response element (ARE), is strategically positioned on the mitochondrial outer membrane where it is able to be an early sensor of mitochondrial ROS escape [208]. Superoxide dismutase produces hydrogen peroxide and oxygen from superoxide, (4.17). Because of the abundant expression of SOD, hydrogen peroxide is rapidly produced from superoxide resulting in an "entangling" of the effects associated with these two ROS. Oxidative stress attributed to O_2^- production is often the result of its subsequent conversion to secondary products (i.e., H_2O_2 and ONO_2^-), the reactivity associated with these species, and their derived radicals.

Although superoxide is generated in the largest quantities within mitochondria, three different forms of SOD are expressed in high levels in erythrocytes and cytosol (SOD1), mitochondria (SOD2), and the extracellular medium (SOD3) [209–211]. Cytosolic SOD1 and the extracellular SOD3 are characterized by the requirement for the transition metal ions Cu^{1+} and Zn^{2+}, whereas mitochondrial SOD2 is an Mn^{2+} metalloprotein [212]. SOD2 is transcribed by the mitochondrial DNA, whereas the other two are coded by nuclear DNA. Under normal conditions, cytosolic superoxide is generated by NADPH dependent oxidases or xanthine oxidase [57], which catalyzes the catabolic breakdown of xanthine to uric acid in the liver and is implicated in superoxide production [213]. Xanthine oxidase is found in retina, corneal epithelium, skin, milk fat, kidney and other tissues [53, 63, 64, 201, 213–216].

Dismutation of superoxide (4.17) is a highly favorable reaction having an equilibrium constant on the order of 10^{20} [154]. The rate of the uncatalyzed reaction is rapid (4.16) but because it is second order, the half-life is hundredths of seconds at mM concentrations and increases to hours at nM concentrations. The SOD-catalyzed reaction has a reported rate constant of $\sim 7 \times 10^9\ M^{-1}\,s^{-1}$ and is among the fastest of all enzymatic processes, limited only by the collision frequency [217]. Because its half-life can be long at low concentrations, in the range of seconds to minutes, superoxide has the potential to act at points that are remote from its place of production. This half-life makes its function as a signaling molecule possible. It can pass through channels in biological membranes, particularly damaged membranes [218]. Dismutation of superoxide will generate hydrogen peroxide with its attendant oxidative reactivity and an ability to generate hydroxyl radicals. Catalase protects against formation of hydroxyl radical from H_2O_2. Although it is reported in the literature that peroxide oxidizes superoxide to produce singlet oxygen and hydroxyl radical in the Haber-Weiss reaction, (4.28), measurements of the reaction rate demonstrate that it cannot compete with the rate of O_2^- reaction with SOD or nitric oxide under *in vivo* conditions [165, 187]. When $^{\bullet}NO$ is present, superoxide reacts at diffusion-controlled rates, generating peroxynitrite.

Superoxide is a good reducing agent with a comparable strength to that of dithionite, $E^{\circ\prime} = -0.6$ v. In aqueous environments, superoxide's properties arise from its rapid dismutation to form peroxide, which is a strong oxidant [154]. The protonation of superoxide produces the uncharged hydrogen dioxide radical ($HO_2^{\bullet}$, pK_a near 4.7), the conjugate weak acid of superoxide, (4.15). The protonation of superoxide may be of real importance to biological systems [219]. At physiological pH, this neutral form of superoxide would represent about 0.4 % of the total superoxide. Although a small percentage, long-lived neutral $HO_2^{\bullet}$ might be vastly more soluble in membranes and readily diffuse through and across membranes, but evidence is limited. Within lysozomes, where the physiological pH is approximately 5, $HO_2^{\bullet}$ would represent almost 40 % of superoxide. The ability for lysosomal production of superoxide has been reported in the vacuoles of hemocytes of mollusks, renal LLC-PK1 cells treated with gentamicin, and in the hippocampal neuronal cell line, HT22 [220–222]. An electron spin resonance study demonstrated that superoxide can cross natural biological plasma membranes prepared from erythrocyte ghosts but not those prepared from egg-derived phosphatidylcholine [218]. Diffusion of superoxide across membrane boundaries is not sufficiently enhanced by the formation of neutral $HO_2^{\bullet}$ radical at normal cellular pH to be able to be detectable in pure synthetic membranes.

Hydrogen Peroxide ($t_{1/2}$ ~ 4 min)

Hydrogen peroxide, a potent oxidant, is produced by the rapid dismutation of superoxide and is a substrate for many enzymatic systems including the glutathione peroxidases, cytochrome c peroxidases, catalases, haloperoxidases, thyroid peroxidase, lactoperoxidase, prostaglandin H synthase (COX), and myeloperoxidases [6, 78, 197, 223–227]. Hydrogen peroxide is an important signaling molecule associated with NF-κB and mitogen-activated protein (MAP) kinase pathways [223]. Its long lifetime (~4 min) and neutrality enable it to be an effective intercellular signal [176]. Hydrogen peroxide itself reacts relatively slowly with substrates but is readily activated by the transition metal ion-catalyzed Fenton reaction, involving either iron (II) or copper (I), (4.23a) and (4.23b), to produce the extremely reactive hydroxyl radical, (•OH) [157, 167, 228, 229]. Peroxidases produce a range of potent oxidizers from H_2O_2. A prime example is formation of hypochlorite by neutrophils during respiratory burst [230]. Because hydrogen peroxide readily diffuses through membranes and many membrane lipids are unsaturated, they are readily susceptible to oxidation by hydroxyl radical [231]. The chain reaction of hydroxyl radical with lipids can generate large numbers of lipid hydroperoxides within cell membranes, (4.26)–(4.27b), disrupting properties and functions [231]. COX activity is triggered by the action of peroxide and results in prostaglandin production [78].

Peroxy Radical, ROO• ($t_{1/2}$ = ~7 s)

Lipid hydroperoxy radicals are generated by reaction of a lipid carbon free radical with oxygen, (4.7) and (4.27a). Although these alkyl peroxy radicals are more stable than the hydroxyl radical, they may react by abstracting H from additional lipids, (4.27b), electron transfer from abundant reducing agents (*Red*), such as glutathione or ascorbate, producing the alkyl peroxide, (4.39), and direct addition reactions with alkenes (4.40).

$$LOO^{\bullet} + Red \rightarrow LOO^{-} + Ox \tag{4.39}$$

$$LOO^{\bullet} + H_2C = CH - R \rightarrow LOO - CH_2 - {}^{\bullet}CHR \tag{4.40}$$

Hydroxyl Radical ($t_{1/2}$ = 1 × 10^{-8} s)

Once generated, the hydroxyl radical has a lifetime on the order of 10 ns in the aqueous cellular environment and its ability to diffuse through cellular media is limited to about 60 Å, approximately the width of a bilipid membrane [172]. The extremely reactive nature of the hydroxyl radical is due to the

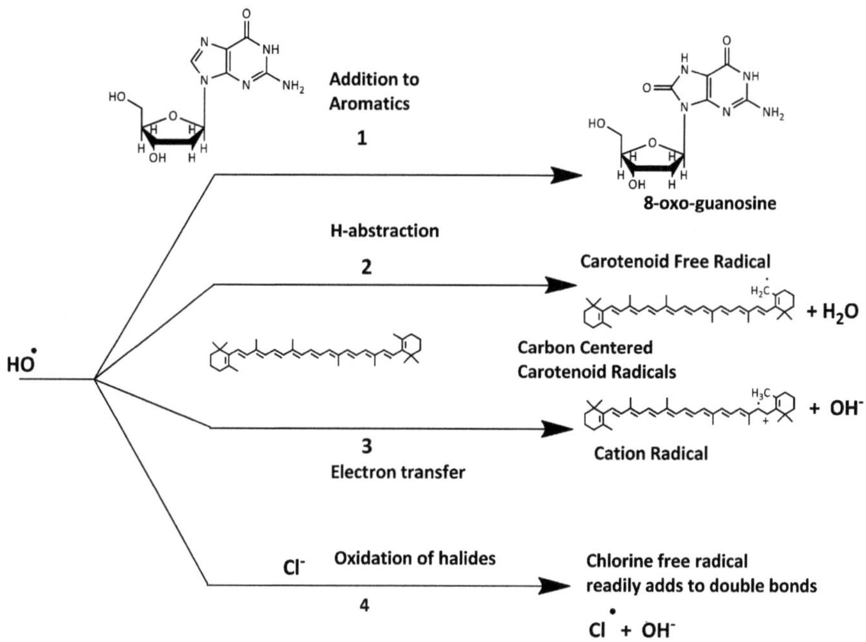

Scheme 4.3

favorability of the processes in which it participates. The primary diffusion-controlled reactive options for hydroxyl radical are: (1) hydrogen abstraction; (2) addition to aromatic rings, including purines and pyrimidines in DNA; and (3) oxidation of a variety of abundant species including halide ions, carotenoids, and other antioxidants (Scheme 4.3) [232]. Hydroxyl radical can also react with protein, lipid, and carbohydrates via similar processes.

Abstraction of a hydrogen from a carotenoid produces a carbon-centered radical that can be much longer lived than the hydroxyl radical [180, 181, 233]. Lifetimes of carbon-centered free radicals vary over a wide range and resonance in aromatic and conjugated radicals is an important contributor to stability. The ability of these alkyl radicals to diffuse from their point of generation and react with ground-state molecular oxygen to produce peroxy radicals (4.7) poses a threat to cellular systems that are otherwise relatively remote from active oxygen metabolism [234, 235]. The carotenoid radical is not sufficiently reactive to add oxygen at physiological partial pressures and thus disrupts the pro-oxidative mechanism [236]. Chlorine radicals may be generated by direct reaction of Cl^- with $HO^•$, (4.41), and may generate new carbon free radicals by addition to double bonds or abstraction of a hydrogen atom [237–239].

$$HO^• + Cl^- \rightarrow Cl^• + OH^- \tag{4.41}$$

Nitric Oxide ($t_{1/2}$ = 0.002–10 s)

The path leading to the discovery that free radical nitric oxide is the endothelium-derived relaxing factor was laid by Furtchgott in 1980 and lead to a Nobel Prize in 1998 [35, 240–244]. Nitric oxide is generated from the oxidation of the L-arginine guanidium group by nitric oxide synthase [166]. Three isoforms of this enzyme are expressed: neuronal or nNOS (NOS1), endothelial or eNOS (NOS2), and inducible or iNOS (NOS3) [245]. The latter is inducible by ROS whereas the other two are constitutive. The iNOS form also appears to be expressed continuously in some cell types, airway epithelium, and basal skin keratinocytes [246]. Some pathogenic bacteria (gram positive) also express a nitric oxide synthase, which regulates bacterial SOD transcription and serves an important role in protection from phagocytosis and action of antibiotics, many of which result in production of high levels of ROS [247–249]. In *Staphylococcus aureus,* the presence of the yellow carotenoid pigment confers added virulence by protecting the bacteria from oxidative stress [250]. In humans, the generation of $^{\bullet}NO$ by the endothelial form, NOS3, is important for regulation of vascular dilation [251]. NOS1 and NOS3 can be inhibited by the oxidized cholesterol metabolite, secosterol aldehyde, which is produced under pathogenic conditions such as atherosclerosis, potentially compromising vascular function in the aging brain [252]. Nitric oxide also plays a critical role in cognitive function of the brain and the events involved in the formation of memory [253]. Although nitric oxide is a free radical, its reaction chemistry is surprisingly benign and it can be quite long-lived, as great as 10 s in tissues but lower, as short as 0.002 ms, in vascular medium where it rapidly reacts with oxyhemoglobin to form nitrate ion preventing it from traveling in the blood stream (4.42) [35]. $^{\bullet}NO$ is soluble in water as well as lipids and it diffuses readily through cell membranes to effectively act as a signal of local cellular status without influencing remote tissues by vascular transport.

$$^{\bullet}NO + HbO_2 \rightarrow NO_3^- + metHb \tag{4.42}$$

At ambient oxygen partial pressures, nitric oxide rapidly reduces molecular oxygen producing NO_2, a reactive secondary free radical, see (4.43) [254].

$$2^{\bullet}NO + O_2 \rightarrow 2^{\bullet}NO_2 \tag{4.43}$$

Nitrogen Dioxide ($t_{1/2}$ ~ 10 μs)

Nitrogen dioxide is capable of abstracting a hydrogen from phenols such as tyrosine leading to nitration, (4.38) [255], which can inactivate native enzymatic function and is a critical redox balance sensor. In the event of imbalanced radical production, formation of nitro-tyrosine can also be pathogenic [35].

Peroxynitrite ($t_{1/2}$ = 0.05–1 s)

Peroxynitrite, formed from superoxide ion and nitric oxide, (4.29) [256], owes its toxicity more to the formation of secondary ROS/RNS than to its direct action as an oxidizing agent [35, 255, 257]. As much as 50 % of the superoxide produced in the cell will react with $^{\bullet}NO$ to form peroxynitrite, [258], which may serve as a protective mechanism against the toxic consequences of superoxide and its by-products [34, 169, 255]. Peroxynitrite formation is extremely sensitive to the superoxide concentration, which is controlled by expression of SOD and sensitive to O_2 levels [35]. Under inflammatory conditions, concentrations of nitric oxide and superoxide can increase by nearly 1,000-fold and formation of peroxynitrite can be 1,000,000 times greater than under normal resting conditions [35].

As described earlier, peroxynitrite is a weak base and the protonated form slowly decomposes to produce hydroxyl radical and nitrogen dioxide, (4.31) and (4.32). In the presence of physiological levels of CO_2, ca. 1 mM, a diffusion-controlled reaction occurs between peroxynitrite and CO_2 leading to the production of the nitrating and oxidizing species, $^{\bullet}NO_2$ and $CO_3^{\bullet-}$, see (4.30) [255]. At physiological CO_2 levels, few biological molecules are able to compete with CO_2 to intercept peroxynitrite;

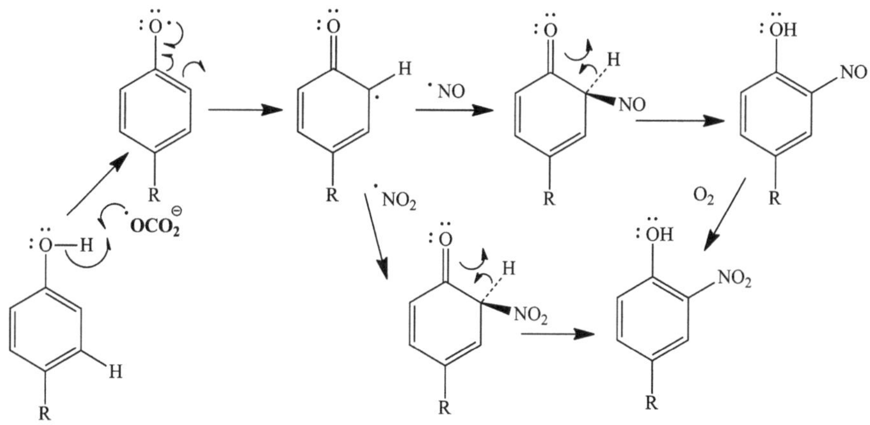

Scheme 4.4

thus, it reacts directly with a very limited number of biological molecules. $^{\bullet}NO_2$ and $CO_3^{\bullet-}$ are long-lived radicals, (1,500 ms $CO_3^{\bullet-}$; 10 μs for $^{\bullet}NO_2$) especially when compared to such species as the hydroxyl radical [255]. The carbonate anion radical is an oxy-radical that is resonance-stabilized. $CO_3^{\bullet-}$and $^{\bullet}NO_2$ can both behave as oxidants and react with substrates either by direct electron transfer or by abstraction of a hydrogen atom, particularly from phenolics. The nitration of tyrosine in the presence of CO_2 occurs with greater selectivity in product formation than in its absence, producing predominantly 3-nitro-tyrosine because $CO_3^{\bullet-}$ primarily reacts to abstract H and is less prone toward direct addition to the ring in contrast to $HO^{\bullet}$ [259]. Scheme 4.4 illustrates the mechanism of nitration of tyrosine by $^{\bullet}NO$ or $^{\bullet}NO_2$, where $^{\bullet}NO_2$ radical is also a nitrating agent. Oxygen transfer from the carbonate anion radical to guanine is also rapid and site-selective [260]. Nitration can be a step in signal transduction but may also be pathogenic [35]. Elevated concentrations of nitro-tyrosine have been identified and correlated with over 50 human diseases. Nitrosylation of tyrosine affects the pK_a of the phenolic OH and alters protein interactions and function [41, 261].

Carotenoid nitration occurs by a similar mechanistic process as seen in Scheme 4.5.

Carotenoids and ROS Regulation

Many types of ROS are widely generated within various organelles, cells, and tissues and carotenoids may be involved in ROS/RNS regulation. The unifying structural feature shared by carotenoids is the extended conjugation of the polyene chain (Fig. 4.2). Although carotenoids are often classified as provitamin A or non-provitamin A, an alternative grouping is based on the structural presence of oxygen functional groups on the ionone ring system, i.e., xanthophylls. Fucoxanthin and astaxanthin consumption and abundance are low but they are commercially significant and may have unique actions [123, 262–268]. Provitamin A carotenoids were recognized in the early part of the twentieth century [269, 270]. The significance of vitamin A to human health served as a motivating factor for much of the research directed toward understanding the chemistry of β-carotene and its structurally related provitamin A congenors during the twentieth century.

Seventy years passed between the discovery that β-carotene could be metabolized to produce vitamin A [270] and the characterization of the β, β-carotene-15,15′-monooxygenase (BCMO1) in mammals responsible for this reaction [142]. Reports suggesting critical or essential functions for the non-provitamin A carotenoids began to appear in the literature during the final two decades of the

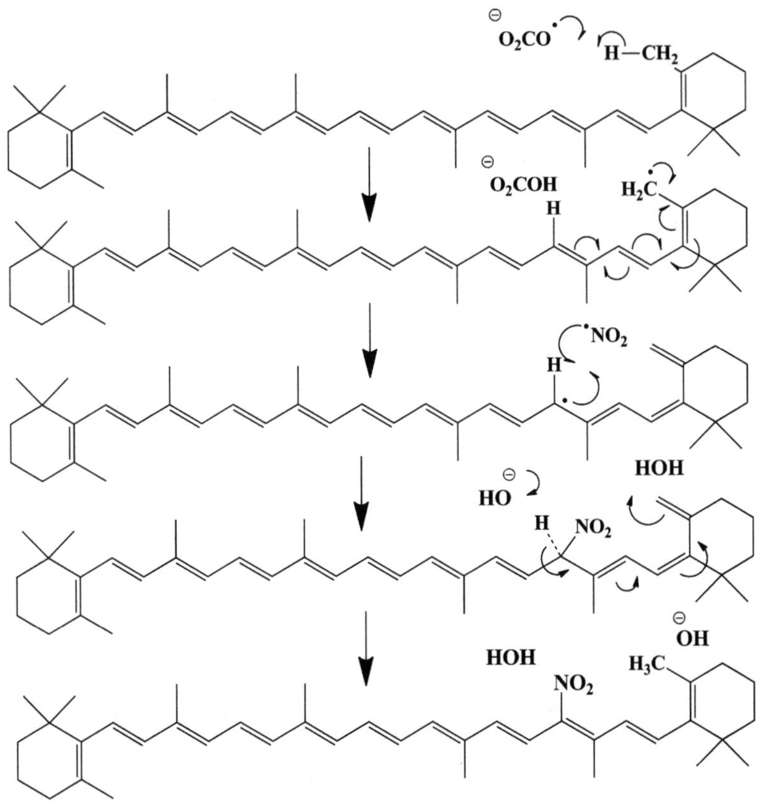

Scheme 4.5

twentieth century and accelerated into the twenty-first century [103, 271–273]. Most prominent among these are the demonstrations that lutein and zeaxanthin accumulate at high levels in the retina where their role in protection of the retina from age-related macular degeneration appears to be significant as discussed in Chap. 13 [137, 274–277]. The potential for lycopene and other carotenoids to influence carcinogenesis as discussed in Chap. 12, particularly in prostate, has also stimulated intensive investigation of the mechanisms of action for the non-provitamin A carotenoids [95, 278, 279]. Astaxanthin, β-cryptoxanthin, and fucoxanthin are also current research foci [73, 267, 280–283]. Carotenoids appear to be nonspecifically accumulated in tissues but important exceptions are lycopene in prostate [121] and lutein and zeaxanthin in retina [275, 277, 284]. Serum concentrations of β-cryptoxanthin are anomalously high relative to estimates of dietary intake [285].

Interactions of Carotenoids with ROS/RNS

As outlined above, two major sources of ROS involve the generation of singlet oxygen by photochemical sensitization and the production of superoxide by NADPH oxidase and related enzymatic processes. Singlet oxygen and superoxide production can ultimately lead to the formation of hydrogen peroxide and lipid hydroperoxides that react primarily via formation of hydroxyl and hydroperoxyl radicals. These species may trigger inflammation through the activation of NF-κB or a related mechanism [18].

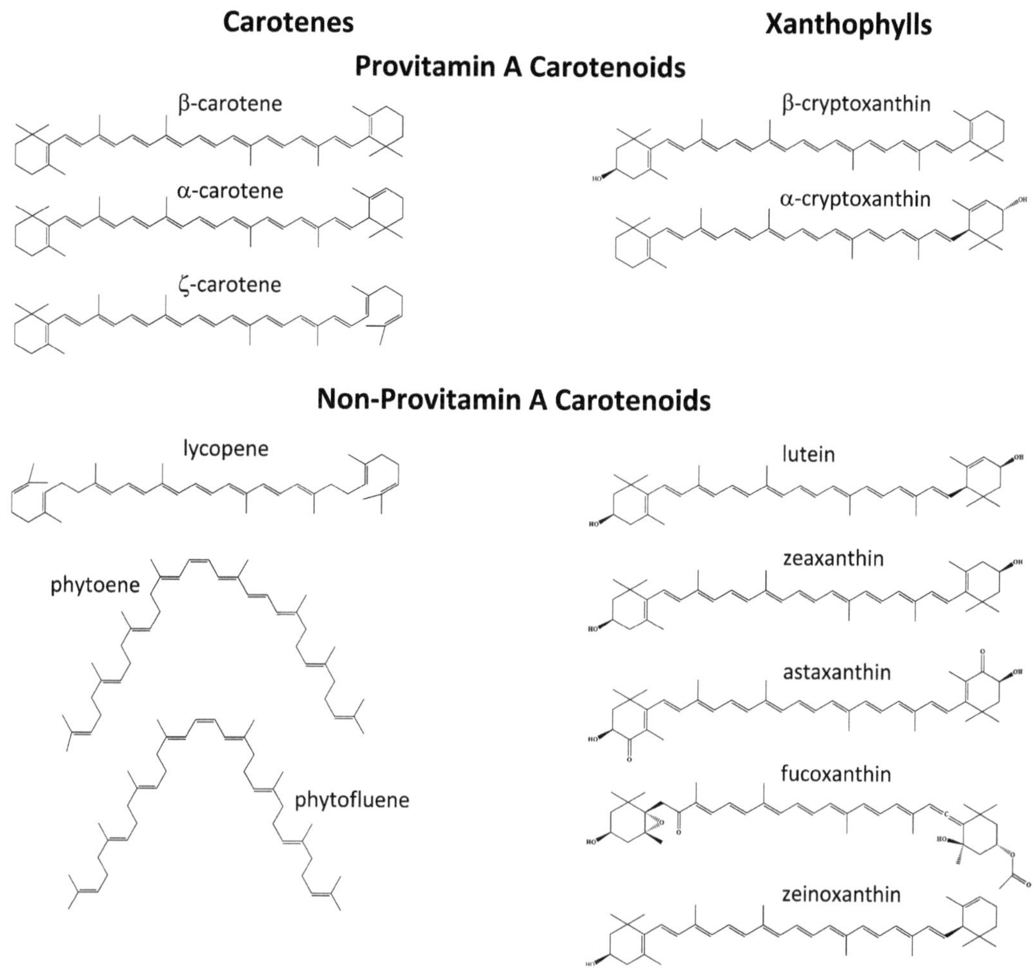

Fig. 4.2 The structural characteristics of the predominant carotenoids observed in human serum vary principally in the end-groups. Hydrocarbon carotenes are shown on the *left* and divided between provitamin A (*top left*) and non-provitamin A (*bottom left*) carotenoids. Xanthophylls possess at least one oxygen functional group and are grouped on the *right* as pro vitamin A (*top right*) and non-provitamin A (*bottom right*) xanthophylls. Although found in very low concentrations in human serum, zeinoxanthin and α-cryptoxanthin isomers of β-cryptoxanthin have been included because there exists some confusion in the literature regarding the names of these structures [99]

The mechanism of singlet oxygen generation in tissues exposed to short wavelength light, particularly, cornea, lens, retina, and skin, is favored by high levels of oxygen as well as elevated levels of luminance. Upon absorption of light, sensitizers initially populate a short-lived singlet excited state, see Scheme 4.2. Rapid relaxation of the "hot" vibrational states within the singlet electronic level dissipates excess energy and for efficient sensitizers, intersystem-crossing follows in ns. Triplet excited states are long-lived with half-lives that range from 10^{-3} to 10^{-6} s allowing time for energy transfer to oxygen. Many naturally abundant sensitizers have measured quantum yields, Φ, for the generation of singlet oxygen that are in the range of 0.5–1.0, i.e., between 50 and 100 % of the absorbed photons generate singlet oxygen by energy transfer [286].

Mechanistically, the presence of carotenoids may diminish the levels of singlet oxygen and its cytotoxic effects in three ways: (1) direct absorption of light decreasing the number of high energy triplet excited state sensitizers, (2) efficient quenching of triplet sensitizers prior to their interaction

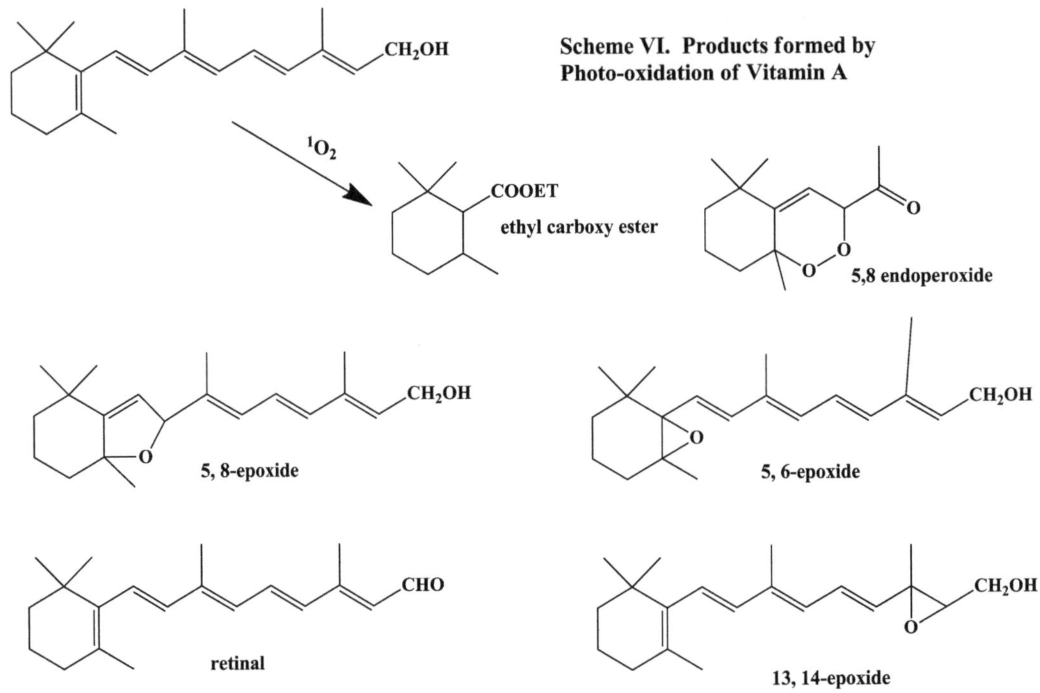

Scheme 4.6

with oxygen (4.44), and (3) direct interaction with singlet oxygen, (4.45) [113, 287]. Carotenoids absorb light with an exceptionally large absorption coefficient ensuring that they absorb a large fraction of the incident photons relative to other molecules. Carotenoids can only reduce the rate of production of excited state sensitizer molecules when the carotenoid concentration is sufficiently high and mechanically positioned within the light path between the source and the sensitizer. This is the arrangement present in the human macula [137, 138]. Carotenoid excited states are also very efficient in their ability to relax to the ground-state by a mechanism involving inter-conversion of excited state energy to vibrational kinetic energy and dissipation of heat through collision with the surrounding medium (4.46). In this way, carotenoids can efficiently quench triplet excited states of most sensitizers via a mechanism of energy transfer.

$$^{1}\mathrm{Car} + {}^{3}\mathrm{Sens}^{*} \rightarrow {}^{3}\mathrm{Car}^{*} + {}^{1}\mathrm{Sens} \quad \text{Quenching of Sensitizers} \tag{4.44}$$

$$\mathrm{Car} + {}^{1}\mathrm{O}_2^{*} \rightarrow {}^{3}\mathrm{Car}^{*} + {}^{3}\mathrm{O}_2 \quad k = 10^{9}\,\mathrm{M}^{-1}\mathrm{s}^{-1} \quad \text{Singlet Oxygen Quenching} \tag{4.45}$$

$$^{3}\mathrm{Car}^{*} \rightarrow {}^{1}\mathrm{Car} + \text{heat} \quad \text{Non - destructive Relaxation} \tag{4.46}$$

Via this mechanism, carotenoids dissipate the excess energy from the excited state sensitizer or singlet oxygen and divert chemical potential available to generate ROS by an efficient, catalytic process, (4.44)–(4.46). By-products of photo-oxidation of carotenoids resulting from reaction with singlet oxygen include *apo*-carotenals produced by double bond cleavage, as well as epoxides and endo peroxides. The photochemical reactions of vitamin A (Scheme 4.6) illustrate the products that arise from singlet oxygen reaction with double bonds [288]. Excited state carotenoid energy levels are positioned to enable them to effectively quench triplet states of sensitizers reducing the production of singlet oxygen [287, 289]. The carotenoid concentration, at or above 10^{-6} M, is a critical factor controlling the efficiency of sensitizer quenching.

Plants, quenching within leaves. Light-generated singlet oxygen is a source of toxicity in photosynthetic plants and the participation of zeaxanthin in the xanthophyll cycle is a mechanism by which toxic ROS generation is moderated at high illumination levels [98, 290]. Zeaxanthin accumulation in organisms lacking a functional xanthophyll cycle demonstrates that it protects against photo-initiated oxidative damage by intercepting and quenching singlet oxygen and/or its reactive oxygen by-products protecting the photosynthetic system [98, 113]. Notably, such plants tolerate higher oxygen levels than non-zeaxanthin accumulating plants.

Animals and humans, quenching within skin. Carotenoids at μM concentrations absorb a small percentage of incident light depending on the wavelength and concentration. Average molar concentrations of carotenoids in skin are in the range of 10^{-7} to 10^{-6} M [291]. Based on Beer's law, an (optimistic) estimate for light absorption in the skin at 450 nm would be on the order of 0.014 absorbance units, assuming a uniform concentration of 10^{-6} M β-carotene and a thickness of 0.1 cm [291]. The resultant transmittance of this tissue would be ~97 %, i.e., only 3 % of the incident light would be intercepted prior to potential interaction with intracellular sensitizers residing behind this layer. Although a measurable reduction of light levels can occur in skin, the filtering of the light intensity by carotenoids is likely to produce very modest protection from singlet oxygen, <3 %. The threshold intensity using a UV lamp needed to produce a detectable erythemal response was reported to be ~0.15 $\mathrm{J\,cm^{-2}}$ for subjects with low carotenoid levels in skin (~10^{-7} M) versus ~0.25 $\mathrm{J\,cm^{-2}}$ for those with higher concentrations ($5–6\times10^{-7}$ M) [291]. These differences should not produce a significant decrease in blue light transmission through the dermal layer. Carotenoids interfered with the action of singlet oxygen after its generation or reduced the inflammatory response via events subsequent to light absorption exerting protection against erythema in skin.

Humans, macular pigment and light absorption. Concentrations of lutein and zeaxanthin within the inner layers of the retina range between 10^{-3} and 10^{-4} M [137, 292, 293]. A typical thickness of the inner layers of the macula is close to 50 μm and the effective absorbance at 450 nm ranges between 0.2 and 0.8 AU. The transmittance of the macular pigment in the retina of a typical individual would range from 32 to 63 %. Macular pigment is therefore absorbing about 50 % of the incident blue light (λ=450 nm) capable of sensitizing the production of singlet oxygen and provides a substantial level of protection to retinal tissue against damage due to the photochemical generation of singlet oxygen. During supplementation studies, macular pigment optical density in the fovea increased from 0.4 to 0.65 AU with a corresponding decrease in transmittance from 0.4 to 0.22 and a 45 % reduction in the intensity of blue light reaching the underlying outer segments of the photoreceptors and retinal pigment epithelium. Light absorption by the macular pigment clearly provides substantial protection against photosensitized $^1O_2$ production.

In resupplementation studies conducted on macaques raised on a carotenoid and omega-3 fatty acid free diet, significant increases of carotenoid levels in the maculae and improved protection against photic lesions induced by exposure to laser light at 488 nm were observed. Since optical density increases were small, ~0.03 AU corresponding to a 7 % reduction in the transmittance of light at this wavelength, the authors concluded that the majority of the observed protection against lesion formation must be attributed to the photochemical mechanisms, i.e., quenching effects and interception of ROS, as opposed to absorption of light [150].

The lipophilic nature of carotenoids necessitates their localization primarily within membranes and lipid vesicles or bound to proteins. Carotenoids are almost certainly carried by both intra- and extracellular proteins, which may be specific or nonspecific carriers [294]. In human serum, carotenoids are transported by HDL and LDL, which transport different proportions of carotenes and xanthophylls likely due to polarity differences [96, 107, 295, 296]. Specific binding proteins are involved in transport and/or localization of ocular xanthophylls, i.e., lutein and zeaxanthin [297]. The light harvesting complex of higher plants specifically binds four carotenoids and evidence supports their

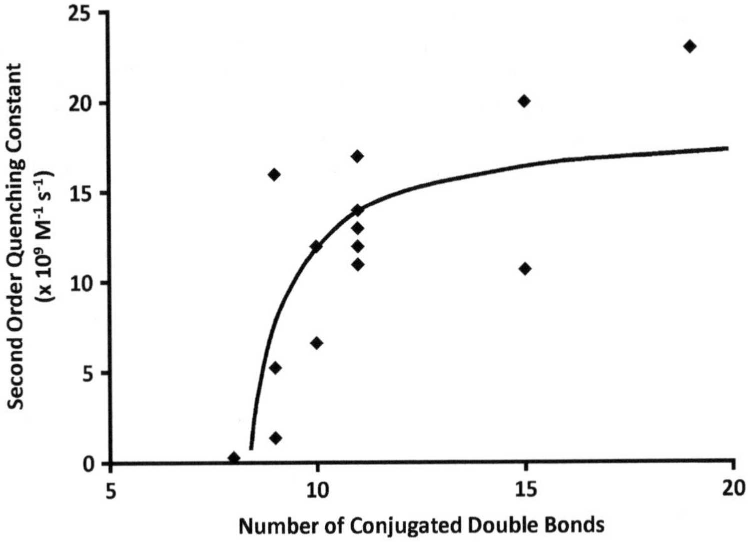

Fig. 4.3 The second order rate constant for singlet oxygen quenching by carotenoids increases logarithmically with increasing length of conjugation (based on data from [233, 302])

functions of antioxidant action, structural stabilization of the protein, regulation of the efficiency of energy capture, and ancillary antenna functions [111, 298]. The importance that carotenoid accumulation within various cellular structures and binding to proteins has in modulating carotenoid antioxidant actions are difficult to assess but are clearly significant. High levels of carotenoids must exist near ROS sources if they are to be functionally relevant. When overall concentrations of carotenoids in a tissue or cell are low, as they are in the human lens (~10^{-8} M), localization within a smaller compartment may have significant consequences [299, 300]. The xanthophylls present in the lens may be concentrated within the small volume of the living layer of epithelial cells on the anterior surface [299, 301]. Xanthophyll intake has been correlated to a reduction in the risk for extraction of cataract [90, 91]. Risk of cataract is increased by exposure to high light levels that increase the exposure of the lens to $^1O_2$.

The extended conjugation of the polyene system of carotenoids accounts for the low lying pi antibonding molecular orbitals that are populated in the excited state. The separation between the ground and singlet excited states varies somewhat between carotenoids with the principal absorption maxima varying from ~430 to 480 nm. Photogenerated excited state sensitizers and singlet oxygen are efficiently quenched by carotenoids because the energy in these excited state species is modestly larger than that of the carotenoid triplet-excited states. Thus quenching is a thermodynamically favored process. These overall processes are quantum mechanically spin-allowed and thus the rates are high. The efficiency of carotenoid quenching of $^1O_2$ as measured by comparison of the second order rate constants shows that rate generally increases with the extent of conjugation (Fig. 4.3).

In Fig. 4.3, the rate constant k_q initially increases rapidly with the number of conjugated double bonds but levels off at larger values, following the trend in energy difference between the ground- and excited state [303]. Although fast, the rates of reactions of unsaturated fatty acids with singlet oxygen are relatively slow ($k \sim 10^5$ M^{-1}s^{-1}), see step a in Scheme 4.1, when compared with the diffusion-limited rate of quenching $^1O_2$ by carotenoids, (4.45) ($k \sim 10^9$ M^{-1}s^{-1}) [148, 287]. Sensitizer quenching by both carotenoids and molecular oxygen are of comparable rates. Comparing these rate constants might lead to the conclusion that sensitizer quenching by carotenoids should result in significant reduction of singlet oxygen production. Under normal, physiological conditions, β-carotene quenching of the sensitizer cannot compete with molecular oxygen, (4.9), because the concentration of dissolved molecular oxygen is fairly high (~1.4×10^{-3} M at 150 mmHg, 3.7×10^{-4} M at 40 mmHg characteristic of the partial pressure of O_2 at the cellular level) compared to that of carotenoids (~10^{-6}) [289]. Therefore, the antioxidant action of β-carotene is due principally to quenching of the relatively long-lived $^1O_2$ prior to its reaction with other substrates. β-Carotene can quench as many as 2,500 molecules of singlet oxygen prior to degradation [304]. This leads to an estimate that chemical inactivation of singlet oxygen (i.e., involving degradation of the carotenoid) occurs in only 0.4–0.04 % of the carotenoid-singlet oxygen interactions [289, 304].

The competitive opportunity for carotenoids to effectively quench singlet oxygen prior to oxidative reaction with lipids is reasonably high. Oxygen's solubility is greatest in lipophilic membranes. The partition coefficient of O_2, $K_p = [O_2]_{lipid}/[O_2]_{water}$, is between 3 and 5 and so $^1O_2$ concentrates within membranes [305]. Membrane systems also have a greater abundance of unsaturated fatty acids that can readily react with $^1O_2$. Thus lipid solubility places carotenoids in the environment that is sensitive to singlet oxygen damage and has high singlet oxygen concentrations. Within membranes, nonpolar carotenoids, e.g., β-carotene, tend to be oriented parallel to the surface, whereas xanthophylls with polar hydroxyl groups tend to span the membrane exposed to the polar, aqueous media [306, 307]. While β-carotene is uniformly distributed, xanthophylls are localized in membrane regions with greater proportions of unsaturated fatty acids and excluded from lipid rafts dominated by cholesterol and saturated fatty acids [308]. The greater concentration of xanthophylls within those domains results in greater protection from singlet oxygen relative to identical concentrations of β-carotene. The membranes of the photoreceptors are among those most rich in unsaturated fatty acids within the human body [309].

Carotenoid Protection Against Superoxide

As described above, superoxide is a major product of oxygen metabolism and has a number of important functions (e.g., indicator of oxygen tension regulating vasodilation/contraction). O_2^{1-} is not exceptionally reactive, but it is efficiently transformed into more reactive secondary ROS. To protect against secondary ROS, a system of antioxidants is essential. The ability to limit the deleterious actions of these ROS enables biological systems to capitalize on the rapid signaling capability and toxicity associated with O_2^{1-}, e.g., in macrophages. Investigation of the direct interaction of carotenoids with superoxide indicates that they form a carotenoid-superoxide adduct [84, 310, 311]. However, recently Martinez et al. reported theoretical calculations showing that electron transfer from superoxide to carotenoids may be favored in nonpolar environments but disfavored in aqueous media [312, 313]. These authors reported a difference in the ability of carotenoids to act as electron acceptors for superoxide with astaxanthin predicted to be a much better acceptor than lycopene or β-carotene. Recently, water-soluble derivatives of astaxanthin were synthesized and reported to effectively scavenge superoxide. The mechanism(s) of this reaction and/or the carotenoid by-products were not identified [264, 268]. Whether these synthetic carotenoids are reacting directly with superoxide or with secondary ROS that are rapidly produced from superoxide needs to be resolved. Superoxide participates in an electron transfer to hydroxyl radical, (4.47), a reaction that generates singlet oxygen as a by-product [187].

$$^{\bullet}OH + O_2^{1-} \rightarrow {}^1O_2 + OH^{1-} \tag{4.47}$$

Free transition-metal ions (Fe^{3+}/Cu^{2+}) also contribute to $^1O_2$ formation, (4.20a) and (4.20b). Iron released in lysosomes during degradation of proteins contributes to radical formation and may lead to degradation of the lysosomal membrane [314]. Cellular iron concentrations are normally low, but promote increased inflammation when bound iron is released exacerbating oxidative stress [315]. In synovial fluid of rheumatoid patients and normal cerebrospinal fluid, the measured levels of unbound iron can be sufficiently high (μmol L^{-1}) and an important contributor to pro-oxidative processes [157, 316–321]. Markers for ROS production are also associated with temporomandibular joint disease and associated with increased iron levels [322].

Damage to DNA by Oxidative Reactions

Many age-related diseases involve damage to DNA and particularly mitochondrial DNA (mt-DNA) [37]. Mt-DNA replication is orchestrated by mt-DNA polymerase-g (POLG). Defective POLG lacking the ability to proofread and correct the replicated sequences leads to high levels of mutations that accumulate in mt-DNA and is associated with rapid aging in mice carrying this POLG defect [323]. Lifespans of such mice are greatly reduced and they exhibit many pathological conditions comparable to those in aging humans [324]. Humans with POLG mutations may suffer from Parkinsonism and other diseases typical of aging. In mice and *Drosophila,* over-expression of mitochondrial antioxidant proteins MnSOD, catalase, and/or methionine sulphoxide reductase are protective against O_2^-, H_2O_2, and their by-products and are associated with increased longevity [325–327]. Reduced levels of mt-DNA oxidation were observed in addition to reductions in pathologies including arteriosclerosis and cardiac damage. In humans, oxidative damage to DNA has been associated with cognitive decline during aging [328]. G/C-rich promoter sequences, which are uniquely susceptible to oxidation, may accumulate unrepaired errors due to oxidation. In experiments on neuroblastoma-derived cells, small interfering RNA reduced the expression of F1-ATPase and resulted in damage to promoter DNA, but the effect was partly reversed by vitamin E. Collectively, evidence that mt-DNA damage is responsible for unregulated ROS generation and consequent pathological conditions is compelling [37].

Lin and Beal state that mitochondrial generation and metabolism of ROS is so complex that therapeutic treatment with a single or small selection of antioxidants is too simplistic an approach to produce more than modest success in the treatment of oxidative stress-induced diseases [37]. This is not an indictment of the role and importance of antioxidants so much as a recognition of the need for a multi-pronged approach to the reduction of oxidative stress. As expressed earlier, it is the multilayered nature of the antioxidant protection system, including carotenoids, that makes it difficult to demonstrate the unambiguous actions of carotenoids against ROS *in vivo.* A single antioxidant will rarely be sufficient to address any incompetency in the antioxidant system. The build-up of DNA errors associated with lowered levels of the antioxidant proteins and rapid ROS production clearly require a pro-active, multi-faceted approach. Early and consistent intake of dietary antioxidants may contribute to a reduction in the accumulation of DNA errors.

Carotenoid Radical Anions

The generation of carotenoid radical anions has been explored for selected carotenoids and *apo*-carotenoids [84, 311]. Carotenoid radical anions are quite stable in acetonitrile but they are rapidly protonated in the presence of protic solvents such as water and methanol (4.48a) and (4.48b). Reaction of carotenoids with O_2^- occurs favorably only in lipophilic environments to form the carotenoid radical anions that are resonance-stabilized [84, 233]. The product of the carotenoid radical anion is unlikely to be a significant contributor to the oxidation of superoxide.

$$\mathrm{Car} + \mathrm{O}_2^- \rightarrow \mathrm{Car}^{\bullet -} + \mathrm{O}_2 \tag{4.48a}$$

$$\mathrm{Car}^{\bullet -} + \mathrm{H}^+ \rightarrow \mathrm{CarH}^{\bullet} \tag{4.48b}$$

Carotenoid Cation Radicals

The carotenoid cation radical is rapidly generated by transfer of an electron from a carotenoid to a variety of radicals and oxidants that are produced by oxidative processes *in vivo* (Fig. 4.4). Particularly, hydroxyl, peroxy, and carbonate radicals all readily react with carotenoids via electron transfer to produce carotenoid cation radicals, see (4.49), (4.50), and (4.51a). Truscott and coworkers have demonstrated that carotenoid cation radicals, once generated, can be subsequently reduced by a host of natural reductants (e.g., ascorbate, glutathione) [84]. Carotenoid cation radicals ($CAR^{\bullet+}$) effectively interrupt radical chain reactions because the $CAR^{\bullet+}$ is very stable with a half-life on the order of minutes. Carotenoids are readily regenerated by electron transfer from abundant natural antioxidants, including other carotenoids, ascorbate, glutathione (as well as other thiols), and tocopherols [89]. The carotenoid is able to function as a true catalyst enhancing the rate of radical decomposition by glutathione and other cellular reductants. Hydrogen abstraction, as suggested by (4.51b) would lead to formation of a neutral carotenoid radical that would be highly delocalized and could readily react with either $^{\bullet}NO$ or $^{\bullet}NO_2$ leading to nitrated products.

$$\mathrm{Car} + \mathrm{HO}^{\bullet} \rightarrow \mathrm{Car}^{+} + \mathrm{HO}^{-} \tag{4.49}$$

$$\mathrm{Car} + \mathrm{ROO}^{\bullet} \rightarrow \mathrm{Car}^{\bullet+} + \mathrm{ROO}^{-}\mathrm{R} = \mathrm{H}, \quad \text{alkyl} \tag{4.50}$$

$$\mathrm{Car} + \mathrm{CO}_3^{\bullet-} \rightarrow \mathrm{Car}^{\bullet+} + \mathrm{CO}_3^{2-} \quad \text{electron transfer} \tag{4.51a}$$

$$\mathrm{Car} + \mathrm{CO}_3^{\bullet-} \rightarrow \mathrm{Car}^{\bullet} + \mathrm{HOCO}_2^{1-} \quad \mathrm{H-abstraction} \tag{4.51b}$$

The measured oxidation potentials for carotenoids differ very little, but oxygen substitution in the carotenoid influences the trend in the oxidation potential and carotenoids that are more oxygen-rich, such as astaxanthin, are less readily oxidized due to the electron withdrawing action of the oxygen atoms [329].

Reaction of Carotenoids with Peroxynitrite

The rapid reaction of nitric oxide with superoxide ensures that peroxynitrite is often present when superoxide is generated in significant quantities *in vivo* [235]. The products formed during reaction of carotenoids with peroxynitrite (and the peroxynitrite-derived ROS) have been studied *in vitro* [330–332]. Studies to test the ability of carotenoids to protect LDL against degradation by peroxynitrite show that exposure to peroxynitrite results in loss of carotenes carried by LDL. All carotenoids tested, efficiently scavenged peroxynitrite preventing the formation of fluorescent rhodamine 123 from non-fluorescent dihydrorhodamine 123, an indicator sensitive to peroxynitrite and H_2O_2 *in vivo* [333–335]. The more polar xanthophylls, i.e., lutein, zeaxanthin, and β-cryptoxanthin, while effective did not scavenge peroxynitrite as efficiently as lycopene, β-carotene, and α-carotene. The observed order of reactivity of the carotenoids was lycopene>α-carotene>β-carotene>β-cryptoxanthin>zeaxanthin>lutein. The authors noted that xanthophylls were as effective in reacting with peroxynitrite as biothiols, such as glutathione, cysteine, and thiol groups within proteins [336]. While the authors did not identify the mechanism or products formed in peroxynitrite reactions with carotenoids, they clearly observed by HPLC that numerous carotenoid-derived products were present in solution after reaction. Carotenoids likely react with ROS derived from ONO_2^- and not peroxynitrite itself.

Etoh and coworkers have investigated the reaction of astaxanthin, β-carotene, fucoxanthin, capsanthin, and retinol in the presence of peroxynitrite and have identified a large number of nitro-carotenoids, nitro-*apo*-carotenoids, and degradation products formed in these reactions [330–332].

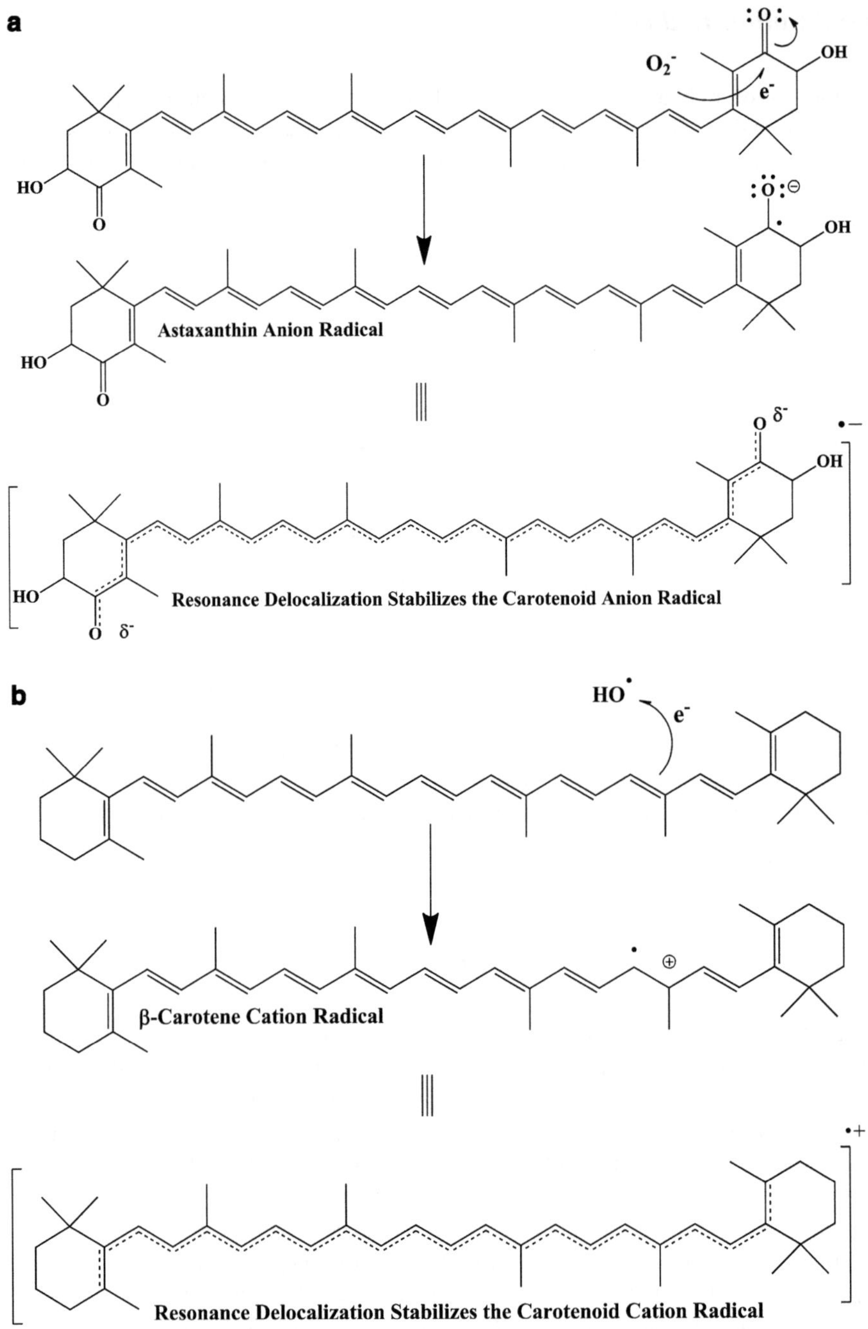

Fig. 4.4 (**a**) Reduction of carotenoids by superoxide is possible in nonpolar environments producing the carotenoid radical anion. Presence of oxygen functional groups, particularly keto groups on the ionone ring, stabilize the resulting anion as seen for astaxanthin in this example. Delocalization of both the charge and the unpaired electron contributes to the stability of these species. (**b**) Oxidation by radicals (e.g., $HO^{\bullet}$, $CO_3^{\bullet-}$ or $ROO^{\bullet}$) can produce a long-lived and much less reactive carotenoid cation radical that is resonance stabilized

Using NMR techniques many of the nitro-carotenoids and nitro-*apo*-carotenoids were shown to exist as *cis*- and s-*cis* isomers. Substitution by the sterically demanding and strongly electron-withdrawing nitro group on the polyene chain alters the relative stability of *cis*- relative to *trans*-isomers and conformers. 14′-s-*cis*-15′-nitro-astaxanthin was the most abundant product formed by the reaction of astaxanthin with peroxynitrite [330]. Cleavage of astaxanthin formed 13-*apo*-astaxanthinone, 12′-*apo*-astaxanthinal, and 12′-*apo*-15′-nitro-astaxanthinal [331]. Capsanthin reacts with peroxynitrite to form predominantly (14′Z)-15′-nitro-capsanthin and 12-nitro-capsanthin but also *apo*-capsanthins. Similarly, fucoxanthin yields the products (14Z)-15-nitro-fucoxanthin, (11Z)-11-nitro-fucoxanthin, and (14Z, 9′Z)-15-nitro-fucoxanthin [332].

The stoichiometry of degradation is an important factor in understanding the effectiveness of the role of carotenoids in controlling peroxynitrite-induced oxidative stress. Identifying the oxidation products observed *in vitro* provides insight into their possible reactivity *in vivo* and may help establish the extent of reactivity of carotenoids with peroxynitrite and peroxynitrite-derived ROS in natural systems. An investigation of the ability of capsanthin and fucoxanthin to inhibit nitration of tyrosine *in vitro* demonstrated that they reduced nitration by about 10 %, almost the same as observed for γ-tocopherol [332]. The mechanism by which the inhibition of tyrosine nitration occurs in the presence of carotenoids is proposed to involve competition for the nitrating agent and will result in depletion of carotenoids, which contrasts with those processes in which the carotenoid inactivates ROS via a catalytic series of events. In additional studies, nitro-capsanthins and nitro-fucoxanthins inhibited proliferation of human carcinoma cells in culture and were able to reduce mouse skin carcinogenesis *in vivo* [332]. This observation may indicate that it is the further degradation of these nitro-carotenoids by cleavage and consequent signaling action that is involved in antioxidant protection. Carotenoids are likely reacting with $CO_3^{\bullet-}$, $^{\bullet}NO_2$, and $^1O_2$ generated from decomposition of ONO_2^- (4.13) and (4.17).

Involvement of Carotenoids in Oxidation Signaling Pathways

Extensive research has focused on the ability of antioxidants to directly inhibit molecular or cellular damage by ROS and RNS. These studies have provided an understanding of the important mechanisms by which the build-up of undesirable, high concentrations of free radicals occurs and how its pathogenic consequences can be ameliorated by the presence of carotenoids and other antioxidants. Particularly important may be the formation of carotenoid cation radicals [233]. Recent work has provided evidence that ROS/RNS are important physiologically and at low concentrations serve a role as cellular messengers [39]. $^{\bullet}NO$ serves a critically important role as the endothelium-derived relaxing factor. Superoxide, peroxide, and other ROS can trigger the commencement of apoptosis and activate protein kinases. ROS are also involved in the regulation of protein phosphatases, transcription factors such as NF-κB, and heat shock protein transcription factor. The involvement of retinal in the regulation of transcription events suggests the possibility that other *apo*-carotenals might act in a similar, albeit limited way.

Carotenoids are able to react directly and thereby modulate ROS/RNS actions, which have a regulatory function in a number of pathways [18].

Nuclear Factor κB

NF-κB is found in many tissues and cell types and plays a key role in the immune system [337]. It may be responsible for pathogenesis in many diseases that involve an inflammatory component, including ROS/RNS production [39]. NF-κB activates transcription of a number of genes associated with inflammatory processes; these include tumor necrosis factor-α (TNF-α), several cytokines, and inducible nitric oxide synthase [39]. In the cytosol, NF-κB is present as a heterodimer composed of two subunits, p65 (also known as RelA) and p50 (also known as NF-κB1). Normally, in unstimulated cells, an inactivating protein, IκB is bound to the dimer masking the positively charged nuclear locating sequence present on p65 and p50. This prevents transport of the dimer into the nucleus where it serves a regulatory role in protein transcription. A number of triggers induce ROS production, including phorbol esters, cigarette smoke, and inflammatory agents, which activate NF-κB [18]. Potent antioxidants, particularly *N*-acetylcysteine, inhibit NF-κB activation [69, 338]. The presence of ROS within cells triggers phosphorylation of two serine hydroxyl groups of IκB and subsequently, IκB is ubiquitinated and degraded. Once the IκB masking inhibitor is removed, the NF-κB heterodimer (p65/p50) is free to bind to the nuclear receptor responsible for its transport into the nucleus. Within the nucleus, NF-κB binds to DNA, activating transcription events. This binding event is dependent upon reduction, within the nucleus, of cysteine 62 of p50 by thioredoxin. Thioredoxin is itself induced by ROS and DNA binding by NF-κB [339, 340]. Moderately oxidized LDL induces activation of NF-κB, i.e., through IκB degradation [338]. The resulting cytokines produced following NF-κB activation of transcription events in the nucleus act as intercellular signals initiating the more extensive events of the inflammatory processes within tissues, i.e., IL-1 and TNF-α also activate NF-κB reinforcing the response in a positive feedback mechanism. TNF-α specifically initiates the steps of apoptotic cell death and cachexia. Upregulation of iNOS by NF-κB results in elevated levels of •NO and potentiates reaction between superoxide and nitric oxide to form peroxynitrite. NF-κB activation is associated with AIDS, atherosclerosis, rheumatoid arthritis, osteoporosis, asthma, renal disease, Alzheimer's disease, chronic obstructive pulmonary disease, and ischemic–reperfusion injury [39]. Cancer pathogenesis has also been associated with NF-κB activation [39, 72, 341–343].

Palozza has reported that β-carotene can induce ROS production in cancer cells and that sustained elevation of NF-κB accompanied this observation [18, 344–346]. In this case, the role of β-carotene was suggested to be that of a pro-oxidant. Carotenoid oxidation products may be involved in signaling, leading to the activation of transcription events as opposed to participation in a pro-oxidant free radical chain reaction. In this study, very high concentrations of β-carotene resulted in increased ROS levels and increased NF-κB activation, whereas lowering β-carotene concentrations restored ROS production to more normal levels, and decreased NF-κB activation. In a study of rats supplemented with very high levels of β-carotene (250–500 mg kg^{-1}), cytochrome p450 levels were increased 2- to 3.6-fold and large amounts of ROS were detected by EPR using spin traps. (Note: A comparable dose in a 70 kg human would correspond to 17.5–35 g/day and is far beyond any pharmacological dose!) This observation is also consistent with the potential role for high doses of β-carotene to act as an inducer of ROS production [135].

Lycopene treatment of human hepatoma cells, reduced activation of NF-κB and also inhibited matrix metalloproteinase-9 levels [347]. Matrix metalloproteinases are associated with angiogenesis and metastasis. In macrophages treated with gliadin (a mitogenic wheat glycoprotein) and the cytokine interferon-gamma, lycopene inhibited activation of NF-κB and lowered nitric oxide synthase and COX2 levels, suggesting that lycopene may constitute an effective means of reducing pro-inflammatory responses in celiac disease [348]. In additional studies of activated macrophages, β-carotene and astaxanthin also inhibited NF-κB [349, 350]. A partial explanation of the pro-oxidant action of β-carotene might be ascribable to the formation and action of carotenoid cleavage products that are sensitive to both carotenoid and total ROS/RNS levels. The authors of these studies have not reported the metabolic products generated from the carotenoids in these systems.

Cyclooxygenases (COX1 and COX2)

COX1 is a constitutive oxygenase and is responsible for the conversion of arachidonic acid to form prostaglandins, which are essential to normal cell activity [351]. COX1 catalyzes the formation of prostacyclin, an anti-thrombogenic cytokine [352]. COX2 is induced by NF-κB in response to ROS. Modulation of ROS levels by carotenoids through activation of NF-κB poses a mechanism for regulation of COX2 upregulation.

Activator Protein 1 Transcription Factor, AP-1

In mammalian cells, activator protein-1, like NF-κB is induced by ROS and is a heterodimeric transcription factor composed of the proteins, c-Fos and c-Jun. Its functions include regulation of gene expression that controls differentiation, proliferation, and apoptosis [353]. This transcription factor is noted to be particularly sensitive to oxidative stress [337]. It is post-transcriptionally modified ensuring it is transported to and acts in neighboring cells [354]. Lycopene and β-carotene downregulate AP-1 [18]. In contrast, ferrets exposed to cigarette smoke and/or pharmacological doses of β-carotene, retinoic acid concentrations in lung tissue were lowered by induction of cytochrome p450 enzymes while levels of AP-1 increased [355]. Induction of cytochrome p450 by β-carotene is a notable observation in light of the still common perception that β-carotene and carotenoids are universally benign dietary nutrients, even at elevated levels of consumption. Low doses of β-carotene reversed the decrease of retinoic acid demonstrating a dose dependent relationship of the action of β-carotene on these pathways leading to cytochrome p450 production [143]. These results are suggestive of a mechanism accounting for the observation of increased rates of lung cancer during human trials with high doses of β-carotene in smokers [129, 356].

The acyclic oxidation products derived from lycopene, either enzymatically or by ROS oxidation, may be active as inhibitors of cell growth in human cancer cells [357]. In an investigation of the influence of the lycopene cleavage product, *acyclo*-retinoic acid, on cell growth in human mammary cancer cells, *acyclo*-retinoic acid interacted with retinoic acid receptor weakly, ~100 times less effective than retinoic acid. Since the ability of lycopene-derived *acyclo*-retinoic acid to inhibit cell growth was found to be similar to that of retinoic acid, *acyclo*-retinoic acid most likely exerts its influence on cell growth through a different family of nuclear transcription receptors [358]. *Acyclo*-retinoic acid has not been detected in biological tissues and Sharoni has suggested it may not be a significant active metabolite of lycopene *in vivo* [134]. Additional lycopene metabolites have been observed in animals, i.e., *apo*-10′-lycopenal in ferrets and *apo*-8′-lycopenal in rats [359, 360]. These also may be involved in the cell regulatory apparatus.

Beta-Carotene Monooxygenase 1 and Beta-Carotene Dioxygenase 2

β-Carotene dioxygenase 2 (BCDO2) is less substrate specific, cleaving both carotenes and xanthophylls, predominantly at the 9,10 position, than BCMO1 which only cleaves carotenoids with a β-ionone ring and exclusively at the 15,15′ double bond. Studies with knockout mice demonstrate that the absence of BCMO1 not only removes the ability to metabolize β-carotene to produce retinal but also represses carotenoid absorption through its influence on the expression of SR-B1 [361]. The gene for BCDO2 is found in the mitochondrial proteome and immunostaining of BCDO2 shows that it is co-localized with cytochrome c oxidase within mitochondria [362]. In BCDO2-deficient mice, large amounts of xanthophyll metabolites produced by lutein and zeaxanthin supplementation accumulated in several tissues. These metabolites were identified as keto- and dehydro-carotenoids and were not observed in similarly treated wild-type mice [362]. The authors noted that BCDO2−/− knockout mice and BCDO2+/− heterozygous mice supplemented with xanthophylls develop liver steatosis, whereas wild-type mice or unsupplemented BCDO2−/− did not. In the BCDO2−/− knockout mice supplemented with xanthophylls, mitochondria exhibited a ninefold increase in MnSOD levels (a marker for mitochondrial dysfunction) relative to wild-type animals. BCDO2 may serve a detoxifying role protecting mitochondria from the ability of high carotenoids to depolarize the mitochondrial membrane.

The Antioxidant Response Element

The ARE is an essential component of the cellular antioxidant defense system and is activated by the transcription factor NrF2 [nuclear transcription factor (erythroid-derived 2)] [363]. The genes encoded by ARE activation include many of the phase II antioxidant enzymes, such as NAD(P)H quinone oxidoreductase 1, glutathione *S*-transferase, hemeoxygenase-1, peroxiredoxin 1, and thioredoxin. This suite of antioxidative defense enzymes blankets a range of ROS generating and interception mechanisms. NrF2 is a short-lived protein with a half-life of about 20 min. Under normal, resting conditions, NrF2 is bound to the cysteine-rich represser protein, Keap1, within the cytoplasm, which targets NrF2 for ubiquitation and proteasomal degradation [364]. An oxidative stress sensor, Keap1 functions as an adaptor for Cul3-Based E3 ligase to regulate proteasomal degradation of NrF2 [364]. Keap1 is sensitive to ROS production which triggers Keap1 dissociation from NrF2. After release of Keap1, NrF2 is transported into the nucleus where it forms a heterodimer with small Maf (small Maf proteins confer DNA binding specificity to NrF2 and related proteins) [365]. NrF2:Maf binds to the ARE, upregulating the proteins described above, which are transcribed by nuclear DNA. This contrasts with the proteins BCDO2 and SOD2, which are mitochondrial in origin [141, 327]. The NrF2:Keap1 complex appears to be tethered to the mitochondrial outer membrane via a mitochondrial protein, PGAM5. Localization at the mitochondrial outer membrane makes the NrF2:Keap1 complex ideally positioned to detect mitochondrial ROS release [208]. ROS exposure interferes with NrF2 degradation and results in upregulation of ARE.

Skepticism has been expressed as to the potential of intact hydrophobic carotenoids to interact effectively with Keap1 and activate NrF2 [134]. Although inducers of NrF2 action are varied, they can function as electrophiles. Sharoni has suggested that the *apo*-carotenoids produced by ROS carotenoid cleavage might function as effective NrF2 activators. Partially oxidized lycopene derivatives were able to activate the ARE in human hepatocellular carcinoma cells whereas intact lycopene had a negligible effect [19]. The aldehydes and dialdehydes formed from lycopene, but not the acids, have ARE activity. The intact carotenoids phytoene, phytofluene, β-carotene, and astaxanthin did not influence ROS in a manner consistent with activation of ARE. *Apo*-carotenal cleavage products of these carotenoids may be able to upregulate transcription of ARE proteins.

Summary and Conclusions

The ROS/RNS produced by biological systems originate as a natural consequence of oxygen reduction during aerobic metabolism [1, 2, 4, 5, 113]. Radicals such as NO and O_2^- are of critical physiological importance and function as reporters of the metabolic status of cells and cellular systems [2, 5, 6]. The occurrence of excess or unregulated ROS/RNS produces undesirable oxidative stress and must be regulated to prevent pathogenesis [35–39]. Deactivation of ROS is accomplished by the action of a variety of antioxidants and enzyme systems that are accumulated and localized at effective concentrations within the cell and specific cellular compartments where ROS levels are likely to be highest and pose the greatest threat [38, 39]. Dynamic responses within the cell to the production of ROS/RNS are essential to physiologic feedback mechanisms designed to regulate levels [2, 3, 19, 20, 35, 132, 364]. Although the number of ROS/RNS produced *in vivo* is large, those which are principally and directly responsible for oxidative damage include singlet oxygen, hydroxyl radical, alkyl radicals, carbonate radical, hydroperoxy radical, and alkyl peroxy radicals [5, 6, 31–33, 113]. These are produced from the larger group of longer-lived ROS/RNS including, but not exclusively superoxide, hydrogen peroxide, nitric oxide, and peroxynitrite. The ability of hydroxyl and carbonate radicals to diffuse within the cell is limited by their extremely high chemical reactivity [32, 35–37, 165, 259]. The hydroxyl radical as well as most alkyl radicals can diffuse no more than approximately 100 Å prior to its reaction with proteins, lipids, or other cellular components [31, 161, 164]. The more stable ROS/RNS as well as cytokines and mitogens, have the ability to diffuse across longer distances and activate oxidative processes at locations remote from their generation [33].

Carotenoids react directly with the most reactive radicals and carotenoid cation radicals are a typical product with such species as the hydroxyl radical [18, 19, 88, 113, 132, 138]. Because carotenoids are lipophilic, they concentrate principally in membranes and lipophilic structures within the cell poised to react with radicals that are generated by redox active proteins. The preferential tendency of carotenoids to concentrate in membrane regions having high levels of unsaturated fatty acids can provide significant protection to these essential lipid components [306]. Carotenoid cation radicals are long-lived because of their extensive conjugation and can be regenerated by glutathione, ascorbate, and/or tocopherol creating a catalytic cycle whereby a single carotenoid can effectively react with hundreds, if not thousands of potentially damaging ROS [84, 233, 302]. Evidence is strong that carotenoids in the skin and retina are protective against light-induced production of singlet oxygen and a host of reactive radicals [87, 114–120]. β-Carotene will quench an estimated 2,500 singlet oxygen molecules for each one that reacts by chemical addition [292, 304].

The variety of naturally occurring carotenoids *in vivo* presents an opportunity for their recruitment within the regulatory system as signal molecules [18–20, 88, 89, 113, 141, 142, 149, 361]. The most widely recognized of these is β-carotene, which serves as a source of retinal that regulates many cellular events through the retinoic acid receptors [18, 93, 361]. β-Carotene and the related provitamin A carotenoids are exclusively the substrates for BCMO1 and data indicate that retinoic acid endogenously produced by BCMO1 is functionally distinct in its actions from preformed vitamin A absorbed from the diet [141, 361]. Evidence is now strong, and growing, that other *apo*-carotenals formed by oxidative cleavage of carotenoids function to influence protein transcription associated with ROS production, peroxisomal activity, and synthesis and transport of cytokines and mitogenic proteins [18–20]. Nonspecific BCDO2, capable of cleaving numerous carotenoids at the 9,10 position, is a mitochondrial protein responsible for production of high levels of *apo*-carotenals. The lycopene cleavage products *acyclo*-retinoic acid, *apo*-10′-lycopenal, and *apo*-8′-lycopenal are involved in the cell regulatory apparatus [139, 358–360]. The ability to inhibit cell cycle progression appears to be a component of the involvement of carotenoids in the events of cancer pathogenesis [93].

The concern that carotenoids may act as pro-oxidants by participating in and propagating free radical reactions by the addition of oxygen to carotenoid radicals is minimal. Carotenoid radicals react very sluggishly to form peroxide except when the partial pressure of O_2 and carotenoid concentrations are well above physiological conditions [124, 126]. At least some carotenoid derived *apo*-carotenals formed by oxidative cleavage can lead to upregulation of proteins and signal molecules responsible for increased radical production [18].

The actions or activity of specific carotenoids and the products formed under oxidative stress needs to be better understood. Despite this limitation, during the past decade work has progressed remarkably along these lines, particularly in assessing the dynamics of the interplay of ROS and transcription. The full extent to which carotenoids are functionally significant in the maintenance of cellular redox homeostasis, as yet, remains incompletely understood. The involvement of *apo*-carotenoids in regulation of transcription of the redox-related pathways and the differences that are now being observed among dietary carotenoids in producing these species suggest their importance to overall health and the prevention or modulation of disease initiation and progression, particularly diseases that are inflammatory.

References

1. Novo E, Parola M. Redox mechanisms in hepatic chronic wound healing and fibrogenesis. Fibrogenesis Tissue Repair. 2008;1(1):5.
2. Palmer HJ, Paulson KE. Reactive oxygen species and antioxidants in signal transduction and gene expression. Nutr Rev. 1997;55(10):353–61.
3. Valko M, et al. Free radicals, metals and antioxidants in oxidative stress-induced cancer. Chem Biol Interact. 2006;160(1):1–40.
4. Raedschelders K, Ansley DM, Chen DD. The cellular and molecular origin of reactive oxygen species generation during myocardial ischemia and reperfusion. Pharmacol Ther. 2012;133(2):230–55.
5. Apel K, Hirt H. Reactive oxygen species: metabolism, oxidative stress, and signal transduction. Annu Rev Plant Biol. 2004;55:373–99.
6. Gechev TS, et al. Reactive oxygen species as signals that modulate plant stress responses and programmed cell death. Bioessays. 2006;28(11):1091–101.
7. Brown GC, Borutaite V. There is no evidence that mitochondria are the main source of reactive oxygen species in mammalian cells. Mitochondrion. 2012;12(1):1–4.
8. Breusing N, Grune T. Biomarkers of protein oxidation from a chemical, biological and medical point of view. Exp Gerontol. 2010;45(10):733–7.
9. Ivashchenko O, et al. Intraperoxisomal redox balance in mammalian cells: oxidative stress and interorganellar cross-talk. Mol Biol Cell. 2011;22(9):1440–51.
10. Gabaldon T. Peroxisome diversity and evolution. Philos Trans R Soc Lond B Biol Sci. 2010;365(1541):765–73.
11. Turrens JF. Superoxide production by the mitochondrial respiratory chain. Biosci Rep. 1997;17(1):3–8.
12. Brand MD. The sites and topology of mitochondrial superoxide production. Exp Gerontol. 2010;45(7–8):466–72.
13. Brand MD, et al. Mitochondrial superoxide: production, biological effects, and activation of uncoupling proteins. Free Radic Biol Med. 2004;37(6):755–67.
14. Miwa S, Brand MD. The topology of superoxide production by complex III and glycerol 3-phosphate dehydrogenase in Drosophila mitochondria. Biochim Biophys Acta. 2005;1709(3):214–9.
15. Schwarzlander M, et al. Confocal imaging of glutathione redox potential in living plant cells. J Microsc. 2008;231(2):299–316.
16. Mates JM. Effects of antioxidant enzymes in the molecular control of reactive oxygen species toxicology. Toxicology. 2000;153(1–3):83–104.
17. Sies H. Oxidative stress: oxidants and antioxidants. Exp Physiol. 1997;82(2):291–5.
18. Palozza P, Catalano A, Simone R. Carotenoids as modulators of molecular pathways involved in cell proliferation and apoptosis. In: Landrum JT, editor. Carotenoids: physical, chemical, and biological functions and properties. Boca Raton: CRC; 2010. p. 465–84.
19. Ben-Dor A, et al. Carotenoids activate the antioxidant response element transcription system. Mol Cancer Ther. 2005;4(1):177–86.
20. Sharoni Y, et al. Carotenoids and transcription. Arch Biochem Biophys. 2004;430(1):89–96.
21. Fraticelli A, et al. Hydrogen peroxide and superoxide modulate leukocyte adhesion molecule expression and leukocyte endothelial adhesion. Biochim Biophys Acta. 1996;1310(3):251–9.
22. Van Antwerpen VL, et al. Plasma levels of beta-carotene are inversely correlated with circulating neutrophil counts in young male cigarette smokers. Inflammation. 1995;19(4):405–14.
23. Dahlen SE, et al. Leukotrienes promote plasma leakage and leukocyte adhesion in postcapillary venules: *in vivo* effects with relevance to the acute inflammatory response. Proc Natl Acad Sci USA. 1981;78(6):3887–91.
24. Prasadam I, Crawford R, Xiao Y. Aggravation of ADAMTS and matrix metalloproteinase production and role of ERK1/2 pathway in the interaction of osteoarthritic subchondral bone osteoblasts and articular cartilage chondrocytes—possible pathogenic role in osteoarthritis. J Rheumatol. 2012;39:621–34.
25. Blake DR, Winyard PG, Marok R. The contribution of hypoxia-reperfusion injury to inflammatory synovitis: the influence of reactive oxygen intermediates on the transcriptional control of inflammation. Ann N Y Acad Sci. 1994;723:308–17.

26. Yang D, et al. Synthetic fluorescent probes for imaging of peroxynitrite and hypochlorous acid in living cells. Methods Mol Biol. 2010;591:93–103.
27. Yee DJ, et al. Fluorogenic metabolic probes for direct activity readout of redox enzymes: selective measurement of human AKR1C2 in living cells. Proc Natl Acad Sci USA. 2006;103(36):13304–9.
28. Brandes RP, Janiszewski M. Direct detection of reactive oxygen species *ex vivo*. Kidney Int. 2005;67(5):1662–4.
29. Baier J, et al. Direct detection of singlet oxygen generated by UVA irradiation in human cells and skin. J Invest Dermatol. 2007;127(6):1498–506.
30. Del Rio D, Stewart AJ, Pellegrini N. A review of recent studies on malondialdehyde as toxic molecule and biological marker of oxidative stress. Nutr Metab Cardiovasc Dis. 2005;15(4):316–28.
31. Bolin C, Cardozo-Pelaez F. Assessing biomarkers of oxidative stress: analysis of guanosine and oxidized guanosine nucleotide triphosphates by high performance liquid chromatography with electrochemical detection. J Chromatogr B Analyt Technol Biomed Life Sci. 2007;856(1–2):121–30.
32. Olinski R, et al. Oxidative DNA damage in cancer patients: a cause or a consequence of the disease development? Mutat Res. 2003;531(1–2):177–90.
33. Naik E, Dixit VM. Mitochondrial reactive oxygen species drive proinflammatory cytokine production. J Exp Med. 2011;208(3):417–20.
34. Pryor WA. Oxy-radicals and related species: their formation, lifetimes, and reactions. Annu Rev Physiol. 1986;48: 657–67.
35. Pacher P, Beckman JS, Liaudet L. Nitric oxide and peroxynitrite in health and disease. Physiol Rev. 2007;87(1): 315–424.
36. Halliwell B. Free radicals, antioxidants, and human disease: curiosity, cause, or consequence? Lancet. 1994;344(8924):721–4.
37. Lin MT, Beal MF. Mitochondrial dysfunction and oxidative stress in neurodegenerative diseases. Nature. 2006;443(7113):787–95.
38. Rao AV, Rao LG. Carotenoids and human health. Pharmacol Res. 2007;55(3):207–16.
39. Winyard PG, Blake DR. Antioxidants, redox-regulated transcription factors, and inflammation. Adv Pharmacol. 1997;38:403–21.
40. Halliwell B. Role of free radicals in the neurodegenerative diseases: therapeutic implications for antioxidant treatment. Drugs Aging. 2001;18(9):685–716.
41. Greenacre SA, Ischiropoulos H. Tyrosine nitration: localisation, quantification, consequences for protein function and signal transduction. Free Radic Res. 2001;34(6):541–81.
42. Wolin MS, Ahmad M, Gupte SA. Oxidant and redox signaling in vascular oxygen sensing mechanisms: basic concepts, current controversies, and potential importance of cytosolic NADPH. Am J Physiol Lung Cell Mol Physiol. 2005;289(2):L159–73.
43. Dowling DK, Simmons LW. Reactive oxygen species as universal constraints in life-history evolution. Proc Biol Sci. 2009;276(1663):1737–45.
44. Foyer CH, Noctor G. Redox sensing and signalling associated with reactive oxygen in chloroplasts, peroxisomes and mitochondria. Physiol Plant. 2003;119:355–64.
45. Yamamizo C, et al. Rewiring mitogen-activated protein kinase cascade by positive feedback confers potato blight resistance. Plant Physiol. 2006;140(2):681–92.
46. Doke N. Involvement of superoxide anion generation in the hypersensitive response of potato tuber tissue to infection with an incompatible race of Phytophthora infestans and the hyphal wall components. Physiol Plant Pathol. 1983;23:345–57.
47. Kawasaki T, et al. The small GTP-binding protein rac is a regulator of cell death in plants. Proc Natl Acad Sci USA. 1999;96(19):10922–6.
48. Oracz K, et al. ROS production and protein oxidation as a novel mechanism for seed dormancy alleviation. Plant J. 2007;50(3):452–65.
49. Gapper C, Dolan L. Control of plant development by reactive oxygen species. Plant Physiol. 2006;141(2): 341–5.
50. Schopfer P, et al. Evidence that hydroxyl radicals mediate auxin-induced extension growth. Planta. 2002;214(6): 821–8.
51. Schopfer P. Hydroxyl radical-induced cell-wall loosening *in vitro* and *in vivo*: implications for the control of elongation growth. Plant J. 2001;28(6):679–88.
52. Schopfer P, Plachy C, Frahry G. Release of reactive oxygen intermediates (superoxide radicals, hydrogen peroxide, and hydroxyl radicals) and peroxidase in germinating radish seeds controlled by light, gibberellin, and abscisic acid. Plant Physiol. 2001;125(4):1591–602.
53. Kelley EE, et al. Hydrogen peroxide is the major oxidant product of xanthine oxidase. Free Radic Biol Med. 2010;48(4):493–8.
54. Moilanen E, et al. Nitric oxide synthase is expressed in human macrophages during foreign body inflammation. Am J Pathol. 1997;150(3):881–7.

55. Gao X, et al. Role of TNF-alpha-induced reactive oxygen species in endothelial dysfunction during reperfusion injury. Am J Physiol Heart Circ Physiol. 2008;295(6):H2242–9.
56. Gao Y, et al. Preservation of cGMP-induced relaxation of pulmonary veins of fetal lambs exposed to chronic high altitude hypoxia: role of PKG and Rho kinase. Am J Physiol Lung Cell Mol Physiol. 2008;295(5):L889–96.
57. Heitzer T, et al. Increased NAD(P)H oxidase-mediated superoxide production in renovascular hypertension: evidence for an involvement of protein kinase C. Kidney Int. 1999;55(1):252–60.
58. Kasten TP, et al. Potentiation of osteoclast bone-resorption activity by inhibition of nitric oxide synthase. Proc Natl Acad Sci USA. 1994;91(9):3569–73.
59. Brandi ML, et al. Bidirectional regulation of osteoclast function by nitric oxide synthase isoforms. Proc Natl Acad Sci USA. 1995;92(7):2954–8.
60. Huang L, et al. Nitroglycerin enhances proliferation and osteoblastic differentiation in human mesenchymal stem cells via nitric oxide pathway. Acta Pharmacol Sin. 2008;29(5):580–6.
61. Ralston SH, et al. Nitric oxide: a cytokine-induced regulator of bone resorption. J Bone Miner Res. 1995;10(7):1040–9.
62. Taskiran D, et al. Nitric oxide mediates suppression of cartilage proteoglycan synthesis by interleukin-1. Biochem Biophys Res Commun. 1994;200(1):142–8.
63. Jarasch ED, et al. Localization of xanthine oxidase in mammary-gland epithelium and capillary endothelium. Cell. 1981;25(1):67–82.
64. Ozer N, et al. Simple, high-yield purification of xanthine oxidase from bovine milk. J Biochem Biophys Methods. 1999;39(3):153–9.
65. Silanikove N, Shapiro F. Distribution of xanthine oxidase and xanthine dehydrogenase activity in bovine milk: physiological and technological implications. Int Dairy J. 2007;17:1188–94.
66. Weinmann A, et al. Tetrahydrobiopterin is present in high quantity in human milk and has a vasorelaxing effect on newborn rat mesenteric arteries. Pediatr Res. 2011;69(4):325–9.
67. Ufer C, Wang CC. The roles of glutathione peroxidases during embryo development. Front Mol Neurosci. 2011;4:12.
68. Moon HJ, et al. Antioxidants, like coenzyme Q10, selenite, and curcumin, inhibited osteoclast differentiation by suppressing reactive oxygen species generation. Biochem Biophys Res Commun. 2012;418(2):247–53.
69. Antonicelli F, et al. Nacystelyn inhibits oxidant-mediated interleukin-8 expression and NF-kappaB nuclear binding in alveolar epithelial cells. Free Radic Biol Med. 2002;32(6):492–502.
70. Piao S, Cha YN, Kim C. Taurine chloramine protects RAW 264.7 macrophages against hydrogen peroxide-induced apoptosis by increasing antioxidants. J Clin Biochem Nutr. 2011;49(1):50–6.
71. Botting RM. Cyclooxygenase: past, present and future. A tribute to John R. Vane (1927–2004). J Therm Biol. 2006;31:208–19.
72. Simone RE, et al. Lycopene inhibits NF-kB-mediated IL-8 expression and changes redox and PPAR gamma signalling in cigarette smoke-stimulated macrophages. PLoS One. 2011;6(5):e19652.
73. Kim YJ, Kim YA, Yokozawa T. Protection against oxidative stress, inflammation, and apoptosis of high-glucose-exposed proximal tubular epithelial cells by astaxanthin. J Agric Food Chem. 2009;57(19):8793–7.
74. Lesnefsky EJ, et al. Mitochondrial dysfunction in cardiac disease: ischemia–reperfusion, aging, and heart failure. J Mol Cell Cardiol. 2001;33(6):1065–89.
75. Lesnefsky EJ, et al. Hydrogen peroxide decreases effective refractory period in the isolated heart. Free Radic Biol Med. 1991;11(6):529–35.
76. Lenaz G, et al. Mitochondrial respiratory chain super-complex I–III in physiology and pathology. Biochim Biophys Acta. 2010;1797(6–7):633–40.
77. Gryglewski RJ. Prostacyclin among prostanoids. Pharmacol Rep. 2008;60(1):3–11.
78. Hemler ME, Cook HW, Lands WE. Prostaglandin biosynthesis can be triggered by lipid peroxides. Arch Biochem Biophys. 1979;193(2):340–5.
79. Hamberg M, et al. Isolation and structure of two prostaglandin endoperoxides that cause platelet aggregation. Proc Natl Acad Sci USA. 1974;71(2):345–9.
80. Halliwell B, Gutteridge JMC. Free radicals in biology and medicine. 2nd ed. Oxford, UK: Clarendon; 1989.
81. Wrona M, et al. Cooperation of antioxidants in protection against photosensitized oxidation. Free Radic Biol Med. 2003;35(10):1319–29.
82. Wrona M, Rozanowska M, Sarna T. Zeaxanthin in combination with ascorbic acid or alpha-tocopherol protects ARPE-19 cells against photosensitized peroxidation of lipids. Free Radic Biol Med. 2004;36(9):1094–101.
83. Foyer CH, Noctor G. Ascorbate and glutathione: the heart of the redox hub. Plant Physiol. 2011;155(1):2–18.
84. Edge R, et al. Studies of carotenoid one-electron reduction radicals. Arch Biochem Biophys. 2007;458(2):104–10.
85. Mortensen A, Skibsted L, Truscott TG. The interaction of dietary carotenoids with radical species. Arch Biochem Biophys. 2001;385:13–9.
86. Brash DE, Havre PA. New careers for antioxidants. Proc Natl Acad Sci USA. 2002;99(22):13969–71.

87. Stahl W, Sies H. Bioactivity and protective effects of natural carotenoids. Biochim Biophys Acta. 2005;1740(2):101–7.
88. Krinsky NI. Function. In: Isler O, editor. Carotenoids. Basel: Birkhauser; 1971. p. 669–716.
89. Krinsky NI, Johnson EJ. Carotenoid actions and their relation to health and disease. Mol Aspects Med. 2005;26(6):459–516.
90. Brown L, et al. A prospective study of carotenoids intake and risk of cataract extraction in US men. Am J Clin Nutr. 1999;70:517–24.
91. Chasan-Taber L, et al. A prospective study of carotenoid and vitamin A intakes and risk of cataract extraction in US women. Am J Clin Nutr. 1999;70:509–16.
92. Seddon JM, Cote J, Rosner B. Progression of age-related macular degeneration: association with dietary fat, trans unsaturated fat, nuts, and fish intake. Arch Ophthalmol. 2003;121(12):1728–37.
93. Tang XH, Gudas LJ. Retinoids, retinoic acid receptors, and cancer. Annu Rev Pathol. 2011;6:345–64.
94. Aust O, et al. Lycopene oxidation product enhances gap junctional communication. Food Chem Toxicol. 2003;41(10):1399–407.
95. Bowen P. Lycopene oxidation, uptake, and activity in human prostate cell cultures. In: Landrum JT, editor. Carotenoids: physical, chemical, and biological functions and properties. Boca Raton: CRC; 2010. p. 437–64.
96. Harrison EH. Mechanisms of intestinal absorption of carotenoids: insights from *in vitro* systems. In: Landrum JT, editor. Carotenoids: physical chemical and biological functions and properties. Boca Raton: CRC; 2010. p. 367–79.
97. Sparrow J, Kim SR. The carotenoids of macular pigment and bisretinoid lipfuscin precursors in photoreceptor outer segments. In: Landrum JT, editor. Carotenoids: physical, chemical and biological functions and properties. Boca Raton: CRC; 2010. p. 355–63.
98. Baroli I, et al. Zeaxanthin accumulation in the absence of a functional xanthophyll cycle protects *Chlamydomonas reinhardtii* from photooxidative stress. Plant Cell. 2003;15(4):992–1008.
99. Britton G, Liaaen-Jensen S, Pfander H, editors. Handbook of carotenoids. Basel: Birkhauser; 2004. p. 670.
100. Frank HA, et al. Carotenoids in photosynthesis: structure and photochemistry. Pure Appl Chem. 1991;63:109–14.
101. Britton G. The biochemistry of natural pigments. Cambridge: Cambridge University Press; 1983.
102. McGraw KJ, Blount J. Control and function of carotenoid coloration in birds: selected case studies. In: Landrum JT, editor. carotenoids: physical, chemical, and biological functions and properties. Boca Raton: CRC; 2010. p. 487–510.
103. Schiedt K. New aspects of carotenoid metabolism in animals. Carotenoids: chemistry and biology. New York: Plenum; 1990. p. 247–68.
104. Brush AH. Carotenoids in wild and captive birds. In: Bauernfeind JC, editor. Carotenoids as colorants and vitamin A precursors. New York: Academic; 1981. p. 539–62.
105. Schiedt K. Absorption and metabolism of carotenoids in birds, fish and crustaceans. In: Britton G, Liaaen-Jensen S, Pfander H, editors. Biosynthesis and metabolism. Basel: Birkhauser; 1998. p. 285–358.
106. Landrum JT, Callejas D, Alvarez-Calderon F. Specific accumulation of lutein within the epidermis of butterfly larvae. In: Landrum JT, editor. Carotenoids: physical, chemical, and biological functions and properties. Boca Raton: CRC; 2010. p. 525–35.
107. Kotake-Nara E, Nagao A. Absorption and metabolism of xanthophylls. Mar Drugs. 2011;9(6):1024–37.
108. Chaudiere J, Ferrari-Iliou R. Intracellular antioxidants: from chemical to biochemical mechanisms. Food Chem Toxicol. 1999;37(9–10):949–62.
109. Mares-Perlman JA, et al. Serum carotenoids and tocopherols and severity of nuclear and cortical opacities. Invest Ophthalmol Vis Sci. 1995;36:276–88.
110. Burton GW, Joyce A, Ingold KU. Is vitamin E the only lipid-soluble, chain-breaking antioxidant in human blood plasma and erythrocyte membranes? Arch Biochem Biophys. 1983;221(1):281–90.
111. Ruban AV, Johnson MP. Xanthophylls as modulators of membrane protein function. Arch Biochem Biophys. 2010;504(1):78–85.
112. Betterle N, et al. Dynamics of zeaxanthin binding to the photosystem II monomeric antenna protein Lhcb6 (CP24) and modulation of its photoprotection properties. Arch Biochem Biophys. 2010;504(1):67–77.
113. Krinsky NI. Singlet oxygen in biological systems. Trends Biochem Sci. 1977;2:35–8.
114. Stahl W, Sies H. Carotenoids in systematic protection against sunburn. In: Krinsky NI, Mayne ST, Sies H, editors. Carotenoids in health and disease. New York: Marcel Dekker; 2004. p. 491–502.
115. Mathews-Roth M. Techniques for studying photoprotective function of carotenoid pigments. In: Packer L, editor. Methods enzymol. New York: Academic; 1992. p. 479–84.
116. Mathews-Roth MM. Beta-carotene therapy for erythropoietic protoporphyria and other photosensitivity diseases. Biochimie. 1986;68(6):875–84.
117. Mathews-Roth MM. Treatment of the cutaneous porphyrias. Clin Dermatol. 1998;16(2):295–8.
118. Wingerath T, Sies H, Stahl W. Xanthophyll esters in human skin. Arch Biochem Biophys. 1998;355(2):271–4.

119. Mathews-Roth MM. Photoprotection by carotenoids. J Ethnopharmacol. 1988;22:315.
120. Roberts RL, Green J, Lewis B. Lutein and zeaxanthin in eye and skin health. Clin Dermatol. 2009;27(2): 195–201.
121. Liu A, et al. Absorption and subcellular localization of lycopene in human prostate cancer cells. Mol Cancer Ther. 2006;5(11):2879–85.
122. Lademann J, et al. Carotenoids in human skin. Exp Dermatol. 2011;20(5):377–82.
123. Nishino H, et al. Cancer prevention by carotenoids. Arch Biochem Biophys. 2009;483(2):165–8.
124. Burton GW. Antioxidant action of carotenoids. J Nutr. 1989;119(1):109–11.
125. Burton GW, Ingold KU. β-Carotene: an unusual type of lipid antioxidant. Science. 1984;224:569–73.
126. Beutner S, et al. Quantitative assessment of antioxidant properties of natural colorants and phytochemicals: carotenoids, flavonoids, phenols and indigoid. The role of β-carotene in antioxidant functions. J Sci Food Agric. 2001;81:559–68.
127. Lowe GM, Vlismas K, Young AJ. Carotenoids as prooxidants? Mol Aspects Med. 2003;24(6):363–9.
128. Blumberg J, Block G. The alpha-tocopherol, beta-carotene cancer prevention study in Finland. Nutr Rev. 1994;52(7):242–5.
129. Albanes D, et al. Alpha-Tocopherol and beta-carotene supplements and lung cancer incidence in the alpha-tocopherol, beta-carotene cancer prevention study: effects of base-line characteristics and study compliance. J Natl Cancer Inst. 1996;88(21):1560–70.
130. Omenn GS, et al. The carotene and retinol efficacy trial (CARET) to prevent lung cancer in high-risk populations: pilot study with asbestos-exposed workers. Cancer Epidemiol Biomarkers Prev. 1993;2(4):381–7.
131. Wang XD, et al. Retinoid signaling and activator protein-1 expression in ferrets given beta-carotene supplements and exposed to tobacco smoke. J Natl Cancer Inst. 1999;91(1):60–6.
132. Linnewiel K, et al. Structure activity relationship of carotenoid derivatives in activation of the electrophile/antioxidant response element transcription system. Free Radic Biol Med. 2009;47(5):659–67.
133. Sharoni AM, et al. Comparative transcriptome analysis of AP2/EREBP gene family under normal and hormone treatments, and under two drought stresses in NILs setup by Aday Selection and IR64. Mol Genet Genomics. 2012;287(1):1–19.
134. Sharoni Y, et al. Carotenoids and apocarotenoids in cellular signaling related to cancer: a review. Mol Nutr Food Res. 2012;56(2):259–69.
135. Paolini M, et al. Induction of cytochrome P450 enzymes and over-generation of oxygen radicals in beta-carotene supplemented rats. Carcinogenesis. 2001;22(9):1483–95.
136. Goodwin TW. Carotenoids their comparative biochemistry. New York: Chemical Publishing Co. Inc; 1954. p. 356.
137. Landrum JT, Bone RA. Lutein, zeaxanthin, and the macular pigment. Arch Biochem Biophys. 2001;385:28–40.
138. Krinsky NI, Landrum JT, Bone RA. Biologic mechanisms of the protective role of lutein and zeaxanthin in the eye. Annu Rev Nutr. 2003;23:171–201.
139. Schalch W, Bone RA, Landrum JT. The functional role of xanthophylls in primate retina. In: Landrum JT, editor. Carotenoids: physical, chemical and biological functions and properties. Boca Raton: CRC; 2010. p. 257–82.
140. Palozza P, Calviello G, Bartoli GM. Prooxidant activity of beta-carotene under 100 % oxygen pressure in rat liver microsomes. Free Radic Biol Med. 1995;19(6):887–92.
141. Lobo GP, et al. Mammalian carotenoid-oxygenases: key players for carotenoid function and homeostasis. Biochim Biophys Acta. 2012;1821(1):78–87.
142. Kiefer C, et al. Identification and characterization of a mammalian enzyme catalyzing the asymmetric oxidative cleavage of provitamin A. J Biol Chem. 2001;276(17):14110–6.
143. Prakash P, et al. Beta-carotene and beta-apo-14′-carotenoic acid prevent the reduction of retinoic acid receptor beta in benzo[a]pyrene-treated normal human bronchial epithelial cells. J Nutr. 2004;134(3):667–73.
144. Mik EG, et al. Quantitative determination of localized tissue oxygen concentration *in vivo* by two-photon excitation phosphorescence lifetime measurements. J Appl Physiol. 2004;97(5):1962–9.
145. Meyron-Holtz EG, Ghosh MC, Rouault TA. Mammalian tissue oxygen levels modulate iron-regulatory protein activities *in vivo*. Science. 2004;306(5704):2087–90.
146. Yu DY, Cringle SJ. Oxygen distribution and consumption within the retina in vascularised and avascular retinas and in animal models of retinal disease. Prog Retin Eye Res. 2001;20(2):175–208.
147. Steinbeck MJ, Khan AU, Karnovsky MJ. Intracellular singlet oxygen generation by phagocytosing neutrophils in response to particles coated with a chemical trap. J Biol Chem. 1992;267(19):13425–33.
148. Min DB. Chemistry and reaction of singlet oxygen in foods. Compr Rev Food Sci Food Saf. 2002;1:58–72.
149. Landrum JT, Bone RA. Mechanistic evidence for eye diseases and carotenoids. In: Krinsky NI, Mayne ST, Sies H, editors. Carotenoids in health and disease. New York: Marcel Dekker; 2004. p. 445–72.
150. Barker II FM, et al. Nutritional manipulation of primate retinas. V: Effects of lutein, zeaxanthin, and n-3 fatty acids on retinal sensitivity to blue-light-induced damage. Invest Ophthalmol Vis Sci. 2011;52(7):3934–42.
151. Cunningham ML, et al. Superoxide anion is generated from cellular metabolites by solar radiation and its components. J Free Radic Biol Med. 1985;1(5–6):381–5.

152. Gao Q, Wolin MS. Effects of hypoxia on relationships between cytosolic and mitochondrial NAD(P)H redox and superoxide generation in coronary arterial smooth muscle. Am J Physiol Heart Circ Physiol. 2008;295(3):H978–89.
153. Grivennikova VG, Vinogradov AD. Generation of superoxide by the mitochondrial Complex I. Biochim Biophys Acta. 2006;1757(5–6):553–61.
154. Sawyer DT, Valentine JS. How super is superoxide? Acc Chem Res. 1981;14:393–400.
155. Kramer ML, et al. Prion protein binds copper within the physiological concentration range. J Biol Chem. 2001;276(20):16711–9.
156. Neumann PZ, Sass-Kortsak A. The state of copper in human serum: evidence for an amino acid-bound fraction. J Clin Invest. 1967;46(4):646–58.
157. Halliwell B, Gutteridge JM. Oxygen toxicity, oxygen radicals, transition metals and disease. Biochem J. 1984;219(1):1–14.
158. Koster JF, Slee RG. Ferritin, a physiological iron donor for microsomal lipid peroxidation. FEBS Lett. 1986;199(1):85–8.
159. Eiserich JP, et al. Formation of nitrating and chlorinating species by reaction of nitrite with hypochlorous acid. A novel mechanism for nitric oxide-mediated protein modification. J Biol Chem. 1996;271(32):19199–208.
160. Halliwell B, Wasil M, Grootveld M. Biologically significant scavenging of the myeloperoxidase-derived oxidant hypochlorous acid by ascorbic acid. Implications for antioxidant protection in the inflamed rheumatoid joint. FEBS Lett. 1987;213(1):15–7.
161. Pierre JL, Fontecave M. Iron and activated oxygen species in biology: the basic chemistry. Biometals. 1999;12(3): 195–9.
162. Wardman P, Candeias LP. Fenton chemistry: an introduction. Radiat Res. 1996;145(5):523–31.
163. Ho YS, et al. Mice lacking catalase develop normally but show differential sensitivity to oxidant tissue injury. J Biol Chem. 2004;279(31):32804–12.
164. Beckman JS. Oxidative damage and tyrosine nitration from peroxynitrite. Chem Res Toxicol. 1996;9(5):836–44.
165. Koppenol WH. The Haber-Weiss cycle—70 years later. Redox Rep. 2001;6(4):229–34.
166. Moncada S, Higgs A. The L-arginine-nitric oxide pathway. N Engl J Med. 1993;329(27):2002–12.
167. Gutteridge JM, Halliwell B. Free radicals and antioxidants in the year 2000. A historical look to the future. Ann N Y Acad Sci. 2000;899:136–47.
168. Gold V, Hughes ED, Ingold CK. (1950) Kinetics and mechanism of aromatic nitration. Part V. Nitration by acyl nitrates, particularly benzoyl nitrate. J Chem Soc. 1950;2467–73.
169. Pryor WA, et al. Free radical biology and medicine: it's a gas, man! Am J Physiol Regul Integr Comp Physiol. 2006;291(3):R491–511.
170. Tompkins AJ, et al. Mitochondrial dysfunction in cardiac ischemia-reperfusion injury: ROS from complex I, without inhibition. Biochim Biophys Acta. 2006;1762(2):223–31.
171. Hutchinson F. The distance that a radical formed by ionizing radiation can diffuse in a yeast cell. Radiat Res. 1957;7(5):473–83.
172. Roots R, Okada S. Estimation of life times and diffusion distances of radicals involved in x-ray-induced DNA strand breaks of killing of mammalian cells. Radiat Res. 1975;64(2):306–20.
173. Thomas DD, et al. The biological lifetime of nitric oxide: implications for the perivascular dynamics of NO and O_2. Proc Natl Acad Sci USA. 2001;98(1):355–60.
174. Ford E, Hughes MN, Wardman P. Kinetics of the reactions of nitrogen dioxide with glutathione, cysteine, and uric acid at physiological pH. Free Radic Biol Med. 2002;32(12):1314–23.
175. Forni L, Bahnemann D, Hart EJ. Mechanism of the hydroxide ion-initiated decomposition of ozone in aqueous solution. J Phys Chem. 1982;86:255–9.
176. Dringen R, Hamprecht B. Involvement of glutathione peroxidase and catalase in the disposal of exogenous hydrogen peroxide by cultured astroglial cells. Brain Res. 1997;759(1):67–75.
177. Sies H, Krinsky NI. The present status of antioxidant vitamins and beta-carotene. Am J Clin Nutr. 1995;62(6 Suppl):1299S–300.
178. Svingen BA, Powis G. Pulse radiolysis studies of antitumor quinones: radical lifetimes, reactivity with oxygen, and one-electron reduction potentials. Arch Biochem Biophys. 1981;209(1):119–26.
179. Pryor WA, et al. The radicals in cigarette tar: their nature and suggested physiological implications. Science. 1983;220(4595):425–7.
180. Deng Y, et al. Effects of polyene chain length and acceptor substituents on the stability of carotenoid radical cations. J Phys Chem B. 2000;104:5651–6.
181. Khaled M, Hadjipetrou A, Kispert L. Electrochemical and electron paramagnetic resonance studies of carotenoid cation radicals and dications: effect of deuteration. J Phys Chem. 1990;94:5164–9.
182. Kim SR, et al. Mechanisms involved in A2E oxidation. Exp Eye Res. 2008;86(6):975–82.
183. Sparrow JR, Boulton M. RPE lipofuscin and its role in retinal pathobiology. Exp Eye Res. 2005;80(5):595–606.

184. Kim SR, et al. Photooxidation of A2-PE, a photoreceptor outer segment fluorophore, and protection by lutein and zeaxanthin. Exp Eye Res. 2006;82(5):828–39.
185. Redmond RW, Gamlin JN. A compilation of singlet oxygen yields from biologically relevant molecules. Photochem Photobiol. 1999;70(4):391–475.
186. Harvey JN. Understanding the kinetics of spin-forbidden chemical reactions. Phys Chem Chem Phys. 2007;9(3): 331–43.
187. Khan AU, Kasha M. Singlet molecular oxygen in the Haber-Weiss reaction. Proc Natl Acad Sci USA. 1994;91(26):12365–7.
188. Di Mascio P, et al. Singlet molecular oxygen production in the reaction of peroxynitrite with hydrogen peroxide. FEBS Lett. 1994;355(3):287–9.
189. Martinez GR, et al. Peroxynitrite does not decompose to singlet oxygen ((1)Delta (g)O(2)) and nitroxyl (NO(-)). Proc Natl Acad Sci USA. 2000;97(19):10307–12.
190. Miyamoto S, et al. Direct evidence of singlet molecular oxygen generation from peroxynitrate, a decomposition product of peroxynitrite. Dalton Trans. 2009;29:5720–9.
191. Pfeiffer S, et al. Metabolic fate of peroxynitrite in aqueous solution. Reaction with nitric oxide and pH-dependent decomposition to nitrite and oxygen in a 2:1 stoichiometry. J Biol Chem. 1997;272(6):3465–70.
192. Gunston FD. Chemical properties. In: Gunston FD, Harwood JL, Padley FB, editors. The lipid handbook. New York: Chapman and Hill; 1986. p. 449–84.
193. Hayashi S, Yasui H, Sakurai H. Essential role of singlet oxygen species in cytochrome P450-dependent substrate oxygenation by rat liver microsomes. Drug Metab Pharmacokinet. 2005;20(1):14–23.
194. Kerver ED, et al. *In situ* detection of spontaneous superoxide anion and singlet oxygen production by mitochondria in rat liver and small intestine. Histochem J. 1997;29(3):229–37.
195. Gaeta LM, et al. Determination of superoxide dismutase and glutathione peroxidase activities in blood of healthy pediatric subjects. Clin Chim Acta. 2002;322(1–2):117–20.
196. Ono T, et al. Xanthine oxidase is one of the major sources of superoxide anion radicals in blood after reperfusion in rats with forebrain ischemia/reperfusion. Brain Res. 2009;1305:158–67.
197. Furtmuller PG, et al. Mechanism of reaction of myeloperoxidase with hydrogen peroxide and chloride ion. Eur J Biochem. 2000;267(19):5858–64.
198. Reeves EP, et al. Killing activity of neutrophils is mediated through activation of proteases by K^+ flux. Nature. 2002;416(6878):291–7.
199. Zhao W, et al. Effect of carotenoids on the respiratory burst of rat peritoneal macrophages. Biochim Biophys Acta. 1998;1381(1):77–88.
200. Fridovich I. Hypoxia and oxygen toxicity. Adv Neurol. 1979;26:255–9.
201. Fox NE, van Kuijk FJ. Immunohistochemical localization of xanthine oxidase in human retina. Free Radic Biol Med. 1998;24(6):900–5.
202. Tapner MJ, et al. Toxicity of low dose azathioprine and 6-mercaptopurine in rat hepatocytes. Roles of xanthine oxidase and mitochondrial injury. J Hepatol. 2004;40(3):454–63.
203. Gladden JD, et al. Novel insights into interactions between mitochondria and xanthine oxidase in acute cardiac volume overload. Free Radic Biol Med. 2011;51(11):1975–84.
204. Li ZY, et al. Mitochondrial ROS generation for regulation of autophagic pathways in cancer. Biochem Biophys Res Commun. 2011;414(1):5–8.
205. Richter C, Park JW, Ames BN. Normal oxidative damage to mitochondrial and nuclear DNA is extensive. Proc Natl Acad Sci USA. 1988;85(17):6465–7.
206. Chance B, Sies H, Boveris A. Hydroperoxide metabolism in mammalian organs. Physiol Rev. 1979;59(3): 527–605.
207. Lesnefsky EJ, et al. Mitochondrial electron transport and aging in the heart. Adv Cell Aging Gerontol. 2002;11: 201–32.
208. Lo SC, Hannink M. PGAM5 tethers a ternary complex containing Keap1 and Nrf2 to mitochondria. Exp Cell Res. 2008;314(8):1789–803.
209. Cao X, et al. Structures of the G85R variant of SOD1 in familial amyotrophic lateral sclerosis. J Biol Chem. 2008;283(23):16169–77.
210. Lee HP, et al. Early induction of oxidative stress in mouse model of Alzheimer disease with reduced mitochondrial superoxide dismutase activity. PLoS One. 2012;7(1):e28033.
211. Okado-Matsumoto A, Fridovich I. Subcellular distribution of superoxide dismutases (SOD) in rat liver: Cu, Zn-SOD in mitochondria. J Biol Chem. 2001;276(42):38388–93.
212. Miao L, St Clair DK. Regulation of superoxide dismutase genes: implications in disease. Free Radic Biol Med. 2009;47(4):344–56.
213. Ardan T, Kovaceva J, Cejkova J. Comparative histochemical and immunohistochemical study on xanthine oxidoreductase/xanthine oxidase in mammalian corneal epithelium. Acta Histochem. 2004;106(1):69–75.

214. Deliconstantinos G, Villiotou V, Stavrides JC. Alterations of nitric oxide synthase and xanthine oxidase activities of human keratinocytes by ultraviolet B radiation. Potential role for peroxynitrite in skin inflammation. Biochem Pharmacol. 1996;51(12):1727–38.
215. Lalanne M, Willemot J. Xanthine oxidase from mouse skeletal muscle purification and kinetic studies. Int J Biochem. 1975;6:479–84.
216. Khoury W, et al. Mannitol attenuates kidney damage induced by xanthine oxidase-associated pancreas ischemia-reperfusion. J Surg Res. 2010;160(1):163–8.
217. Heinrich P, Löffler G, Petrides PE. Biochemie und Pathobiochemie. 8th ed. Berlin: Springer-Lehrbuch; 2007.
218. Mao GD, Poznansky MJ. Electron spin resonance study on the permeability of superoxide radicals in lipid bilayers and biological membranes. FEBS Lett. 1992;305(3):233–6.
219. De Grey AD. HO_2*: the forgotten radical. DNA Cell Biol. 2002;21(4):251–7.
220. Winston GW, et al. Production of reactive oxygen species by hemocytes from the marine mussel, *Mytilus edulis*: lysosomal localization and effect of xenobiotics. Comp Biochem Physiol C Pharmacol Toxicol Endocrinol. 1996;113(2):221–9.
221. Kubota C, et al. Constitutive reactive oxygen species generation from autophagosome/lysosome in neuronal oxidative toxicity. J Biol Chem. 2010;285(1):667–74.
222. Denamur S, et al. Role of oxidative stress in lysosomal membrane permeabilization and apoptosis induced by gentamicin, an aminoglycoside antibiotic. Free Radic Biol Med. 2011;51(9):1656–65.
223. Wood ZA, Poole LB, Karplus PA. Peroxiredoxin evolution and the regulation of hydrogen peroxide signaling. Science. 2003;300(5619):650–3.
224. Taylor L, Menconi MJ, Polgar P. The participation of hydroperoxides and oxygen radicals in the control of prostaglandin synthesis. J Biol Chem. 1983;258(11):6855–7.
225. Singh AK, et al. Structural evidence for the order of preference of inorganic substrates in mammalian heme peroxidases: crystal structure of the complex of lactoperoxidase with four inorganic substrates, SCN, I, Br and Cl. Int J Biochem Mol Biol. 2011;2(4):328–39.
226. Toppo S, et al. Catalytic mechanisms and specificities of glutathione peroxidases: variations of a basic scheme. Biochim Biophys Acta. 2009;1790(11):1486–500.
227. Brigelius-Flohe R. Tissue-specific functions of individual glutathione peroxidases. Free Radic Biol Med. 1999;27(9–10):951–65.
228. Freinbichler W, et al. The detection of hydroxyl radicals *in vivo*. J Inorg Biochem. 2008;102(5–6):1329–33.
229. Gutteridge JM. Reactivity of hydroxyl and hydroxyl-like radicals discriminated by release of thiobarbituric acid-reactive material from deoxy sugars, nucleosides and benzoate. Biochem J. 1984;224(3):761–7.
230. Chapman AL, et al. Chlorination of bacterial and neutrophil proteins during phagocytosis and killing of *Staphylococcus aureus*. J Biol Chem. 2002;277(12):9757–62.
231. Costa D, et al. Hydrogen peroxide scavenging activity by non-steroidal anti-inflammatory drugs. Life Sci. 2005;76(24):2841–8.
232. Halliwell B. Antioxidants: the basics—What they are and how to evaluate them. In: Sies H, editor. Antioxidants in disease: mechanisms and therapy. San Diego: Academic; 1997. p. 3–17.
233. Edge R, Truscott TG. Properties of carotenoid radicals and excited states and their potential role in biological systems. In: Landrum JT, editor. Carotenoids: physical, chemical, and biological functions and properties. Boca Raton: CRC; 2010. p. 283–307.
234. Ouedraogo GD, Redmond RW. Secondary reactive oxygen species extend the range of photosensitization effects in cells: DNA damage produced via initial membrane photosensitization. Photochem Photobiol. 2003;77(2): 192–203.
235. Sies H, Stahl W. Vitamins E and C, beta-carotene, and other carotenoids as antioxidants. Am J Clin Nutr. 1995;62(6 Suppl):1315S–21.
236. El-Agamey A, McGarvey DJ. Evidence for a lack of reactivity of carotenoid addition radicals towards oxygen: a laser flash photolysis study of the reactions of carotenoids with acylperoxyl radicals in polar and non-polar solvents. J Am Chem Soc. 2003;125(11):3330–40.
237. Halliwell B. Oxygen and nitrogen are pro-carcinogens. Damage to DNA by reactive oxygen, chlorine and nitrogen species: measurement, mechanism and the effects of nutrition. Mutat Res. 1999;443(1–2):37–52.
238. Hollenberg PF, Rand-Meir T, Hager LP. The reaction of chlorite with horseradish peroxidase and chloroperoxidase. Enzymatic chlorination and spectral intermediates. J Biol Chem. 1974;249(18):5816–25.
239. Hawkins CL, Davies MJ. Hypochlorite-induced damage to proteins: formation of nitrogen-centered radicals from lysine residues and their role in protein fragmentation. Biochem J. 1998;332(Pt 3):617–25.
240. Martin W, Robert F. Furchgott, Nobel laureate (1916–2009)—a personal reflection. Br J Pharmacol. 2009;158(3):633–7.
241. Furchgott RF. Nitric oxide: from basic research on isolated blood vessels to clinical relevance in diabetes. An R Acad Nac Med (Madr). 1998;115(2):317–31.

242. Furchgott RF, Zawadzki JV. The obligatory role of endothelial cells in the relaxation of arterial smooth muscle by acetylcholine. Nature. 1980;288(5789):373–6.
243. Palmer RM, Ferrige AG, Moncada S. Nitric oxide release accounts for the biological activity of endothelium-derived relaxing factor. Nature. 1987;327(6122):524–6.
244. Ignarro LJ, et al. Endothelium-derived relaxing factor produced and released from artery and vein is nitric oxide. Proc Natl Acad Sci USA. 1987;84(24):9265–9.
245. Xu W, et al. Mapping of the genes encoding human inducible and endothelial nitric oxide synthase (NOS2 and NOS3) to the pericentric region of chromosome 17 and to chromosome 7, respectively. Genomics. 1994;21(2):419–22.
246. Brennan PA, Moncada S. From pollutant gas to biological messenger: the diverse actions of nitric oxide in cancer. Ann R Coll Surg Engl. 2002;84(2):75–8.
247. Gusarov I, Nudler E. NO-mediated cytoprotection: instant adaptation to oxidative stress in bacteria. Proc Natl Acad Sci USA. 2005;102(39):13855–60.
248. Gusarov I, et al. Endogenous nitric oxide protects bacteria against a wide spectrum of antibiotics. Science. 2009;325(5946):1380–4.
249. Kohanski MA, et al. A common mechanism of cellular death induced by bactericidal antibiotics. Cell. 2007;130(5):797–810.
250. Liu GY, et al. *Staphylococcus aureus* golden pigment impairs neutrophil killing and promotes virulence through its antioxidant activity. J Exp Med. 2005;202(2):209–15.
251. Vallance P, Chan N. Endothelial function and nitric oxide: clinical relevance. Heart. 2001;85(3):342–50.
252. Lai YL, et al. Inhibition of endothelial- and neuronal-type, but not inducible-type, nitric oxide synthase by the oxidized cholesterol metabolite secosterol aldehyde: implications for vascular and neurodegenerative diseases. J Clin Biochem Nutr. 2012;50(1):84–9.
253. Steinert JR, et al. Nitric oxide is an activity-dependent regulator of target neuron intrinsic excitability. Neuron. 2011;71(2):291–305.
254. Cotton FA, Wilkinson G. Advanced inorganic chemistry. 5th ed. New York: Wiley. A Wiley-Interscience publication; 1988. p. xvii, 1455.
255. Squadrito GL, Pryor WA. Oxidative chemistry of nitric oxide: the roles of superoxide, peroxynitrite, and carbon dioxide. Free Radic Biol Med. 1998;25(4–5):392–403.
256. Augusto O, et al. Nitrogen dioxide and carbonate radical anion: two emerging radicals in biology. Free Radic Biol Med. 2002;32(9):841–59.
257. Wattanapitayakul SK, et al. Endothelial dysfunction and peroxynitrite formation are early events in angiotensin-induced cardiovascular disorders. FASEB J. 2000;14(2):271–8.
258. Estevez AG, Jordan J. Nitric oxide and superoxide, a deadly cocktail. Ann N Y Acad Sci. 2002;962:207–11.
259. Santos CX, Bonini MG, Augusto O. Role of the carbonate radical anion in tyrosine nitration and hydroxylation by peroxynitrite. Arch Biochem Biophys. 2000;377(1):146–52.
260. Shafirovich V, et al. The carbonate radical is a site-selective oxidizing agent of guanine in double-stranded oligonucleotides. J Biol Chem. 2001;276(27):24621–6.
261. Halliwell B, Zhao K, Whiteman M. Nitric oxide and peroxynitrite. The ugly, the uglier and the not so good: a personal view of recent controversies. Free Radic Res. 1999;31(6):651–69.
262. Miki W. Biological functions and activities of animal carotenoids. Pure Appl Chem. 1991;63:141–6.
263. Lee DH, Kim CS, Lee YJ. Astaxanthin protects against MPTP/MPP+-induced mitochondrial dysfunction and ROS production *in vivo* and *in vitro*. Food Chem Toxicol. 2011;49(1):271–80.
264. Cardounel AJ, et al. Direct superoxide anion scavenging by a disodium disuccinate astaxanthin derivative: relative efficacy of individual stereoisomers versus the statistical mixture of stereoisomers by electron paramagnetic resonance imaging. Biochem Biophys Res Commun. 2003;307(3):704–12.
265. Jackson HL, et al. Synthesis, characterization, and direct aqueous superoxide anion scavenging of a highly water-dispersible astaxanthin-amino acid conjugate. Bioorg Med Chem Lett. 2004;14(15):3985–91.
266. Otton R, et al. Astaxanthin ameliorates the redox imbalance in lymphocytes of experimental diabetic rats. Chem Biol Interact. 2010;186(3):306–15.
267. Yonekura L, et al. Keto-carotenoids are the major metabolites of dietary lutein and fucoxanthin in mouse tissues. J Nutr. 2010;140(10):1824–31.
268. Nadolski G, et al. The synthesis and aqueous superoxide anion scavenging of water-dispersible lutein esters. Bioorg Med Chem Lett. 2006;16(4):775–81.
269. Pitt GAJ. Vitamin A. In: Isler O, editor. Carotenoids. Basek: Birkhauser; 1971. p. 717–42.
270. Karrer P, Morf R, Schopp K. Zur Kenntnis des Vitamins-A aus Fischtranen II. Helv Chim Acta. 1931;14:1036.
271. Krinsky NI. Carotenoids in medicine. In: Krinsky NI, Mathews-Roth MM, Taylor RF, editors. Carotenoids: chemistry and biology. New York: Plenum; 1987. p. 279–91.
272. Sies H, Stahl W. Non-nutritive bioactive constituents of plants: lycopene, lutein and zeaxanthin. Int J Vitam Nutr Res. 2003;73(2):95–100.

273. Bertram JS, et al. Diverse carotenoids protect against chemically induced neoplastic transformation. Carcinogenesis. 1991;12(4):671–8.
274. Bone RA, et al. Macular pigment in donor eyes with and without AMD: a case-control study. Invest Ophthalmol Vis Sci. 2001;42:235–40.
275. Bone RA, Landrum JT, Tarsis SL. Preliminary identification of the human macular pigment. Vision Res. 1985;25:1531–5.
276. Handelman GJ, et al. Carotenoids in the human macula and whole retina. Invest Ophthalmol Vis Sci. 1988;29:850–5.
277. Bone RA, et al. Analysis of the macular pigment by HPLC: retinal distribution and age study. Invest Ophthalmol Vis Sci. 1988;29:843–9.
278. Kotake-Nara E, et al. Carotenoids affect proliferation of human prostate cancer cells. J Nutr. 2001;131(12):3303–6.
279. Nishino H, et al. Cancer prevention by natural carotenoids. Biofactors. 2000;13(1–4):89–94.
280. Sugawara T, et al. Brown algae fucoxanthin is hydrolyzed to fucoxanthinol during absorption by Caco-2 human intestinal cells and mice. J Nutr. 2002;132(5):946–51.
281. Yoshiko S, Hoyoku N. Fucoxanthin, a natural carotenoid, induces G1 arrest and GADD45 gene expression in human cancer cells. *In Vivo*. 2007;21(2):305–9.
282. Palozza P, Krinsky NI. Astaxanthin and canthaxanthin are potent antioxidants in a membrane model. Arch Biochem Biophys. 1992;297(2):291–5.
283. Liu C, et al. beta-Cryptoxanthin supplementation prevents cigarette smoke-induced lung inflammation, oxidative damage, and squamous metaplasia in ferrets. Cancer Prev Res (Phila). 2011;4(8):1255–66.
284. Bone RA, et al. Distribution of lutein and zeaxanthin stereoisomers in the human retina. Exp Eye Res. 1997;64:211–8.
285. Landrum JT, Bone RA, Herrero C. Astaxanthin, β-carotene, lutein, and zeaxanthin. In: Meskin MS et al., editors. Phytochemicals in nutrition and health. Boca Raton: CRC; 2002. p. 173–91.
286. DeRosa MC, Crutchley RJ. Photosensitized singlet oxygen and its applications. Coord Chem Rev. 2002;233–234:351–71.
287. Foote CS, Chang YC, Denny RW. Chemistry of singlet oxygen. X. Carotenoid quenching parallels biological protection. J Am Chem Soc. 1970;92:5216–8.
288. Crank G, Pardijanto MS. Photo-oxidations and photosensitized oxidations of vitamin A and its palmitate ester. J Photochem Photobiol A Chem. 1995;85:93–100.
289. Foote CS, Denny RW. Chemistry of singlet oxygen. VII. Quenching by β-carotene. J Am Chem Soc. 1968;90:6233–5.
290. Johnson MP, Zia A, Ruban AV. Elevated ΔpH restores rapidly reversible photoprotective energy dissipation in Arabidopsis chloroplasts deficient in lutein and xanthophyll cycle activity. Planta. 2012;235(1):193–204.
291. Alaluf S, et al. Dietary carotenoids contribute to normal human skin color and UV photosensitivity. J Nutr. 2002;132(3):399–403.
292. Snodderly DM, Auron JD, Delori FC. The macular pigment. II. Spatial distribution in primate retinas. Invest Ophthalmol Vis Sci. 1984;25:674–85.
293. Landrum JT, et al. A one year study of the macular pigment: the effect of 140 days of a lutein supplement. Exp Eye Res. 1997;65:57–62.
294. Reboul E, Borel P. Proteins involved in uptake, intracellular transport and basolateral secretion of fat-soluble vitamins and carotenoids by mammalian enterocytes. Prog Lipid Res. 2011;50(4):388–402.
295. Harrison EH. Mechanisms involved in the intestinal absorption of dietary vitamin A and provitamin A carotenoids. Biochim Biophys Acta. 2012;1821(1):70–7.
296. Clevidence BA, Bieri JG. Association of carotenoids with human plasma carotenoids. In: Packer L, editor. Methods Enzymol. San Diego: Academic; 1993. p. 33–46.
297. Bhosale P, et al. Identification and characterization of a pi isoform of glutathione S-transferase (GSTP1) as a zeaxanthin-binding protein in the macula of the human eye. J Biol Chem. 2004;47:49447–54.
298. Ruban AV. Identification of carotenoid in photosyntheic proteins: xanthophylls of the light harvesting antenna. In: Landrum JT, editor. Carotenoids: physical, chemical and biological functions and properties. Boca Raton: CRC; 2010. p. 113–36.
299. Yeum K-J, et al. Fat-soluble nutrient concentrations in different layers of human cataractous lens. Curr Eye Res. 1999;19:502–5.
300. Yeum K-J, et al. Measurement of carotenoids, retinoids, and tocopherols in human lenses. Invest Ophthalmol Vis Sci. 1995;36:2756–61.
301. Landrum JT, et al. A preliminary study of the stereochemistry of human lens zeaxanthin. Invest Ophthalmol Vis Sci. 1997;38:S1026.
302. Edge R, Truscott TG. Carotenoid radicals and interaction of carotenoids with active oxygen species. In: Frank HA et al., editors. The photochemistry of carotenoids. Dordrecht: Kluwer; 1999. p. 223–34.

303. Vetter W, et al. Spectroscopic methods. In: Isler O, editor. Carotenoids. Basel: Birkhause; 1971. p. 190–266.
304. Krasnovskii AA, Pamonava LJ. Interaction of singlet oxygen with carotenoids: rate constants of physical and chemical quenching. Biophysics. 1983;28:769–74.
305. Moller M, et al. Direct measurement of nitric oxide and oxygen partitioning into liposomes and low density lipoprotein. J Biol Chem. 2005;280(10):8850–4.
306. Subczynski WK, Widomska J. EPR spin labeling in carotenoid-membrane interactions. In: Landrum JT, editor. Carotenoids: physical, chemical and biochemical functions and properties. Boca Raton: CRC; 2010. p. 189–212.
307. Gruszecki WI. Carotenoids in lipid membranes. In: Landrum JT, editor. Carotenoids: physical, chemical and biochemical functions and properties. Boca Raton: CRC; 2010. p. 19–30.
308. Wisniewska A, Subczynski WK. Distribution of macular xanthophylls between domains in a model of photoreceptor outer segment membranes. Free Radic Biol Med. 2006;41(8):1257–65.
309. Neuringer M, Anderson GJ, Connor WE. The essentiality of n-3 fatty acids for the development and function of the retina and brain. Annu Rev Nutr. 1988;8:517–41.
310. Conn PF, et al. Carotene-oxygen radical interactions. Free Radic Res Commun. 1992;16(6):401–8.
311. Konovalova TA, et al. EPR spin trapping detection of carbon-centered carotenoid and beta-ionone radicals. Free Radic Biol Med. 2000;28(7):1030–8.
312. Galano A, Vargas R, Martinez A. Carotenoids can act as antioxidants by oxidizing the superoxide radical anion. Phys Chem Chem Phys. 2010;12(1):193–200.
313. Martinez A, et al. Donator acceptor map for carotenoids, melatonin and vitamins. J Phys Chem A. 2008;112(38):9037–42.
314. Nohl H, Gille L. Lysosomal ROS formation. Redox Rep. 2005;10(4):199–205.
315. Klausner RD, Rouault TA, Harford JB. Regulating the fate of mRNA: the control of cellular iron metabolism. Cell. 1993;72(1):19–28.
316. Carroll GJ, et al. Ferritin concentrations in synovial fluid are higher in osteoarthritis patients with HFE gene mutations (C282Y or H63D). Scand J Rheumatol. 2010;39(5):413–20.
317. Kaur H, et al. Hydroxyl radical generation by rheumatoid blood and knee joint synovial fluid. Ann Rheum Dis. 1996;55(12):915–20.
318. Gutteridge JM. Thiobarbituric acid-reactivity following iron-dependent free-radical damage to amino acids and carbohydrates. FEBS Lett. 1981;128(2):343–6.
319. Gutteridge JM. The role of superoxide and hydroxyl radicals in phospholipid peroxidation catalysed by iron salts. FEBS Lett. 1982;150(2):454–8.
320. Gutteridge JM, Rowley DA, Halliwell B. Superoxide-dependent formation of hydroxyl radicals in the presence of iron salts. Detection of 'free' iron in biological systems by using bleomycin-dependent degradation of DNA. Biochem J. 1981;199(1):263–5.
321. Gutteridge JM, Rowley DA, Halliwell B. Superoxide-dependent formation of hydroxyl radicals and lipid peroxidation in the presence of iron salts. Detection of 'catalytic' iron and anti-oxidant activity in extracellular fluids. Biochem J. 1982;206(3):605–9.
322. Lee MC, et al. Evidence of reactive oxygen species generation in synovial fluid from patients with temporomandibular disease by electron spin resonance spectroscopy. Redox Rep. 2004;9(6):331–6.
323. Park CB, Larsson NG. Mitochondrial DNA mutations in disease and aging. J Cell Biol. 2011;193(5):809–18.
324. Trifunovic A. Mitochondrial DNA and ageing. Biochim Biophys Acta. 2006;1757(5–6):611–7.
325. Ruan H, et al. High-quality life extension by the enzyme peptide methionine sulfoxide reductase. Proc Natl Acad Sci USA. 2002;99(5):2748–53.
326. Schriner SE, et al. Extension of murine life span by overexpression of catalase targeted to mitochondria. Science. 2005;308(5730):1909–11.
327. Sun J, et al. Induced overexpression of mitochondrial Mn-superoxide dismutase extends the life span of adult *Drosophila melanogaster*. Genetics. 2002;161(2):661–72.
328. Lu T, et al. Gene regulation and DNA damage in the ageing human brain. Nature. 2004;429(6994):883–91.
329. Cantrell A, Truscott TG. Carotenoids and radicals; interactions with other nutrients. In: Krinsky NI, Mayne ST, Sies H, editors. Carotenoids in health and disease. New York: Marcel Dekker; 2004. p. 31–52.
330. Hayakawa T, et al. Reaction of astaxanthin with peroxynitrite. Biosci Biotechnol Biochem. 2008;72(10):2716–22.
331. Suzuki R, et al. Reaction of retinol with peroxynitrite. Biosci Biotechnol Biochem. 2007;71(10):2596–9.
332. Tsuboi M, et al. Nitrocapsanthin and nitrofucoxanthin, respective products of capsanthin and fucoxanthin reaction with peroxynitrite. J Agric Food Chem. 2011;59(19):10572–8.
333. Panasenko OM, et al. Interaction of peroxynitrite with carotenoids in human low density lipoproteins. Arch Biochem Biophys. 2000;373(1):302–5.
334. Pannala AS, et al. Interaction of peroxynitrite with carotenoids and tocopherols within low density lipoprotein. FEBS Lett. 1998;423(3):297–301.
335. Henderson LM, Chappell JB. Dihydrorhodamine 123: a fluorescent probe for superoxide generation? Eur J Biochem. 1993;217(3):973–80.

336. Arteel GE, Briviba K, Sies H. Protection against peroxynitrite. FEBS Lett. 1999;445(2–3):226–30.
337. Baeuerle PA, Henkel T. Function and activation of NF-kappa B in the immune system. Annu Rev Immunol. 1994;12:141–79.
338. Liao F, et al. Genetic control of inflammatory gene induction and NF-kappa B-like transcription factor activation in response to an atherogenic diet in mice. J Clin Invest. 1993;91(6):2572–9.
339. Matthews JR, et al. Thioredoxin regulates the DNA binding activity of NF-kappa B by reduction of a disulphide bond involving cysteine 62. Nucleic Acids Res. 1992;20(15):3821–30.
340. Wei SJ, et al. Thioredoxin nuclear translocation and interaction with redox factor-1 activates the activator protein-1 transcription factor in response to ionizing radiation. Cancer Res. 2000;60(23):6688–95.
341. Kaarniranta K, Salminen A. NF-kappa B signaling as a putative target for omega-3 metabolites in the prevention of age-related macular degeneration (AMD). Exp Gerontol. 2009;44(11):685–8.
342. Hwang JR, et al. Upregulation of CD9 in ovarian cancer is related to the induction of TNF-alpha gene expression and constitutive NF-kappa B activation. Carcinogenesis. 2012;33(1):77–83.
343. Ruparel SB, et al. Role of NF-kB in prostate cancer progression. Proc Am Assoc Cancer Res. 2006;47:Abstract #5337.
344. Palozza P, et al. Induction of cell cycle arrest and apoptosis in human colon adenocarcinoma cell lines by beta-carotene through down-regulation of cyclin A and Bcl-2 family proteins. Carcinogenesis. 2002;23(1):11–8.
345. Palozza P, et al. Regulation of cell cycle progression and apoptosis by beta-carotene in undifferentiated and differentiated HL-60 leukemia cells: possible involvement of a redox mechanism. Int J Cancer. 2002;97(5):593–600.
346. Palozza P, et al. Beta-carotene regulates NF-kappa B DNA-binding activity by a redox mechanism in human leukemia and colon adenocarcinoma cells. J Nutr. 2003;133(2):381–8.
347. Huang CS, et al. Lycopene inhibits matrix metalloproteinase-9 expression and down-regulates the binding activity of nuclear factor-kappa B and stimulatory protein-1. J Nutr Biochem. 2007;18(7):449–56.
348. Cui Y, et al. beta-Carotene induces apoptosis and upregulates peroxisome proliferator-activated receptor gamma expression and reactive oxygen species production in MCF-7 cancer cells. Eur J Cancer. 2007;43(17):2590–601.
349. Bai SK, et al. beta-Carotene inhibits inflammatory gene expression in lipopolysaccharide-stimulated macrophages by suppressing redox-based NF-κB activation. Exp Mol Med. 2005;37(4):323–34.
350. Lee SJ, et al. Astaxanthin inhibits nitric oxide production and inflammatory gene expression by suppressing I(kappa)B kinase-dependent NF-κB activation. Mol Cells. 2003;16(1):97–105.
351. Smith WL, Urade Y, Jakobsson PJ. Enzymes of the cyclooxygenase pathways of prostanoid biosynthesis. Chem Rev. 2011;111(10):5821–65.
352. Moncada S, et al. An enzyme isolated from arteries transforms prostaglandin endoperoxides to an unstable substance that inhibits platelet aggregation. Nature. 1976;263(5579):663–5.
353. Ameyar M, Wisniewska M, Weitzman JB. A role for AP-1 in apoptosis: the case for and against. Biochimie. 2003;85(8):747–52.
354. Ozolins TR, Hales BF. Post-translational regulation of AP-1 transcription factor DNA-binding activity in the rat conceptus. Mol Pharmacol. 1999;56(3):537–44.
355. Liu C, Russell RM, Wang XD. Exposing ferrets to cigarette smoke and a pharmacological dose of beta-carotene supplementation enhance *in vitro* retinoic acid catabolism in lungs via induction of cytochrome P450 enzymes. J Nutr. 2003;133(1):173–9.
356. Omenn GS, et al. The beta-carotene and retinol efficacy trial (CARET) for chemoprevention of lung cancer in high risk populations: smokers and asbestos-exposed workers. Cancer Res. 1994;54(7 Suppl):2038s–43.
357. Nara E, et al. Acyclic carotenoids and their oxidation mixtures inhibit the growth of HL-60 human promyelocytic leukemia cells. Nutr Cancer. 2001;39(2):273–83.
358. Ben-Dor A, et al. Effects of acyclo-retinoic acid and lycopene on activation of the retinoic acid receptor and proliferation of mammary cancer cells. Arch Biochem Biophys. 2001;391(2):295–302.
359. Hu KQ, et al. The biochemical characterization of ferret carotene-9′,10′-monooxygenase catalyzing cleavage of carotenoids *in vitro* and *in vivo*. J Biol Chem. 2006;281(28):19327–38.
360. Gajic M, et al. Apo-8′-lycopenal and apo-12′-lycopenal are metabolic products of lycopene in rat liver. J Nutr. 2006;136(6):1552–7.
361. Lobo GP, et al. ISX is a retinoic acid-sensitive gatekeeper that controls intestinal beta, beta-carotene absorption and vitamin A production. FASEB J. 2010;24(6):1656–66.
362. Amengual J, et al. A mitochondrial enzyme degrades carotenoids and protects against oxidative stress. FASEB J. 2011;25(3):948–59.
363. Kim J, Cha YN, Surh YJ. A protective role of nuclear factor-erythroid 2-related factor-2 (Nrf2) in inflammatory disorders. Mutat Res. 2010;690(1–2):12–23.
364. Kobayashi A, et al. Oxidative stress sensor Keap1 functions as an adaptor for Cul3-based E3 ligase to regulate proteasomal degradation of Nrf2. Mol Cell Biol. 2004;24(16):7130–9.
365. Motohashi H, et al. Small Maf proteins serve as transcriptional cofactors for keratinocyte differentiation in the Keap1-Nrf2 regulatory pathway. Proc Natl Acad Sci USA. 2004;101(17):6379–84.

Chapter 5
Kinetic Studies with Carotenoids

Guangwen Tang

Key Points

- This chapter reviews the recent progress on kinetic studies with carotenoids.
- Through the development of advanced isotopic techniques and HPLC methods, many kinetic studies with carotenoids on humans have been performed. These studies were reviewed and categorized in mass balance kinetics in humans, factors that affect β-carotene kinetic characters, dynamic products from β-carotene kinetic studies, kinetics with lycopene, xanthophyll kinetics, and interaction of mixtures.
- These kinetic studies with carotenoids provide detailed physiological information on utilization of these nutrients in humans.
- This kinetic information facilitates our understanding of the dynamics of these carotenoids in human health.

Keywords Carotenoids • Kinetics • β-carotene • Lutein/zeaxanthin • Lycopene • Isotope techniques • Absorption • Metabolism

Introduction

Carotenoids, an important group of colorful food components closely related to our diets and health, were discovered over 200 years ago. However, kinetic studies with carotenoids in humans were reported only recently. Challenges exist in conducting kinetic studies of carotenoids due to low levels in human circulation. That is, it is not an easy task to study the absorption and metabolism of a physiological dose of carotenoids. Subjects were administered radioisotopes of carotenoids or near pharmacological doses of nonradioactive synthetic carotenoids. Recently, physiological doses of carotenoids labeled with stable isotopes were used for kinetic studies.

G. Tang, Ph.D. (✉)
Carotenoids and Health Laboratory, Jean Mayer USDA Human Nutrition Research Center on Aging,
Friedman School of Nutrition Science and Policy, Tufts University, 711 Washington Street, Boston, MA 02111, USA
e-mail: guangwen.tang@tufts.edu

S.A. Tanumihardjo (ed.), *Carotenoids and Human Health*, Nutrition and Health,
DOI 10.1007/978-1-62703-203-2_5, © Springer Science+Business Media New York 2013

In the 1960s, two radioisotope studies of β-carotene were conducted to study bioavailability and bioconversion to vitamin A [1, 2], in which β-[^{14}C] carotene doses from 6–52 μCi were administered to lymph-cannulated hospitalized patients. In lymph, β-carotene peaked at 3 and 4 h after the dose and 8–17% of the dose appeared, of which 1.7–27.9% was intact β-carotene and 60–70% was in the form of retinyl esters.

In the late 1980s, with the development of HPLC technology, Brown et al. studied carotenoids from foods (broccoli, carrots, or tomato juice) or from purified β-carotene in capsules (12 or 30 mg) and followed the blood response for 11 days [3]. A controlled, low-carotenoid diet was fed in a cross-over design. Maximum plasma concentrations of β-carotene occurred 24–48 h after dosing with β-carotene (12 or 30 mg) or carrots (29 mg β-carotene and 9 mg α-carotene in 270 g carrots). However, single intakes of broccoli or tomato juice did not change plasma carotenoids. Furthermore, kinetic studies with carotenoids have used high or pharmacologic doses, such as 120 and 126 mg [4, 5] of synthetic β-carotene. Later, β-carotene doses given at levels of 15–40 mg [6–8] were reported.

In the 2000s, a sensitive tracer method used β-[^{14}C]-carotene coupled with accelerator mass spectrometry (AMS) detection [9] and applied it to a series of kinetic characteristics of β-carotene in humans [10, 11]. AMS is an isotope ratio instrument that measures $^{14}C/^{12}C$ to parts per quadrillion (10^{-15}). The extremely low detection limits allowed the use of low radioactive doses, in which radiation exposure was comparable to natural cosmic rays in a single day [12]. AMS is an excellent tool for defining the *in vivo* dynamics of β-carotene and related compounds at physiological concentrations.

Here, recent progress in kinetic studies with carotenoids is reviewed to understand the dynamics of carotenoid absorption and metabolism in humans.

Blood Response Kinetics

From acute dose kinetic studies with β-carotene in humans, β-carotene in circulation reached a first peak at 4 h (AMS method, 11), 5 h (stable isotope method, 6), 5.5 h [9], 6 h (range 4–12 h, $n=8$, HPLC method, 13), and the maximum peak at 8 h (AMS method, 9). From these studies, more than two rises of β-carotene concentration in the circulation were observed in the first 24 h following the intake of β-carotene [9–13]. The first rise was due to the direct intestinal uptake of β-carotene through passive diffusion into the enterocyte, where the absorbed β-carotene was incorporated into chylomicrons, then released to circulation. The circulating β-carotene was delivered to the liver, cleared by hepatic tissues, and released to circulation forming the second rise of β-carotene in plasma. This second rise is also called hepatic re-secretion of β-carotene with VLDL. In addition, the second rise of β-carotene may relate to the further release of β-carotene from the intestine due to the intake of the second meal after the labeled dose of β-carotene. The long-term plasma kinetics showed that the half-life of β-carotene decay was 40 days and the turnover time was 58 days [9].

Mass Balance Kinetics in Humans

Carotenoids go through absorption, conversion, distribution, and further metabolism in various parts of the body at different times, making mass balance studies challenging. However, the sensitive, robust AMS technique using physiological amounts of radio-isotope labeled carotenoids has simplified this complex kinetic process and made it feasible to study mass balance and metabolism. A study using AMS on one male subject found that 42.6% of the labeled β-carotene dose (0.306 mg, 200 nCi of ^{14}C-β-carotene purified from labeled spinach) was absorbed and 57.4% of the dose was recovered from the feces and <1% was eliminated from the urine in early (0–6 h) urine collections [9].

In a test–retest study using AMS, two female subjects absorbed 57% (subject #1) and 52% (subject #2) of the labeled β-carotene dose (1 nmol, 100 nCi of all-*trans* [10,10′,11,11′-^{14}C]-β-carotene). Urine excretion was 31 and 26% of the dose, which was 2.2–2.4 times higher than fecal excretion [10]. In another study in a male subject using AMS and labeled β-carotene, 65% of administered dose (1.01 nmol, 100 nCi of all-*trans* [10,10′,11,11′-^{14}C]-β-carotene) was absorbed, ~35% was recovered from the first feces after the dose, and 1.1% of the dose was eliminated in the urine [11]. From these studies, about 60% of a physiological dose of β-carotene will be absorbed and utilized by the human body.

Factors Affect β-Carotene Kinetic Characters

The kinetic characteristics of β-carotene are variable under different conditions. The absorption and metabolism is affected by the intake of dietary vitamin A [10]. In the test–retest study on two female subjects conducted by Lemke et al., they found that vitamin A supplementation (3,000 retinol equivalents/day for 21 days) was associated with increased apparent absorption of the β-carotene dose, that is, test versus retest values rose from 57 to 74% (Subject 1) and from 52 to 75% (Subject 2). Further, vitamin A supplements led to a ~10-fold reduction in urinary excretion. As an effect of the increased absorption of the labeled β-carotene dose, the molar vitamin A value of the dose for the retest increased from 0.62 mol (Subject 1) to 0.85 mol and from 0.54 mol (Subject 2) to 0.74 mol vitamin A equivalents to 1 mol β-carotene.

High dietary doses of β-carotene will limit its absorption and conversion to vitamin A. This was studied by Novotny et al. [7], who conducted a randomized crossover feeding study on seven volunteers (four men and three women). The volunteers consumed two doses of deuterium-labeled β-carotene (20 and 40 mg) on two occasions. The plasma AUC (area under the curve) for β-carotene-d8 increased twofold from the 20 to the 40 mg dose. However, the AUC calculations for plasma labeled retinol plus retinyl esters did not increase to the same magnitude as the increase in β-carotene dose. That is, plasma AUC for retinol plus retinyl ester increased by only 36% from the 20 to the 40 mg dose. Therefore, the sum of the AUC values for β-carotene plus retinol and retinyl esters increased 47% from the low to high dose. In other words, β-carotene conversion to vitamin A decreases as the dietary dose increases. This dose-dependent effect of the bioavailability of dietary β-carotene was in accord with previous reports [5, 8, 14].

These results show that when consuming large amounts of β-carotene, the efficiency of β-carotene conversion to vitamin A in humans is reduced to avoid possible vitamin A toxicity, implying that β-carotene is a safer source to provide vitamin A.

Dynamic Products from Kinetic Characteristics

Dietary β-carotene is a safe and important source of vitamin A. The conversion of β-carotene to vitamin A is mainly in the intestine. However, other human tissues or organs can convert β-carotene to vitamin A. The oxygenase in humans to cleave β-carotene to vitamin A is the β-carotene monooxygenase (BCO1) [15–17]. Post-absorptive conversion of β-carotene to vitamin A has been observed in several studies, from 19 to 34%, when intake of β-carotene is 2.5–6.0 mg [18–20].

A related, widely distributed cleavage enzyme (BCO2) that cleaves β-carotene to β-*apo*-carotenals was identified and characterized [21, 22]. Its cleavage products were identified using AMS. Ho et al. reported [11] that on day 3 after a labeled β-carotene dose (1.01 nmol, 100 nCi of all-*trans*

[10,10′,11,11′-^{14}C]-β-carotene), two large ^{14}C peaks appeared in plasma: one matched the retention time of β-*apo*-8′-carotenal and the other did not match any of the reference standards used. Therefore, excentral cleavage of ingested β-carotene occurs in vivo in humans and the delayed appearance of ^{14}C-β-*apo*-8′-carotenal in plasma suggested that the excentral cleavage occurred after the ^{14}C-β-carotene was absorbed through the small intestine, a post-β-carotene absorption conversion. The biological significance of this needs further investigation.

Kinetics with Lycopene

A physiological pharmacokinetic model was developed for a lycopene study in humans [23]. Tomato beverage formulation in five graded doses (10, 30, 60, 90, or 120 mg) was used for the study ($n=5$ per dose level). The study data were analyzed using a model that was comprised of seven compartments: gastrointestinal tract, enterocytes, chylomicrons, plasma lipoproteins, fast-turnover liver, slow-turnover tissues, and a delay compartment before the enterocytes. For all five dose levels, the percent absorption at the 10 mg dose (33.9 ± 8.1%) was significantly greater than at the higher doses; however, the amount of lycopene absorbed (mg) was not statistically different (mean: 4.69 ± 0.55 mg) between doses, suggesting a possible saturation of absorptive mechanisms. This kinetic study also showed that most individuals may be able to absorb modest quantities of lycopene (2–6 mg) within the dose range investigated in this study, but in the majority of the population, lycopene absorption may plateau at less than 6 mg, with high accumulators representing only a small fraction. That is, lycopene over the same dose range in the present experiment displayed reduced absorption efficiencies with increasing dose. The wide range of lycopene absorption observed in this study (1.78–14.28 mg) could also have important implications for using lycopene supplements in human health [23].

A kinetic study using stable isotope labeled lycopene was conducted to compare bioavailability of two deuterated sources, synthetic or natural lycopene [24]. Two subjects (one male and one female) consumed hydroponically grown tomatoes containing deuterium-enriched lycopene [80–84 g wet weight tomato containing 16.3 (~8.8 mg) and 17.4 (~9.5 mg) μmol lycopene, respectively] and two subjects (one male and one female) consumed 11 μmol (6.0 mg) synthetic $^{2}H_{10}$ lycopene in 6 g corn oil. The study results showed that enrichment response of synthetic lycopene reached 33.9 ± 1.7 nmol day/μmol lycopene in the dose, whereas that of lycopene from the tomato dose was 11.8 ± 0.3 nmol day/μmol lycopene in the dose. This study provided evidence that the bioavailability of synthetic lycopene in oil appeared to be about three times higher than that of lycopene from steamed and pureed tomatoes.

Xanthophyll Kinetics

Xanthophylls are oxygenated carotenoids. The xanthophylls lutein and zeaxanthin, have shown a protective effect on two common eye diseases of aging, cataract and macular degeneration [25]. More data regarding xanthophyll kinetics are needed.

A kinetic study [26] using intrinsically labeled spinach (two subjects, 200 g with 18.8 mg lutein) and collard greens (two subjects, 193–214 g with 9.8 mg or 15.4 mg lutein) reported that the maximum levels of enrichment for lutein were 38–67% and peaked at 13 or 24 h after the intake of the labeled vegetables.

Another study [27] used chronic supplementation and a range of lutein doses (2.4–30 mg/day), as well as a high zeaxanthin dose (30 mg/day). The serum and macular pigment were analyzed in a series of experiments. Serum lutein concentrations reached a plateau that was correlated with dose ($r=0.82$,

$P<0.001$). Plateau concentrations ranged from 2.8×10^{-7} to 2.7×10^{-6} mol/L. Zeaxanthin was less well-absorbed than an equal lutein dose, resulting in plateaus of $\sim5\times10^{-7}$ mol/L. The rate of increase in macular pigment optical density was correlated with the plateau concentration of carotenoids in the serum ($r=0.58$, $P<0.001$) but not with the pre-supplementation optical density ($r=0.13$, $P=0.21$). The mean rate of increase was $(3.42\pm0.80)\times10^5$ mAU/day per unit concentration (mol/L) of carotenoids in the serum.

Another chronic supplementation study [28] used 20 mg lutein ester (equivalent to 10 mg/day free lutein) to seven patients with early age-related maculopathy (ARM) and six age-matched controls for 18–20 weeks. No differences were detected between ARM sufferers and controls showing that lutein supplementation may help people with established ARM to build up macular pigment optical density.

Further, an intervention study [29] with a crossover design in healthy men ($n=10$) administered one of four lutein doses (lutein supplement, lutein ester supplement, spinach, and lutein-enriched egg) for 9 days. All lutein doses provided 6 mg lutein except for the lutein ester, which provided 5.5 mg lutein equivalents. Subjects completed all four treatments of the study in random order. Serum samples were collected from fasting subjects on day -14, 1 (baseline), 2, 3, and 10 and analyzed for changes in lutein concentration. The baseline and dose-adjusted lutein response in serum was significantly higher after egg consumption than after lutein, lutein ester, and spinach consumption on day 10. Therefore, lutein bioavailability from egg is higher than that from other sources such as lutein in oil or lutein ester in oil supplements, and spinach, which did not differ. This finding is important for dietary recommendations in that foods with various matrices may have different bioavailability.

Another study [30] compared the relative serum response during supplementation with free lutein (12.2 mg) and lutein esters [27 mg (13.5 mg lutein equivalents)] on 72 volunteers (23–52 years). Subjects were matched for gender, age, and BMI and randomized to treatment. Fasting blood was obtained at baseline and after 7, 14, 21, and 28 days. Absolute changes in serum lutein, per mg daily dose, were significantly greater from free lutein than esterified after 21 days ($P=0.0012$) and remained after 28 days ($P=0.0011$), while subject age, gender, BMI, and serum lipids did not affect serum response.

A recent study administered 12 mg/day lutein to 11 subjects (60–80 year) for 4 months [31] and evaluated serum concentrations and macular pigment optical density (MPOD). The supplement resulted in an increase in serum lutein from baseline at 2 and 4 months ($P<0.001$), and MPOD increased eccentrically at 3.0° ($P<0.01$).

A study on plasma kinetics of zeaxanthin [32] was conducted by giving 20 healthy volunteers either 1 mg (1.76 μmol) or 10 mg (17.6 μmol) zeaxanthin per day as beadlets for 42 days. Zeaxanthin concentrations increased 4- to 20-fold from 0.048 ± 0.026 μmol/L at baseline to 0.20 ± 0.07 and 0.92 ± 0.28 μmol/L with 1 and 10 mg zeaxanthin, respectively. The dose-normalized bioavailability of zeaxanthin after the 10 mg dose was 40% lower ($P<0.001$) than after the 1 mg dose. After 17 days of dosing, >90% of steady-state concentrations were reached, which was compatible with an effective half-life for accumulation of 5 days. The terminal elimination half-life was 12 ± 7 days ($n=20$).

A similar study on plasma kinetics of lutein [33] was conducted by giving 19 healthy volunteers daily oral doses as beadlets of either 4.1 mg ($n=8$), 20.5 mg ($n=8$), or 0 mg ($n=3$) lutein for 42 days. The lutein supplement contained 8.3% zeaxanthin relative to lutein (100%). Plasma lutein concentrations increased from 0.14 to 0.52 ± 0.13 for the group taking 4.1 mg lutein/day and to 1.45 ± 0.69 μmol/L for the group taking 20.5 mg lutein per day. Dose-normalized lutein bioavailability in the group taking 20.5 mg was ~60% of that in the group taking 4.1 mg per day. Kinetic disposition half-life did not differ significantly between groups. On average, dosing for 18 days was required to reach >90% fraction of the steady-state concentration, which is consistent with an effective half-life for accumulation of ~5.6 day. Lutein was well-tolerated and did not affect the concentrations of other carotenoids.

These kinetic studies demonstrate that the bioavailability of the dose is level dependent and dose intakes <20 mg/day will not affect other carotenoids in the circulation.

Interaction of Mixtures of Carotenoids

The interaction between pharmacological doses of carotenoids and the consequences of this interaction are not equally distributed [34]. For example, ingestion of a combined dose of β-carotene and canthaxanthin resulted in antagonism between β-carotene and canthaxanthin, but canthaxanthin did not affect β-carotene in circulation.

From food sources, mixtures of carotenoids did not affect overall absorption. An experiment with chronic intakes of vegetables and supplements assessed whether vegetable-borne carotenoids (lycopene, lutein, and β-carotene) compete for intestinal absorption and whether this affects the plasma status of carotenoids after a 3-week intervention [35]. During 3-week periods separated by 3-week washouts, 20 women were supplemented with either 96 g tomato purée/day (14.98 mg lycopene + 1.50 mg β-carotene), 92 g cooked chopped spinach/day (11.93 mg lutein + 7.96 mg β-carotene), 96 g tomato purée/day + 92 g chopped spinach/day, 96 g tomato purée/day + 2 lutein pills (12 mg lutein), or 92 g chopped spinach/day + 1 lycopene pill (15 mg lycopene). Plasma carotenoids were measured before and after each supplementation period. The subjects also participated in postprandial experiments in which they ingested meals containing double amounts of the supplements described above. Carotenoids were measured in chylomicrons to assess the interaction of carotenoids on absorption.

Adding a second carotenoid to a meal that provided a first carotenoid diminished the chylomicron response to the first carotenoid. However, cosupplementation with a second carotenoid of a diet supplemented with a first carotenoid did not diminish the medium-term plasma response to the first carotenoid. Therefore, consumption of carotenoids from different vegetable sources does not diminish plasma carotenoid concentrations in the medium-term, despite the finding in postprandial testing of competitive inhibitory interactions among different carotenoids.

In summary, kinetic studies with carotenoids provide detailed physiological information on utilization of these compounds in humans. This kinetic information facilitates our understanding of the dynamics of these carotenoids in human health.

References

1. Goodman DS, Blomstrand R, Werner B, Huang HS, Shiratori T. The intestinal absorption and metabolism of vitamin A and β-carotene in man. J Clin Invest. 1966;45:1615–23.
2. Blomstrand R, Werner B. Studies on the intestinal absorption of radioactive β-carotene and vitamin A in man. Conversion of β-carotene into vitamin A. J Clin Lab Invest. 1967;19:339–45.
3. Brown ED, Micozzi MS, Craft NE, Bieri JG, Beecher G, Edwards BK, Rose A, Taylor PR, Smith Jr JC. Plasma carotenoids in normal men after a single ingestion of vegetables or purified β-carotene. Am J Clin Nutr. 1989; 49(6):1258–65.
4. Johnson EJ, Russell RM. Distribution of orally administered beta-carotene among lipoproteins in healthy men. Am J Clin Nutr. 1992;56:128–35.
5. Tang G, Qin J, Dolnikowski G, Russell RM. Vitamin A equivalence of β-carotene in a woman as determined by a stable isotope reference method. Eur J Nutr. 2000;39:7–11.
6. Novotny JA, Ducker SR, Zech LA, Clifford AJ. Compartmental analysis of the dynamics of β-carotene metabolism in an adult volunteer. J Lipid Res. 1995;36:1825–38.
7. Novotny JA, Harrison DJ, Pawlosky R, Flanagan VP, Harrison EH, Kurilich AC. β-carotene conversion to vitamin A decreases as the dietary dose increases in humans. J Nutr. 2010;140:915–8.
8. Hickenbottom SJ, Follett JR, Lin Y, Dueker SR, Burri BJ, Neidlinger TR, Clifford AJ. Variability in conversion of β-carotene to vitamin A in men as measured by using a double-tracer study design. Am J Clin Nutr. 2002;75(5):900–7.
9. Dueker SR, Lin Y, Buchholz BA, Schneider PD, Lamé MW, Segall HJ, Vogel JS, Clifford AJ. Long-term kinetic study of β-carotene, using accelerator mass spectrometry in an adult volunteer. J Lipid Res. 2000;41:1790–800.

10. Lemke SL, Dueker SR, Follett JR, Lin Y, Carkeet C, Buchholz BA, Vogel JS, Clifford AJ. Absorption and retinol equivalence of β-carotene in humans is influenced by dietary vitamin A intake. J Lipid Res. 2003;44:1591–600.
11. Ho CC, de Moura FF, Kim S-H, Clifford AJ. Excentral cleavage of β-carotene in vivo in a healthy man. Am J Clin Nutr. 2007;85:770–7.
12. Vogel JS, Turteltaub KW. Accelerator mass spectrometry as a bioanalytical tool for nutritional research. Adv Exp Med Biol. 1998;445:397–410.
13. Kostic D, White WS, Olson JA. Intestinal absorption, serum clearance, and interactions between lutein and β-carotene when administered to human adults in separate or combined oral doses. Am J Clin Nutr. 1995;62:604–10.
14. Lin Y, Dueker SR, Burri BJ, Neidlinger TR, Clifford AJ. Variability of the conversion of beta-carotene to vitamin A in women measured by using a double-tracer study design. Am J Clin Nutr. 2000;71:1545–54.
15. Olson JA, Hayaishi O. The enzymatic cleavage of β-carotene into vitamin A by soluble enzymes of rat liver and intestine. Proc Natl Acad Sci U S A. 1965;54:1364–70.
16. Goodman DS, Huang HS, Kanai M, Shiratori T. The enzymatic conversion of all-trans β-carotene into retinal. J Biol Chem. 1967;242:3543–4.
17. Lindqvist A, Andersson S. Biochemical properties of purified recombinant human β-carotene 15,15′-monooxygenase. J Biol Chem. 2002;277:23942–8.
18. Tang G, Qin J, Dolnikowski GG, Russell RM. Short-term (intestinal) and long-term (postintestinal) conversion of β-carotene to retinol in adults as assessed by a stable-isotope reference method. Am J Clin Nutr. 2003;78:259–66.
19. Wang ZX, Zhao XF, Yin SA, Russell RM, Tang G. β-carotene-vitamin A equivalence in Chinese adults assessed by an isotope dilution technique. Br J Nutr. 2004;91:121–3.
20. Wang J, Wang Y, Wang Z, Li L, Qin J, Lai W, Fu Y, Russell RM, Grusak MA, Tang G, Yin S. Vitamin A equivalent of spirulina β-carotene in Chinese adults assessed by stable isotope dilution and reference techniques. Am J Clin Nutr. 2008;87:1730–7.
21. Kiefer C, Hessel S, Lampert JM, et al. Identification and characterization of a mammalian enzyme catalyzing the asymmetric oxidative cleavage of provitamin A. J Biol Chem. 2001;276:14110–6.
22. Lindqvist A, He Y-G, Andersson S. Cell type-specific expression of β-carotene 9′,10′-monooxygenase in human tissues. J Histochem Cytochem. 2005;53:1403–12.
23. Diwadkar-Navsariwala V, Novotny JA, Gustin DM, Sosman JA, Rodvold KA, Crowell JA, Stacewicz-Sapuntzakis M, Bowen PE. A physiological pharmacokinetic model describing the disposition of lycopene in healthy men. J Lipid Res. 2003;44:1927–39.
24. Tang G, Ferreira ALA, Grusak MA, Qin J, Dolnikowski GG, Russell RM, Krinsky NI. Bioavailability of synthetic and biosynthetic deuterated lycopene in humans. J Nutr Biochem. 2005;16(4):229–35.
25. Mares-Perlman JA, Millen AE, Ficek TL, Hankinson SE. The body of evidence to support a protective role for lutein and zeaxanthin in delaying chronic disease. Overview. J Nutr. 2002;132:518S–24.
26. Lienau A, Glaser T, Tang G, Dolnikowski GG, Grusak MA, Albert K. Bioavailability of lutein in humans from intrinsically labeled vegetables determined by LC-APCI-MS. J Nutr Biochem. 2003;11:663–70.
27. Bone RA, Landrum JT, Guerra LH, Ruiz CA. Lutein and zeaxanthin dietary supplements raise macular pigment density and serum concentrations of these carotenoids in humans. J Nutr. 2003;133:992–8.
28. Koh H-H, Murray IJ, Nolanc D, Carden D, Feather J, Beatty S. Plasma and macular responses to lutein supplement in subjects with and without age-related maculopathy: a pilot study. Exp Eye Res. 2004;79:21–7.
29. Chung HK, Rasmussen HM, Johnson EJ. Lutein bioavailability is higher from lutein-enriched eggs than from supplements and spinach in men. J Nutr. 2004;134:1887–93.
30. Norkus EP, Norkus KL, Dharmarajan TS, Schierle J, Schalch W. Serum lutein response is greater from free lutein than from esterified lutein during 4 weeks of supplementation in healthy adults. J Am Coll Nutr. 2010;29:575–85.
31. Johnson EJ, Chung H-Y, Caldarella SM, Snodderly DM. The influence of supplemental lutein and docosahexaenoic acid on serum, lipoproteins, and macular pigmentation. Am J Clin Nutr. 2008;87(5):1521–9.
32. Hartmann D, Thürmann PA, Spitzer V, Schalch W, Manner B, Cohn W. Plasma kinetics of zeaxanthin and 3′-dehydro-lutein after multiple oral doses of synthetic zeaxanthin. Am J Clin Nutr. 2004;79(3):410–7.
33. Thürmann PA, Schalch W, Aebischer J-C, Tenter U, Cohn W. Plasma kinetics of lutein, zeaxanthin, and 3-dehydro-lutein after multiple oral doses of a lutein supplement. Am J Clin Nutr. 2005;82(1):88–97.
34. White WS, Stacewicz-Sapuntzakis M, Erdman Jr JW, Bowen PE. Pharmacokinetics of beta-carotene and canthaxanthin after ingestion of individual and combined doses by human subjects. J Am Coll Nutr. 1994;13:665–71.
35. Tyssandier V, Cardinault N, Caris-Veyrat C, Amiot M-J, Grolier P, Bouteloup C, Azais-Braesco V, Borel P. Vegetable-borne lutein, lycopene, and β-carotene compete for incorporation into chylomicrons, with no adverse effect on the medium-term (3-wk) plasma status of carotenoids in humans. Am J Clin Nutr. 2002;75(3):526–34.

Chapter 6
Carotenoid Bioavailability: Influence of Dietary Lipid and Fiber

Shellen R. Goltz and Mario G. Ferruzzi

Key Points

- Consistent with observed nutritive and health promoting roles of dietary carotenoids, interest in factors that impact their bioavailability has grown.
- The intestinal absorption of carotenoids is a complex, multistep process including (1) release from the food matrix, (2) incorporation into bile salt–lipid micelles, (3) uptake by intestinal epithelial cells, and (4) packaging into chylomicrons with secretion into the lymphatic system.
- Co-consumption of dietary lipids may be one of the most effective stimulators of carotenoid absorption *in vivo* considering their fat-soluble nature and the role of triacylglycerols in several steps of carotenoid intestinal absorption.
- The presence of dietary fiber reduces the bioavailability of carotenoids by mechanisms related to sequestration of bile acids and reduction of cholesterol intestinal re-absorption.
- In light of current dietary guidelines that recommend a reduction of fat and an increase in dietary fiber intake, critical evaluation of the impact of these dietary components on carotenoid bioavailability is warranted.

Keywords Carotenoid • Bioavailability • Triacylglycerol • Fiber • Dietary Guidelines • Micellarization • Chylomicron • *In vivo* • *In vitro*

Introduction

The role of carotenoids as nutritive and disease preventative plant pigments has stimulated interest in these dietary compounds. Consistent with these interests, the 2010 Dietary Guidelines for Americans recommends that adults consume at least 4½ cups of carotenoid rich fruits and vegetables per day, as part of a balanced diet promoting health [1]. However, the average American adult consumes only about 2.6 cups each day [1] and this poor level of consumption is further compounded by the poor efficiency of carotenoid absorption from foods [2]. These findings have highlighted the need to better

S.R. Goltz, Ph.D., R.D. • M.G. Ferruzzi, Ph.D. (✉)
Department of Food Science, Purdue University, 745 Agriculture Mall Drive, West Lafayette, IN 47907, USA

Department of Nutrition Science, Purdue University, 700 W. State St., West Lafayette, IN 47907, USA
e-mail: sgoltz@purdue.edu; mferruzz@purdue.edu

S.A. Tanumihardjo (ed.), *Carotenoids and Human Health*, Nutrition and Health,
DOI 10.1007/978-1-62703-203-2_6, © Springer Science+Business Media New York 2013

understand factors that can positively influence carotenoid absorption from commonly consumed fruits and vegetables.

Carotenoid absorption is dependent upon many factors including chemical species, nature of the food matrices; interactions with macro-, micro-, and phytonutrients; type and extent of food processing and preparation; as well as the nutritional, pathophysiological, and genetic factors of individuals [2, 3]. Considering the fat-soluble nature of carotenoids, it is recognized that co-consumption of lipid in the form of triacylglycerols (TAG) is one of the most effective stimulators of carotenoid absorption *in vivo*. Interestingly, the presence of dietary fiber, soluble fiber in particular, may reduce the bioavailability of carotenoids by mechanisms related to their lipophilic nature and similar to those involved in sequestration of bile acids and reduction of cholesterol intestinal re-absorption. In light of current dietary guidelines that recommend a reduction of fat and an increase in dietary fiber intake [1], critical evaluation of the impact of these dietary components on carotenoid bioavailability is warranted. This chapter describes current knowledge of the impact of these two critical dietary components (lipid, in the form of TAG, and fiber) on carotenoid bioavailability in humans.

Bioaccessibility and Bioavailability of Carotenoids

The intestinal absorption of carotenoids is a complex, multistep process including (1) release from the food matrix, (2) incorporation into bile salt–lipid micelles, (3) uptake by intestinal epithelial cells, and (4) packaging into chylomicrons with secretion into the lymphatic system [2, 3] (Fig. 6.1). The term *bioaccessibility* is often used to describe the first two steps, release and micellarization, and thus represents the fraction of carotenoids from a meal available for subsequent uptake by the intestinal epithelia [4, 5]. *Bioavailability* is used to describe the proportion of carotenoids from a meal that are absorbed, present in circulation and available for utilization, metabolism, or storage by the organism [6]. Both dietary lipid, as TAG, and fiber appear to have effects at multiple steps in this process.

Step 1—Digestion: Release from the food matrix

Prior to intestinal absorption, carotenoids must first be released from plant tissues and food matrices [7, 8]. Mechanical breakdown of the food matrix begins during mastication and continues in the stomach, where the combination of grinding, gastric churning, and enzymatic hydrolysis of lipids and proteins promotes the release of carotenoids [9]. During these steps, co-consumed dietary fats and oils aid in extraction as well as in generation of a crude emulsion favoring the solubilization of carotenoids in an otherwise aqueous environment of the gastric chyme [5, 9, 10].

Step 2—Incorporation into bile salt–lipid micelles

As chyme, containing a crude lipid emulsion, is transferred from the stomach to the duodenum, it is followed by release of bile from the gall bladder into the small intestinal lumen. Further digestion by pancreatic enzymes continues in the small intestine including conversion of TAG to monoglycerides, diglycerides and free fatty acids by pancreatic lipase [11]. The combination of bile, free fatty acids, monoglycerides, and phospholipids facilitates the formation of bile salt–lipid micelles and vesicles in which carotenoids, and other fat-soluble compounds are solubilized [12]. Solubilization of carotenoids in mixed micelles is a critical step for absorption, providing a vehicle for carotenoids and other fat-soluble compounds to maintain solubility in the aqueous environment of the gut lumen. Solubility in micelles facilitates passage through the unstirred water layer prior to uptake by intestinal epithelial cells.

The concentration of bile salts and products of lipid digestion (e.g., mono- and diglycerides) is a critical factor affecting the efficiency of carotenoid transfer from the gastric lipid droplets to the micelles in the duodenum. When bile salt concentrations are below the critical micellar concentration

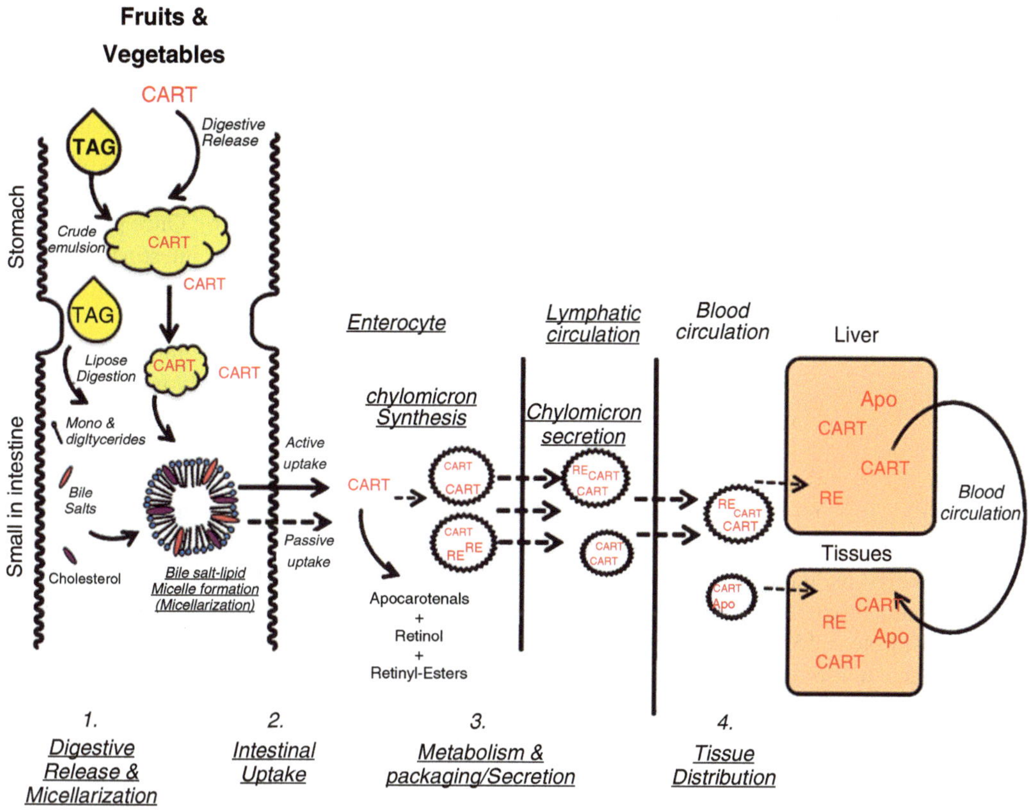

Fig. 6.1 Schematic of carotenoid absorption. Key steps in the absorption of carotenoids include release from the food matrix and association of carotenoids with bulk lipid in a crude emulsion during gastric digestion. Following small intestinal digestion of TAG, carotenoids are partitioned into bile salt–lipid micelles (micellarization). These initial steps which include release from the food matrix and micellarization are termed *bioaccessibility* and refer to the fraction of carotenoids from a food available for subsequent intestinal absorption. Micellarized carotenoids are then absorbed by intestinal epithelial cells through active and passive processes. Intracellularly, carotenoids are then packaged into chylomicrons, and secreted into the lymphatic system. *Bioavailability* encompasses all of these processes and defines the fraction of carotenoids from a food absorbed by the body and made available for subsequent tissue distribution, metabolism and utilization. Co-consumption of dietary lipids and fibers is believed to both positively and negatively impact carotenoid absorption, respectively, at both preabsorptive (bioaccessibility) and absorptive stages. *Abbreviations*: *CART* carotenoid, *RE* retinyl-esters, *Apo* apocarotenals

(CMC), little to no transfer of carotenoids to mixed micelles is observed [13, 14]. These findings suggest that dietary TAGs serve four purposes in facilitating carotenoid bioaccessibility—(1) facilitating carotenoid extraction from the food matrix, (2) maintaining carotenoid solubility in crude emulsions during the transfer of gastric chyme to the small intestine, (3) promoting bile flow from the gall bladder to the small intestine thereby allowing for adequate micelle formation, and (4) serving as structural components of mixed micelles in the intestinal lumen [9, 15].

The efficiency of transfer from gastric chyme to mixed micelles is believed to be impacted by the nature of the carotenoid species. For example, the polarity of individual carotenoid species is known to influence both the rate of transfer and the location in the mixed micelles. In gastric chyme, apolar carotenes are incorporated into the TAG-rich core and cannot be appreciably transferred until TAG hydrolysis. In contrast, polar xanthophylls predominate in the phospholipid-rich emulsion surface and are therefore more readily transferred to mixed micelles in the duodenum [9, 10, 14]. Although carotenoid hydrophobicity causes differential solubility in the emulsified lipid droplets, solubility within the micelles is believed to be generally similar among all carotenoid species [10].

Step 3—Uptake by intestinal epithelia

Carotenoids incorporated into newly formed micelles must pass diffusively through the unstirred water layer prior to uptake by the intestinal epithelia. At the epithelial surface, micelles are disrupted and carotenoids are released along with fatty acids, monoglycerides, phospholipids, and other partially hydrolyzed lipids which constitute mixed micelle structure and content [16]. Once presented to the epithelial surface, the mechanism by which carotenoids are transferred into intestinal epithelial cells is believed to occur through a combination of passive and facilitated diffusion including involvement of transporters such as the class B-type 1 scavenger receptor (SR-B1) [17–22].

Carotenoid structure and the presence of other components may influence the rate and extent of uptake by the intestinal epithelia. Apolar carotenoids appear to be more efficiently transferred from micelles into epithelial cells compared to polar carotenoid species [23]. Additionally, phospholipids may impact absorption as assessed in rodent and intestinal cell culture models [23–26]; however, the extent of impact in humans remains to be explored.

Following uptake by the enterocyte, carotenoids are transferred intracellularly through the cytosol and to organelles. While the mechanisms of intracellular transport are not fully understood, several possibilities exist including involvement of fatty acid binding protein (FABP) [18]. Additionally, provitamin A carotenoids (α-, β-carotene and β-cryptoxanthin) are subject to symmetric cleavage by cytosolic β-carotene 15,15′ monooxygenase (BCO1) forming retinal and subsequently retinol [27]. Both pro- and non-provitamin A carotenoids can also be cleaved asymmetrically by β-carotene monooxygenase 2 (BCO2) forming several apocarotenal species [28, 29]. Therefore, following uptake by the intestinal epithelia, both native carotenoid species and their metabolites generated through the action of BCO1 and BCO2 are available for subsequent systemic distribution.

Step 4—Packaging into chylomicrons and secretion into the lymphatic system

Following intestinal uptake, intact carotenoids and their metabolites are subsequently transferred to the Golgi apparatus where, along with retinyl esters and other fat-soluble compounds, they are assembled into chylomicron particles [15]. Once formed, chylomicrons are secreted into the intracellular space and subsequently secreted into the lymphatic system to the thoracic duct, emptied into the blood stream via the subclavian vein, and transported to the liver for further processing and packaging for extrahepatic tissue distribution. Chylomicron secretion can be stimulated more effectively by TAG with certain chain lengths and degrees of saturation [30, 31], which suggests that lipid source, not just the presence of lipid, may play a role in carotenoid absorption.

Impact of Dietary Lipid on Bioavailability *In Vivo*

Considering the prominent role of dietary lipid in both pre-absorptive (extraction and micellarization) and absorptive events (uptake and chylomicron production), significant efforts have been made to study the influence of both quantitative and qualitative meal lipid profiles on carotenoid absorption *in vivo*. While several human studies have been conducted, results remain difficult to directly compare due to differences in food matrices, carotenoid species, and clinical methodologies applied.

Methodologies Applied in Assessing Carotenoid Bioavailability In Vivo

Methods applied in the investigation of carotenoid bioavailability in humans include: deuterium-labeled vitamin A, oral-fecal balance, serum or plasma response, chylomicron isolation, and isolation of the triglyceride rich lipoprotein fraction (TRL). However, the most common methods are serum or plasma response and chylomicron or TRL response following chronic or acute ingestion of carotenoid-rich meals or dietary supplements.

In the serum or plasma response method, changes in serum or plasma carotenoid concentrations are measured at multiple time points following ingestion of a carotenoid containing food or supplement. This method is most often used to measure the response following chronic intake of carotenoid rich foods after circulating carotenoids reach steady state (~9–10 days) [32]. While useful, this approach is limited by the requirement for lengthy wash out periods (1–2 weeks) to reduce circulating endogenous carotenoid levels in a manner sufficient to see effects from a subsequent dietary intervention.

When assessing the acute response following a single carotenoid dose, chylomicron or TRL response is often used. These plasma fractions contain predominantly newly absorbed carotenoids [6] with only minor presence of hepatic VLDL. In this method, chylomicrons or TRL fractions are isolated from fresh plasma via ultracentrifugation at multiple time points following ingestion of a single test meal or supplemental dose. Peak absorption of carotenoids occurs between 3 and 6 h after consumption and carotenoid levels return to baseline levels typically by 9–12 h after consumption [30, 33].

Impact of Lipid Quantity on Carotenoid Absorption in Humans

Key studies investigating the relationship between dietary lipid quantity and carotenoid absorption are summarized in Table 6.1. Early efforts focused on the impact of fats and oils on the absorption of provitamin A carotenoids in vitamin A deficient or at-risk populations. Jayarajan et al. [34] found that consumption of spinach with either 5 or 10 g of groundnut oil improved vitamin A concentrations in rural Indian preschool aged children relative to the group receiving 0 g oil. Similarly, Takyi [35] found that addition of 1.3 or 5.1 g shea butter and groundnut oil to stews containing dark green leafy vegetables significantly improved serum retinol concentrations in Ghanaian children by 23.4% and 26.5%, respectively. Ribaya-Mercado et al. [36] also found that serum concentrations of β-carotene, α-carotene, and β-cryptoxanthin from boiled vegetables were similarly improved in Filipino schoolchildren when consumed over 9 weeks with either 2.4, 5, or 10 g fat at each meal. These studies support the notion that minimal levels of co-consumed lipid are needed for effective carotenoid absorption and bioconversion. While interesting, these studies were generally conducted in vitamin A-deficient populations, which may have reduced the potential impact of the higher co-consumed lipid levels [37].

Several groups subsequently evaluated the effect of dietary lipid quantity on carotenoid bioavailability in healthy subjects with a focus on both provitamin A and non-provitamin A carotenoid species. Roodenburg et al. [38] compared the absorption of α- and β-carotene (8 mg total) or lutein esters (8 mg) from supplements consumed with either low-fat (3 g) or high-fat (36 g) spreads. Fasting blood samples taken before and after a 7-day intervention period demonstrated that plasma α- and β-carotene concentrations were not significantly higher after eating the high-fat spread compared to the low-fat spread (Fig. 6.2). These results further suggested that as little as 3–5 g fat might be adequate for absorption of these carotenoids [38]. However, plasma lutein concentrations were significantly higher after consuming the high-fat spread, indicating that the amount of fat required for optimal absorption differs by carotenoid species and/or form (free vs. esterified). Similar results were noted following consumption of fresh vegetable salads with 0, 12, or 24 g fat from avocados [39]. In this study, 12 g of co-consumed lipid was sufficient for the absorption of α- and β-carotene, whereas 24 g of lipid was required to significantly enhance plasma lutein levels.

Increasing meal lipid amount also improves acute postprandial carotenoid absorption. Brown et al. [33] evaluated the amount of fat required to optimize absorption of carotenoids from raw vegetables by topping salads with fat-free (0 g), low fat (6 g), or high fat (28 g) canola oil-based dressing. While

Table 6.1 Impact of lipid amount on carotenoid bioavailability in human subjects

Study	*n*	Nutritional status	Carotenoid type and amount	TG type and amount	Methodology	Duration	Results
Brown et al. [33]	7	Healthy	*Raw* salad (247 g): 5.875 mg lutein, 0.163 mg zeaxanthin, 4.4 mg α-carotene, 12.224 mg β-carotene, 8.613 mg lycopene	Canola oil made into dressing (0, 6, 28 g dietary fat)	Chylomicron response	3 Separate testing days, 12 h each	Negligible absorption without added lipids. Significantly greater absorption between 0 and 6 g and also between 6 and 28 g for all carotenoids
Goltz et al. [40]	29	Healthy	*Raw* salad (262 g): 4.2 mg lutein, 6.9 mg zeaxanthin, 3.1 mg α-carotene, 6.3 mg β-carotene, 4.4 mg all-*trans* lycopene	Canola oil, soybean oil, or butter (3, 8, 20 g dietary fat)	TRL response	3 Separate testing days, 10 h each	20 g Promoted significantly higher absorption of lutein, zeaxanthin, β-carotene, and lycopene compared to 3 and 8 g. No significant differences detected between 3 and 8 g
Unlu et al. [39]	8	Healthy	*Raw* salad: (220 g): 6 mg lutein, 7 mg α-carotene, 12 mg β-carotene	Avocado (0, 12, 24 g dietary fat)	TRL response	3 Separate testing days, 10 h each	Absorption of α- and β-carotene significantly higher with 12 g vs. 0 g. No difference between 12 and 24 g. Absorption of lutein significantly higher with 24 g vs. 0 g
Dimitrov et al. [82]	10	Healthy	β-Carotene *supplements* (45 mg/day)	Meals (6 g/day or 70 g/day)	Plasma response	21 days	Consumption of high fat meals resulted in significantly higher plasma β-carotene levels in shorter time
Roodenburg et al. [38]	60	Healthy	α- and β-carotene *supplements* OR lutein *supplements* (8 mg/day)	Low-fat spread (3 g) plus low-fat meal (5 g) *OR* high fat spread (36 g) plus low-fat meal (5 g)	Plasma response	Two separate 7-day periods	No difference in plasma α- and β-carotene between groups. Plasma lutein concentrations increased significantly with 36 g

Jayarajan et al. [34]	48	17% Deficient in vitamin A; not evenly distributed between groups	*Cooked* spinach (1.2 mg β-carotene/day)	Groundnut oil (0, 5, or 10 g/day)	Serum response	4 weeks	Serum vitamin A significantly increased in all groups compared to baseline. Differences between 5 and 10 g not significant
Prince and Frisoli [32]	3	Healthy	β-Carotene *supplements* (51 mg/day)	Haagen-Daz vanilla swiss almond ice cream (0 or 200 g fat)	Serum response	2 Separate interventions; monitored for 168 h (0 g) or 640 h (200 g)	Serum β-carotene undetectable without lipid; increased 2.5-fold with 200 g lipid
Takyi [35]	519	75% Low or deficient in vitamin A	Stews with *cooked* cassava or kapok leaves (400 RE/day = 2.4 mg β-carotene/4.8 mg mixed carotene)	*Group #1*: Shea butter (5.1 g) plus groundnut oil for stew prep (1.3 g) *Group #2*: Groundnut oil (1.3 g)	Serum response	3 months	Serum retinol increased significantly from baseline in both groups (26.5% in group #1 and 23.4% in group #2)
Ahuja et al. [83]	21	Healthy	Meals including *cooked* tomato soup and tomato paste (19.5 mg/day)	Olive oil (16 or 35 g/day)	Serum response	10 days each	No significant difference in serum lycopene levels between groups
Ribaya-Mercado et al. [36]	104	35% Low liver vitamin A; 19% low serum vitamin A	*Boiled* vegetables (4.2 mg provitamin A carotenoids, mainly β-carotene)	Coconut oil (2.4, 5, or 10 g)	Stable-isotope-dilution	5 days/week for 9 weeks	Similar increases in serum β-carotene, α-carotene, and β-cryptoxanthin between all groups

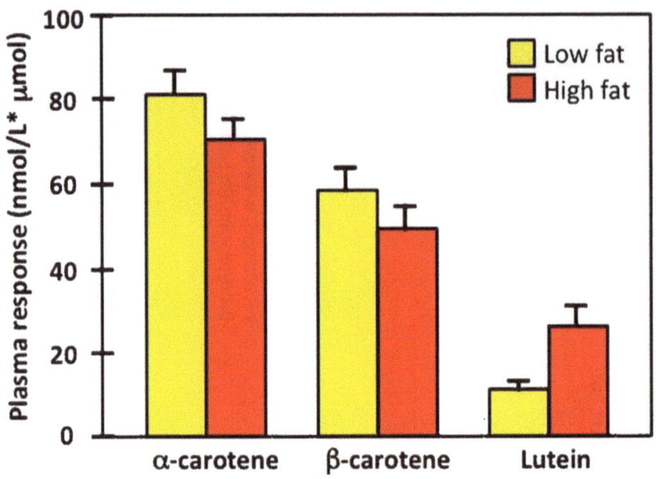

Fig. 6.2 Low amounts of dietary lipid are adequate for the absorption of purified α- and β-carotene supplements, whereas absorption of lutein esters requires larger amounts of lipid. Mean (±SE) plasma α- and β-carotene concentrations were similar in subjects consuming low-fat (3 g) and high-fat (36 g) meals. Plasma lutein concentrations were significantly higher when consumed with high-fat compared to low-fat meals ($P<0.001$). Adapted from Roodenburg et al. [38]

fat-free dressing provided minimal carotenoid absorption, 6 and 28 g salad dressings improved carotene and lycopene chylomicron postprandial response in a dose-dependent manner. Most surprising was the substantial increase in absorption with the high-fat level suggesting additional benefit to absorption (Fig. 6.3). Similarly, Unlu et al. [39] demonstrated that adding 12 g oil in the form of avocado enhanced carotene and lycopene postprandial TRL response relative to the 0 g control. However, no difference was noted between 12 and 24 g fat levels. Recently, the impact of both TAG amount (3, 8, and 20 g) and source (butter, canola oil, and soybean oil) on carotenoid bioavailability from raw vegetable salads was measured in humans. While source had minor impacts on absorption, 20 g TAG, regardless of source, promoted significantly higher absorption of lutein, zeaxanthin, β-carotene, and lycopene compared to 3 and 8 g [40]. Significant increases in carotenoid absorption were not detected between the low (3 g) and moderate (8 g) doses of lipid suggesting that low to intermediate levels of fat can greatly improve carotenoid absorption but higher levels can provide additional improvement in bioavailability.

Although it is difficult to compare studies using different methodologies (i.e., serum/plasma response vs chylomicron/TRL isolation), other factors that may have influenced the results from these studies should still be evaluated. Supplemental sources are generally more readily absorbed than those from whole and raw food systems [41]. Therefore, more co-consumed lipid may be required to improve extraction and micellarization of carotenoids from food matrices relative to presolubilized/emulsified supplements as provided by Roodenburg et al. [38]. Furthermore, the lipid:carotenoid ratio present in the gut lumen is likely just as important as overall lipid load. These often vary dramatically between studies (Table 6.2). For example Brown et al. [33], Unlu et al. [39], and Goltz et al. [40] provided three times the dose of total carotenoids compared to Roodenburg et al. [38]. Considering that the relative mass fraction of absorbed carotenoids decreases when the carotenoid amount increases [10], additional fat may be required to improve micellarization and subsequent intestinal absorption/secretion at higher carotenoid amounts.

Considering the complexity in comparing these key studies, defining an optimal dietary lipid amount remains challenging. Furthermore, it is unclear if carotenoid absorption continues to increase

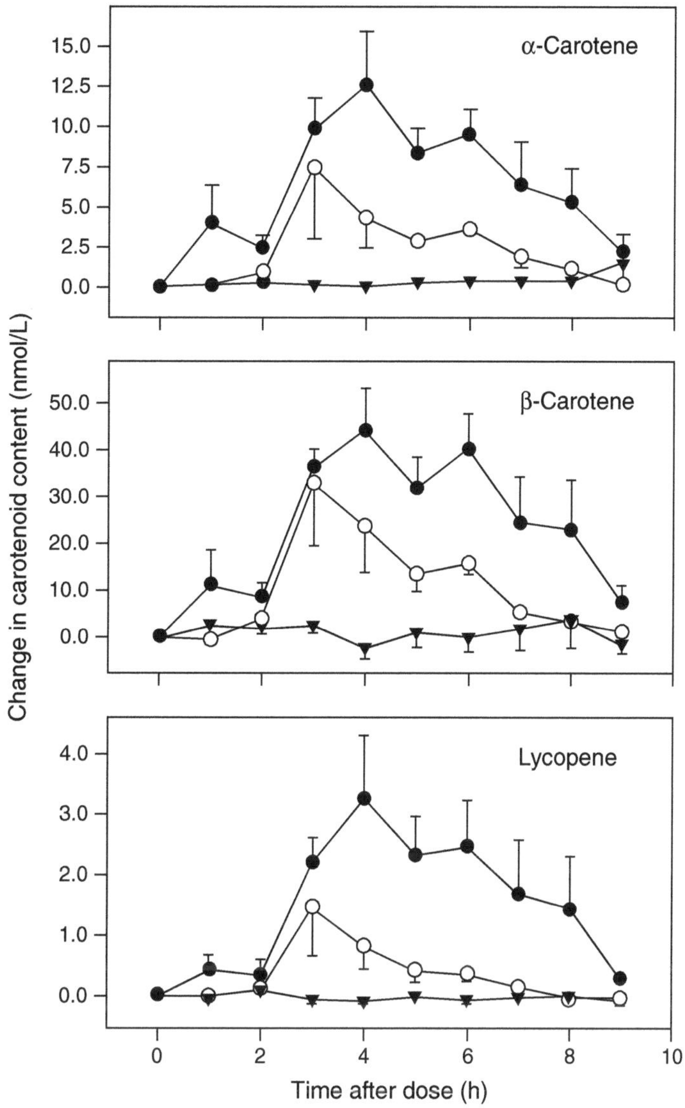

Fig. 6.3 Amount of oil in salad dressing impacts postprandial absorption of α-carotene, β-carotene, and lycopene from raw vegetables compared to baseline content. Subjects ingested a fresh vegetable salad with dressing containing 0 (▼), 6 (○), or 28 (●) g canola oil. Changes in chylomicron content (mean ± SE) of each carotenoid was greater for salads consumed with full-fat dressing compared to reduced-fat dressing ($P=0.02$) and for reduced-fat dressing compared to fat-free dressing ($P=0.04$). (Reprinted with permission from Brown et al. [33])

linearly with higher fat intakes. In human subjects, the highest amount of dietary lipids that has been evaluated is 200 g; however, incremental doses of TAG were not provided, making it difficult to determine if absorption occurs in a dose-dependent manner [32]. Several animal studies support the notion of a direct relationship between meal lipid content and carotenoid bioavailability. Cannulated rats fed emulsions of canthaxanthin, a polar carotenoid, with increasing amounts of olive oil (10, 30, 50, 70, 90 mg/h for 12 h) resulted in a linear increase [42]. In Mongolian gerbils fed vitamin-A free purified basal diets with added orange-fleshed sweet potato powder and 3, 6, or 12% fat, a positive linear relationship was observed between fat and β-carotene bioefficacy [43]. In a separate study using Mongolian gerbils, when dietary fat was increased from 10 to 30% of total energy from fat, conversion of β-carotene to vitamin A was enhanced [44]. Taken together with clinical findings, these results suggest that higher levels of co-consumed lipid would enhance carotenoid absorption.

Table 6.2 Impact of lipid source on carotenoid bioavailability in human subjects

Study	*n*	Nutritional status	Carotenoid type and amount	TG type and amount	Methodology	Duration	Results
Borel et al. [30]	16	Healthy	β-Carotene *supplements* (120 mg)	MCT or LCT (40 g)	Chylomicron response	2 Separate testing days, 12 h each	Lower concentration of chylomicron β-carotene and retinyl palmitate when β-carotene consumed with MCT compared to LCT. Consuming β-carotene with MCT did not impair the intestinal conversion of β-carotene into vitamin A
Hu et al. [55]	11	Healthy	β-Carotene *supplements* (25 mg)	Sunflower oil OR beef tallow (60 g)	Chylomicron response	2 Separate testing days, 10 h each, and monitored for 528 h	Lower amounts of β-carotene and retinyl palmitate incorporated into TRLs when consumed with PUFA-rich sunflower oil compared to SFA-rich beef tallow
Goltz et al. [40]	29	Healthy	*Raw* salad (262 g): 4.2 mg lutein, 6.9 mg zeaxanthin, 3.1 mg α-carotene, 6.3 mg β-carotene, 4.4 mg all-*trans* lycopene	Canola oil, soybean oil, or butter (3, 8, 20 g dietary fat)	TRL response	3 Separate testing days, 10 h each	Absorption was higher with MUFA-rich canola oil compared to PUFA-rich soybean oil for all carotenoids except lycopene. SFA-rich butter promoted the least amount of absorption for all carotenoid species
Lee et al. [54]	6	Healthy	Tomato soup and canned tomatoes (46 mg lycopene)	Olive oil OR sunflower oil (20 mL)	Plasma response	2 Separate 7-day periods	No significant difference between consumption of tomato products with olive oil or sunflower oil

Impact of Qualitative Lipid Profile on Carotenoid Bioavailability

The close association between carotenoid and lipid absorption raises the additional possibility that the source and qualitative fatty acid profile of dietary lipid may affect carotenoid absorption. Postprandial lipemia in animal and human models is dependent on qualitative lipid profile. For example, certain saturated fatty acids (SFA) increase postprandial lipemia compared to monounsaturated fatty acids (MUFA) [45] and polyunsaturated fatty acids (PUFA) [46–48]. Slower rates of triacylglycerol clearance after SFA consumption may be responsible for these trends. In contrast, SFAs from butter reduce lipemic responses compared with olive and sunflower oils, likely due to the abundance of short and medium chain fatty acids in this SFA source as well as its reduced digestibility [49]. Yet, Tholstrup et al. showed that even long chain SFAs reduce postprandial lipemia compared to MUFA and PUFA, again suggesting that both chain length and degree of saturation influence absorption of fatty acids and potentially carotenoids [50].

The extent to which differences in lipid profiles influence carotenoid absorption has been the subject of several human studies highlighted in Table 6.2. Additional animal studies have been conducted to augment these findings. Comparison of SFA-, MUFA-, and PUFA-rich lipids on β-carotene absorption in Wistar Kyoto rats was completed by Alam et al. [51]. While no difference was noted in serum β-carotene following 6 weeks of supplemental dosing with coconut oil (SFA-rich), olive oil (MUFA-rich), or safflower oil (PUFA-rich), hepatic β-carotene levels were the highest in rats fed olive and safflower oils, suggesting that these oils promote β-carotene absorption [51].

Additional animal studies support the notion that MUFA-rich lipids promote greater carotenoid absorption compared to PUFA-rich lipids overall. β-Carotene absorption was higher in cannulated rats when infused with oleic acid ($C_{18:1}$) compared to linoleic acid ($C_{18:2}$) or linolenic acid ($C_{18:3}$) [18]. Similarly, concentrations of polar xanthophylls were elevated in plasma and eyes from rats fed powdered *Commelina benghalensis* L., an Indian green leafy vegetable, with MUFA-rich olive oil compared to PUFA-rich sunflower oil [52].

The impact of lipid source on absorption of more hydrophobic carotenoid species is more complicated. A twofold increase in lycopene absorption was reported when cannulated rats were infused with an emulsion containing MUFA-rich olive oil in place of PUFA-rich corn oil [53]. However, no significant differences were observed in lycopene absorption by human subjects consuming tomato products with either MUFA-rich olive oil or PUFA-rich sunflower oil [54] suggesting minimal difference in absorption of aploar lycopene with altered meal lipid profile. Similarly, absorption of carotenoids by human subjects consuming raw vegetable salads was higher when co-consumed with MUFA-rich canola oil compared to PUFA-rich soybean oil for lutein, zeaxanthin, α-carotene, and β-carotene but not lycopene [40]. Collectively these findings suggest that MUFA-rich lipids may enhance carotenoid absorption to a greater extent than PUFA-rich lipids, especially for the more polar carotenoid species.

Many theories have been proposed to explain the reduction of carotenoid absorption by PUFA compared to MUFA. The first concerns the fatty acid binding protein (FABP), which has been implicated in the intracellular transfer of β-carotene as well as fatty acids [18]. Because FABP binds more readily to fatty acids with more unsaturated sites, β-carotene may be affected by competitive binding to FABP when consumed with PUFA-rich soybean oil compared to MUFA-rich canola oil. Therefore, a greater degree of fatty acid unsaturation in co-consumed lipid may decrease transport of carotenoids to chylomicrons. Another possibility includes potential differences in micelle size when MUFA vs. PUFA are consumed. Micelles containing PUFA are larger in size, resulting in slower diffusion through the unstirred water layer and decreased rates of absorption [53]. Finally, carotenoids ingested with PUFA may be more susceptible to oxidation and less available for absorption [53].

The impact of SFA on carotenoid absorption is also complex. Goltz et al. [40] reported that postprandial carotenoid absorption was lower when salads were co-consumed with SFA-rich butter compared to MUFA-rich canola or PUFA-rich soybean oil. Yet, Hu et al. [55] reported that postprandial absorption of β-carotene in humans from supplements was enhanced when co-consumed with 60 g SFA-rich beef tallow compared to 60 g PUFA-rich sunflower oil. While differences in matrices (raw vegetables compared to supplements) may have affected these outcomes, physiochemical differences between the SFA sources likely played a larger role. Beef tallow contains a high amount of oleic acid, a MUFA, which as discussed, may enhance carotenoid absorption. While butter, an oil-in-water emulsion, is poorly emulsified in the gut and may have limited ability to aid in carotenoid extraction from the food matrix and micellarization [49]. Additionally, butter contains appreciable amounts of short and medium chain triglycerides (MCT) which induce a relatively low lipemic response following ingestion [49]. Borel et al. [30] demonstrated that a lower lipemic response does translate to a reduction in postprandial β-carotene absorption, an effect that was attributed to the distribution of MCTs through the portal circulation and little chylomicron secretion. It was also suggested that β-carotene may have lower solubility in micelles composed of MCT than LCT, leading to lower intestinal absorption.

Overall, the results from these studies suggest that MUFA-rich lipids may enhance carotenoid absorption to a greater extent than PUFA-rich lipids but the effect of SFA and MCT requires clarification. The potential for a stronger effect of lipid source on polar carotenoid species compared to apolar carotenes is apparent. In any case, the conflicting results suggest that the relationship between qualitative lipid profile and carotenoid absorption is complex and remains to be further explored.

Mechanisms by Which Dietary Lipid Modulates Carotenoid Bioavailability

In addition to clinical investigations, several model systems have been used to dissect specific mechanisms by which co-consumed lipid modulates carotenoid absorption. Of the many systems applied in carotenoid research, the *in vitro* digestion and Caco-2 cell culture models are most often applied individually or as coupled systems to predict carotenoid bioaccessibility and to draw correlations with observations from human trials. These methods are not only used because they are cost and time efficient, but they also enhance clinical evaluations by providing the ability to test specific hypotheses related to mechanistic aspects of carotenoid release, micellarization, intestinal uptake, and chylomicron packaging and secretion [56].

Pre-absorptive Impact of Meal Lipid Profile on Carotenoid Release and Micellarization

In vitro digestion models, based on the porcine enzyme system, have been applied in the evaluation of factors impacting carotenoid digestive stability and efficiency of micellarization. Micellarization, as described previously, if considered to be a precursor to absorption and in combination with extraction/release and stability to digestive conditions, constitutes the concept of bioaccessibility. Good correlations have been established between micellarization efficiency *in vitro* and absorption in humans [57]. Other similarities exist as well. For example, the presence of TAG and bile salts are both required for micellarization of carotenoids [56]. Additionally, micellarization of xanthophylls including lutein and zeaxanthin is consistently more efficient than carotenes or lycopene [56, 58, 59]. However, the amount and source of TAG appears to have modest effects on carotenoid bioaccessibility *in vitro*. Huo et al. [59] reported that only small amounts of lipid (0.5–1%) were required to promote effective micellarization of α-carotene (14–17%), β-carotene (10–20%), and lycopene (1–5%)

from a mixed salad meal. Further, micellarization appears directly impacted by fatty acyl chain length ($C_{18:1}>C_{8:0}>C_{4:0}$) but not degree of unsaturation for C18 fatty acids [59]. Using identical digestion conditions, Kohut et al. [60] reported modest differences in micellarization efficiency of carotenes, lycopene, and xanthophylls from mixed green salads digested with either MUFA-rich canola oil, PUFA-rich soybean oil or SFA-rich vegetable shortening. These results suggest that only modest amounts of lipid, regardless of source, may be required to potentiate efficient carotenoid micellarization from food. Therefore, differences observed *in vivo* are more likely a result of absorptive and post-absorptive effects.

Impact of Meal Lipid Profile on Intestinal Uptake and Transport

The Caco-2 cell line is widely applied in the investigation of mechanisms of intestinal transport for many bioactive compounds including minerals [61–63], flavonoids [64–66], and drugs [67–69]. Originated from colonic adenocarcinoma, these cells spontaneously differentiate post-confluency to exhibit enterocyte-like cells [70]. This characteristic has made them suitable for investigation of mechanisms of carotenoid intestinal transport as well as factors that modulate intestinal absorption.

Uptake of micellerized carotenoids by differentiated monolayers of Caco-2 cells is generally proportional to media content and thus factors impacting micellarization have a direct impact on the quantity absorbed by Caco-2 cells [58]. This model has been applied to intestinal uptake of carotenoids from mixed vegetables digested with different lipid profiles. Interestingly, uptake of lutein and β-carotene by Caco-2 cells does not appear to be significantly impacted by chain length (trioctanoin and triolein) of co-digested TAG [59] suggesting intestinal uptake is not critically impacted by meal lipid profile.

More recently, media composition and culture conditions have been established that favor chylomicron synthesis and secretion by Caco-2 monolayers. Presence of oleic acid appears to stimulate chylomicron synthesis in Caco-2 monolayers [21, 31, 71] and suggests that fatty acyl composition of mixed micelles may impact post-absorptive packaging and transport of carotenoids through chylomicrons to a greater extent than pre-absorptive micellarization and intestinal uptake. Utilizing these models, a more detailed investigation of the impact of TAG amount and type on carotenoid transport is now underway [72]. To date, these efforts appear to support the *in vivo* observations that MUFA and PUFA are more effective than SFA in promoting carotenoid bioavailability and that differences in absorption are occurring at the level of epithelial processing and chylomicron secretion rather than through pre-absorptive modulations. Future research is required to systematically evaluate the impact of both amount and type of dietary lipid on carotenoid intestinal uptake and transport to better understand factors that may potentiate carotenoid bioavailability *in vivo*.

Dietary Fiber as a Modulator of Carotenoid Bioavailability

In addition to recommendations for a reduction of overall fat as a portion of calories, the 2010 Dietary Guidelines have listed dietary fiber in their list of, "nutrients of concern" because American adults consume only 40% of recommended amounts. Increasing intake of dietary fiber is associated with reduce risks of cardiovascular disease, diabetes, and obesity, and improved gastrointestinal health [1]. However, evidence exists that increasing certain types of dietary fiber may negatively impact carotenoid bioavailability (Fig 6.4).

The effect of dietary fiber has primarily focused on β-carotene absorption and conversion in animal models. Erdman et al. [73] reported that select purified dietary fiber sources reduced bioavailability

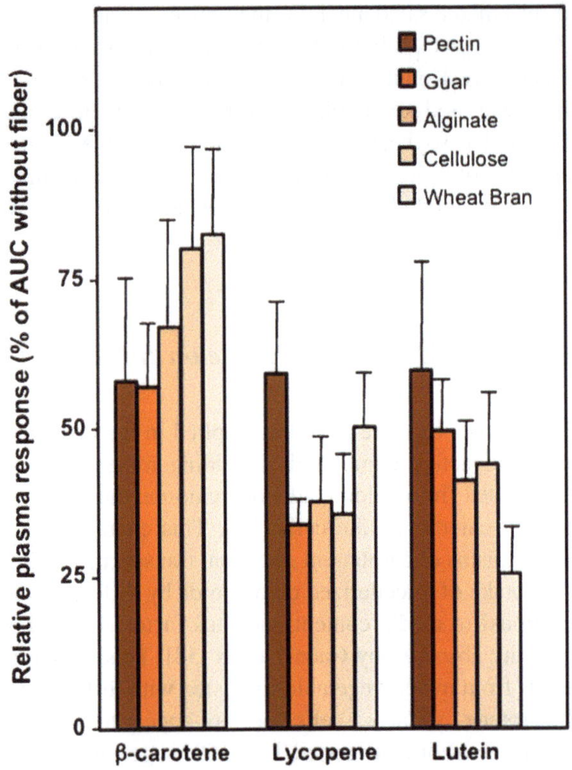

Fig. 6.4 Dietary fiber negatively impacts the bioavailability of carotenoids from dietary supplements. Mean plasma AUC_{24h} for β-carotene was reduced in subjects who consumed dietary supplements containing carotenoids along with a standard meal and water-soluble fibers pectin, guar, and alginate ($P<0.05$). Water insoluble fibers, cellulose, and wheat bran, as well as the water-soluble fibers reduced the absorption of lycopene and lutein ($P<0.05$). Adapted from Riedl et al. [75]

and bioconversion of this carotenoid in young chicks. Specifically, hemicelluloses, lignin, and citrus pectin, but not polygalacturonic acid reduced the percentage of β-carotene converted to vitamin A in the liver compared to controls. Further, the greatest reduction in liver vitamin A was seen with the pectin group. A second experiment within the same study indicated that β-carotene bioavailability and utilization was proportional to pectin methoxyl content [73].

The negative effects of pectin on β-carotene utilization have subsequently been observed in mammalian models. Deming et al. [44] reported a reduction in hepatic vitamin A with a corresponding increase in hepatic β-carotene stores in 4–5-week-old Mongolian gerbils fed diets containing citrus pectin. These data suggest that pectin may serve to reduce bioconversion rather than absorption. Rock and Swendseid [74] demonstrated that these findings were similar to results in humans where co-consumed pectin was found to reduce bioavailability of acute doses of purified β-carotene. In a separate study, both soluble fibers (pectin, guar, and alginate) and insoluble fibers (cellulose and wheat bran) at 8–10 g/day significantly reduced bioavailability of lycopene and lutein, in humans. However, only the soluble fibers were found to significantly reduce β-carotene bioavailability [75].

While only limited data exist, pectin and other soluble fibers appear to affect utilization of carotenoids, particularly provitamin A conversion, more strongly than absorption. Examining the effect that soluble fibers have on lipid metabolism may help to explain the mechanisms by which carotenoid bioavailability is reduced. Soluble fibers are known to bind bile acids resulting in increased fecal excretion of bile acids and total fat [76–78]. Physical properties of these fibers also increase the viscosity and volume of chyme in the gastrointestinal tract while reducing the concentration of phospholipids [79–81]. Together, these changes may disturb micelle formation and by extension, reduce the bioaccessible carotenoid content available for intestinal absorption and subsequent incorporation into chylomicrons [80]. Therefore, while co-consumed dietary lipids appear to impact carotenoid bioavailability most prominently at the level of chylomicron synthesis and secretion, the influence of dietary fiber on bioavailability appears to be exerted primarily during pre-absorptive stages. Additional research is needed to clarify the exact mechanism and extent of fiber effects on carotenoid bioavailability.

Conclusion

Dietary lipids and fibers exert direct effects on the absorption of carotenoids from fruits, vegetables, and dietary supplements. Considering that dietary guidelines focus on altering both total fat and fiber consumption, it remains critical to understand the potential influence these changes may have on carotenoid absorption. While lipid is a positive promoter of carotenoid absorption, the fine details on the impact of qualitative and quantitative lipid profiles continue to be explored. The possibility that a low dose of a "heart healthy" MUFA-rich oil as strong potentiator of carotenoid absorption merits further investigation. Similarly, many questions remain regarding the impact of fiber on carotenoid absorption. While believed to be a negative effector, the current body of studies has primarily focused on the effect of single, purified fiber sources on carotenoid absorption using animal models. Results of ongoing and future clinical investigations focused on lipid, fiber, and the interactions between these macro- and micronutrients will provide the foundation for assessing the potential impact of the 2010 Dietary Guidelines on bioavailability of carotenoids.

References

1. United States Department of Health and Human Services, U.S.D.A., and United States Dietary Guidelines Committee. *Report of the Dietary Guidelines Advisory Committee on the Dietary Guidelines for Americans, 2010.* 2010.
2. Yonekura L, Nagao A. Intestinal absorption of dietary carotenoids. Mol Nutr Food Res. 2007;51(1):107–15.
3. Yeum KJ, Russell RM. Carotenoid bioavailability and bioconversion. Annu Rev Nutr. 2002;22:483–504.
4. Stahl W, et al. Bioavailability and metabolism. Mol Aspects Med. 2002;23(1–3):39–100.
5. Tyssandier V, et al. Processing of vegetable-borne carotenoids in the human stomach and duodenum. Am J Physiol Gastrointest Liver Physiol. 2003;284(6):G913–23.
6. Parker RS, et al. Bioavailability of carotenoids in human subjects. Proc Nutr Soc. 1999;58(1):155–62.
7. Poor CL, et al. The accumulation of α- and β-carotene in serum and tissues of preruminant calves fed raw and steamed carrot slurries. J Nutr. 1993;123(7):1296–304.
8. Dietz JM, Sri Kantha S, Erdman Jr JW. Reversed phase HPLC analysis of α- and β-carotene from selected raw and cooked vegetables. Plant Foods Hum Nutr. 1988;38(4):333–41.
9. Furr HC, Clark RM. Intestinal absorption and tissue distribution of carotenoids. Nutr Biochem. 1997;8:364–77.
10. Borel P, et al. Carotenoids in biological emulsions: solubility, surface-to-core distribution, and release from lipid droplets. J Lipid Res. 1996;37(2):250–61.
11. Thomson AB, et al. Lipid absorption: passing through the unstirred layers, brush-border membrane, and beyond. Can J Physiol Pharmacol. 1993;71(8):531–55.
12. Hernell O, Staggers JE, Carey MC. Physical-chemical behavior of dietary and biliary lipids during intestinal digestion and absorption. 2. Phase analysis and aggregation states of luminal lipids during duodenal fat digestion in healthy adult human beings. Biochemistry. 1990;29(8):2041–56.
13. Hofmann AF. The function of bile salts in fat absorption. The solvent properties of dilute micellar solutions of conjugated bile salts. Biochem J. 1963;89:57–68.
14. Tyssandier V, Lyan B, Borel P. Main factors governing the transfer of carotenoids from emulsion lipid droplets to micelles. Biochim Biophys Acta. 2001;1533(3):285–92.
15. Nagao A. Absorption and function of dietary carotenoids. Forum Nutr. 2009;61:55–63.
16. Erdman Jr JW, Bierer TL, Gugger ET. Absorption and transport of carotenoids. Ann N Y Acad Sci. 1993;691:76–85.

17. El-Gorab MI, Underwood BA, Loerch JD. The roles of bile salts in the uptake of β-carotene and retinol by rat everted gut sacs. Biochim Biophys Acta. 1975;401(2):265–77.
18. Hollander D, Ruble Jr PE. β-carotene intestinal absorption: bile, fatty acid, pH, and flow rate effects on transport. Am J Physiol. 1978;235(6):E686–91.
19. Scita G, Aponte GW, Wolf G. Uptake and cleavage of β-carotene by cultures of rat small intestinal cells and human lung fibroblasts. Methods Enzymol. 1993;214:21–32.
20. Moore AC, Gugger ET, Erdman Jr JW. Brush border membrane vesicles from rats and gerbils can be utilized to evaluate the intestinal uptake of all-*trans* and 9-*cis* β-carotene. J Nutr. 1996;126(11):2904–12.
21. During A, et al. Carotenoid uptake and secretion by CaCo-2 cells: β-carotene isomer selectivity and carotenoid interactions. J Lipid Res. 2002;43(7):1086–95.
22. van Bennekum A, et al. Class B scavenger receptor-mediated intestinal absorption of dietary β-carotene and cholesterol. Biochemistry. 2005;44(11):4517–25.
23. Sugawara T, et al. Lysophosphatidylcholine enhances carotenoid uptake from mixed micelles by Caco-2 human intestinal cells. J Nutr. 2001;131(11):2921–7.
24. Baskaran V, Sugawara T, Nagao A. Phospholipids affect the intestinal absorption of carotenoids in mice. Lipids. 2003;38(7):705–11.
25. Lakshminarayana R, et al. Enhanced lutein bioavailability by lyso-phosphatidylcholine in rats. Mol Cell Biochem. 2006;281(1–2):103–10.
26. Raju M, et al. Influence of phospholipids on β-carotene absorption and conversion into vitamin A in rats. J Nutr Sci Vitaminol (Tokyo). 2005;51(4):216–22.
27. Parker RS. Absorption, metabolism, and transport of carotenoids. FASEB J. 1996;10(5):542–51.
28. Glover J, Redfearn ER. The mechanism of the transformation of β-carotene into vitamin A in vivo. Biochem J. 1954;58(331st Meeting):xv–xvi.
29. Wang XD, et al. Retinoic acid can be produced from excentric cleavage of β-carotene in human intestinal mucosa. Arch Biochem Biophys. 1992;293(2):298–304.
30. Borel P, et al. Chylomicron β-Carotene and retinyl palmitate responses are dramatically diminished when men ingest β-carotene with medium-chain rather than long-chain triglycerides. J Nutr. 1998;128(8):1361–7.
31. van Greevenbroek MM, et al. Effects of saturated, mono-, and polyunsaturated fatty acids on the secretion of apo B containing lipoproteins by Caco-2 cells. Atherosclerosis. 1996;121(1):139–50.
32. Prince MR, Frisoli JK. β-Carotene accumulation in serum and skin. Am J Clin Nutr. 1993;57(2):175–81.
33. Brown MJ, et al. Carotenoid bioavailability is higher from salads ingested with full-fat than with fat-reduced salad dressings as measured with electrochemical detection. Am J Clin Nutr. 2004;80(2):396–403.
34. Jayarajan P, Reddy V, Mohanram M. Effect of dietary fat on absorption of β carotene from green leafy vegetables in children. Indian J Med Res. 1980;71:53–6.
35. Takyi EE. Children's consumption of dark green, leafy vegetables with added fat enhances serum retinol. J Nutr. 1999;129(8):1549–54.
36. Ribaya-Mercado JD, et al. Carotene-rich plant foods ingested with minimal dietary fat enhance the total-body vitamin A pool size in Filipino schoolchildren as assessed by stable-isotope-dilution methodology. Am J Clin Nutr. 2007;85(4):1041–9.
37. Ribaya-Mercado JD, et al. Bioconversion of plant carotenoids to vitamin A in Filipino school-aged children varies inversely with vitamin A status. Am J Clin Nutr. 2000;72(2):455–65.
38. Roodenburg AJ, et al. Amount of fat in the diet affects bioavailability of lutein esters but not of α-carotene, β-carotene, and vitamin E in humans. Am J Clin Nutr. 2000;71(5):1187–93.
39. Unlu NZ, et al. Carotenoid absorption from salad and salsa by humans is enhanced by the addition of avocado or avocado oil. J Nutr. 2005;135(3):431–6.
40. Goltz SG, et al. Meal triacylglycerol profile modulates carotenoid post-prandial absorption in humans. FASEB J. 2011;25:975.10.
41. Goltz SR, et al. Meal triacylglycerol profile modulates postprandial absorption of carotenoids in humans. Mol Nutr Food Res. 2012;56(6):866–77.
42. Clark RM, Furr HC. Absorption of canthaxanthin by the rat is influenced by total lipid in the intestinal lumen. Lipids. 2001;36(5):473–5.
43. Mills JP, et al. Sweet potato β-carotene bioefficacy is enhanced by dietary fat and not reduced by soluble fiber intake in Mongolian gerbils. J Nutr. 2009;139(1):44–50.
44. Deming DM, et al. Amount of dietary fat and type of soluble fiber independently modulate postabsorptive conversion of β-carotene to vitamin A in Mongolian gerbils. J Nutr. 2000;130(11):2789–96.
45. Roche HM, et al. The effect of test meal monounsaturated fatty acid: saturated fatty acid ratio on postprandial lipid metabolism. Br J Nutr. 1998;79(5):419–24.
46. Harris WS, et al. Reduction of postprandial triglyceridemia in humans by dietary n-3 fatty acids. J Lipid Res. 1988;29(11):1451–60.

47. Weintraub MS, et al. Dietary polyunsaturated fats of the W-6 and W-3 series reduce postprandial lipoprotein levels. Chronic and acute effects of fat saturation on postprandial lipoprotein metabolism. J Clin Invest. 1988;82(6):1884–93.
48. Lai HC, Ney DM. Corn oil, palm oil and butterfat fractions affect postprandial lipemia and lipoprotein lipase in meal-fed rats. J Nutr. 1995;125(6):1536–45.
49. Mekki N, et al. Butter differs from olive oil and sunflower oil in its effects on postprandial lipemia and triacylglycerol-rich lipoproteins after single mixed meals in healthy young men. J Nutr. 2002;132(12):3642–9.
50. Tholstrup T, et al. Effect of 6 dietary fatty acids on the postprandial lipid profile, plasma fatty acids, lipoprotein lipase, and cholesterol ester transfer activities in healthy young men. Am J Clin Nutr. 2001;73(2):198–208.
51. Alam BS, Brown LR, Alam SQ. Influence of dietary fats and vitamin E on plasma and hepatic vitamin A and β-carotene levels in rats fed excess β-carotene. Nutr Cancer. 1990;14(2):111–6.
52. Lakshminarayana R, et al. Lutein and zeaxanthin in leafy greens and their bioavailability: olive oil influences the absorption of dietary lutein and its accumulation in adult rats. J Agric Food Chem. 2007;55(15):6395–400.
53. Clark RM, et al. A comparison of lycopene and astaxanthin absorption from corn oil and olive oil emulsions. Lipids. 2000;35(7):803–6.
54. Lee A, Thurnham DI, Chopra M. Consumption of tomato products with olive oil but not sunflower oil increases the antioxidant activity of plasma. Free Radic Biol Med. 2000;29(10):1051–5.
55. Hu X, Jandacek RJ, White WS. Intestinal absorption of β-carotene ingested with a meal rich in sunflower oil or beef tallow: postprandial appearance in triacylglycerol-rich lipoproteins in women. Am J Clin Nutr. 2000;71(5):1170–80.
56. Garrett DA, Failla ML, Sarama RJ. Development of an *in vitro* digestion method to assess carotenoid bioavailability from meals. J Agric Food Chem. 1999;47(10):4301–9.
57. Reboul E, et al. Bioaccessibility of carotenoids and vitamin E from their main dietary sources. J Agric Food Chem. 2006;54(23):8749–55.
58. Chitchumroonchokchai C, Schwartz SJ, Failla ML. Assessment of lutein bioavailability from meals and a supplement using simulated digestion and Caco-2 human intestinal cells. J Nutr. 2004;134(9):2280–6.
59. Huo T, et al. Impact of fatty acyl composition and quantity of triglycerides on bioaccessibility of dietary carotenoids. J Agric Food Chem. 2007;55(22):8950–7.
60. Kohut AR, et al. The impact of lipid quantity and type on carotenoid bioaccessibility from vegetables. FASEB J. 2007;21:A350.
61. Boato F, et al. Red grape juice inhibits iron availability: application of an *in vitro* digestion/Caco-2 cell model. J Agric Food Chem. 2002;50(23):6935–8.
62. Mesias M, Seiquer I, Navarro MP. Influence of diets rich in Maillard reaction products on calcium bioavailability. Assays in male adolescents and in Caco-2 cells. J Agric Food Chem. 2009;57(20):9532–8.
63. Kim EY, Pai TK, Han O. Effect of bioactive dietary polyphenols on zinc transport across the intestinal Caco-2 cell monolayers. J Agric Food Chem. 2011;59(8):3606–12.
64. Brand W, et al. Metabolism and transport of the citrus flavonoid hesperetin in Caco-2 cell monolayers. Drug Metab Dispos. 2008;36(9):1794–802.
65. Shulman M, et al. Enhancement of naringenin bioavailability by complexation with hydroxypropoyl-β-cyclodextrin. PLoS One. 2011;6(4):e18033.
66. Liu Y, Hu M. Absorption and metabolism of flavonoids in the Caco-2 cell culture model and a perused rat intestinal model. Drug Metab Dispos. 2002;30(4):370–7.
67. Flanagan SD, et al. Contributions of saturable active secretion, passive transcellular, and paracellular diffusion to the overall transport of furosemide across adenocarcinoma (Caco-2) cells. J Pharm Sci. 2002;91(4):1169–77.
68. Hu M, et al. Mechanisms of transport of quinapril in Caco-2 cell monolayers: comparison with cephalexin. Pharm Res. 1995;12(8):1120–5.
69. Lo Y, Liu F, Cherng J. Effect of PSC 833 liposomes and intralipid on the transport of epirubicin in Caco-2 cells and rat intestines. J Control Release. 2001;76(1–2):1–10.
70. Hidalgo IJ, Raub TJ, Borchardt RT. Characterization of the human colon carcinoma cell line (Caco-2) as a model system for intestinal epithelial permeability. Gastroenterology. 1989;96(3):736–49.
71. Moberly JB, et al. Oleic acid stimulation of apolipoprotein B secretion from HepG2 and Caco-2 cells occurs post-transcriptionally. Biochim Biophys Acta. 1990;1042(1):70–80.
72. Chitchumroonchokchai C, et al. Dietary fats with increased ratio of unsaturated to saturated fatty acids enhance absorption of carotenoid and vitamin E by increasing both efficiency of micellarization and lipoprotein secretion. FASEB J. 2010;24:539.3.
73. Erdman Jr JW, Fahey Jr GC, White CB. Effects of purified dietary fiber sources on β-carotene utilization by the chick. J Nutr. 1986;116(12):2415–23.
74. Rock CL, Swendseid ME. Plasma β-carotene response in humans after meals supplemented with dietary pectin. Am J Clin Nutr. 1992;55(1):96–9.
75. Riedl J, et al. Some dietary fibers reduce the absorption of carotenoids in women. J Nutr. 1999;129(12):2170–6.

76. Kay RM, Judd PA, Truswell AS. The effect of pectin on serum cholesterol. Am J Clin Nutr. 1978;31(4):562–3.
77. Kay RM, Truswell AS. Effect of citrus pectin on blood lipids and fecal steroid excretion in man. Am J Clin Nutr. 1977;30(2):171–5.
78. Vahouny GV, Cassidy MM. Dietary fibers and absorption of nutrients. Proc Soc Exp Biol Med. 1985;180(3):432–46.
79. Phillips DR. The effect of guar gum in solution on diffusion of cholesterol mixed micelles. J Sci Food Agric. 1986;37:548–52.
80. Judd PA, Truswell AS. The hypocholesterolaemic effects of pectins in rats. Br J Nutr. 1985;53(3):409–25.
81. Gallaher D, Schneeman BO. Intestinal interaction of bile acids, phospholipids, dietary fibers, and cholestyramine. Am J Physiol. 1986;250(4 Pt 1):G420–6.
82. Dimitrov NV, et al. Bioavailability of β-carotene in humans. Am J Clin Nutr. 1988;48(2):298–304.
83. Ahuja KD, et al. Effects of olive oil and tomato lycopene combination on serum lycopene, lipid profile, and lipid oxidation. Nutrition. 2006;22(3):259–65.

Chapter 7
Host Factors That Affect Carotenoid Metabolism

Georg Lietz

Key Points

- Host factors can affect the nutrient status by influencing the ability to absorb, convert, and metabolize dietary carotenoids. Factors such as gender, body fat and genetic variation, play an important role in this process.
- The recent discoveries of specific carotenoid binding proteins such as StARD3 and GSTP1, as well as the existence of a diet-responsive regulatory network influencing intestinal carotenoid uptake via the gatekeeper ISX, further highlights the complex interaction between nutrient intake and nutrient status.
- The occurrence of the low responder phenotype can partly be explained through genetic variations in key enzymes and proteins involved in carotenoid uptake and metabolism.
- This chapter explores the importance of host factors affecting absorption, conversion, secretion, and tissue uptake of carotenoids using lutein and β-carotene as examples of two classes of carotenoids.

Keywords Host factors • Dietary carotenoids • StaRD3 • GSTP1 • BCMO1 • Low responder phenotype • Diet responsive regulatory network • Nutrient intake • Nutrient status

Introduction

Dietary carotenoids follow the same absorptive pathways as dietary lipids and are transported in the bloodstream exclusively by lipoproteins, with the adipose tissue being their main storage site [1]. Several studies have observed the existence of high interindividual variability in carotenoid absorption and plasma status [2–8]. Host-related factors may explain many of the observed differences in serum and tissue responses to dietary carotenoids, although other factors such as the food matrix and absorption modifiers (see Chap. 6) can also affect interindividual variations even under strict experimental conditions.

G. Lietz, Dipl.oec.troph., Ph.D. (✉)
School of Agriculture, Food and Rural Development (AFRD), Human Nutrition Research Centre, Newcastle University, Kings Road, Agriculture Building, Newcastle upon Tyne, NE1 7RU, UK
e-mail: georg.lietz@newcastle.ac.uk

S.A. Tanumihardjo (ed.), *Carotenoids and Human Health*, Nutrition and Health,
DOI 10.1007/978-1-62703-203-2_7, © Springer Science+Business Media New York 2013

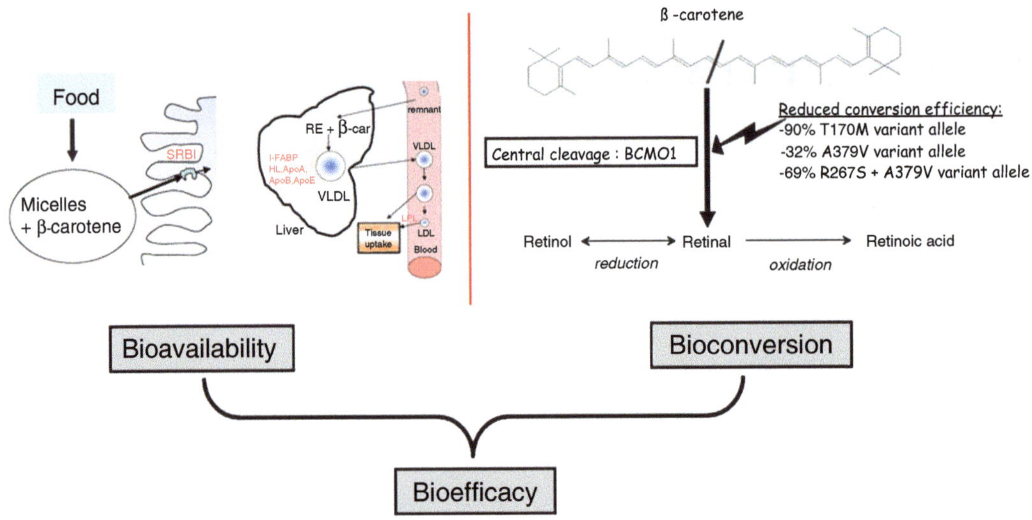

Fig. 7.1 Bioavailability, bioconversion, and bioefficacy of provitamin A carotenoids

The pharmacological terms bioavailability, bioconversion, and bioefficacy are commonly used in carotenoid metabolism. Bioavailability is defined as the fraction of an ingested carotenoid that is available for utilization or storage, whereas bioconversion is defined as the fraction of an absorbed provitamin A carotenoid which is cleaved to the active metabolite retinol. Bioefficacy is defined as the combination of bioavailability and bioconversion, therefore representing the fraction of the nutrient absorbed and converted to the active metabolite in the body [9] (Fig. 7.1). Variation in bioavailability and bioefficacy of dietary carotenoids can be caused by impaired intestinal absorption, impaired conversion to vitamin A, inefficient incorporation into chylomicrons or accelerated clearance due to atypical lipoprotein metabolism [10] (Fig. 7.2). Finally, specific transport proteins for carotenoids such as the steroidogenic acute regulatory domain (StARD3) protein for lutein [11] and glutathione *S*-transferase (GSTP1) for zeaxanthin [12] as well as tissue-specific uptake [13] could potentially contribute to the observed large interindividual variation. This chapter elaborates on the importance of host factors affecting absorption, conversion, secretion, and tissue uptake of carotenoids using lutein and β-carotene as two examples of an oxygenated and a hydrocarbon carotenoid, respectively.

The Low Responder/Low Converter Phenotype

Depending on the carotenoid, the definition of the low responder phenotype has been associated with different tissue or plasma concentrations leading to some confusion in the literature. For β-carotene, the definition of the low responder phenotype has been used to describe a low or nonincrease in plasma β-carotene concentrations after dosing [2–4, 14], or in relation to provitamin A conversion efficiency [8, 15]. On the other hand, studies investigating provitamin A activity have demonstrated that approximately 45% of the Western population have a low conversion efficiency, which has lead to the definition of the low converter phenotype [6, 8, 15, 16]. Controversial earlier studies concluded that variations in responses between subjects may be caused by differences in absorption and transport of β-carotene rather than by differing conversion efficiency [2, 4]. However, more recent studies

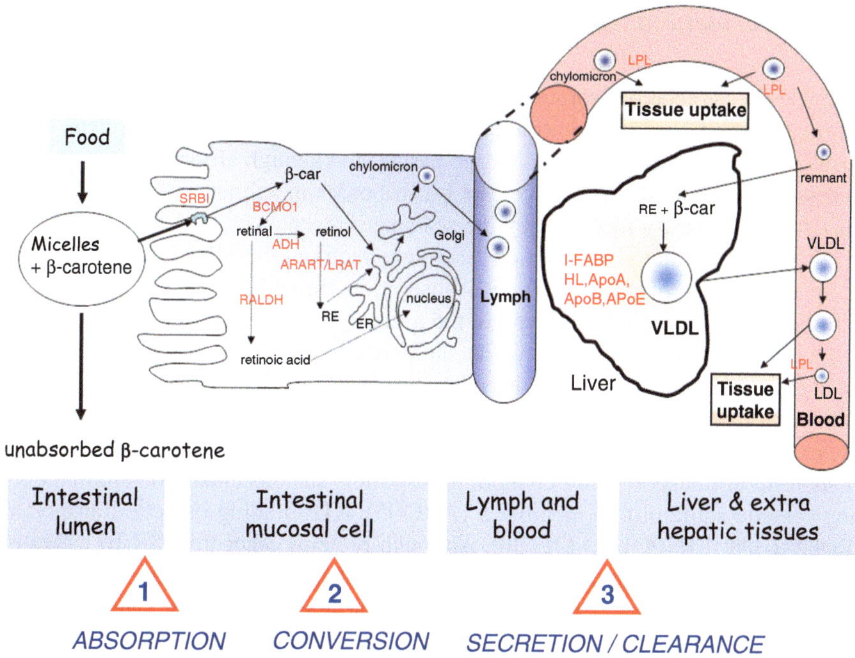

Fig. 7.2 Key regulatory proteins influencing carotenoid status. This diagram illustrates the influence of key regulatory genes on carotenoid absorption, conversion to vitamin A, incorporation into chylomicrons and their subsequent clearance. *ADH* alcohol dehydrogenases, *ARAT* acyl-CoA:retinol acyltransferase, *ER* endoplasmic reticulum, *LPL* lipoprotein lipase, *LRAT* lecithin-retinol acyltransferase, *RALDH* retinaldehyde dehydrogenase, *RE retinyl ester.* Reproduced from [10] with permission

using stable isotopes concluded that both absorption and conversion of ingested β-carotene to vitamin A contributed to the variable plasma response to ingested β-carotene [6, 8, 15, 16]. Interestingly, low responders and low converters were observed after ingestion of a pharmacological dose of β-carotene with interindividual variations of newly absorbed β-carotene and retinyl palmitate/β-carotene ratios ranging from 53 to 60%, respectively [17]. Furthermore, low responders also display a lower conversion efficiency compared to normal responders.

For lutein, the low responder phenotype in most studies refers to macular pigment optical density (MPOD) measurements before and after lutein supplementation [18–20] and is defined as the "retinal responder" phenotype, although one study also refers to plasma lutein nonresponders as "blood nonresponders" [19]. Retinal nonresponders showed no increases in MPOD after consuming 12 mg lutein for 6 months indicating that intestinal malabsorption is not responsible for the lack of macular response to lutein supplementation [20]. Interestingly, retinal responders tended to be female and to have lower serum lutein concentrations, lower MPOD, and greater retinal thickness at baseline, whereas age, frequency of lighter irises, or smoking was not significantly different between retinal responders or nonresponders [18]. Furthermore, MPOD is lower in subjects with body fat >27% [21]. Body fat is of particular interest because adipose tissue is a major storage tissue for lutein providing a "sink" for lutein, which makes this carotenoid less available to other tissues. Changes in the macular pigment density is negatively correlated with lutein concentration of the adipose tissue in women, but positively in men [22–24]. This suggests that factors such as gender, body fat, and low levels of lutein in serum and retina may indicate which subject is likely to be classified as a retinal responder.

Regulation of Carotenoid Absorption

At the intestinal level, carotenoid absorption is dependent on three steps: (1) absorption at the enterocyte brush border membrane, (2) enzymatic conversion of a fraction of absorbed β-carotene into retinal or *apo*-carotenals, and (3) secretion of chylomicron particles. Although absorption was thought to be a passive process with simple diffusion over the brush border membrane following a concentration gradient, this process is partly mediated by the scavenger receptor class B type I (SR-BI) [25–28]. During et al. [25] showed that absorption of β-carotene required the SR-BI intestinal transporter by demonstrating a 60% decrease in β-carotene absorption through inhibition of SR-BI transport. Likewise, the SR-BI transporter is involved in the absorption process of lutein [27]. The functional role for SR-BI is consistent with the finding that an SR-BI homolog is essential for cellular uptake of carotenoids in *Drosophila*, because flies with a genetic ninaD knockout become completely blind due to the inability to absorb β-carotene [29]. Expressed at high levels in the intestine, the SR-BI transporter is also involved in the process of cholesterol absorption leading to the suggestion that β-carotene, lutein, and cholesterol transport share common transporters such as cluster determinant 36 (CD36), ATP binding cassette subfamily G member 5 (ABCG5), ATP-binding cassette transporter A1, and Niemann Pick C1-like 1 (NPC1L1) [25, 30]. Although proteins other than SR-BI affect carotenoid absorption (i.e., CD36, ABCG5, and NPC1L1), there is little evidence to date to support their role in carotenoid uptake at the enterocyte. For example, only a near significant association between plasma lutein and the Q640E variant in ABCG5 was observed in a human intervention study [31], whereas the involvement of CD36 in β-carotene uptake has only been confirmed in mouse adipocytes [32] and no evidence for the role of NPC1L1 in carotenoid uptake exists to date [30].

Other indications that specific epithelial transporters are involved in carotenoid absorption across the brush border membrane come from the observations that β-carotene isomers are discriminated during absorption [33]. Human studies have consistently reported that all-*trans*-β-carotene is preferentially accumulated over 9-*cis* in total plasma and the postprandial triacylglycerol-rich lipoprotein plasma fraction [34–37]. The intestinal *cis–trans* isomerization of 9-*cis* to all-*trans* β-carotene occurs in the enterocyte since a significant accumulation of ^{13}C-all-*trans* β-carotene occurred in plasma of subjects who ingested only ^{13}C-9-*cis* β-carotene [36]. However, the enzyme responsible for this isomeration has to date not been identified.

Importantly, humans, but not rodents, absorb significant amounts of intact β-carotene [38] as only a fraction of absorbed β-carotene is oxidatively cleaved in a centric or eccentric fashion by the β-carotene 15,15′-monooxygenase (BCMO1) or the β-carotene 9′,10′-dioxygenase (BCDO2), respectively [39, 40]. The regulation of this process is described in detail below.

In contrast to carotenoids, dietary preformed retinol enters intestinal cells by diffusion [41]. Although both retinyl esters formed from cleavage of carotenoids in the enterocyte and intact absorbed carotenoids are transported to the lymph in chylomicrons, recent data show that the efflux of preformed retinol is partly facilitated by the basolateral ATP-binding cassette transporter A1, indicating that 19% of preformed retinol could be delivered to the liver via the portal circulation, therefore circumventing the apoB-dependent pathway [41]. Interestingly, carotenoid efflux occurs exclusively via their secretion in chylomicrons [41]. Upon entering the bloodstream chylomicrons undergo immediate lipolysis by lipoprotein lipases to produce chylomicron remnants [42]. Importantly, intestinal absorption and release of dietary carotenoid on chylomicra follows the same time-course as that of other dietary lipids. However, due to their redistribution into different lipoprotein particles, carotenoids seems to reach their maximum plasma concentration slower compared to triacylglycerol or retinyl esters after an oral test dose [14]. This effect differs depending on the carotenoid species, since hydrocarbon carotenes (e.g., β-carotene) are transported primarily on LDL plus VLDL, whereas the xanthophylls (e.g., lutein) are distributed approximately equally between HDL and LDL in human serum [14].

Potential Causes for the Low Converter Phenotype

Several studies have reported high interindividual variation in the ability to convert provitamin A carotenoids; 4.5- to 8-fold differences have been reported [5] between the highest and lowest converter. The enzyme responsible for provitamin A conversion into two retinal is BCMO1, and approximately 95% of retinoids arising from β-carotene are produced by this pathway *in vivo* [43]. Studies using BCMO1 knock-out mice have provided evidence for the fundamental role of this enzyme in producing vitamin A from dietary β-carotene [44–46]. Between 35 and 88% of absorbed β-carotene is cleaved into all-*trans* retinal, with the rest being secreted as intact β-carotene [39]. The rate of intact β-carotene absorption is between 3 and 55% [6, 8]. All-*trans* retinal can be oxidized irreversibly to retinoic acid by retinal dehydrogenase or reduced reversibly to retinol by a retinal reductase [39]. BCMO1 has high specificity towards the double bonds at the 15,15′-position of carotenoids but quite broad specificity towards carotenoids containing at least one unsubstituted β-ionone ring [47–51]. BCMO1 substrate specificity decreases in the order: β-carotene > β-cryptoxanthin > β-*apo*-8′-carotenal > β-*apo*-4′-carotenal > α-carotene > γ-carotene [48]. In human tissues, BCMO1 is expressed at high levels in intestinal mucosa, liver and kidney [51]. The expression/activity of BCMO1 in extra-intestinal tissues has been linked to the capacity of these tissues to directly convert locally stored carotenoids into vitamin A [52]. Indeed, recent isotope studies indicated that post-intestinal conversion of vitamin A accounted for up to 30% of the total converted retinol over the period of 52 days [16]. Thus, observed variations in cleavage efficiency between individual could be caused by two aspects: (a) by factors influencing the expression and activity of intestinal BCMO1 and (b) by variations in post-intestinal conversion of provitamin A carotenoids.

Although BCDO2 cleaves β-carotene at the 9,10 double bond forming β-*apo*-10-carotenal and β-ionone, it does not rescue BCMO1 deficiency and can therefore not substantially contribute to the production of retinoids in mammals [40]. However, BCDO2 plays an important role in protecting against carotenoid-induced mitochondrial dysfunction and has a broader substrate specificity than BCMO1 [53, 54] (please see review [40] for more details).

Tissue Uptake, Distribution, and Metabolic Effects

Although relative tissue concentrations in human liver, kidney, and lung are qualitatively similar to those in serum, the human macular pigment consists of lutein, zeaxanthin, and meso-zeaxanthin to the exclusion of other carotenoids [55]. In the fovea, the carotenoid concentration approaches 1 mM, and decreases more than 100-fold just a few millimeters from the foveal center [11, 56]. Interestingly, the specific uptake of lutein and zeaxanthin to millimolar concentrations into macular retina appears to be unique to humans and fellow primates [11]. Understanding the biochemical mechanisms underlying the selective uptakes of lutein and zeaxanthin into the human macula let to the discovery of GSTP1 as the macular zeaxanthin-binding protein [12] and StARD3 as a lutein-binding protein in the macula of the primate retina [11]. Furthermore, although not implicated in lutein transport in enterocytes, CD36 was postulated as a potential candidate for a surface receptor and transport protein that could interact with StARD3 to mediate lutein uptake from the serum and transfer into the macula [11, 57]. Thus, unraveling the biochemical regulation of xanthophyll uptake into the retina is fundamental in providing key insights into the role of macular carotenoids in human ocular health and disease.

Another tissue-specific uptake for lutein may be mammary cells, because milk carotenoid profile changes during lactation from a higher proportion of less polar carotenoids, such as β-carotene, in colostrum to the polar carotenoids, such as lutein, in mature milk [58]. This may be caused by active transport into the mammary cell since lutein is found proportionally more in milk than in plasma, independent of whether plasma carotenoid concentrations are changed during β-carotene supplementation

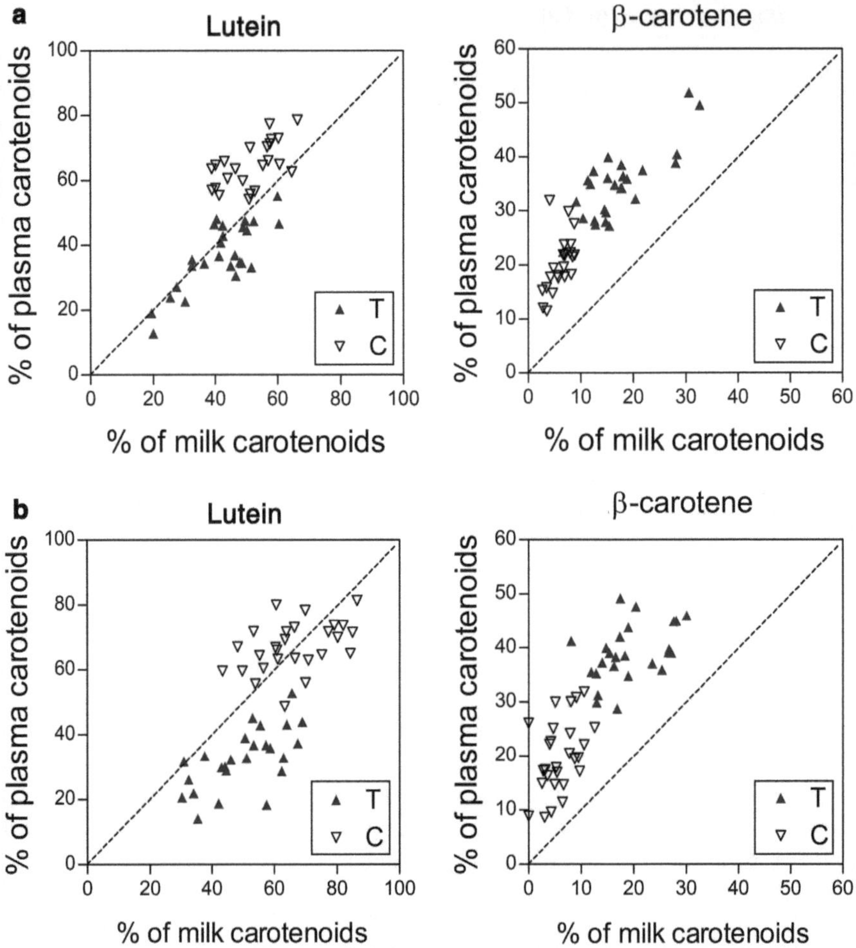

Fig. 7.3 Proportions of lutein and β-carotene in samples of plasma and breast milk obtained simultaneously at 1 month (**a**) and 3 month (**b**) postpartum from Tanzanian women that did (T) or did not (C) receive 2 mg provitamin A/day for 6 months as supplemental red palm oil. In each graph, the *dashed line* indicates equal proportions of carotenoids in milk and plasma. Adapted from [13]

(Fig. 7.3) [13]. Although the exact mechanism of transfer remains to be elucidated, a selective uptake of HDL might be responsible for the change in carotenoid pattern in breast milk compared with plasma. Alternatively, an increase in mammary lipoprotein lipase (LPL) activity may increase catabolism of chylomicron particles, which subsequently increases the formation of discoidal HDL that are directly catabolized by the endothelial lipase [13].

Finally, body mass index was found to be inversely correlated with conversion efficiency [15], suggesting an interrelationship between β-carotene metabolism and adiposity in humans. Indeed, a BCMO1 dependent decrease of PPARγ was observed during β-carotene supplementation in inguinal white adipose tissue [44]. Moreover, body fat mass and leptin serum levels were significantly reduced after β-carotene supplementation in mice with an active BCMO1 enzyme but not in BCMO1 knock-out mice [44]. Furthermore, BCMO1 knock-out mice develop liver steatosis independent of their vitamin A status, indicating that local *de novo* synthesis of retinal or retinoic acid could be key regulatory molecules in the regulation of liver lipid homeostasis [46].

Genetic Variations in Key Enzymes

High interindividual variability in β-carotene metabolism could be caused by genetic variability in key genes involved in provitamin A absorption and conversion [10, 39]. Indeed, the T170M missense mutation in the BCMO1 gene induces a dramatic decrease in enzyme activity *in vitro*, and is associated to hypercarotenemia and hypovitaminosis A in a heterozygote carrier [59]. However, given its very low frequency, this mutation cannot explain the high frequency of the low converter phenotype observed in humans [6, 8, 15, 16]. Screening of the open reading frame of BCMO1 enabled the detection of two common non-synonymous single-nucleotide polymorphisms (R267S; rs12934922 and A379V; rs7501331) with variant allele frequencies of 42% and 24%, respectively [17]. Results of the functional analysis of these SNPs revealed that the recombinant 267S+379V double mutant had a reduced catalytic activity of 57% *in vitro* and assessment of the responsiveness to a pharmacological dose of β-carotene in female volunteers confirmed that carriers of both the 379V and 267S+379V variant alleles had a reduced ability to convert β-carotene by 32% and 69%, respectively [17]. Thus, the observation of high SNP frequencies combined with altered β-carotene metabolism provided a putative explanation for the poor responder phenotype in β-carotene metabolism. Further indication of how genetic variations in key genes can affect β-carotene metabolism comes from a genome-wide association study investigating the effects of common genetic variations on circulating carotenoid levels [60]. This study identified four new SNPs upstream of the BCMO1 gene strongly correlating with increased β-carotene concentrations and reduced non-provitamin A carotenoid levels, such as lutein [60]. Although the authors were unable to test if these SNPs also affected β-carotene conversion efficiency, a recent publication indicated that three out of these four polymorphisms (rs6420424, rs11645428, and rs6564851) reduce the catalytic activity of BCMO1 in female volunteers by 59%, 51%, and 48%, respectively [61]. A number of other polymorphisms potentially affecting the β-carotene low responder phenotype have been identified and are listed in Table 7.1 [10, 30, 62–64]. Polymorphisms known to be present in SR-BI significantly alter fasting plasma β-carotene concentrations [63]. SNPs in other genes involved in lipoprotein metabolism (apoB and LPL) also modulate plasma β-carotene and lutein concentrations, indicating that chylomicron assembly as well as lipoprotein clearance are important factors in determining carotenoid status [62–64]. For more information on genetic variations on carotenoid status, see reviews of Borel [30] and Lietz et al. [39].

Nutrient Status of the Host

Conversion efficiency is also dependent on the vitamin A status of the host [65], caused by the existence of a negative feedback of retinoic acid on BCMO1 mRNA expression [66, 67]. More importantly, a diet-responsive regulatory network exists at the intestinal level which controls β-carotene absorption and vitamin A production by a negative feedback mechanism [68, 69]. The intestine-specific homeodomain transcription factor (ISX) expression is activated by retinoic acid that binds to a specific retinoic acid response element (RARE) within the ISX promoter. Once activated, ISX represses SR-BI and BCMO1 expression, indicating that intestinal vitamin A uptake and production are under negative feedback control via ISX (Fig. 7.4) [68]. Because high retinoic acid concentrations decrease BCMO1 expression via the ISX-driven regulatory network, a production of excess vitamin A and retinoic acid via BCMO1 can be avoided, yet at the same time allows sufficient vitamin A biosynthesis from β-carotene at low cellular retinoic acid concentrations [39].

Table 7.1 Single-nucleotide polymorphisms in genes associated with the low responder, low converter, and retinal nonresponder phenotype

Gene and SNP identification	Polymorphism and predicted change	Evidence for functional effect	References
BCMO1			
R267S (rs12934922)	C/T polymorphism that results in Ala→Val substitution	No effect on BCMO1 activity in vitro and in vivo	[17]
A379V (rs7501331)	A/T polymorphism that results in Arg→Ser substitution	32% Reduced conversion of β-carotene after a pharmacological dose in female volunteers	[17]
T170M (rs119478057)	C/T polymorphism that resulted in Thr→Met substitution	90% Reduced BCMO1 activity compared to wild-type in vitro; causing hypercarotenemia and hypovitaminosis A	[59]
R267S+A379V	A/T and C/T polymorphisms combined with at least one heterozygote each	57% Reduced BCMO1 activity compared to wild-type in vitro 69% Reduced conversion of β-carotene after a pharmacological dose in female volunteers	[17]
5′ Intron (rs6420424)	A/G polymorphism upstream of BCMO1	59% reduced conversion of β-carotene after a pharmacological dose in female volunteers; Variant modulates β-carotene status	[60, 62]
5′ Intron (rs8044334)	G/T polymorphism upstream of BCMO1	Variant modulates β-carotene status	[60, 62]
5′ Intron (rs11645428)	A/G polymorphism upstream of BCMO1	51% Reduced conversion of β-carotene after a pharmacological dose in female volunteers; Variant modulates β-carotene status	[60, 62]
5′ Intron (rs6564851)	G/T polymorphism upstream of BCMO1	48% Reduced conversion of β-carotene after a pharmacological dose in female volunteers; Variant modulates β-carotene and lutein status	[60, 62]
SRBI			
5′ Intron (C→T)	C/T polymorphism in the promoter	Variant modulates β-carotene status, with differences between gender	[63]
ApoB			
–516C>T (rs934197)	C/T polymorphism in the promoter	Variant associated with decreased plasma levels of β-carotene	[63]
CD36			
5′ Intron (rs1761667)	G/A polymorphism in the promoter	GG at rs1761667 locus associated with higher MPOD	[70]
LPL			
S447X (rs328)	C/G polymorphism that results in a truncation of the LPL protein by two amino acids (Ser-Gly) at the carboxyterminal end	Associated with increased plasma HDL cholesterol, reduced plasma triacylglycerol, and decreased concentrations of lutein and β-carotene	[64]

BCMO1 β-carotene 15,15′-monooxygenase, *SRBI* scavenger receptor class B type I, *ApoB* apolipoprotein B, *CD36* cluster determinant 36, *LPL* lipoprotein lipase, *SNP* single-nucleotide polymorphism

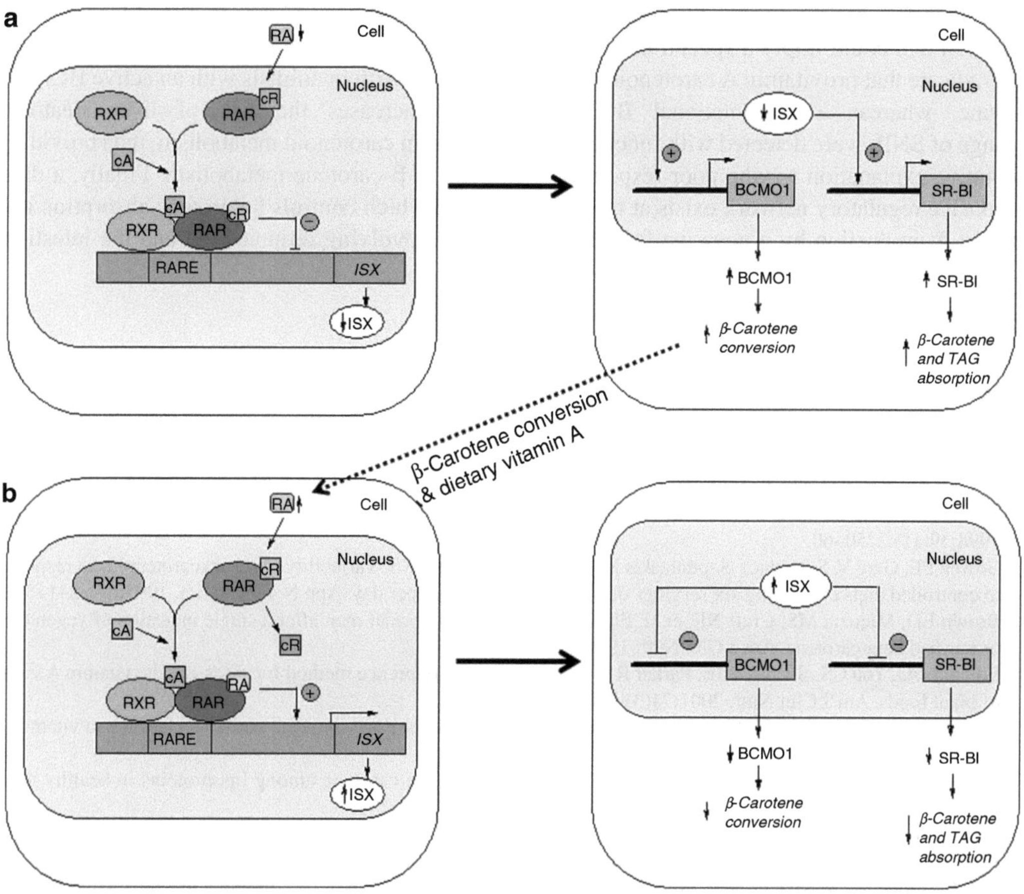

Fig. 7.4 Diet-responsive regulatory network involving the intestine-specific homeodomain transcription factor ISX. (**a**) Vitamin A deficiency: ISX expression is reduced due to low retinoic acid (RA) and RAR concentrations. SRBI and BCMO1 expression are increased significantly in the small intestine. Enhanced SRBI activity facilitates the absorption of various lipids and carotenoids. (**b**) Vitamin A sufficiency: RA derived either from β-carotene conversion or preformed dietary retinoids promote the binding of RARs, therefore inducing ISX expression. Induction of ISX then leads to the repression of intestinal SR-BI and BCMO1 expression. *cR* Co-repressor, *cA* co-activator, *RARE* retinoic acid response element, *RAR* retinoic acid receptor, *RXR* retinoid X receptor, *ISX* intestine-specific homeodomain transcription factor, *SR-BI* intestinal scavenger receptor class B type 1, *BCMO1* β,β-carotene 15,15-monooxygenase 1. Reproduced with permission from [39]

Summary

Absorption and bioconversion to vitamin A of ingested β-carotene contribute to the variable plasma response to ingested β-carotene, leading to the definition of the low responder and the low converter phenotypes. Factors such as gender, body fat, and low retina lutein concentrations may indicate which subjects are likely to be classified as a retinal responder after lutein supplementation. Carotenoid absorption at physiological concentrations is mediated by SR-BI, whereas 95% of provitamin A conversion is achieved by the cytosolic BCMO1. Between 35 and 88% of absorbed β-carotene is cleaved into all-*trans* retinal, and between 3 and 55% of intact β-carotene is bioaccessible from dietary sources. The discovery of GSTP1 as the macular zeaxanthin-binding protein and StARD3 as a lutein-binding protein in the macula of the primate retina is unraveling the biochemical regulation of specific xanthophyll uptake into the retina. Differential carotenoid distributions have been described for the mammary cell and could imply a special need for certain carotenoids during early development. Recent data indicate that provitamin A carotenoids could reduce adiposity in animals with an active BCMO1 enzyme, whereas a nonfunctional BCMO1 enzyme increases the risk of liver steatosis. A range of SNPs were detected with functional significance in carotenoid metabolism, thus providing a putative explanation for the poor responder phenotype in β-carotene metabolism. Finally, a diet-responsive regulatory network exists at the intestinal level which controls β-carotene absorption and vitamin A production by a negative feedback mechanism involving retinoic acid and the intestinal homeobox ISX.

References

1. Parker RS. Carotenoids. 4. Absorption, metabolism, and transport of carotenoids. FASEB J. 1996;10(5):542–51.
2. Borel P, Grolier P, Mekki N, et al. Low and high responders to pharmacological doses of beta-carotene: proportion in the population, mechanisms involved and consequences on beta-carotene metabolism. J Lipid Res. 1998;39(11):2250–60.
3. Bowen PE, Garg V, Stacewicz-Sapuntzakis M, Yelton L, Schreiner RS. Variability of serum carotenoids in response to controlled diets containing six servings of fruits and vegetables per day. Ann N Y Acad Sci. 1993;691:241–3.
4. Brown ED, Micozzi MS, Craft NE, et al. Plasma carotenoids in normal men after a single ingestion of vegetables or purified beta-carotene. Am J Clin Nutr. 1989;49(6):1258–65.
5. Edwards AJ, You CS, Swanson JE, Parker RS. A novel extrinsic reference method for assessing the vitamin A value of plant foods. Am J Clin Nutr. 2001;74(3):348–55.
6. Hickenbottom SJ, Lemke SL, Dueker SR, et al. Dual isotope test for assessing beta-carotene cleavage to vitamin A in humans. Eur J Nutr. 2002;41(4):141–7.
7. Johnson EJ, Russell RM. Distribution of orally administered beta-carotene among lipoproteins in healthy men. Am J Clin Nutr. 1992;56(1):128–35.
8. Lin Y, Dueker SR, Burri BJ, Neidlinger TR, Clifford AJ. Variability of the conversion of beta-carotene to vitamin A in women measured by using a double-tracer study design. Am J Clin Nutr. 2000;71(6):1545–54.
9. van Lieshout M, West CE, van Breemen RB. Isotopic tracer techniques for studying the bioavailability and bioefficacy of dietary carotenoids, particularly beta-carotene, in humans: a review. Am J Clin Nutr. 2003;77(1): 12–28.
10. Lietz G, Hesketh J. A network approach to micronutrient genetics: interactions with lipid metabolism. Curr Opin Lipidol. 2009;20(2):112–20. doi:10.1097/MOL.0b013e3283295ecf.
11. Li B, Vachali P, Frederick JM, Bernstein PS. Identification of StARD3 as a lutein-binding protein in the macula of the primate retina. Biochemistry. 2011;50(13):2541–9.
12. Bhosale P, Larson AJ, Frederick JM, Southwick K, Thulin CD, Bernstein PS. Identification and characterization of a Pi isoform of glutathione S-transferase (GSTP1) as a zeaxanthin-binding protein in the macula of the human eye. J Biol Chem. 2004;279(47):49447–54.
13. Lietz G, Mulokozi G, Henry JC, Tomkins AM. Xanthophyll and hydrocarbon carotenoid patterns differ in plasma and breast milk of women supplemented with red palm oil during pregnancy and lactation. J Nutr. 2006;136(7):1821–7.
14. Furr HC, Clark RM. Intestinal absorption and tissue distribution of carotenoids. J Nutr Biochem. 1997;8(7): 364–77.
15. Tang G, Qin J, Dolnikowski GG, Russell RM. Short-term (intestinal) and long-term (postintestinal) conversion of beta-carotene to retinol in adults as assessed by a stable-isotope reference method. Am J Clin Nutr. 2003;78(2): 259–66.
16. Wang Z, Yin S, Zhao X, Russell RM, Tang G. beta-Carotene-vitamin A equivalence in Chinese adults assessed by an isotope dilution technique. Br J Nutr. 2004;91(1):121–31.
17. Leung WC, Hessel S, Meplan C, et al. Two common single nucleotide polymorphisms in the gene encoding beta-carotene 15,15′-monoxygenase alter beta-carotene metabolism in female volunteers. FASEB J. 2009;23(4):1041–53. doi:fj.08-121962 [pii] 10.1096/fj.08-121962 [doi].
18. Aleman TS, Cideciyan AV, Windsor EAM, et al. Macular pigment and lutein supplementation in ABC44-associated retinal degenerations. Invest Ophthalmol Vis Sci. 2007;48(3):1319–29. doi:10.1167/iovs.06-0764.
19. Hammond BR, Johnson EJ, Russell RM, et al. Dietary modification of human macular pigment density. Invest Ophthalmol Vis Sci. 1997;38(9):1795–801.

20. Trieschmann M, Beatty S, Nolan JM, et al. Changes in macular pigment optical density and serum concentrations of its constituent carotenoids following supplemental lutein and zeaxanthin: the LUNA study. Exp Eye Res. 2007;84(4):718–28.
21. Hammond Jr BR, Ciulla TA, Snodderly DM. Macular pigment density is reduced in obese subjects. Invest Ophthalmol Vis Sci. 2002;43(1):47–50.
22. Thomson LR, Toyoda Y, Delori FC, et al. Long term dietary supplementation with zeaxanthin reduces photoreceptor death in light-damaged Japanese quail. Exp Eye Res. 2002;75(5):529–42.
23. Beatty S, Nolan J, Kavanagh H, O'Donovan O. Macular pigment optical density and its relationship with serum and dietary levels of lutein and zeaxanthin. Arch Biochem Biophys. 2004;430(1):70–6.
24. Nolan J, O'Donovan O, Kavanagh H, et al. Macular pigment and percentage of body fat. Invest Ophthalmol Vis Sci. 2004;45(11):3940–50.
25. During A, Dawson HD, Harrison EH. Carotenoid transport is decreased and expression of the lipid transporters SR-BI, NPC1L1, and ABCA1 is downregulated in Caco-2 cells treated with ezetimibe. J Nutr. 2005;135(10):2305–12. doi:135/10/2305 [pii].
26. During A, Hussain MM, Morel DW, Harrison EH. Carotenoid uptake and secretion by CaCo-2 cells: beta-carotene isomer selectivity and carotenoid interactions. J Lipid Res. 2002;43(7):1086–95.
27. Reboul E, Abou L, Mikail C, et al. Lutein transport by Caco-2 TC-7 cells occurs partly by a facilitated process involving the scavenger receptor class B type I (SR-BI). Biochem J. 2005;387(Pt 2):455–61.
28. van Bennekum A, Werder M, Thuahnai ST, et al. Class B scavenger receptor-mediated intestinal absorption of dietary beta-carotene and cholesterol. Biochemistry. 2005;44(11):4517–25.
29. Kiefer C, Sumser E, Wernet MF, Von Lintig J. A class B scavenger receptor mediates the cellular uptake of carotenoids in Drosophila. Proc Natl Acad Sci U S A. 2002;99(16):10581–6.
30. Borel P. Genetic variations involved in interindividual variability in carotenoid status. Mol Nutr Food Res. 2012;56(2):228–40.
31. Herron KL, McGrane MM, Waters D, et al. The ABCG5 polymorphism contributes to individual responses to dietary cholesterol and carotenoids in eggs. J Nutr. 2006;136(5):1161–5.
32. Moussa M, Gouranton E, Gleize B, et al. CD36 is involved in lycopene and lutein uptake by adipocytes and adipose tissue cultures. Mol Nutr Food Res. 2011;55(4):578–84.
33. Harrison EH. Mechanisms involved in the intestinal absorption of dietary vitamin A and provitamin A carotenoids. Biochim Biophys Acta. 2012;1821(1):70–7.
34. Gaziano JM, Johnson EJ, Russell RM, et al. Discrimination in absorption or transport of beta-carotene isomers after oral supplementation with either all-*trans*-beta-carotene or 9-*cis*-beta-carotene. Am J Clin Nutr. 1995;61(6):1248–52.
35. Johnson EJ, Qin J, Krinsky NI, Russell RM. Concentrations of beta-carotene isomers in serum, breast milk, and buccal mucosa cell after chronic oral doses of all-*trans* (tBC) and 9-*cis* (9cBC) beta-carotene. FASEB J. 1997;11(3):2263.
36. Stahl W, Schwarz W, von Laar J, Sies H. All-*trans* beta-carotene preferentially accumulates in human chylomicrons and very-low-density lipoproteins compared with the 9-*cis* geometrical isomer. J Nutr. 1995;125(8):2128–33.
37. You CS, Parker RS, Goodman KJ, Swanson JE, Corso TN. Evidence of *cis-trans* isomerization of 9-*cis*-beta-carotene during absorption in humans. Am J Clin Nutr. 1996;64(2):177–83.
38. Wang XD, Krinsky NI, Benotti PN, Russell RM. Biosynthesis of 9-*cis*-retinoic acid from 9-*cis*-beta-carotene in human intestinal mucosa in vitro. Arch Biochem Biophys. 1994;313(1):150–5. doi:S0003-9861(84)71371-3 [pii] 10.1006/abbi.1994.1371 [doi].
39. Lietz G, Lange J, Rimbach G. Molecular and dietary regulation of beta, beta-carotene 15,15′-monooxygenase 1 (BCMO1). Arch Biochem Biophys. 2010;502(1):8–16. doi:10.1016/j.abb.2010.06.032.
40. von Lintig J. Colors with functions: elucidating the biochemical and molecular basis of carotenoid metabolism. Annu Rev Nutr. 2010;30:35–56. doi:10.1146/annurev-nutr-080508-141027.
41. During A, Harrison EH. Mechanisms of provitamin A (carotenoid) and vitamin A (retinol) transport into and out of intestinal Caco-2 cells. J Lipid Res. 2007;48(10):2283–94. doi:M700263-JLR200 [pii] 10.1194/jlr.M700263-JLR200 [doi].
42. Norum KR. Dietary fat and blood lipids. Nutr Rev. 1992;50(4 Pt 2):30–7.
43. Barua AB, Olson JA. beta-Carotene is converted primarily to retinoids in rats in vivo. J Nutr. 2000;130(8):1996–2001.
44. Amengual J, Gouranton E, van Helden YG, et al. beta-Carotene reduces body adiposity of mice via BCMO1. PLoS One. 2011;6(6):e20644. doi:10.1371/journal.pone.0020644.
45. Fierce Y, de Morais Vieira M, Piantedosi R, Wyss A, Blaner WS, Paik J. *In vitro* and *in vivo* characterization of retinoid synthesis from beta-carotene. Arch Biochem Biophys. 2008;472(2):126–38.
46. Hessel S, Eichinger A, Isken A, et al. CMO1 deficiency abolishes vitamin A production from beta-carotene and alters lipid metabolism in mice. J Biol Chem. 2007;282(46):33553–61.

47. Grolier P, Duszka C, Borel P, AlexandreGouabau MC, AzaisBraesco V. *In vitro* and *in vivo* inhibition of beta-carotene dioxygenase activity by canthaxanthin in rat intestine. Arch Biochem Biophys. 1997;348(2):233–8.
48. Kim YS, Oh DK. Substrate specificity of a recombinant chicken beta-carotene 15,15′-monooxygenase that converts beta-carotene into retinal. Biotechnol Lett. 2009;31(3):403–8. doi:10.1007/s10529-008-9873-4 [doi].
49. Lakshmanan MR, Chansang H, Olson JA. Purification and properties of carotene 15,15′-dioxygenase of rabbit intestine. J Lipid Res. 1972;13(4):477–82.
50. Lakshmanan MR, Pope JL, Olson JA. The specificity of a partially purified carotenoid cleavage enzyme of rabbit intestine. Biochem Biophys Res Commun. 1968;33(2):347–52. doi:0006-291X(68)90791-2 [pii].
51. Lindqvist A, Andersson S. Biochemical properties of purified recombinant human beta-carotene 15,15′-monooxygenase. J Biol Chem. 2002;277(26):23942–8.
52. Lindqvist A, Andersson S. Cell type-specific expression of beta-carotene 15,15′-mono-oxygenase in human tissues. J Histochem Cytochem. 2004;52(4):491–9.
53. Amengual J, Lobo GP, Golczak M, et al. A mitochondrial enzyme degrades carotenoids and protects against oxidative stress. FASEB J. 2011;25(3):948–59. doi:10.1096/fj.10-173906.
54. Mein JR, Dolnikowski GG, Ernst H, Russell RM, Wang XD. Enzymatic formation of *apo*-carotenoids from the xanthophyll carotenoids lutein, zeaxanthin and beta-cryptoxanthin by ferret carotene-9′,10′-monooxygenase. Arch Biochem Biophys. 2011;506(1):109–21. doi:10.1016/j.abb.2010.11.005.
55. Bone RA, Cains A, Friedes LM, Landrum JT, Vidal I, Zamor J. Distribution of the macular carotenoids zeaxanthin, meso-zeaxanthin and lutein in the human retina. Invest Ophthalmol Vis Sci. 1993;34(4):1199.
56. Bone RA, Landrum JT. Distribution of macular pigment components, zeaxanthin and lutein, in human retina. Methods Enzymol. 1992;213:360–6.
57. Tserentsoodol N, Gordiyenko NV, Pascual I, Lee JW, Fliesler SJ, Rodriguez IR. Intraretinal lipid transport is dependent on high density lipoprotein-like particles and class B scavenger receptors. Mol Vis. 2006;12:1319–33.
58. Schweigert FJ, Bathe K, Chen F, Buscher U, Dudenhausen JW. Effect of the stage of lactation in humans on carotenoid levels in milk, blood plasma and plasma lipoprotein fractions. Eur J Nutr. 2004;43(1):39–44.
59. Lindqvist A, Sharvill J, Sharvill DE, Andersson S. Loss-of-function mutation in carotenoid 15,15′-monooxygenase identified in a patient with hypercarotenemia and hypovitaminosis A. J Nutr. 2007;137(11):2346–50.
60. Ferrucci L, Perry JR, Matteini A, et al. Common variation in the beta-carotene 15,15′-monooxygenase 1 gene affects circulating levels of carotenoids: a genome-wide association study. Am J Hum Genet. 2009;84(2):123–33. doi:S0002-9297(09)00010-X [pii] 10.1016/j.ajhg.2008.12.019 [doi].
61. Lietz G, Oxley A, Leung W, Hesketh J. Single nucleotide polymorphisms upstream from the beta-carotene 15,15′-monoxygenase gene influence provitamin A conversion efficiency in female volunteers. J Nutr. 2011;142(1):161S–5. doi:10.3945/jn.111.140756.
62. Borel P, Moussa M, Reboul E, et al. Human fasting plasma concentrations of vitamin E and carotenoids, and their association with genetic variants in apo C-III, cholesteryl ester transfer protein, hepatic lipase, intestinal fatty acid binding protein and microsomal triacylglycerol transfer protein. Br J Nutr. 2009;101(5):680–7.
63. Borel P, Moussa M, Reboul E, et al. Human plasma levels of vitamin E and carotenoids are associated with genetic polymorphisms in genes involved in lipid metabolism. J Nutr. 2007;137(12):2653–9. doi:137/12/2653 [pii].
64. Herbeth B, Gueguen S, Leroy P, Siest G, Visvikis-Siest S. The lipoprotein lipase serine 447 stop polymorphism is associated with altered serum carotenoid concentrations in the Stanislas Family Study. J Am Coll Nutr. 2007;26(6): 655–62.
65. Ribaya-Mercado JD, Solon FS, Solon MA, et al. Bioconversion of plant carotenoids to vitamin A in Filipino school-aged children varies inversely with vitamin A status. Am J Clin Nutr. 2000;72(2):455–65.
66. Bachmann H, Desbarats A, Pattison P, et al. Feedback regulation of beta, beta-carotene 15,15′-monooxygenase by retinoic acid in rats and chickens. J Nutr. 2002;132(12):3616–22.
67. Takitani K, Zhu CL, Inoue A, Tamai H. Molecular cloning of the rat beta-carotene 15,15′-monooxygenase gene and its regulation by retinoic acid. Eur J Nutr. 2006;45(6):320–6. doi:10.1007/s00394-006-0601-3 [doi].
68. Lobo GP, Hessel S, Eichinger A, et al. ISX is a retinoic acid-sensitive gatekeeper that controls intestinal beta, beta-carotene absorption and vitamin A production. FASEB J. 2010;24(6):1656–66. doi:fj.09-150995 [pii] 10.1096/fj.09-150995 [doi].
69. Seino Y, Miki T, Kiyonari H, et al. Isx participates in the maintenance of vitamin A metabolism by regulation of beta-carotene 15,15′-monooxygenase (Bcmo1) expression. J Biol Chem. 2008;283(8):4905–11. doi:M707928200 [pii] 10.1074/jbc.M707928200 [doi].
70. Borel P, de Edelenyi FS, Vincent-Baudry S, et al. Genetic variants in BCMO1 and CD36 are associated with plasma lutein concentrations and macular pigment optical density in humans. Ann Med. 2011;43(1):47–59.

Chapter 8
Host Factors: Gender and Body Composition

Joseph Dever

Key Points

- The intake and biological fate of carotenoids are influenced by a complex array of environmental and genetic factors.
- This chapter focuses on the impact of gender and body composition on carotenoid bioprocessing.
- Colorful bird and fish species provide the most spectacular examples of gender-specific patterns in carotenoid metabolism and accumulation; such gender differences in humans are more subtle.
- Women tend to consume more dietary carotenoids and have higher circulating carotenoid concentrations than men.
- Some studies suggest that estrogen status may modulate carotenoid utilization in humans, but these observations require further clarification.
- A higher body mass index has been correlated to lower serum carotenoid concentrations. This effect is probably mediated by several mechanisms.

Keywords Carotenoids • Gender Differences • Intake • Serum Concentrations • Body Mass Index

Introduction

Carotenoid intake, absorption, transport, and storage in humans as well as other animals are influenced by a wide range of host-related factors. These include, but are certainly not limited to, expression levels of metabolic enzymes such as carotenoid monooxygenase 1 and 2, serum lipoprotein homeostasis, and fatty tissue prevalence. Such factors are impacted by environmental modulators including the type of diet consumed and individual genetics. Thus, the biological fate of carotenoids is complex and multifaceted.

The focus of this chapter is on the impact of gender and body composition on carotenoid bioprocessing. The discussion is initiated using some dramatic examples of gender-specific utilization of carotenoids for coloration in some male birds and fish. Much is known about the mechanisms that govern these processes, some of which may be informative when considering the potential gender differences in human carotenoid bioprocessing. In addition, gender-specific carotenoid metabolism within these species has been useful in deciphering some of the physiological roles of carotenoids, notably their impact on the immune system.

J. Dever, Ph.D. (✉)
University of Wisconsin-Madison, Department of Nutritional Sciences, 1415 Linden Drive, Madison, WI 53706, USA
e-mail: jtdever@gmail.com

S.A. Tanumihardjo (ed.), *Carotenoids and Human Health*, Nutrition and Health,
DOI 10.1007/978-1-62703-203-2_8, © Springer Science+Business Media New York 2013

Next, epidemiological studies in humans are examined that have provided some correlative evidence for gender-specific patterns in carotenoid intake, circulating concentrations, tissue distribution, and utilization. While detailed mechanistic insights into their etiology are lacking, some differences may be due to the specific biochemical effects of sex hormones as suggested by studies demonstrating a modulation of carotenoid levels in women during different phases of the menstrual cycle. Finally, the importance of body composition in shaping carotenoid metabolism and biodistribution patterns in humans is examined.

Carotenoids as Gender-Specific Colorants in Birds and Fish

The prevalence of carotenoids in nature is nothing short of prolific. Their first biological use probably occurred early in evolution by primitive bacteria to stabilize cell membranes [1]. Upon the emergence of photosynthesis, carotenoids became further utilized as both light-harvesting and antioxidant pigments. Within eukaryotes and multicellular animals, carotenoids serve as lipophilic antioxidants but are also a key component of the colorful pigmentation found in everything from sponges and crustaceans to many vertebrates including fish, amphibians, reptiles, and birds. Some of these species utilize dramatic, gender-specific colorations as a central component of reproductive signaling. Because carotenoids are an essential part of these pigments, distinct gender differences in carotenoid bioprocessing have evolved. For example, during mating season, avian males may sequester dietary carotenoids for sexual display whereas females and their offspring maintain less conspicuous coloration patterns, perhaps to avoid notice by potential predators (Fig. 8.1). Thus, birds serve as especially transparent examples of gender-specific carotenoid metabolism in the animal kingdom.

The underlying mechanisms that govern gender-specific patterns in carotenoid sequestration in birds and fish have been extensively examined. The overarching theme that emerges is the crucial role of sex hormones, including testosterone and estradiol, in regulating carotenoid utilization by particular physiological systems and accumulation in specific physiological compartments. In Arctic Char, a salmonid fish species, sexual maturation coincides with selective accumulation of carotenoids in the skin and gonads [2]. Implants of 11-ketotestosterone in this species led to a reduction of astaxanthin and canthaxanthin concentrations in the plasma and fillets and increased levels of these carotenoids in liver and skin directly demonstrating the ability of this particular sex hormone to regulate carotenoid metabolism [3]. Similar processes are at work in avian species. Treatment of male and female diamond doves with testosterone and dihydrotestosterone increased the hue and size of their characteristic red eye ring which contains high levels of lutein esters [4]. Treatment with estradiol had no effect but did increase circulating lipoprotein levels. This suggested that carotenoid sequestration in the eye ring may be conferred by androgen-dependent upregulation of carotenoid-specific cellular transporters in the eye-ring tissue rather than increased overall circulation of carotenoids by lipoproteins. In male zebra finches, testosterone levels were positively linked to increased beak coloration [5]; however, in contrast to diamond doves, testosterone was also associated with lipoprotein upregulation concomitant with increased serum levels of carotenoids. Female zebra finches also exhibited increased beak color upon testosterone administration but without upregulation of serum lipoproteins suggestive of a mechanism of carotenoid sequestration more similar to diamond doves [6]. Collectively, these studies demonstrate that, while sex hormones play a major role in regulating gender-dependent carotenoid pigmentation, the exact interaction is species, gender, age, and tissue specific.

Animals with distinct gender differences in carotenoid bioprocessing also serve to illustrate the role of carotenoids in certain physiological processes, notably the immune system. In general, higher testosterone levels correlate to decreased immune function; however, this trend appears to be somewhat abrogated in species that utilize carotenoids to develop colorful traits. In one study, nonbreeding male zebra finches had higher circulating carotenoid levels than females and mounted a stronger

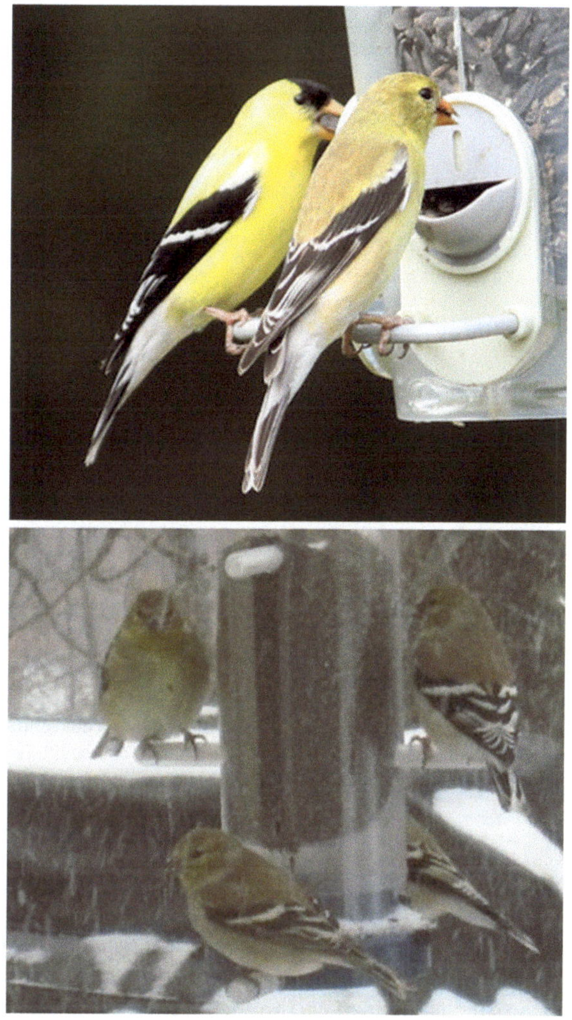

Fig. 8.1 Gender differences in feather carotenoid accumulation in the American Goldfinch lead to a much brighter yellow hue in males compared with females in the spring and summer months (*top* photograph by Leslie Morrison, reprinted with permission). During winter, males and females are nearly indistinguishable from each other (*bottom* photograph by Robert Dever, reprinted with permission)

humoral immune response when challenged with phytohemagglutinin [7]. Both male and female finches supplemented with dietary carotenoids showed an improved humoral immune response compared with non-supplemented birds. Another study in carotenoid-supplemented nestling great tits (*Parus major*) noted that the carotenoids commonly used for coloration in that species (lutein and zeaxanthin) were not as immunoenhancing as carotenoids not utilized for coloration (β-carotene) suggesting that individual carotenoids have specific immunological effects [8]. Thus, while male birds with a higher degree of coloration may be more sexually attractive to prospective females, it remains unclear if increased coloration correlates to increased immunocompetence.

Carotenoid-Related Gender Differences in Humans

Gender clearly plays a dramatic role in carotenoid bioprocessing in many species of wildlife; however, the story is more subtle in humans. Whereas in our own species carotenoid-based coloration is not relevant, gender-related differences with regard to carotenoid intake and bioprocessing have been detected (Fig. 8.2).

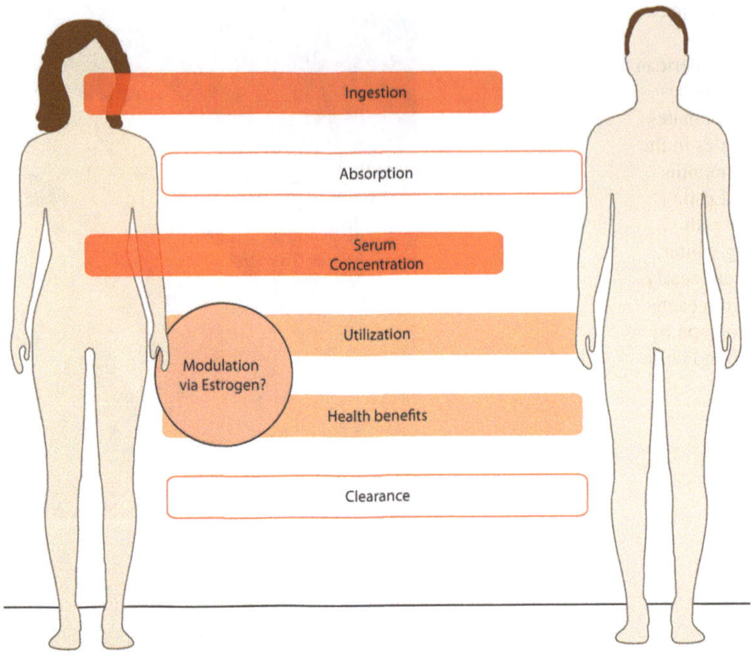

Fig. 8.2 Gender-specific trends in human carotenoid intake and metabolism. On average, women consume more dietary carotenoids and have higher serum carotenoid concentrations than men. Some evidence suggests that estrogen status in women may affect carotenoid utilization and health benefits. There is currently no evidence for the existence of gender differences in human carotenoid absorption and clearance

Many epidemiological studies have been undertaken over the past 30 years to clarify the overall relationship between carotenoids and health and to develop a more thorough understanding of factors that impact carotenoid intake, circulation, and utilization in various subsets of the population. In cohorts including men and women, gender comparisons have been extrapolated. Such studies comprise the current understanding of carotenoid-related gender differences in humans; however, it is important to exercise some caution in interpreting such correlative data. First, total carotenoid intake is often measured using dietary questionnaires and thus can be prone to inaccuracies and/or assumptions even under the best study circumstances. Second, measurement of serum carotenoids which typically include β-carotene, α-carotene, β-cryptoxanthin, lutein, zeaxanthin, and lycopene is notoriously difficult due to methodological variation and carotenoid degradation during sample processing, even when state-of-the-art analytical technology is utilized. Third, the inherently high level of human genetic and environmental diversity can confound results or trends emerging from different carotenoid-based studies.

Finally, while the observed correlations between carotenoids and gender are in some cases compelling, information on the potential mechanisms driving them is generally quite limited. The reported modulation of carotenoid levels in women during different phases of the menstrual cycle does hint at a possible regulatory role for sex hormones [9, 10]. In addition, men and women naturally differ in their body composition. This, combined with observations that body mass index (BMI) and waist circumference impact carotenoid biodistribution patterns, makes it a potentially relevant factor when considering the underlying etiology of any carotenoid-based gender difference.

Gender and Carotenoid Intake

One consistently reported carotenoid-related gender difference in humans has been that of intake. Multiple human studies suggest that women, on average, consume greater amounts of carotenoids than men. In one study examining the impact of various physiologic and lifestyle factors on serum carotenoid concentrations in a randomized cohort of Americans over the age of 43 years, men reported consuming 17% less β-carotene, 18% less α-carotene, 30% less β-cryptoxanthin, and 25% less lutein+zeaxanthin compared with women through a National Cancer Institute Diet History Questionnaire [11]. Lycopene consumption was similar between men and women. A nearly identical gender trend in carotenoid consumption was detected in a cohort of older Americans (age 67–93 years) based on their answers to a Willett 126-item food frequency questionnaire [12]. In a cohort of nearly 600 Dutch men and women (age 20–59 years), men reported consuming, on average, 10% less vegetables and 20% less fruit compared with women [13] via a semiquantitative food frequency questionnaire, and this translated into a lower calculated intake of β- and α-carotene for the males. In addition to the diversity of dietary questionnaires utilized in studies, each relied on separate databases to estimate the total carotenoid content of the diet. This particular gender trend thus has additional strength because of its detection using multiple methodologies.

In contrast to the aforementioned investigations, there have been some studies where gender differences in carotenoid intake were not apparent. While comparing the effectiveness of two types of food questionnaires, no difference in carotenoid intake could be detected between 162 healthy men and women recruited by the Arizona Cancer Center [14]. In a comprehensive study comprising over 36,000 people from ten different European countries, men and women reported consuming similar amounts of β-carotene; however, region-specific analysis of the overall cohort did reveal differences in male and female β-carotene intake in some areas [15].

In summary, women may consume more dietary carotenoids than men, but variation exists within particular population subgroups due to the types of food available and the dietary customs in particular regions. Regiospecific changes in overall food consumption patterns over time are likely to modulate this presumably dynamic carotenoid-related gender trend.

Gender and Carotenoid Serum Concentrations

Differences in the consumption of carotenoids by men and women also correlate with differences in their circulating carotenoid concentrations. In studies where carotenoid intake by men was significantly lower than that of women [11–13], circulating serum levels of the less-ingested carotenoids in men were also lower. Fitting with this trend, a recent large-scale investigation in >15,000 US adults (>20 years old) found that men comprised only 41% of individuals with serum α-carotene concentrations of 6–8 μg/dL and 35% of those with >9 μg/dL circulating α-carotene [16]. Likewise, in a study where no gender differences in carotenoid intake were detected [14], similar serum carotenoid concentrations in men and women were observed. These results imply that intake is an important predictor of serum carotenoid concentrations. Furthermore, with few notable exceptions, the reported correlation coefficients between carotenoid intake and circulating concentrations in men and women have been similar. This suggests, albeit indirectly, that the overall absorption and clearance of carotenoids do not significantly differ between the two genders. This assertion, however, is far from proven as, to date, virtually no mechanistic studies have been undertaken to directly investigate the role of gender on carotenoid bioavailability and clearance in humans. If such trends are to be detected, it will require targeted studies with high statistical power to overcome the wide variability inherent to carotenoid metabolism.

Gender- and Carotenoid-Related Health Benefits

It is well known that increased intake of carotenoid-containing fruits and vegetables is associated with a lower risk of many age-related diseases. Much research has centered around β-carotene; however, other major carotenoids, notably α-carotene [16], are now being investigated for their potential health benefits (see Chap. 11). While such effects apply to both men and women, there is evidence that the health-imparting properties of carotenoids may be modulated via gender-specific mechanisms. A study of over 2,000 individuals found that low dietary intake of lycopene was associated with an increased risk of rectal cancer in women (odds ratio of 1.5–1.7), but not men (odds ratio of 0.9) [17]. Women participants were then further divided into estrogen-positive (premenopausal) and estrogen-negative (postmenopausal with no hormone replacement therapy) groups. In the estrogen-negative cohort, lower β-carotene and lycopene intake were associated with a two- and threefold higher risk, respectively, of rectal cancer compared with women in the estrogen-positive cohort. Consistent with these results, data collected from a representative sample of >2,500 US adults over the age of 65 years revealed a strong association between low total serum carotenoid concentrations and all-cause mortality in women, but not men [18]. These two studies suggest that increased carotenoid intake may be especially important in postmenopausal women for disease prevention. They also imply a potentially important, but presently unclarified, mechanistic role for estrogen in the regulation of carotenoid bioactivity.

Carotenoids and the Menstrual Cycle

Further evidence that estrogen and other sex hormones modulate carotenoid bioprocessing comes from observations that circulating carotenoid concentrations fluctuate during different phases of the menstrual cycle. In a carefully designed and well-controlled study [9], serum carotenoid concentrations were measured at menses, early and late follicular, and midluteal phases in 12 women placed on a carotenoid-controlled diet for two complete menstrual cycles. Individual carotenoids were found to vary in distinct patterns throughout the cycle, but all were at their lowest concentrations during the menses phase. β-Carotene concentrations increased 10% and peaked during the late-follicular phase, while α-carotene did not fluctuate. Lutein/zeaxanthin, anhydrolutein, and lycopene increased 10%, 30%, and 12%, respectively, and peaked during the luteal phase. Serum retinol concentrations were also increased during the luteal phase. In a separate analysis [10], carotenoid concentrations within each of the major lipoprotein fractions were measured during menstrual phases. All carotenoids were found to primarily reside within the LDL fraction. From the early to late-follicular phase, α- and β-carotene concentrations increased approximately 10% in the LDL fraction, yet were not lower in any other fraction. From the late-follicular to the luteal phase, carotenoid concentrations decreased in the LDL fraction and increased slightly in the VLDL ± IDL fraction. Some fluctuation of carotenoid concentrations was also detected in the HDL_2 fraction.

Collectively, these data suggest that carotenoid transport and distribution are affected or even regulated by the natural fluctuations in estradiol, luteinizing hormone, and progesterone associated with the menstrual cycle; however, the physiological ramifications of these changes remain unclear. Carotenoids are known to be absorbed into the reproductive tissue including the ovaries in cats [19] and dogs [20] and may have some biological role, perhaps as a source of vitamin A, during particular phases of the female reproductive cycle. Further studies will be necessary to verify and decipher the implications of these trends.

Carotenoids and Body Composition

The body composition of an individual, specifically the amount and distribution of adipose tissue, plays a critical role in the distribution and possibly metabolism of carotenoids. Whereas the underlying mechanisms driving gender-related carotenoid trends are mostly unknown, some biochemical and physiological details have been identified that may at least partially explain the effects of body composition on carotenoid biological concentrations. It is worth noting that, due to the natural differences of the body compositions of men and women, the impacts of gender and body composition on carotenoid bioprocessing are intrinsically linked.

Body Composition and Carotenoid Concentrations

The most notable and well-documented physiological effect of body composition with regard to carotenoids centers on their physiological concentrations. Multiple observations suggest a strong, inverse relationship between adiposity and carotenoid concentrations in both serum and the adipose tissue itself. In a population-based sample of 400 individuals, increased BMI was associated with a decrease in serum α-carotene, β-carotene, and β-cryptoxanthin [11]. In a European cohort of over 1,000 middle-aged and elderly participants, a 5 kg/m^2 increase in BMI and a 10 cm increase in waist circumference were predictive of a 15–30% decrease in adipose tissue carotenoid concentrations [21]. In a small cohort of healthy men and women, higher BMI, percent body fat, and fat mass correlated to lower plasma carotenoid concentrations in women aged 60–80 years [22]. BMI, percent body fat, waist circumference, and waist-to-hip ratio were correlated to lower serum β-carotene concentrations in 276 women, but the association was less apparent in men [23]. In a multiracial cohort, serum carotenoids were 22% lower in individuals with a BMI >30 kg/m^2 compared to those with a BMI <22 [24]. Two investigations correlated obesity to lower serum concentrations of all carotenoids, except lycopene in children and adolescents [25, 26].

The consistency of these associations among population cohorts that span both age and ethnicity adds to their strength. Lower carotenoid concentrations in obese individuals may be a contributing factor to increased risk for cardiovascular disease and cancer. Individuals with the lowest serum concentrations of α-carotene, the increased presence of which is linked to a lower risk of death, also have the highest BMI [16]. Decreased β-carotene concentrations in adipose tissue were also correlated to an increased risk of myocardial infarction in a Costa Rican cohort [27].

Potential Mechanisms

Multiple factors likely contribute to the lower carotenoid concentrations present in individuals with more body fat (Fig. 8.3). First, it is possible that obese individuals simply ingest less carotenoids per kg body weight. Two studies in particular found that individuals with a high BMI did not report consuming more carotenoids than individuals with a low BMI [11, 24]. Thus, in obese individuals, the physiological carotenoid pool may simply be more dilute.

A second explanation for the lower carotenoid concentrations in humans with a higher BMI may relate to the increased overall levels of oxidative stress that are associated with obesity, which, in turn, could result in carotenoid oxidation and depletion [28]. Higher serum carotenoid concentrations have been associated with lower levels of the oxidative stress markers 8-hydroxy-2′-deoxyguanosine [29] and malondialdehyde-thiobarbituric acid [30], but the biological significance of carotenoid depletion by excessive free radicals in obese individuals is not clear.

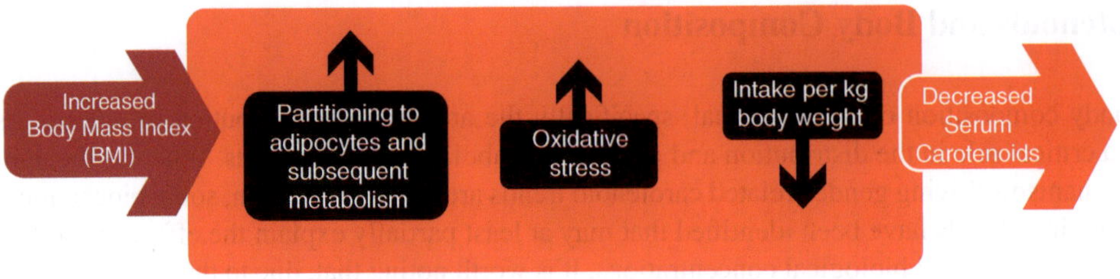

Fig. 8.3 Potential mechanisms contributing to lower serum carotenoid concentrations in individuals with a higher BMI

Finally, adipocytes not only readily absorb but also utilize and metabolize carotenoids. More body fat may thus lead to increased partitioning of carotenoids out of serum and into adipocytes concomitant with a higher rate of carotenoid clearance. Carotenoid metabolism in adipocytes is at least partially accomplished via the carotenoid monooxygenases. For example, β-carotene metabolism results in formation of two molecules of retinal by carotenoid monooxygenase 1, which can be converted to retinoic acid [31], or multiple asymmetric β-apocarotenals by carotenoid monooxygenase 2, some of which have been shown to regulate adipogenesis [32]. Other major carotenoids, including α-carotene and β-cryptoxanthin, are likely to produce additional novel metabolites that may have unique biological activities. The characterization of such metabolites and their effects in adipose tissue is an active area of research.

Conclusions

The biological fate of ingested carotenoids is influenced by a wide range of variables, both environmental and genetic. The most dramatic examples of gender-specific carotenoid utilization occur in bird and fish species where carotenoid-based coloration patterns serve as sexual attractants. Sex hormones are primarily responsible for regulating these gender-specific effects.

In humans, increased dietary consumption of carotenoids by women compared with men has been documented. This phenomenon is more pronounced in some regions than others. Gender differences in carotenoid intake are likely the major cause of the higher serum carotenoid concentrations typically detected in women. The apparent health benefits of carotenoids may be manifested through mechanisms affected by gender-specific hormones.

Finally, high BMI and overall adiposity correlate strongly with low carotenoid concentrations in the serum and adipose tissue. This may be due to the overall dilution of the physiological carotenoid pool in obese individuals, increased clearance of carotenoids via free radical oxidation, or increased absorption and metabolism of carotenoids within adipocytes, but other mechanisms are likely involved. Future studies may clarify these processes and determine their biological significance.

Acknowledgments We thank Sara Tiner for her major role in the creation of the figures in this chapter.

References

1. McGraw KJ. Mechanisms of carotenoid-based coloration. In: Hill GE, McGraw KJ, editors. Bird coloration, Mechanisms and measurements, vol. 1. Cambridge, MA: Harvard University Press; 2006. p. 177–243.
2. Bjerkeng B. Carotenoid pigmentation of salmonid fishes—recent progress. In: Cruz-Suarez LE, Ricque-Marie D, Tapia-Salazar M, Olvera-Novoa MA, Civera-Cerecedo R, editors. Avances en Nutricion Acuicola. Merida,

Yucatan: Avances en Nutricion Acuicola V. Memorias del V Simposium Internacional de Nutricion Acuicola; 2000 Nov 19–22.

3. Bjerkeng B, Hamre J, Hatlen B, Wathne E. Influence of 11-ketotestosterone, 17 α-estradiol, and 3,5,3′-triiodo-*L*-thyronine on distribution and metabolism of carotenoids in Arctic charr, *Salvelinus alpines L.*. Fish Physiol Biochem. 1999;21:353–64.
4. Casagrande S, Dijkstra C, Tagliavini J, Goerlich VC, Groothuis TG. Differential effects of testosterone, dihydrotestosterone and estradiol on carotenoid deposition in an avian sexually selected signal. J Comp Physiol A. 2011;197:1–13.
5. McGraw KJ, Correa SM, Adkins-Regan E. Testosterone upregulates lipoprotein status to control sexual attractiveness in a colorful songbird. Behav Ecol Sociobiol. 2006;60:117–22.
6. McGraw KJ. Sex steroid dependence of carotenoid-based coloration in female zebra finches. Physiol Behav. 2006;88(4–5):347–52.
7. McGraw KJ, Ardia DR. Sex differences in carotenoid status and immune performance in zebra finches. Evol Ecol Res. 2005;7:251–62.
8. Fitze PS, Tschirren B, Gasparini J, Richner H. Carotenoid-based plumage colors and immune function: is there a trade-off for rare carotenoids? Am Nat. 2007;169(S1):S137–44.
9. Forman MR, Beecher GR, Muesing R, Lanza E, Olson B, Campbell WS, McAdam P, Raymond E, Schulman JD, Graubard BI. The fluctuation of plasma carotenoid concentrations by phase of the menstrual cycle: a controlled diet study. Am J Clin Nutr. 1996;64(4):559–65.
10. Forman MR, Johnson EJ, Lanza E, Graubard BI, Beecher GR, Muesing R. Effect of menstrual cycle phase on the concentration of individual carotenoids in lipoproteins of premenopausal women: a controlled dietary study. Am J Clin Nutr. 1998;67(1):81–7.
11. Brady WE, Mares-Perlman JA, Bowen P, Stacewicz-Sapuntzakis M. Human serum carotenoid concentrations are related to physiologic and lifestyle factors. J Nutr. 1996;126(1):129–37.
12. Tucker KL, Chen H, Vogel S, Wilson PW, Schaefer EJ, Lammi-Keefe CJ. Carotenoid intakes, assessed by dietary questionnaire, are associated with plasma carotenoid concentrations in an elderly population. J Nutr. 1999;129(2):438–45.
13. Jansen MC, Van Kappel AL, Ocké MC, Van't Veer P, Boshuizen HC, Riboli E, Bueno-de-Mesquita HB. Plasma carotenoid levels in Dutch men and women, and the relation with vegetable and fruit consumption. Eur J Clin Nutr. 2004;58(10):1386–95.
14. Ritenbaugh C, Peng YM, Aickin M, Graver E, Branch M, Alberts DS. New carotenoid values for foods improve relationship of food frequency questionnaire intake estimates to plasma values. Cancer Epidemiol Biomarkers Prev. 1996;5(11):907–12.
15. Jenab M, Salvini S, van Gils CH, Brustad M, Shakya-Shrestha S, Buijsse B, Verhagen H, Touvier M, Biessy C, Wallström P, Bouckaert K, Lund E, Waaseth M, Roswall N, Joensen AM, Linseisen J, Boeing H, Vasilopoulou E, Dilis V, Sieri S, Sacerdote C, Ferrari P, Manjer J, Nilsson S, Welch AA, Travis R, Boutron-Ruault MC, Niravong M, Bueno-de-Mesquita HB, van der Schouw YT, Tormo MJ, Barricarte A, Riboli E, Bingham S, Slimani N. Dietary intakes of retinol, beta-carotene, vitamin D and vitamin E in the European Prospective Investigation into Cancer and Nutrition cohort. Eur J Clin Nutr. 2009;63 Suppl 4:S150–78.
16. Li C, Ford ES, Zhao G, Balluz LS, Giles WH, Liu S. Serum α-carotene concentrations and risk of death among US Adults: the Third National Health and Nutrition Examination Survey Follow-up Study. Arch Intern Med. 2011;171(6):507–15.
17. Murtaugh MA, Ma KN, Benson J, Curtin K, Caan B, Slattery ML. Antioxidants, carotenoids, and risk of rectal cancer. Am J Epidemiol. 2004;159(1):32–41.
18. Shardell MD, Alley DE, El-Kamary SS, Hicks GE, Miller RR, Magaziner J, Langenberg P, Hochberg MC, Ferrucci L. Sex differences in the relationship of serum carotenoid levels with mortality risk among older US adults: the Third National Health and Nutrition Examination Survey (NHANES III). J Womens Health. 2009;18(10):1492.
19. Chew BP, Weng BB, Kim HW, Wong TS, Park JS, Lepine AJ. Uptake of beta-carotene by ovarian and uterine tissues and effects on steroidogenesis during the estrous cycle in cats. Am J Vet Res. 2001;62(7):1063–7.
20. Weng BC, Chew BP, Wong TS, Park JS, Kim HW, Lepine AJ. Beta-carotene uptake and changes in ovarian steroids and uterine proteins during the estrous cycle in the canine. J Anim Sci. 2000;78(5):1284–90.
21. Virtanen SM, van't Veer P, Kok F, Kardinaal AF, Aro A. Predictors of adipose tissue carotenoid and retinol levels in nine countries. The EURAMIC Study. Am J Epidemiol. 1996;144(10):968–79.
22. Yeum KJ, Booth SL, Roubenoff R, Russell RM. Plasma carotenoid concentrations are inversely correlated with fat mass in older women. J Nutr Health Aging. 1998;2(2):79–83.
23. Wallström P, Wirfält E, Lahmann PH, Gullberg B, Janzon L, Berglund G. Serum concentrations of beta-carotene and alpha-tocopherol are associated with diet, smoking, and general and central adiposity. Am J Clin Nutr. 2001;73(4):777–85.
24. Andersen LF, Jacobs Jr DR, Gross MD, Schreiner PJ, Dale Williams O, Lee DH. Longitudinal associations between body mass index and serum carotenoids: the CARDIA study. Br J Nutr. 2006;95(2):358–65.

25. Ford ES, Gillespie C, Ballew C, Sowell A, Mannino DM. Serum carotenoid concentrations in US children and adolescents. Am J Clin Nutr. 2002;76(4):818–27.
26. Neuhouser ML, Rock CL, Eldridge AL, Kristal AR, Patterson RE, Cooper DA, Neumark-Sztainer D, Cheskin LJ, Thornquist MD. Serum concentrations of retinol, alpha-tocopherol and the carotenoids are influenced by diet, race and obesity in a sample of healthy adolescents. J Nutr. 2001;131(8):2184–91.
27. Kabagambe EK, Furtado J, Baylin A, Campos H. Some dietary and adipose tissue carotenoids are associated with the risk of nonfatal acute myocardial infarction in Costa Rica. J Nutr. 2005;135(7):1763–9. Erratum in: J Nutr. 2005;135(10):2497.
28. Bloomer RJ, Fisher-Wellman KH. Systemic oxidative stress is increased to a greater degree in young, obese women following consumption of a high fat meal. Oxid Med Cell Longev. 2009;2(1):19–25.
29. Thomson CA, Stendell-Hollis NR, Rock CL, Cussler EC, Flatt SW, Pierce JP. Plasma and dietary carotenoids are associated with reduced oxidative stress in women previously treated for breast cancer. Cancer Epidemiol Biomarkers Prev. 2007;16(10):2008–15.
30. Dixon ZR, Shie FS, Warden BA, Burri BJ, Neidlinger TR. The effect of a low carotenoid diet on malondialdehyde-thiobarbituric acid (MDA-TBA) concentrations in women: a placebo-controlled double-blind study. J Am Coll Nutr. 1998;17(1):54–8.
31. Lobo GP, Amengual J, Li HN, Golczak M, Bonet ML, Palczewski K, von Lintig J. Beta, beta-carotene decreases peroxisome proliferator receptor gamma activity and reduces lipid storage capacity of adipocytes in a beta, beta-carotene oxygenase 1-dependent manner. J Biol Chem. 2010;285(36):27891–9.
32. Ziouzenkova O, Orasanu G, Sukhova G, Lau E, Berger JP, Tang G, Krinsky NI, Dolnikowski GG, Plutzky J. Asymmetric cleavage of beta-carotene yields a transcriptional repressor of retinoid X receptor and peroxisome proliferator-activated receptor responses. Mol Endocrinol. 2007;21(1):77–88.

Section II
Carotenoids and Human Health

Chapter 9
Carotenoid Metabolism and Health in Pregnancy and Lactation

Kerry Schulze and Parul Christian

Key Points

- Carotenoids derived entirely from the mother are important sources of provitamin A for the fetus and the young infant, making adequate carotenoid intake in pregnancy and lactation critical.
- Carotenoids may also be important for maternal health and birth outcomes, but research in humans is limited, especially beyond β-carotene.
- Carotenoids in breast milk can confer numerous health benefits beyond providing a good source of vitamin A to replete infant stores.
- Evidence that carotenoids via diet, supplementation, or other means can impact birth size, fetal health, and maternal or infant survival is limited.
- Research which examines the function of carotenoids beyond that of provitamin A in pregnancy and lactation is urgently needed.
- At present, promoting intake of diets rich in carotenoids during pregnancy and lactation can proceed in parallel while research on elucidating the functional importance of carotenoids during these life stages is pursued.

Keywords Pregnancy • Lactation • Carotenoids • β-carotene • Vitamin A • Placenta • Colostrum • Breast milk • Infant

Introduction

Carotenoids are complex plant-derived compounds known to have important roles in human health, as reviewed elsewhere in this book. Carotenoids are best known for their function as antioxidants, while some also act as precursors for vitamin A (e.g., β-carotene, α-carotene, β-cryptoxanthin). Other roles for carotenoids are less well-delineated, but include immune-enhancing activity and effects on reproductive capacity. These alternative roles may be associated with antioxidant function, provitamin A activity, or both, or may work independently of these.

Reproduction is a process that places enhanced nutritional demands on the maternal body. It is also a state in which oxidative stress may be exacerbated and immune function compromised as the body adapts to a role in sharing nutritional resources with the growing offspring, stresses of enhanced

K. Schulze Ph.D. • P. Christian Dr.P.H., Msc. (✉)
Department of International Health, Center for Human Nutrition, Bloomberg School of Public Health, Johns Hopkins University, 615 N. Wolfe Street, W2401, Baltimore, MD 21205, USA
e-mail: pchristi@jhsph.edu; kschulze@jhsph.edu

S.A. Tanumihardjo (ed.), *Carotenoids and Human Health*, Nutrition and Health,
DOI 10.1007/978-1-62703-203-2_9, © Springer Science+Business Media New York 2013

oxygenation of tissues, and tolerating the development of a fetus with distinct antigenic characteristics from the mother. Dietary carotenoids may play a role in protecting mother and offspring during reproductive stress, although much remains to be learned about the role of carotenoids during this important stage of life. This chapter reviews what is currently known about the role of carotenoids in maternal and offspring health during pregnancy and lactation.

Overview of Metabolism

The details of carotenoid metabolism are described elsewhere in this text, but by way of review, information relevant to pregnancy and lactation is provided. The bioavailability of dietary carotenoids is dependent on factors ranging from the food matrix in which they are found, to other dietary factors such as fat content that enhance absorption through micellar formation, to vitamin A status, such that conversion of provitamin A carotenoids like β-carotene to retinol in the enterocyte is enhanced when vitamin A deficiency is present [1]. Carotenoids that are absorbed can also be circulated in lipoprotein fractions, stored in tissues such as liver or adipose, and ultimately converted to retinol/retinal in tissues such as the liver [2]; although in humans, the majority (60–70%) of carotenoid bioconversion to retinol occurs in the enterocyte [3].

During pregnancy and lactation, additional pathways for the transfer or utilization of carotenoids or the retinol that they produce include placenta and breast milk in order to promote preferential transfer of these nutrients to the fetus and the newborn. Additionally, there may be implications for carotenoid intake that strictly benefit the mother over the course of reproduction. The subsequent sections explore the potential roles of carotenoids in pregnancy and lactation, respectively, before summarizing the results of population-based trials of carotenoid supplementation during those life stages.

Pregnancy

Vitamin A, especially its retinoic acid metabolite, has long been known for its critical function during gestation in facilitating proper morphogenesis and organogenesis during the embryonic period. The embryo and subsequently the fetus rely on adequate transfer of retinol from the mother via the placenta. Simple diffusion is known to transfer retinol from the maternal to the fetal compartment, but transfer is also enhanced by retinyl esters being incorporated into maternal chylomicrons [4]. Retinol-binding protein (RBP) receptors have been identified for intracellular transfer of retinol from its complex with RBP [5]. A specific membrane receptor STRA6 which binds to RBP with high affinity to transfer vitamin A from its complex into the cell has been observed to be expressed in the placenta [6].

Maternal serum β-carotene correlates with placental retinol, specifically among women with low serum retinol concentrations (i.e., <15 μg/dL) suggesting that β-carotene may be converted to retinol in the placenta, and that this conversion is influenced by maternal vitamin A status [7]. The cleavage enzyme, β-carotene 15, 15′ monooxygenase, on the fetal side of the amniotic placental membrane can convert carotenoids to retinol. Placental concentrations of carotenoids are not associated with maternal vitamin A status whereas both placental retinol and carotenoids are associated with neonatal retinol concentrations in cord blood [8]. This suggests that preferential transfer of carotenoids to the placenta may occur, although low maternal carotenoid status may still influence neonatal status at birth.

Maternal dietary intake of carotenoid-rich foods and β-carotene supplements are correlated with plasma levels of β-carotene in early pregnancy, at delivery, and in cord blood indicating that maternal diet directly influences the transfer of β-carotene via the placenta to the fetus and the newborn [9].

At delivery, maternal plasma concentration of β-carotene was higher than in the cord blood suggesting that the transfer is well-controlled when maternal intake is high. In this study, maternal β-carotene supplement use was high [9]. In an observational study in Brazil, concentrations of β-carotene were also found to be higher in maternal vs. cord blood, both of which were compromised by tobacco use in the women reflecting an oxidative impact [10]. In rural Nepal, circulating concentrations of carotenoids assessed in pregnancy among women participating in a randomized controlled trial of vitamin A and β-carotene supplementation were found to be low [11]. Among women who were in the β-carotene arm, serum β-carotene, γ-tocopherol, β-cryptoxanthin, and lutein + zeazanthin concentrations were significantly higher post supplementation in pregnancy and at 3 months postpartum relative to women who received a placebo suggesting a sparing of carotenoids due to supplementation.

Carotenoids and Vitamin A Status During Pregnancy

Serum retinol concentration changes in pregnancy vary between well- and undernourished populations. Generally, hemodilution causes declines in concentration during gestation, although this may not represent deficiency. The vitamin A requirement of pregnancy is increased slightly over nonpregnant/non-lactating women from 700 to 770 μg/d [12] and largely confined to the third trimester. In contrast, the requirement is increased to 1,300 μg/d for lactating women. At birth, livers of normal infants generally contain low concentrations of vitamin A, although stores accumulate rapidly over the course of the third trimester. In this respect, birth weight can influence fetal stores and lactation is considered the period for enhancement of infant stores starting with a bolus of carotenoids that a newborn receives at birth via colostrum to boost their low liver stores.

While the small increase in requirement during pregnancy may be of little consequence for healthy populations, for deficient populations subsisting on chronically poor diets this is not the case. Populations "habitually" consuming basal amounts or less of vitamin A are likely to have very poor reserves and, with no improvement in the diets during pregnancy, probably fail to meet the additional vitamin A requirements of pregnancy. Thus, maternal night blindness is common in many deficient populations. Based on low serum retinol concentrations (<0.7 μmol/L), the World Health Organization has estimated that 19 million (15.3%) pregnant women in the world's poorest countries are vitamin A deficient. Moreover, according to Demographic Health Surveys, about 10 million (7.8%) pregnant women are night-blind [13]. Night blindness is a condition generally manifested in later gestation caused by vitamin A deficiency and is associated with an increased risk of anemia, wasting, and increased morbidity [14] and mortality [15].

Little is known about changes in provitamin A carotenoids during pregnancy. Plasma carotenoids, in contrast to vitamin A, are reported to increase in the third trimester even after adjusting for hematocrit, similar to the increase seen with vitamin E. In many populations, β-carotene serves as an important provitamin A source despite its lower bioavailability and bioefficacy [16]. In Nepal, for instance, dark green leafy vegetable and mango consumption in the previous week using a food frequency recall was strongly associated with a lowered odds of night blindness during pregnancy in a matched case–control study [14]. However, in the larger randomized controlled trial in which this study was undertaken, maternal weekly β-carotene supplementation, unlike vitamin A, failed to significantly reduce the risk of night blindness during pregnancy (RR = 0.83, 95% CI: 0.63–1.11) [17]. This was not surprising as in the same trial vitamin A supplementation reduced the prevalence of low serum retinol (<0.7 μmol/L) among pregnant women from 19% in the placebo group to 3%, but β-carotene had only a small impact (14%) (both $p < 0.05$) [18]. Maternal weekly β-carotene supplementation, which was continued during lactation, significantly reduced vitamin A deficiency in infants at 3 months of age by 20%, but this reduction was lower than that achieved with weekly vitamin A (36%) [19]. The weekly dose was 7,000 μg preformed vitamin A (as retinyl palmitate) or 42 mg β-carotene, suggesting that bioconversion of β-carotene to retinol was inefficient despite being in a supplement form. In the same trial, on the other hand, β-carotene supplementation reduced low serum β-carotene concentration (<0.09 μmol/L) from 43% to 27% [18].

In a recent randomized controlled trial in rural northern Bangladesh with a similar design and dosage, β-carotene supplementation modestly reduced the prevalence of low serum retinol (<0.7 μmol/L) in the third trimester of pregnancy from 14.2% to 10.6% compared to the placebo, whereas preformed vitamin A supplementation virtually eliminated its prevalence (1.2%) [20]. However, unlike in Nepal, the difference in the prevalence of low serum β-carotene (<0.09 μmol/L) between the β-carotene and placebo groups was modest, albeit significant (52.4% vs. 45.9%) [20].

Benefits of Carotenoids in Pregnancy

Limited benefits of carotenoid intake have been observed on reproductive health and pregnancy outcome. Outcomes such as birth weight and hypertensive disorders have been examined in some studies, but not systematically. Data on birth weight largely from observational studies have shown mixed results. In a study among 504 women recruited from a clinic in New Zealand, birth weight was lower among those consuming higher levels of β-carotene in their diet after adjusting for other factors [21]. Similarly, in another study, high serum retinol concentrations in late pregnancy were significantly associated with lower birth and placental weights [22].

Several studies have examined maternal carotenoid status during pregnancy and the risk of preeclampsia and hypertension and found equivocal results. In one study, maternal serum carotenoids, including α- and β-carotene, lycopene, and lutein, were assessed three times during pregnancy among diabetic women with and without preeclampsia [23]. In those with preeclampsia, α- and β-carotene were significantly lower during the third trimester and prior to the onset of preeclampsia; although after adjustment, only the β-carotene difference was statistically significant [23]. In a small observational study in the USA, levels of placental β-carotene, lycopene, and canthaxanthin and maternal serum concentrations of β-carotene and lycopene were significantly lower among preeclamptic vs. normal women whereas cord blood levels of these carotenoids were not different between the two groups [24]. Two double-blind, placebo-controlled randomized trials of lycopene supplementation, both conducted in small samples of women recruited from clinics in New Delhi, found contradictory results. One ($n=159$) used daily lycopene at 2 mg and found no difference in the risk of preeclampsia (~18% in both groups) but showed unexpectedly higher rates of preterm labor and low birth weight in the lycopene vs. placebo group [25]. In direct contrast to this trial, the second randomized control trial of lycopene supplementation (2 mg twice a day) among primigravidae ($n=251$) significantly reduced the risk of developing preeclampsia (8.6% vs. 17.7%, $p=0.043$) and intrauterine growth restriction (12% vs. 23.7%, $p=0.033$) [26].

Outcomes in the infants in relation to maternal carotenoid status or intake during pregnancy have also been examined. For example, maternal intake of green and yellow vegetables and β-carotene supplement use in pregnancy were linked to a lower risk of eczema in the offspring (odds ratio, ORs, of 0.41, 95% CI: 0.24–0.71 and ORs of 0.52, 95% CI: 0.30–0.89, respectively in the highest vs. lowest intake group), but not wheeze [27]. Smoking may influence oxidative risk in women during pregnancy and has also been linked with increased risk of wheeze and other allergic conditions in the offspring. Among smoking mothers, plasma as well as breast milk levels of β-carotene were lower compared to those not exposed to smoking perhaps as a result of β-carotene being utilized as an antioxidant [28]. Several cohort studies in Europe have failed to find a link between fruit and vegetable and carotenoid intake during pregnancy and the risk of eczema or wheeze in the offspring [29–31].

Lactation

Maternal Plasma and Milk Carotenoid Content

Milk carotenoid content varies by time of lactation as well as dietary carotenoid status. Over 30 carotenoids, including isomers and metabolic products, have been identified in human milk [32], although 6 (i.e., α- and β-carotene, β-cryptoxanthin, lutein, zeaxanthin, and lycopene) are most commonly assessed and reported. In humans and experimental animals, carotenoids are highest in colostrum (i.e., during the first week of lactation) and total breast milk carotenoid content declines as much as fivefold as lactation progresses [33], even as total lipid content of breast milk increases [34]. Evidence also suggests that colostrum carotenoid content may be influenced by parity, with higher concentrations typical among multiparous mothers [35]. To support the transfer of carotenoids into colostrum, maternal plasma carotenoids may decline in late pregnancy and early lactation, suggesting a specific active mechanism for provision of carotenoids to the mammary gland in early lactation [36].

The carotenoid profile of milk, and its relationship to circulating carotenoids, also changes over the course of lactation. In general, milk carotenoids occur at concentrations 1/3rd to 1/20th that of plasma [32, 36]. Milk concentrations of less polar carotenoids like α- and β-carotene, β-cryptoxanthin, and lycopene are lower relative to maternal plasma than those of polar carotenoids such as lutein and zeaxanthin [36, 37]. Lutein and zeaxanthin concentrations tend to persist over the course of lactation while other carotenoid concentrations decline [36–38]. The mechanism by which carotenoids are transferred into milk is not well-known, although the lower concentrations in milk compared to plasma suggest a mechanism more akin to that of the tocopherols than retinol [2, 39]. The majority of retinol is transferred into breast milk via circulating RBP to maintain breast milk concentrations similar to those of plasma, with an additional variable contribution from chylomicrons in response to dietary vitamin A. Tocopherols and, likely carotenoids, are transferred into milk via the action of lipoprotein lipase on chylomicron and lipid fractions in the mammary gland, releasing some amount into the milk. Lutein and zeaxanthin are associated with both HDL and VLDL/LDL lipid fractions, while less polar carotenoids like α- and β-carotene are primarily associated with the VLDL/LDL fractions. Preferential uptake of HDL at the mammary tissue may be one explanation for the relatively increased breast milk lutein and zeaxanthin concentrations [36].

The responsiveness of plasma and milk carotenoids to doses of β-carotene has been shown in a series of studies. A single 60 mg β-carotene dose given to well-nourished lactating women resulted in a rapid (24 h) threefold (~1.2 μmol/L) increase in plasma β-carotene, declining to near-baseline values by 1 week, while milk β-carotene showed a more delayed (by 2 days) ~threefold (~1.2 nmol/g lipid) increase. A 210 mg dose did not produce a greater effect on either plasma or breast milk β-carotene, however, suggesting absorptive inefficiency above a threshold of intake [40]. Daily 30 mg doses of β-carotene showed no effect on milk β-carotene in women consuming carotenoid-rich diets in early lactation [38], but showed a sustained sixfold increase with a month of supplementation during mature lactation in well-nourished women [41] and a sevenfold increase after just 3 days of supplementation among women with low circulating carotenoids [42]. Doses used in these initial studies were considerably higher than usual dietary intakes [40], but results demonstrated the responsiveness of plasma and milk to carotenoid intake, particularly during mature lactation and with the greatest impact in women with low habitual intake.

Given the link between carotenoid ingestion and plasma and milk carotenoids, it is not surprising that around the world carotenoid content of plasma and breast milk varies, reflecting regional and even seasonal dietary practices. Studies have shown direct correlations between dietary intake of lutein [43] and lycopene [44] and breast milk concentrations. Plasma and breast milk carotenoids are also highly correlated, as shown in a variety of studies and settings [36, 45]. Plasma carotenoid concentrations in lactating women vary dramatically by season, despite relatively stable circulating retinol concentrations, in accordance with the availability of locally produced carotenoid-containing foods [46]. Despite variation in milk carotenoids, a study that compared carotenoid type and content from breast milk samples collected at sites around the world showed that ~60% of human milk carotenoids were provitamin A sources [47], suggesting the potential of breast milk carotenoids to support vitamin A status of infants.

Carotenoids and Vitamin A Status During Lactation

Because provitamin A carotenoids are the most abundant and inexpensive food sources available to support vitamin A status among women in underdeveloped countries, considerable work has gone into examining the potential for interventions of carotenoid-rich foods or supplements to improve vitamin A status of nursing women, and, potentially, their infants. The burden of lactation to the mother's vitamin A status is substantial, in that an estimated 60 times the amount of vitamin A transferred to the fetus during pregnancy is transferred via breast milk in the first 6 months of lactation [48]. Where maternal vitamin A status is poor, breast milk retinol concentrations are lower, and infants of women who are unable to sustain breast milk concentrations of at least 1 μmol/L will be unable to accumulate adequate vitamin A stores during infancy [48]. Despite an observed association of maternal carotenoid intake with vitamin A status during lactation [49], women who rely predominantly on provitamin A carotenoids to maintain vitamin A status may be at higher risk for vitamin A deficiency [50]. To determine the impact of carotenoid-rich food and supplement sources on vitamin A status during lactation, intervention studies have been conducted examining the effects of red palm oil as a natural source of α- and β-carotene; enhanced intakes of β-carotene and other provitamin-rich food sources to improve maternal vitamin A status, enhance breast milk retinol content, and improve infant vitamin A status; or supplementation with purified β-carotene as a potentially safer alternative to a bolus dose of retinyl esters to improve vitamin A status among postpartum women.

Two small studies of red palm oil provided during lactation demonstrated the ability that a carotenoid source has to increase maternal circulating and breast milk α- and β-carotene among women in Tanzania and Honduras [51, 52]. The impact on vitamin A status was less clear, with breast milk retinol concentrations preserved among women provided either red palm oil (~3.5 mg/d total carotenoids) or sunflower oil (0 mg/d carotenoids) for cooking for 6 months compared to women who did not receive cooking oil, in whom milk retinol concentrations declined [51]. The sunflower oil may have provided fat that enhanced the absorption of carotenoids from other sources, and the study also provided information on food preparation that may have made carotenoids from other food sources more bioavailable. The other study was 10 days long, and no change in maternal or infant retinol was observed after women received a total of 90 mg β-carotene as red palm oil [52].

Studies designed to determine the impact of enhancing the diet with carotenoid-rich food sources have not always demonstrated improved vitamin A status among lactating women. In Indonesian women, after a 12-week daily intervention of 3.5 mg β-carotene as either dark green leafy vegetables or a fortified wafer, only women receiving the wafer showed increases in serum and breast milk retinol [53]. Other studies have shown that provitamin A carotenoids (5–6 mg/d) in a fruit matrix were more efficient at improving vitamin A status of lactating women than vegetable matrices, although purified β-carotene or retinol elicited the greatest response to supplementation [54, 55]. In women in Thailand, no difference among intervention groups was observed in maternal serum retinol at the end of a 12-week dietary intervention comparing pure β-carotene in juice (3.6 mg/d) with a low (<0.5 mg/d) or a high (4.7 mg/d) carotenoid diet, although the purified β-carotene seemed to be protective of vitamin A stores compared to the vegetable diets, as assessed by the deuterated retinol dilution method [56]. These data all suggest that the form in which carotenoids are consumed is an important determinant of their efficacy in improving or sustaining vitamin A status during lactation.

Because of the implications for maintaining vitamin A status among lactating women for the good of mother and infant, a trial examining the supplementation of women from 1 to 3 weeks through 9 months postpartum with daily doses of 7.8 mg purified β-carotene in comparison with a single 200,000 IU dose of retinyl palmitate or placebo was conducted in Bangladesh [57]. The 200,000 IU dose represented the recommendation that women be supplemented within 2 months postpartum to enhance vitamin A status during lactation while limiting the possibility that a subsequent pregnancy could be exposed to potential teratogenic effects of high doses of preformed vitamin A [58]. The β-carotene supplementation had only a modest effect on maternal status, with an improved modified relative dose–response test at 6 months postpartum and retinol at 9 months postpartum compared to placebo. However, even the 200,000 IU dose only moderately improved maternal status by these measures, perhaps in part because overt vitamin A deficiency among the women was uncommon and retinol concentrations were typically in the homeostatically controlled range. The persistent β-carotene supplementation improved breast milk retinol compared to the placebo at the end of the study, and suggested a benefit to the infants as assessed by the modified relative dose–response test; even so, over half the infants were vitamin A deficient at the end of the trial by that measure.

Of note, the content of carotenoids provided to mothers in the interventions above, with the exception of the short-term red palm oil study, was in line with usual diets and recommendations for retinol equivalents, as opposed to the higher concentrations used in the dosing studies. Thus, while evidence supports the notion that carotenoids can improve or sustain vitamin A status of mothers during lactation, to date, studies suggest that carotenoids would have to be consumed in greater amounts for a considerable duration of time to adequately maintain the vitamin A status of mothers and infants in populations where vitamin A status is low or marginal.

Other Benefits of Breast Milk Carotenoids

Although previous studies showed modest effects of enhanced carotenoid exposure to the mother on vitamin A status of their infants, breast milk compared to infant formulas offers infants exposure to a greater diversity of carotenoids. Beyond β-carotene, carotenoids have not reliably been identified in a variety of infant formula preparations [33], although lutein and zeaxanthin are in some [59]. These carotenoids may be from adventitious sources, as they were not claimed as constituents of the formulas [59]. Serum lutein concentrations of infants were higher among infants consuming breast milk than those consuming lutein-fortified formulas, with results suggesting that formulas would need to be fortified with 4 times the content of lutein compared to human milk to achieve the same status in infants [60].

The potential health implications of carotenoid exposure to mothers and infants during lactation remain virtually unexplored. Exposure to high concentrations of carotenoids via colostrum may help compensate for low placental transfer of fat-soluble components during pregnancy. This may establish stores, promote immune development, and help infants adjust to the oxidative stress of their new external environment [37].

Lutein and zeaxanthin may have roles in protecting vision, which may have particular relevance for premature infants. These carotenoids are concentrated in the macula lutea and the retina, and may protect the retina from oxidative damage and exposure to short-wavelength light through a filtering effect [61]. While most studies have concentrated on the role of lutein and zeaxanthin in prevention of macular degeneration in the elderly, the potential role of these carotenoids in promoting eye health and proper development in early life is gaining attention [59, 61].

While provitamin A carotenoids and those without provitamin A activity impact immune function in a variety of experimental settings and animal models [62], including lymphocyte proliferation and incident mammary infections in cattle [63], no changes in lymphocyte mitogenic activity were found among either lactating or non-lactating women in a study of 30 mg/d β-carotene supplementation [38].

In a mouse model, supplemental β-carotene increased the number of IgA antibody-secreting cells in mammary and gut tissue and in the stomach contents of the offspring, suggesting enhanced maternal-to-offspring IgA transfer [64]. Conversely, a study in 7-day-old nursing mouse pups demonstrated no impact of milk lycopene enhanced through dietary supplementation on immunization response or neutrophil response to enteropathogen exposure [65]. Specific roles for carotenoids in enhancing immune function of the lactating mother or infant thus remain to be elucidated; although, challenges of using animal models exist due to the differential utilization of carotenoids across species and the choice of biologically relevant doses [39, 65].

Carotenoid exposure during lactation may exclusively benefit the mother. Carotenoid (e.g., lutein and α-carotene) content is inversely related to epithelial cell content, a risk factor for breast cancer, in breast nipple aspirates [66], and is also responsive to dietary intervention with enhanced fruit and vegetable intake [67]. Having experienced lactation is also protective against breast cancer, and there is speculation that the enhanced exposure of the breast tissue to carotenoids during lactation and beyond breast involution may be protective against later development of breast cancer [68]. More work in this area could support this intriguing hypothesis.

Randomized Controlled Trials of β-Carotene Over a Reproductive Cycle

Two randomized controlled trials with a β-carotene-only arm have been conducted among women over the course of a reproductive event. The first was conducted in the terai of Nepal, motivated by the findings of a ~25% reduction in childhood mortality with vitamin A supplementation, high rates of maternal night blindness during pregnancy [69], and an interest in examining the comparability of β-carotene with retinyl palmitate to improve status and outcomes [18]. This cluster-randomized placebo-controlled trial found significant 40% and 49% reductions in pregnancy-related mortality with weekly vitamin A and β-carotene supplementation, respectively. The higher effect of the β-carotene intervention on mortality despite the lower impacts on maternal serum retinol concentration and night blindness incidence has led to speculations regarding the potential antioxidant potential of β-carotene beyond its provitamin activity [18]. In a stratified analysis, β-carotene supplementation, but not vitamin A, benefitted the smokers (RR=0.31, 95% CI: 0.11–0.89) who appeared to experience a higher risk of mortality than the nonsmokers (RR=1.57, 95% CI: 0.80–3.08) [70]. This suggests that β-carotene may have had some antioxidative effect.

In the same trial on a subsample, β-carotene concentrations were assessed in serum and breast milk of the participating women and serum of their infants (Fig. 9.1, West KP Jr, personal communication). These data reveal correlations between maternal serum and breast milk β-carotene concentrations during pregnancy and postpartum and that β-carotene concentrations differ by treatment group. However, breast milk β-carotene and infant β-carotene status is the most strongly correlated, with the correlation being highest in the β-carotene group, whereas maternal serum concentration during mid-pregnancy and infant status appeared to be uncorrelated irrespective of intervention group. This suggests that infant β-carotene status is largely influenced by maternal transfer via breast milk.

Recently, a replicate trial conducted in northern rural Bangladesh which tested the same dosage of weekly vitamin A and β-carotene supplementation during pregnancy found no impact of either intervention on pregnancy-related mortality [20]. A generally better nutritional status, lower risk of maternal mortality, less severe vitamin A deficiency reflected by higher serum retinol concentrations, lower risk of maternal night blindness, and other differences in diet and antenatal care in Bangladesh compared with Nepal may explain the differences, suggesting that context is critical in properly interpreting study findings and their implications. In these same trials, pregnancy and infant outcomes were examined. In Nepal, neither intervention, including β-carotene, had an impact on early neonatal birth size including weight and length [71]. Additionally β-carotene and vitamin A also did not impact fetal

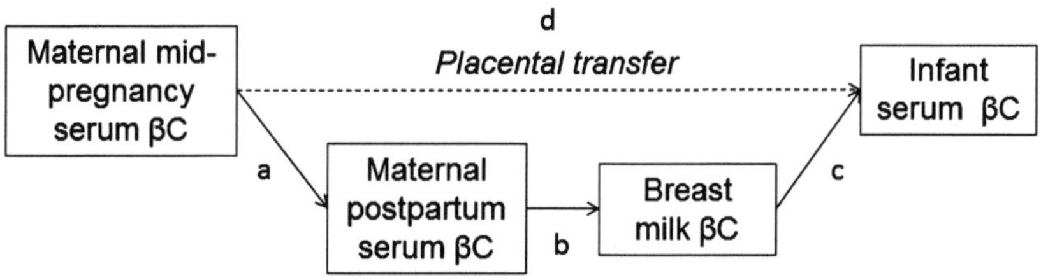

	Correlation coefficients (r)			
Intervention	a	b	c	d
Placebo	.05	.45*	.06	.01
Vitamin A	.04	.64*	.22*	.01
β-carotene	.30*	.63*	.61*	.07

Fig. 9.1 Correlations between maternal serum β-carotene concentrations during pregnancy and the postpartum period, breast milk and infant serum β-carotene at 3 months of age by maternal intervention groups in Nepal. $*p<0.05$, βC = β-carotene

loss, and early infant mortality in either Nepal [19] or Bangladesh [20]. These studies are congruent with the findings of a randomized controlled trial from Indonesia in which β-carotene supplementation during pregnancy in addition to iron-folic acid vs. iron-folic acid alone showed no effect on infant morbidity due to diarrhea or cough [72]. The trial in Nepal, on the other hand, examined treatment effects on self-reported morbidity in women during pregnancy and the postpartum period. β-Carotene (in addition to vitamin A) supplementation reduced the postpartum prevalence of symptoms of diarrhea and night blindness as well as symptoms of high fever [73]. Recently, a longitudinal follow-up of offspring who participated in the maternal vitamin A and β-carotene supplementation trial at 9–13 years of age showed significant improvements in lung function with vitamin A but not with β-carotene [74], although neither supplement reduced the risk of childhood asthma [75].

Conclusions

In conclusion, while observational studies appear to link dietary intake of carotenoids to improvements in health outcomes, data from randomized controlled trials that have examined carotenoids beyond β-carotene are limited. For the infant, breast milk is an important source of carotenoids, especially β-carotene, for providing adequate amounts of vitamin A to support growth and immune function. However, adequate maternal intake of carotenoids during pregnancy, and more importantly during lactation, is essential to meet the requirements of the newborn and the young infant. In pregnancy, inadequate dietary intake of carotenoids, the major source of vitamin A in many regions of the world, and other preformed vitamin A foods can lead to night blindness during pregnancy that is associated with an increased risk of morbidity, mortality, and anemia. During lactation, although preferential transfer of carotenoids in breast milk may occur to provide an adequate supply to the infant, maternal status is likely to influence the supply and in undernourished populations, carotenoid and vitamin A deficiency in infants may exist. Carotenoids in breast milk may confer numerous benefits both to the infant and the woman, but the understanding of this is limited at present.

Future Directions

Carotenoids may have an important antioxidant function in pregnancy and lactation but this role has not been adequately elucidated. A majority of focus on their function during these two physiologic states relates to meeting the vitamin A requirement of the fetus via placental transfer and the young infant via breast milk. In addition, much of the research in this area has been limited to populations from industrialized countries where diets are sufficient in carotenoids and vitamin A supplementation and food fortification are common. Future studies, preferably randomized controlled trials, are needed to examine the effects of food-based or supplementary intakes of carotenoids on reproductive health outcomes, especially the risk of preeclampsia, preterm, premature rupture of membranes, and other conditions of pregnancy. Future research is also needed to better elucidate the impact of carotenoids in pregnancy for enhancing fetal growth and gestational duration using adequately designed experimental studies in human populations. In lactation, it is important to better understand functions of carotenoids, both with regard to their provitamin A activity and their antioxidant properties, in potentially impacting infant health and immune function. Such research is likely to be most relevant in populations whose consumption of fruits and vegetables is inadequate and which harbor a high burden of poor maternal and infant health outcomes. Presently, however, promotion of diets rich in carotenoids during pregnancy and lactation can proceed in parallel alongside the research on elucidating the functional importance of carotenoids during these life stages.

References

1. Lietz G, Lange J, Rimbach G. Molecular and dietary regulation of beta, beta carotene 15, 15'-monooxygenase 1 (BCMO1). Arch Biochem Biophys. 2010;502:8–16.
2. Debier C, Larondelle Y. Vitamins A and E: metabolism, roles and transfer to offspring. Br J Nutr. 2005;93:153–74.
3. Wyss A. Carotene oxygenases, a new family of double bond cleavage enzymes. J Nutr. 2004;134:246S–50S.
4. Marceau G, Gallot D, Lemery D, Sapin V. Metabolism of retinol during mammalian placental and embryonic development. Vitam Horm. 2007;75:97–115.
5. Sundaram M, Sivaprassadaro A, DeSousa MM, Findlay JB. The transfer of retinol from serum retinol-binding protein to cellular retinol-binding protein is mediated by a membrane receptor. J Biol Chem. 1998;273:3336–42.
6. Kawaguchi R, Yu J, Honda J, et al. A membrane receptor for retinol binding protein mediates cellular uptake of vitamin A. Science. 2007;315:820–5.
7. Dimenstein R, Trugo NMF, Donangelo CM, et al. Effect of subadequate maternal vitamin A status on placental transfer of retinol and beta-carotene to the human fetus. Biol Neonate. 1998;69:230–4.
8. Gomes MM, Saunders C, Ramalho A. Placenta: a possible predictor of vitamin A deficiency. Br J Nutr. 2010;103:1340–4.
9. Scaife AR, McNeil G, Campbell DM, Matindale S, Devereux G, Seaton A. Maternal intake of antioxidant vitamins in pregnancy in relation to maternal and fetal plasma levels at delivery. Br J Nutr. 2006;95:771–8.
10. De Barros Silva SS, Rondo PH, Erzinger GS. Beta-carotene concentrations in maternal and cord blood of smokers and non-smokers. Early Hum Dev. 2005;81:313–7.
11. Yamini S, West Jr KP, Wu L, Dreyfuss ML, Yang DX, Khatry SK. Circulating levels of retinol, tocopherol and carotenoid in Nepali pregnant and postpartum women following long-term beta-carotene and vitamin A supplementation. Eur J Clin Nutr. 2001;55:252–9.
12. Institute of Medicine. Dietary reference intakes for vitamin A, vitamin K, arsenic, boron, chromium, copper, iodine, iron, manganese, molybdenum, nickel, silicon, vanadium, and zinc. Washington, DC: National Academy Press; 2001.
13. World Health Organization. Global prevalence of vitamin A deficiency in populations at risk 1995–2005: WHO global database on vitamin A deficiency. 2009, WHO, Geneva. [online], http://www.who.int/vmnis/vitamina/prevalence/en/index.html.
14. Christian P, West Jr KP, Khatry SK, et al. Night blindness of pregnancy in rural Nepal-nutritional and health risks. Int J Epidemiol. 1998;27:231–7.

15. Christian P, West Jr KP, Khatry SK. Maternal night blindness increases risk of mortality in the first 6 months of life among infants in Nepal. J Nutr. 2001;131:1510–2.
16. Tanumihardjo SA, Palacios N, Pixley KV. Provitamin A carotenoid bioavailability: what really matters? Int J Vit Nutr Res. 2010;80:336–50.
17. Christian P, West Jr KP, Khatry SK, et al. Vitamin A or beta-carotene supplementation reduces but does not eliminate maternal night blindness in Nepal. J Nutr. 1998;128:1458–63.
18. West KP Jr, Katz J, Khatry SK et al. Double blind, cluster randomized trial of low dose supplementation with vitamin A of beta carotene on mortality related to pregnancy in Nepal. The NNIPS-2 Study Group. BMJ. 1999 27;318:570–5.
19. Katz J, West Jr KP, Khatry SK, Pradhan EK, LeClerq SC, Christian P, Wu LSF, Adhikari RK, Shrestha SR, Sommer A. Low-dose vitamin A or beta-carotene supplementation does not reduce early infant mortality: A double-masked, randomized, controlled community trial in Nepal. Am J Clin Nutr. 2000;71:1570–6.
20. West Jr KP, Christian P, Labrique AB, et al. Effects of vitamin A or beta carotene supplementation on pregnancy-related mortality and infant mortality in rural Bangladesh: a cluster randomized trial. JAMA. 2011;305:1986–95.
21. Watson PE, McDonald BW. The association of maternal diet and dietary supplement intake in pregnant New Zealand women with infant birth weight. Eur J Clin Nutr. 2010;64:184–93.
22. Mathews F, Youngman L, Neil A. Maternal circulating nutrient concentrations in pregnancy: implications for birth and placental weights of term infants. Am J Clin Nutr. 2004;79:103–10.
23. Azar M, Basu A, Jenkins AJ, et al. Serum carotenoids and fat-soluble vitamins in women with type 1 diabetes and preeclampsia: a longitudinal study. Diabetes Care. 2011;34:1258–64.
24. Palan PR, Mikhail MS, Romney SL. Placental and serum levels of carotenoids in preeclampsia. Obstet Gynecol. 2001;98:459–62.
25. Banerjee S, Jeyaseelan S, Guleria R. Trial of lycopene to prevent pre-eclampsia in healthy primigravidas: results show some adverse effects. J Obstet Gynaecol Res. 2009;35:477–82.
26. Sharma JB, Kumar A, Kumar A, et al. Effect of lycopene on pre-eclampsia and intra-uterine growth retardation in primigravidas. Int J Gynaecol Obstet. 2003;81:257–62.
27. Miyake Y, Sasaki S, Tanaka K, Hirota Y. Consumption of vegetables, fruit, and antioxidants during pregnancy and wheeze and eczema in infants. Allergy. 2010;65:758–65.
28. Orhon FS, Ulukol B, Kahya D, Cengiz B, Başkan S, Tezcan S. The influence of maternal smoking on maternal and newborn oxidant and antioxidant status. Eur J Pediatr. 2009;168:975–81.
29. Litonjua AA, Rifas-Shiman SL, Ly NP, et al. Maternal antioxidant intake in pregnancy and wheezing illness in children at 2 y of age. Am J Clin Nutr. 2006;84:903–11.
30. Sausenthaler S, Koletzko S, Schaaf B, et al. Maternal diet during pregnancy in relation to eczema and allergic sensitization in the offspring at 2 y of age. Am J Clin Nutr. 2007;85:530–7.
31. Willers SM, Wijga AH, Brunekreef B, et al. Maternal food consumption during pregnancy and the longitudinal development of childhood asthma. Am J Respir Crit Care Med. 2008;178:124–31.
32. Khachik F, Spangler CJ, Smith Jr JC, Canfield LM, Steck A, Pfander H. Identification, quantification, and relative concentrations of carotenoids and their metabolites in human milk and serum. Anal Chem. 1997;69:1873–81.
33. Sommerburg O, Meissner K, Nelle M, Lenhartz H, Leichsenring M. Carotenoid supply in breast-fed and formula-fed neonates. Eur J Pediatr. 2000;159:86–90.
34. Macias C, Schweigert FJ. Changes in the concentration of carotenoids, vitamin A, alpha-tocopherol and total lipids in human milk throughout early lactation. Ann Nutr Metab. 2001;45:82–5.
35. Patton S, Canfield LM, Huston GE, Ferris AM, Jensen RG. Carotenoids of human colostrum. Lipds. 1990;25:159–65.
36. Lietz G, Mulokozi G, Henry JC, Tomkins AM. Xanthophyll and hydrocarbon carotenoid patterns differ in plasma and breast milk of women supplemented with red palm oil during pregnancy and lactation. J Nutr. 2006;136: 1821–7.
37. Schweigert FJ, Bathe K, Chen F, Büscher U, Dudenhausen JW. Effect of the stage of lactation in humans on carotenoid levels in milk, blood plasma and plasma lipoprotein fractions. Eur J Nutr. 2004;43:39–44.
38. Gossage C, Deyhim M, Moser-Veillon PB, Douglas LW, Kramer TR. Effect of beta-carotene supplementation and lactation on carotenoid metabolism and mitogenic T lymphocyte proliferation. Am J Clin Nutr. 2000;71:950–5.
39. Rühl R. Effects of dietary retinoids and carotenoids on immune development. Proc Nutr Soc. 2007;66:458–69.
40. Canfield LM, Giuliano AR, Neilson EM, et al. beta-Carotene in breast milk and serum is increased after a single beta-carotene dose. Am J Clin Nutr. 1997;66:52–61.
41. Canfield LM, Giuliano AR, Neilson EM, Blashil BM, Graver EJ, Yap HH. Kinetics of the response of milk and serum beta-carotene to daily beta-carotene supplementation in healthy, lactating women. Am J Clin Nutr. 1998;67:276–83.
42. Canfield LM, Taren DL, Kaminsky RG, Mahal Z. Short-term beta-carotene supplementation of lactating mothers consuming diets low in vitamin A. J Nutr Biochem. 1999;10:532–8.

43. Cena H, Castellazzi AM, Pietri A, Roggi C, Turconi G. Lutein concentration in human milk during early lactation and its relationship with dietary lutein intake. Public Health Nutr. 2009;12:1878–84.
44. Allen CM, Smith AM, Clinton SK, Schwartz SJ. Tomato consumption increases lycopene isomer concentrations in breast milk and plasma of lactating women. J Am Diet Assoc. 2002;102:1257–62.
45. de Azeredo VB, Trugo NM. Retinol, carotenoids, and tocopherols in the milk of lactating adolescents and relationships with plasma concentrations. Nutrition. 2008;24:133–9.
46. Bates CJ, Prentice AM, Paul AA. Seasonal variations in vitamins A, C, riboflavin and folate intakes and status of pregnant and lactating women in a rural Gambian community: some possible implications. Eur J Clin Nutr. 1994;48:660–8.
47. Canfield LM, Clandinin MT, Davies DP, et al. Multinational study of major breast milk carotenoids of healthy mothers. Eur J Nutr. 2003;42:133–41.
48. Stoltzfus RJ, Underwood BA. Breast-milk vitamin A as an indicator of the vitamin A status of women and infants. Bull World Health Organ. 1995;73:703–11.
49. de Pee S, Bloem MW, Gorstein J, et al. Reappraisal of the role of vegetables in the vitamin A status of mothers in Central Java, Indonesia. Am J Clin Nutr. 1998;68:1068–74.
50. da Silva Ribeiro KD, de Araújo KF, de Souza HH, Soares FB, da Costa Pereira M, Dimenstein R. Nutritional vitamin A status in northeast Brazilian lactating mothers. J Hum Nutr Diet. 2010;23:154–61.
51. Lietz G, Henry CJ, Mulokozi G, et al. Comparison of the effects of supplemental red palm oil and sunflower oil on maternal vitamin A status. Am J Clin Nutr. 2001;74:501–9.
52. Canfield LM, Kaminsky RG, Taren DL, Shaw E, Sander JK. Red palm oil in the maternal diet increases provitamin A carotenoids in breastmilk and serum of the mother-infant dyad. Eur J Nutr. 2001;40:30–8.
53. de Pee S, West CE, Muhilal, Karyadi D, Hautvast JG. Lack of improvement in vitamin A status with increased consumption of dark-green leafy vegetables. Lancet. 1995;346:75–81
54. Ncube TN, Greiner T, Malaba LC, Gebre-Medhin M. Supplementing lactating women with puréed papaya and grated carrots improved vitamin A status in a placebo-controlled trial. J Nutr. 2001;131:1497–502.
55. Khan NC, West CE, de Pee S, et al. The contribution of plant foods to the vitamin A supply of lactating women in Vietnam: A randomized controlled trial. Am J Clin Nutr. 2007;85:1112–20.
56. Wasantwisut E, Sungpuag P, Viriyapanich T, et al. Effects of dietary and supplemental β-carotene interventions on total body retinol stores in lactating Thai women. FASEB J. 2000;14:371–3.
57. Rice AL, Stoltzfus RJ, de Francisco A, Chakraborty J, Kjolhede CL, Wahed MA. Maternal vitamin A or beta-carotene supplementation in lactating Bangladeshi women benefits mothers and infants but does not prevent subclinical deficiency. J Nutr. 1999;129:356–65.
58. Sommer A, Davidson FR. Assessment and control of vitamin A deficiency: the Annecy Accords. J Nutr. 2002;132:2845S–50S.
59. Jewell VC, Mayes CB, Tubman TR, Northrop-Clewes CA, Thurnham DI. A comparison of lutein and zeaxanthin concentrations in formula and human milk samples from Northern Ireland mothers. Eur J Clin Nutr. 2004;58:90–7.
60. Bettler J, Zimmer JP, Neuringer M, DeRusso PA. Serum lutein concentrations in healthy term infants fed human milk or infant formula with lutein. Eur J Nutr. 2010;49:45–51.
61. Zimmer JP, Hammond Jr BR. Possible influences of lutein and zeaxanthin on the developing retina. Clin Ophthalmol. 2007;1:25–35.
62. Chew BP, Park JS. Carotenoid action on the immune response. J Nutr. 2004;134:257S–61S.
63. Spears JW, Weiss WP. Role of antioxidants and trace elements in health and immunity of transition dairy cows. Vet J. 2008;176:70–6.
64. Nishiyama Y, Sugimoto M, Ikeda S, Kume S. Supplemental β-carotene increases IgA-secreting cells in mammary gland and IgA transfer from milk to neonatal mice. Br J Nutr. 2011;105:24–30.
65. Adkins B, Contractor N. Immune responses of female BALB/c and C57BL/6 neonatal mice to vaccination or intestinal infection are unaltered by exposure to breast milk lycopene. J Nutr. 2011;14:1326–30.
66. Kato I, Ren J, Visscher DW, Djuric Z. Nutritional predictors for cellular nipple aspirate fluid: Nutrition and Breast Health Study. Breast Cancer Res Treat. 2006;97:33–9.
67. Djuric Z, Chen G, Ren J, et al. Effects of high fruit-vegetable and/or low-fat intervention on breast nipple aspirate fluid micronutrient levels. Cancer Epidemiol Biomarkers. 2007;16:1393–9.
68. Nantais-Smith LM, Covington CY, Nordstrom-Klee BA, et al. Differences in plasma and nipple aspirate carotenoid by lactation status. Nurs Res. 2001;50:172–7.
69. Katz J, Khatry SK, West Jr KP, et al. Night blindness is prevalent during pregnancy and lactation in rural Nepal. J Nutr. 1995;125:2122–7.
70. Christian P, West Jr KP, Katz J, Kimbrough-Pradhan E, LeClerq SC, Khatry SK. Cigarette smoking during pregnancy in rural Nepal. Risk factors and effects of β-carotene and vitamin A supplementation. Eur J Clin Nutr. 2004;58:204–11.
71. Dreyfuss ML, West KP Jr, Katz J, LeClerq SC, Pradhan EK, Adhikari RK et al. Effects of maternal vitamin A or β-carotene supplementation on intrauterine/neonatal and early infant growth in Nepal (abstract). In: Report of the

XVIII International Vitamin A Consultative Group Meeting. Cairo, Egypt, ILSI Research Foundation, Washington DC 1997.

72. Wieringa FT, Dijkhuizen MA, Muhilal, Van der Meer JW. Maternal micronutrient supplementation with zinc and β-carotene affects morbidity and immune function of infants during the first 6 months of life. Eur J Clin Nutr. 2010;64:1072–9
73. Christian P, West Jr KP, Khatry SK, Katz J, Dali SM, LeClerq SC, Kimbrough-Pradhan E, Shrestha SR. The effect of vitamin A and β-carotene supplementation on self-reported illness in pregnant and lactating Nepali women. J Nutr. 2000;130:2675–82.
74. Checkley W, West Jr KP, Wise RA, Baldwin MR, Wu L, LeClerq SC, Christian P, Katz J, Tielsch JM, Khatry SK, Sommer A. Maternal vitamin A supplementation and lung function in offspring. N Engl J Med. 2010;362:1784–94.
75. Checkley W, West Jr KP, Wise RA, Baldwin MR, Wu L, LeClerq SC, Khatry SK, Katz J, Christian P, Tielsch JM, Sommer A. Supplementation with vitamin A early in life and subsequent risk of asthma. Eur Respir J. 2011;38(6):1310–9. 23 Jun 2011 (epub).

Chapter 10
Carotenoids in Early Life

Xiaoming Gong and Lewis P. Rubin

Key Points

- This chapter summarizes the effects of carotenoids in reproduction and provides epidemiological and experimental evidence on decreasing health risks during pregnancy and early postnatal life.
- Retinoic acid, the active derivative of vitamin A, regulates reproduction and embryogenesis. Severe vitamin A deficiency results in infertility impaired reproduction (mostly due to fetal resorption), and may cause congenital malformations.
- A healthy diet that contains sufficient retinoids, carotenoids, and antioxidants protects semen quality and fertility. Low carotenoid status during the periconceptional period or early pregnancy in women is associated with preeclampsia.
- Carotenoids are transferred to the fetus transplacentally and maternal and umbilical cord blood carotenoids are correlated.
- Fetal and early postnatal programming for adult disease risk sheds light on the importance of environment and nutrition on long-term health including the importance of carotenoid and retinoid status during pregnancy and lactation.

Keywords Carotenoids • Development • Eye health • Retina • Lung development • Embryology • Reproductive biology • Placenta

Introduction

Dietary carotenoids and retinoids are essential factors in human health and development. Specifically, they function in a wide range of biological processes, including reproduction, embryonic development, growth, cellular differentiation, immunity, vision, and metabolic control [1, 2]. Adequate or inadequate exposure to these compounds modulates the interplay between heredity and environment from conception through postnatal life and may have long-term effects on child and adult health [3–5]. Deficiencies or low blood and tissue carotenoid levels are associated with the risk of human diseases, including

X. Gong, D.V.M., Ph.D. • L.P. Rubin, M.D. (✉)
Neonatology, Children's Research Institute, University of South Florida, 140 7th Avenue South, 2nd Floor, St. Petersburg, FL 33701, USA
e-mail: lprprb@gmail.com

S.A. Tanumihardjo (ed.), *Carotenoids and Human Health*, Nutrition and Health,
DOI 10.1007/978-1-62703-203-2_10,

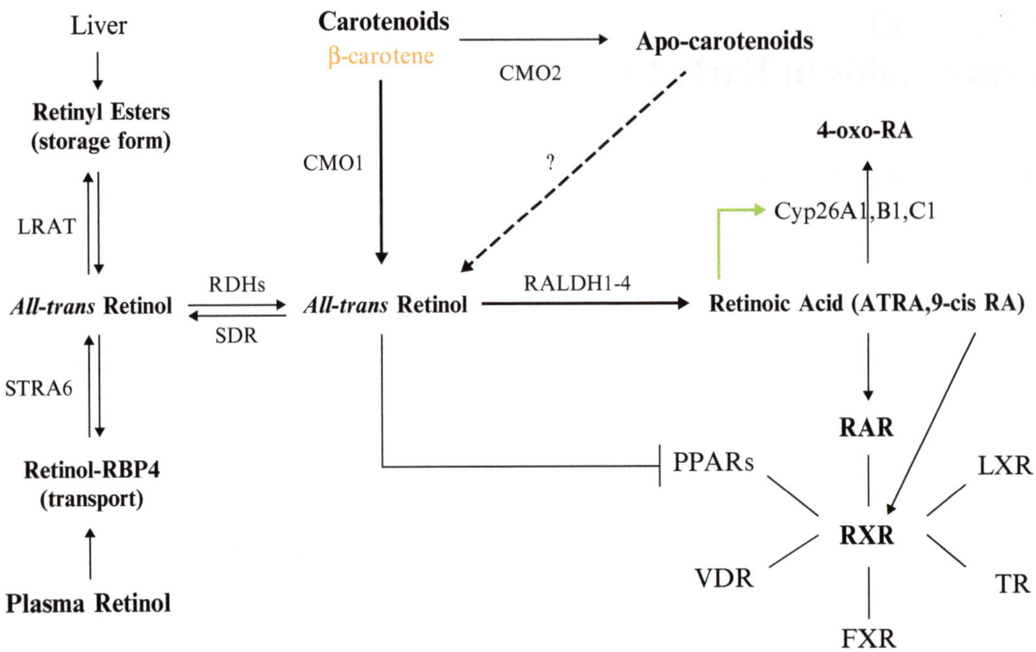

Fig. 10.1 Metabolism and intracellular pathways of carotenoids and retinoids. Carotenoids are obtained from the diet and converted to retinoids or *apo*-carotenoids through carotenoid mono-oxygenases, CMO1 or CMO2. Upon oxidative cleavage, all-*trans* retinal can undergo catalytic reduction/oxidation to form either all-*trans* retinol or all-*trans* retinoic acid (ATRA). All-*trans* retinol can also be obtained from the diet and transported in the blood as a complex with retinol-binding protein (RBP) and transthyretin (TTR). In the liver, retinol is esterified to retinyl esters and stored in stellate cells. In other tissues, all-*trans* retinol is converted to all-*trans* retinal via retinol dehydrogenases (RDH) or short-chain dehydrogenase/reductase (SDR). All-*trans* retinal is metabolized into ATRA in an irreversible reaction catalyzed by retinaldehyde dehydrogenases (RALDHs). ATRA or the 9-*cis* RA isomer activates RAR-RXR heterodimers that specifically bind retinoic acid response elements on DNA for regulation of gene expression. RA, produced in certain cell types, can be released from cells for paracrine and/or autocrine action. RA is further catabolized into 4-oxo- or hydroxyl-RA by the enzymes CYP26 for degradation

reproductive health and fetal life, ranging from infertility to fetal structural defects and long-term diseases [3–5].

Carotenoids are primarily plant-derived polyisoprenoid lipophilic pigments. More than 600 naturally occurring carotenoid compounds have been characterized [1]. Approximately 50–60 of these routinely are consumed in human diets, including lycopene, α-carotene, β-carotene, β-cryptoxanthin, lutein, and zeaxanthin. Correspondingly, carotenoid concentrations are measurable in human plasma and tissues. A critical function for several dietary carotenoids is as precursors to vitamin A (retinol) formation, that is, as provitamin A carotenoids. Other physiological functions ascribed to specific compounds have been associated with their antioxidant properties in lipophilic environments, blue light filtering properties in the retina, and novel effects on gene expression. In these and other instances, carotenoid cleavage products, e.g., *apo*-carotenoids, may account for biological actions.

Carotenoid metabolism is catalyzed by a family of carotenoid cleavage monooxygenases (CMOs). Oxidative cleavage of carotenoids results in a structurally diverse class of compounds known as retinoids and *apo*-carotenoids. The major central cleavage pathway, catalyzed by β-carotene 15,15′-monooxygenase, or CMO1, generates retinoids from provitamin A carotenoids [6–9] such as α-carotene, β-carotene, and β-cryptoxanthin. A second "excentric" pathway for carotenoid metabolism is catalyzed by β-carotene 9′,10′-monooxygenase, or CMO2 [10, 11]. Carotenoid metabolism and some intracellular pathways are summarized in Fig. 10.1.

In this review of carotenoids in early life, we discuss the effects of carotenoids in reproduction and summarize epidemiological and experimental evidence on potential carotenoid effects in decreasing health risks in pregnancy and early postnatal life.

Nutrition in Reproductive Health

A coordinated series of genetic, epigenetic, and cellular processes directs mammalian germ cell differentiation, gametogenesis, ovulation, fertilization, preimplantation, embryo development, implantation, placentation, and parturition. Various stages require the presence of vitamin A and lipid-soluble regulators of oxidative stress. In instances of maternal nutritional insult, timing impacts pregnancy outcomes and developmental programming of health risks in postnatal life.

Maternal nutritional stresses increase glucocorticoid transfer to the conceptus, worsen oxidant stress, and compromise growth. In a classical example of this principle, offspring of women who were exposed to the Dutch Winter Famine of 1944–1945 had different fetal outcomes depending on when starvation occurred in pregnancy. Food restriction in the first trimester of pregnancy was associated with an increased offspring prevalence of coronary heart disease, hyperlipidemia, and obesity decades later [12, 13], whereas famine occurring during late gestation led to decreased glucose tolerance and diabetes mellitus in adult life [14]. Similarly, maternal energy and micronutrient abnormalities increased the risk for several pregnancy-related disorders (e.g., fetal loss, miscarriage, intrauterine growth restriction, preterm birth, and preeclampsia) and congenital anomalies, including congenital diaphragmatic hernia [15]. Furthermore, strong associations between low birth weight and increased risk of adult diseases, including cardiovascular disease, type 2 diabetes, central adiposity, abnormal lipid metabolism, and hypertension, are well-documented [16]. Poor postnatal growth in infancy is also a robust predictor of later adult disease [17].

The β-carotene metabolite, vitamin A, regulates reproduction and embryogenesis through its active derivative, retinoic acid (RA). Severe deficiency of vitamin A results in infertility or impaired reproduction, mostly due to fetal resorption, and causes congenital malformations [18].

Fertility

Mammalian sex is determined genetically, but sex-specific germ cell differentiation is triggered by cues provided in the gonadal microenvironment. During embryogenesis, presumptive ovarian germ cells enter meiosis, thereby committing to oogenesis. In contrast, germ cells in a testicular environment do not enter meiosis until puberty. A key to this sex-specific timing of meiosis entry is the presence or absence of retinoic acid, a bioactive form of vitamin A [19]. Vitamin A is required for normal spermatogenesis [20]; when male rodents are made vitamin A deficient, spermatogenesis ceases. Testes obtained from vitamin A-deficient male mice show only undifferentiated spermatogonia and Sertoli cells within the seminiferous epithelium [21–25], indicating that a lack of vitamin A can prevent further spermatozoa differentiation from this stage. Testes of vitamin A-deficient rats, in contrast, display some preleptotene spermatocytes, suggesting that the severity of the vitamin A-deficiency block in spermatogonial differentiation may be species specific. RA also induces spermatogonial differentiation *in vitro* [26]. These findings implicate the important role for provitamin A carotenoids, as herbivorous mammals obtain vitamin A from metabolism of these dietary carotenoids.

Based on experimental data, a healthy diet that contains sufficient retinoids, carotenoids, and antioxidants protects semen quality and fertility [27]. As is the case for numerous carotenoid-associated effects in development, the fertility effects of certain carotenoids are not restricted to provitamin A activity. A pilot randomized clinical supplementation trial to improve male infertility with astaxanthin, a principal carotenoid in fish and shellfish, showed that this xanthophyll significantly decreased reactive oxygen species (ROS) and secretion of inhibin B by Sertoli cells, indicating potential positive effects on sperm parameters and fertility [28]. Astaxanthin also significantly improved testes weight, sperm count, and sperm head morphology, mitigating cyclophosphamide-induced germ cell chemotoxicity in mice [29]. It is uncertain whether these xanthophyll effects are entirely due to antioxidant action.

Pregnancy, Placenta, and Stress

Maternal nutrition impacts embryo implantation and placental development [30]. The placenta nourishes the fetus throughout pregnancy and regulates fetal growth, metabolism, and redox status. The presence of measurable hepatic vitamin A stores in the newborn indicates that β-carotene or vitamin A is placentally transported during pregnancy [31]. Human placenta expresses CMO1, CMO2, and other enzymes and mediators required for vitamin A metabolism [32–34]; placenta produces retinoids from maternally derived carotenoid precursors [35] and newborn RA levels are associated with variants of genes in the retinol metabolism pathway [36]. A β-carotene-rich diet during pregnancy improves the vitamin A status of women and their infants [37]. Weekly oral supplementation of β-carotene reduced maternal mortality during pregnancy by 49 % in a large trial in Nepal [38].

Placental dysfunction resulting from poor maternal nutrition can lead to intrauterine growth restriction (IUGR) and programming of adult cardiovascular and metabolic disease [39]. Alterations in placental transport functions are associated with pregnancy disorders, including IUGR and preeclampsia [40]. Preeclampsia is a defect of placental trophoblast invasion into the uterine lining that results in maternal hypertension, kidney dysfunction, and poor uteroplacental perfusion. Maternal antioxidants including carotenoids lessen the first trimester placental damage that underlies preeclampsia [41]. Not surprisingly, risk factors for preeclampsia and atherosclerosis are similar and include oxidant stress-inducible endothelial dysfunction. The pathogenesis of preeclampsia involves reduced placental perfusion leading to free radical generation and systemic oxidative damage. This pathway is supported by findings of oxidative stress in blood and tissues of preeclamptic women and elevated serum lipid peroxide levels; in preeclampsia, serum and placental carotenoid levels are decreased compared to samples from women having normal pregnancies [42, 43]. The reductions in maternal and placental antioxidant defenses in preeclampsia result, at least in part, from excessive depletion of antioxidants through the increased generation of oxygen free radicals [44, 45]. The abnormal establishment of the uteroplacental vascular bed in the first trimester leads to increased levels of placental lipid peroxidation, partially via activated placental NADPH oxidase production of superoxide radicals [46].

The importance of carotenoids during pregnancy is highlighted by associations with this major ischemic pregnancy complication. Several studies have assessed carotenoid status during the periconceptional period or early pregnancy in women who later developed preeclampsia [45, 47, 48]. For example, lower placental and maternal circulating β-carotene, lycopene, and canthanxanthin were found in women with preeclampsia [42, 49]. In pregnant women who have type 1 diabetes, low serum α- and β-carotene were associated with subsequent development of preeclampsia [50]. Furthermore, lycopene may prevent preeclampsia as suggested by a prospective cohort study [49]. Oxidant stress and poor uteroplacental perfusion, possibly related to genetic factors, result in preeclampsia in some pregnancies, fetal growth restriction in others, or both conditions. Maternal retinol and lycopene levels have been inversely associated with placental weight at birth [51, 52].

In summary, the antioxidant functions of total carotenoid and several specific (non-provitamin A) carotenoids in pregnancy have been best studied to date. Carotenoids lower oxidative stress by altering free radical production and by ROS scavenging. Moreover, these molecules modify the inflammatory response during placentation.

Embryogenesis and Morphogenesis

Several β-carotene metabolites and enzyme systems that regulate the metabolism of β-carotene, vitamin A, and non-provitamin A carotenoids have been demonstrated in embryos and developing tissues in several species [18, 53, 54]. RA is essential for development of tissues and organs including the hindbrain, spinal cord, heart, eye, skeleton, forelimb buds, lung, pancreas, and genitourinary tract [18, 55]. β-Carotene or vitamin A derivatives (retinoids) are also essential for maintenance of differentiation [18]. The molecular basis for the profound effects of vitamin A on development is largely mediated by the binding of retinoic acid to ligand-activated transcription factors and consequent alterations in gene expression [56]. Not surprisingly, CMO1 activity maintains normal embryonic development when maternal vitamin A supply is limited. Studies in vitamin A-deficient CMO1 null mice indicate that CMO1 is important in embryonic retinoid metabolism, β-carotene serving as the alternative vitamin A source for *in situ* synthesis of retinoids in developing tissues [53]. The critical function of this pathway is highlighted by observations that the absence of CMO1 expression in developing tissues produces a more severe embryonic malformed phenotype when the mice are additionally null for retinol-binding protein (RBP) [53]. More recently, expression of retinaldehyde dehydrogenase (RALDH) mutations that completely eliminate RA synthesis in specific tissues at early stages of development have made it possible to examine the mechanism of RA action in detail [55]. These studies show that RA provides instructive signals for posterior neuroectoderm (hindbrain, spinal cord) and posterior foregut endoderm (pancreas, lung) and a permissive signal for trunk mesoderm (somites, heart, forelimb). At later developmental stages, RA contributes to the development of the eye and other organs. Defects in the forelimb bud, lung, and pancreas appear to be defects in induction of these tissues, as the absence of RA inhibits organogenesis. In contrast, defects in hindbrain, spinal cord, heart, somites, and eye occur after organogenesis has been induced and result from defects in patterning or morphogenesis of these tissues [55]. Several embryonic neurological anomalies are prominent in vitamin A-deficient quail embryos [57].

Carotenoids in Early Life

Carotenoids, in addition to retinoids [58], are transferred to the fetus transplacentally [59]. Umbilical cord blood carotenoid levels obtained at birth reflect the fetoplacental circulation at that time, i.e., carotenoids transferred or metabolized from the maternal circulation. Generally, maternal and umbilical cord blood carotenoids are correlated, albeit lower in the cord [59, 60]. Factors that decrease carotenoid concentrations in nonpregnant adults, such as tobacco smoke, also lower maternal and cord carotenoids, including β-carotene [61]. Daily supplementation with zinc and β-carotene during pregnancy improved plasma retinol concentrations in newborns and in breast milk in a trial in Indonesia [62].

Vitamin A deficiency is associated with defective lung development and decreased immunity and vision after birth. This is because vitamin A metabolites serve as ligands for nuclear receptors (RARs and RXRs) that regulate expression of numerous genes. Clinical trial meta-analyses of vitamin A supplementation in neonates, infants 1–6 months, and children aged 6–59 months indicate a reduction of total and diarrhea-specific mortality in children 6–59 months of age [63, 64].

Carotenoids and Retinoids in Lung Development

Retinoids are critical for lung development and pulmonary alveolar formation [65]. Partially vitamin A-depleted rodent models, in which the fetuses survive longer and later gestational windows can be examined, show that vitamin A is specifically required during midgestation for fetal lung development and neonatal survival [66–69]. All-*trans* RA administration in rodents promotes septation and increases the number of pulmonary alveoli [70–73]. Moreover, RA prevents the inhibition of septation caused by glucocorticoid exposure during alveolization [74]. Although the lung serves as a storage location for retinyl esters [75], levels decrease at birth as retinoids are mobilized [67]. Lipid interstitial cells of the alveolar wall store retinol and also synthesize and secrete RA, thereby suggesting an endogenous source of retinoids for alveolar formation [76]. These lung cells occupy a similar niche and function as the stellate cells in the liver, especially for storage and mobilization of lipids and lipophilic substances [77]. RA also promotes alveolar development via regulation of vascular endothelial growth factor and its receptor-2 [71, 78].

Defects in pulmonary development associated with prenatal vitamin A deficiency in animals can be reversed with early postnatal vitamin A supplementation [79]. Premature infants are susceptible to acute, subacute, and chronic lung injury [80], neonatal chronic lung disease, or bronchopulmonary dysplasia (BPD). Preterm newborns can be retinoid and carotenoid deficient because they have missed the bulk of maternal-fetal transfer that occurs during the third trimester. In the absence of an adequate intake of vitamin A or carotenoids in the postnatal period, these infants often become vitamin A deficient. Two randomized, blinded, placebo-controlled clinical trials [81, 82] showed that vitamin A supplementation from early postnatal life in this population improves vitamin A status and decreases incidence of BPD with its associated morbidities. A recent preliminary report suggests that lutein supplementation in these high-risk newborns also may decrease BPD incidence (Manzoni, P. PAS 2011; 3535.6A, abstract). The potential roles of various carotenoids in protection from lung injury or in lung healing have not yet been thoroughly investigated.

Carotenoids and Retinoids in Immune Development

Vitamin A deficiency affects ~250 million people worldwide and increases the likelihood of childhood mortality due to common respiratory and gastrointestinal infection [83]. Increased disease susceptibilities are, in part, attributable to infection, impaired epithelial barrier function [84, 85], and immunological defects. Responses to mucosal pathogens are impaired when vitamin A stores are low; in experimental systems, vitamin A metabolites support functional maturation of innate immune cells as discussed in Chap. 16 [84, 86]. Immune development in early life involves three retinoid-dependent processes, namely, differentiation of immune-competent cells, thymic selection, and lymphocyte proliferation and expansion. Importantly, recent evidence from a variety of experimental systems and human studies indicates that several non-provitamin A carotenoids also modulate developmental immunity.

Vitamin A-deficient animals exhibit abnormalities in blood and splenic lymphocyte numbers; T cell and, occasionally, B cell populations are reduced and, in general, myeloid lineage cells, especially granulocytes, are increased [87, 88]. The latter observation is consistent with the findings that RA inhibits granulocyte-macrophage colony-stimulating factor production and granulocyte development [89] and reverses the effects of a vitamin A-deficient state *in vivo* [88]. RA signaling also plays a critical role in B lymphoid development. B cells mediate the humoral immune response. After lineage development in bone marrow, naïve B cells enter the circulation and reside in the secondary lymphoid organs, such as lymph nodes, tonsils, and spleen, and become follicular and marginal zone B cells, depending on location, or they recirculate to the bone marrow to reside in sinuses, where they may receive signals from T cells and/or provide surveillance against blood-borne antigens. Vitamin A and RA regulate the maturation and differentiation of B cells, which regulate and often potentiate antibody production. Vitamin A deficiency reduces the number of fetal B cell progenitors, while the pan-RAR antagonist, LE540, inhibits both fetal and adult B lymphopoiesis *in vitro* [90]. RA at physiological concentrations inhibited the proliferation of normal B cell progenitors of both mice and humans [91] and affected multiple stages of B lymphopoiesis and accelerated the generation of B cells [92]. These results suggest that RA provides a microenvironment to sustain B-cell development and maintain a pool for antigen response.

During thymic selection, T cells develop in the thymus through a series of stages defined by the expression of the cell surface markers CD4 and CD8. The development of the human thymus starts before birth and ceases during puberty with involution of the thymus [93]. Vitamin A deficiency is known to be accompanied by immune deficiency and a susceptibility to a wide range of infectious diseases [94, 95]. In vitamin A-deficient animals, a marked atrophy of the thymus and spleen has been observed [96]; on the other hand, retinoids at higher concentrations are toxic and cause involution of lymphoid organs, in particular the thymus [97]. A recent study has shown that retinoic acid-synthesizing enzymes peak at the same time as the RAR response, when thymic cellularity is highest and the T cell selection process, as indicated by a high rate of apoptosis, is most effective [98]. Thymic selection is a direct target of retinoic acid during thymocyte development, and it may be postulated that high maternal dietary intake of vitamin A or provitamin A carotenoids may modify thymic selection processes. To date, effects of carotenoids on thymic selection remain unknown.

A second important process in which retinoids are involved is the proliferation of lymphocyte populations and their response to mitogens [99–101]. In a study of pregnant mice fed control or different retinoid- and carotenoid-enriched (4,500 retinol equivalents/kg) diets from day 1 (conception), increases in the percentage and total number of splenic mononuclear cells were observed on days 3 and 5 with vitamin A (retinyl palmitate) supplementation, while β-carotene supplementation increased $CD3^+$ cell numbers from days 5 to 14. At day 7, increases were found in CD4:CD8 ratios after vitamin A supplementation and T cell:B cell ratios after vitamin A and β-carotene supplementation. In general, IgG levels were not altered by the different diets [102]. These results confirm that supplementation with vitamin A and β-carotene affects immune cell functions during ontogenesis. However, maternal vitamin A supplementation via intraperitoneal injections increases serum IgM and Th2-specific IgG1 levels in the progeny [103]. Furthermore, in a human supplementation study [104], which investigated the effects of β-carotene supplementation during early lactation (days 4–32 postpartum), neither lactation nor β-carotene supplementation affected T-cell proliferation.

T helper cells include the Th1 (cellular immune stimulator via macrophages), Th2 (humoral immune stimulator via B cells), Th17 (immunoregulatory), and Treg (suppressor T cell) subtypes. The Th1:Th2 switch is affected by vitamin A during postnatal development, helping to regulate immunity and response to inflammation [103, 105]. Whether these outcomes are mediated by lymphocyte-mediated effects, or via antigen-presenting cell-mediated effects, is not certain.

The effects of carotenoids are difficult to investigate because of the pronounced differences in carotenoid absorption, kinetics, and metabolism between humans and laboratory rodents [106]. Nevertheless, several presumably non-provitamin A carotenoids also affect T cell polarization. Examples include Treg induction and Th17 inhibition [107], resulting in suppression of inflammation and autoimmunity.

Carotenoids and Retinoids in Visual Development

The retina is the light-sensitive tissue lining the inner surface of the eye. In humans, ocular and neuronal aspects of the visual system are incompletely developed at birth. Postnatal visual development includes maturation of the retina, especially the fovea and macular area, and eyeball growth [108, 109]. At birth, the peripheral retina is more developed than the central retinal structures. The fovea is responsible for central vision and visual acuity; the macula retinal layers mediate color and contrast, visual acuity, and stereoscopic vision. As the central retina matures, photoreceptor number and function increase with the result that central vision sharpens. Functional differentiation starts by 6 weeks and continues up to about 8 months of age [108, 110]. Impaired visual input can lead to abnormal ocular and neural processing (e.g., developmental disorders including anisometropic or strabismic amblyopia).

The xanthophylls lutein and zeaxanthin are highly concentrated in the human eye [111], especially in the macular pigment of the retina and in the lens. The roles of these carotenoids in protection from degenerative eye diseases such as cataracts and retinopathies, especially macular degeneration, are described in Chap. 13. Retinal lutein and zeaxanthin impact the development of the visual system by altering input during a critical/sensitive period of visual development, influencing maturation, and protecting the retina from photo- and oxidant stress.

In fetal, neonatal, and infant development, lutein is the dominant retinal carotenoid, which differs from the adult central retina, in which zeaxanthin-to-lutein ratios across the retina are reversed [112]. Studies from nonhuman primates raised on normal or xanthophyll-free diets [113] demonstrate that, in addition to simply lacking macular pigment, xanthophyll-free monkeys have more drusen-like bodies (indicative of retinal degeneration) within their retinal pigment epithelium (RPE), increased macular hyper-fluorescence, and retinal abnormalities [114]. Some of these findings may be partially attributable to other dietary differences between the groups [115], but one follow-up study [116] on macaques that specifically were deprived of lutein and zeaxanthin (and omega-3 fatty acids in some monkeys) localized the pathological effects to the RPE. The RPE lies between the underlying choroid vasculature and the photoreceptor cell layer, which it nourishes. Some of these retinal changes produced by xanthophyll-depleted diets in monkeys can be reversed if xanthophylls are supplemented later in life [116]. The consequences of carotenoid depletion in young nonhuman primates has some similarities to the human situation of prematurity [117].

The rapid maturation and increased metabolic activity of the developing retina increase tissue susceptibility to hypoxic/oxidant and photo-stress. In animal models [118], poor autoregulation of choroidal blood flow, like the human condition of neonatal retinopathy of prematurity, leads to hyperoxygenation and excess lipid peroxidation. Restricted blood flow (ischemia) induces retinal cellular degeneration. Choi et al. used high intraocular pressure to induce ischemia in rat retinas [119], which stimulated increased production of neuronal nitric oxide synthase (nNOS) which, in turn, generates the oxidative stress mediator, nitric oxide. Lutein reduced the production of nNOS in a dose-dependent manner. Similarly, in rat models, zeaxanthin supplementation inhibited retinal oxidative damage caused by experimental diabetes [120].

Biomarkers of retinal stress, like lipofuscin, show rapid increases in the RPE during the first few years of life suggesting that a large portion of lifetime accumulation of damage may occur early [121, 122]. This retinal damage is elevated when a clearer crystalline lens cannot restrict high energy photon (e.g., blue light) access to the retina and when the retina has lesser antioxidant and photo-stress protection. In humans, lutein and zeaxanthin accumulation in the lens and retina are critical visual protectants. The infant retina and RPE "age" rapidly from increased oxidative and actinic stress and may be more susceptible to blue light damage due to the relative clarity of the young crystalline lens [123]. As crystalline proteins oxidize, the aging lens becomes increasingly yellowed and blocks short-wave light. In contrast, the relatively transparent infant lens transmits more blue light. Perhaps reflecting these needs, human milk contains many antioxidants including lutein [124]. Carotenoid supplementation to preterm infants raised plasma concentrations to the levels observed in mother's milk-fed term infants and decreased inflammation in these preterm infants [60].

One recent area of interest is the potential role of lutein in preventing or lessening severity of neonatal and congenital retinopathies. The major cause of acquired blindness in childhood in developed countries is retinopathy of prematurity (ROP), the pathogenesis of which is hypoxic ischemic injury to the immature retina leading to a proliferative vascular response. Secondary (postnatal) prevention for this retinopathy aims to suppress the retinal oxidant stress and inflammatory responses. Four studies have investigated the relationship between xanthophylls and ROP [60, 125, 126] (Manzoni, P. PAS 2011; 3535.6A, abstract). However, no trial has been adequately designed specifically to test the hypothesis that lutein affects ROP outcomes. Only one study [126] performed a power analysis to test a lutein effect on ROP, but the study ended early; it also assumed that an effect might be maximal with less severe ROP. Intriguingly, the three multicenter trials all showed a trend of decreased ROP severity in the lutein-supplemented groups. Consequently, it remains undetermined whether lutein supplementation can decrease the incidence or severity of ROP in at-risk preterm infants. A reasonable hypothesis is that lutein more likely prevents severe retinopathy. The findings above and experimental data provide a rationale for clinical trials of lutein supplementation in extremely preterm infants targeting multiple eye and visual outcomes.

In embryonic development, the retina and the optic nerve originate as outgrowths of the developing brain. Recent evidence indicates that lutein is by far the most abundant carotenoid found during the first year of life in brain specimens, accounting for nearly 60 % of total brain carotenoids. Overall, xanthophylls are found at greater concentrations in brain tissue than carotenes (Vishwanathan, R. 2011, the 16th international symposium on carotenoids).

Conclusions and Future Directions

Despite considerable progress, further investigations are needed to understand the mechanisms and functions of carotenoids, and especially the non-provitamin A carotenoids, in reproductive health and early life. Discovery of fetal and early postnatal programming for adult disease risk sheds light on the importance of environment and nutrition on long-term health. From early development, an organism's future physiological and even psychological phenotype is informed by the conditions in which it grows. Early blastocyst cell division, implantation, trophoblastic invasion, and subsequent patterning are all orchestrated, in part, by nutritional quantity and quality accessed by the conceptus from the mother via the placenta. Early postnatal micronutrients including carotenoids can be important determinants of antioxidant and antistress protection, organ development, and developmental physiology, especially for vitamin A economy, immunity, vision, and neurodevelopment.

References

1. Olson JA, Krinsky NI. Introduction: the colorful, fascinating world of the carotenoids: important physiologic modulators. FASEB J. 1995;9:1547–50.
2. De Luca LM. Retinoids and their receptors in differentiation, embryogenesis, and neoplasia. FASEB J. 1991;5: 2924–33.
3. McArdle HJ, Ashworth CJ. Micronutrients in fetal growth and development. Br Med Bull. 1999;55:499–510.
4. Ashworth CJ, Antipatis C. Micronutrient programming of development throughout gestation. Reproduction. 2001;122:527–35.
5. Andersen HS, Gambling L, Holtrop G, McArdle HJ. Maternal iron deficiency identifies critical windows for growth and cardiovascular development in the rat postimplantation embryo. J Nutr. 2006;136:1171–7.
6. von Lintig J, Vogt K. Filling the gap in vitamin A research. Molecular identification of an enzyme cleaving beta-carotene to retinal. J Biol Chem. 2000;275:11915–20.
7. Wyss A, Wirtz G, Woggon W, Brugger R, Wyss M, Friedlein A, Bachmann H, Hunziker W. Cloning and expression of beta, beta-carotene 15,15′-dioxygenase. Biochem Biophys Res Commun. 2000;271:334–6.
8. Redmond TM, Gentleman S, Duncan T, Yu S, Wiggert B, Gantt E, Cunningham Jr FX. Identification, expression, and substrate specificity of a mammalian beta-carotene 15,15′-dioxygenase. J Biol Chem. 2001;276:6560–5.
9. von Lintig J, Dreher A, Kiefer C, Wernet MF, Vogt K. Analysis of the blind Drosophila mutant ninaB identifies the gene encoding the key enzyme for vitamin A formation in vivo. Proc Natl Acad Sci U S A. 2001;98:1130–5.
10. Kiefer C, Hessel S, Lampert JM, Vogt K, Lederer MO, Breithaupt DE, von Lintig J. Identification and characterization of a mammalian enzyme catalyzing the asymmetric oxidative cleavage of provitamin A. J Biol Chem. 2001;276:14110–6.
11. Mein JR, Dolnikowski GG, Ernst H, Russell RM, Wang XD. Enzymatic formation of *apo*-carotenoids from the xanthophyll carotenoids lutein, zeaxanthin and beta-cryptoxanthin by ferret carotene-9′,10′-monooxygenase. Arch Biochem Biophys. 2011;506:109–21.
12. Ravelli AC, van Der Meulen JH, Osmond C, Barker DJ, Bleker OP. Obesity at the age of 50 y in men and women exposed to famine prenatally. Am J Clin Nutr. 1999;70:811–6.

13. Roseboom TJ, van der Meulen JH, Osmond C, Barker DJ, Ravelli AC, Schroeder-Tanka JM, van Montfrans GA, Michels RP, Bleker OP. Coronary heart disease after prenatal exposure to the Dutch famine, 1944–45. Heart. 2000;84:595–8.
14. Ravelli AC, van der Meulen JH, Michels RP, Osmond C, Barker DJ, Hales CN, Bleker OP. Glucose tolerance in adults after prenatal exposure to famine. Lancet. 1998;351:173–7.
15. Beurskens LW, Tibboel D, Lindemans J, Duvekot JJ, Cohen-Overbeek TE, Veenma DC, de Klein A, Greer JJ, Steegers-Theunissen RP. Retinol status of newborn infants is associated with congenital diaphragmatic hernia. Pediatrics. 2010;126:712–20.
16. Gluckman PD, Hanson MA, Cooper C, Thornburg KL. Effect of in utero and early-life conditions on adult health and disease. N Engl J Med. 2008;359:61–73.
17. Singhal A, Lucas A. Early origins of cardiovascular disease: is there a unifying hypothesis? Lancet. 2004;363: 1642–5.
18. Clagett-Dame M, DeLuca HF. The role of vitamin A in mammalian reproduction and embryonic development. Annu Rev Nutr. 2002;22:347–81.
19. Bowles J, Koopman P. Retinoic acid, meiosis and germ cell fate in mammals. Development. 2007;134:3401–11.
20. Livera G, Rouiller-Fabre V, Pairault C, Levacher C, Habert R. Regulation and perturbation of testicular functions by vitamin A. Reproduction. 2002;124:173–80.
21. Wang Z, Kim KH. Vitamin A-deficient testis germ cells are arrested at the end of S phase of the cell cycle: a molecular study of the origin of synchronous spermatogenesis in regenerated seminiferous tubules. Biol Reprod. 1993;48:1157–65.
22. Morales A, Cavicchia JC. Spermatogenesis and blood-testis barrier in rats after long-term vitamin A deprivation. Tissue Cell. 2002;34:349–55.
23. van Pelt AM, de Rooij DG. Synchronization of the seminiferous epithelium after vitamin A replacement in vitamin A-deficient mice. Biol Reprod. 1990;43:363–7.
24. Griswold MD, Bishop PD, Kim KH, Ping R, Siiteri JE, Morales C. Function of vitamin A in normal and synchronized seminiferous tubules. Ann N Y Acad Sci. 1989;564:154–72.
25. Hirota Y, Kurohmaru M, Matsumoto M, Hayashi Y. Stage-synchronization of the seminiferous tubules after vitamin A replacement in vitamin A deficient golden hamsters. J Vet Med Sci. 1994;56:439–42.
26. Zhou Q, Li Y, Nie R, Friel P, Mitchell D, Evanoff RM, Pouchnik D, Banasik B, McCarrey JR, Small C, Griswold MD. Expression of stimulated by retinoic acid gene 8 (Stra8) and maturation of murine gonocytes and spermatogonia induced by retinoic acid *in vitro*. Biol Reprod. 2008;78:537–45.
27. Eskenazi B, Kidd SA, Marks AR, Sloter E, Block G, Wyrobek AJ. Antioxidant intake is associated with semen quality in healthy men. Hum Reprod. 2005;20:1006–12.
28. Comhaire FH, El Garem Y, Mahmoud A, Eertmans F, Schoonjans F. Combined conventional/antioxidant "Astaxanthin" treatment for male infertility: a double blind, randomized trial. Asian J Androl. 2005;7:257–62.
29. Tripathi DN, Jena GB. Astaxanthin inhibits cytotoxic and genotoxic effects of cyclophosphamide in mice germ cells. Toxicology. 2008;248:96–103.
30. Cross JC, Mickelson L. Nutritional influences on implantation and placental development. Nutr Rev. 2006;64:S12–8. discussion S72–91.
31. Ross AC, Gardner EM. The function of vitamin A in cellular growth and differentiation, and its roles during pregnancy and lactation. Adv Exp Med Biol. 1994;352:187–200.
32. Lindqvist A, He YG, Andersson S. Cell type-specific expression of beta-carotene 9′,10′-monooxygenase in human tissues. J Histochem Cytochem. 2005;53:1403–12.
33. Marceau G, Gallot D, Lemery D, Sapin V. Metabolism of retinol during mammalian placental and embryonic development. Vitam Horm. 2007;75:97–115.
34. Quadro L, Hamberger L, Gottesman ME, Colantuoni V, Ramakrishnan R, Blaner WS. Transplacental delivery of retinoid: the role of retinol-binding protein and lipoprotein retinyl ester. Am J Physiol Endocrinol Metab. 2004;286:E844–51.
35. Dimenstein R, Trugo NM, Donangelo CM, Trugo LC, Anastacio AS. Effect of subadequate maternal vitamin-A status on placental transfer of retinol and beta-carotene to the human fetus. Biol Neonate. 1996;69:230–4.
36. Manolescu DC, El-Kares R, Lakhal-Chaieb L, Montpetit A, Bhat PV, Goodyer P. Newborn serum retinoic acid level is associated with variants of genes in the retinol metabolism pathway. Pediatr Res. 2010;67:598–602.
37. Radhika MS, Bhaskaram P, Balakrishna N, Ramalakshmi BA. Red palm oil supplementation: a feasible diet-based approach to improve the vitamin A status of pregnant women and their infants. Food Nutr Bull. 2003;24:208–17.
38. West Jr KP, Katz J, Khatry SK, LeClerq SC, Pradhan EK, Shrestha SR, Connor PB, Dali SM, Christian P, Pokhrel RP, Sommer A. Double blind, cluster randomised trial of low dose supplementation with vitamin A or beta carotene on mortality related to pregnancy in Nepal. The NNIPS-2 Study Group. BMJ. 1999;318:570–5.
39. Jansson T, Myatt L, Powell TL. The role of trophoblast nutrient and ion transporters in the development of pregnancy complications and adult disease. Curr Vasc Pharmacol. 2009;7:521–33.

40. Jansson N, Pettersson J, Haafiz A, Ericsson A, Palmberg I, Tranberg M, Ganapathy V, Powell TL, Jansson T. Down-regulation of placental transport of amino acids precedes the development of intrauterine growth restriction in rats fed a low protein diet. J Physiol. 2006;576:935–46.
41. Eason E. The use of first trimester ultrasound. J Obstet Gynaecol Can. 2004;26:17–8. Author reply 18.
42. Palan PR, Mikhail MS, Romney SL. Placental and serum levels of carotenoids in preeclampsia. Obstet Gynecol. 2001;98:459–62.
43. Williams MA, Woelk GB, King IB, Jenkins L, Mahomed K. Plasma carotenoids, retinol, tocopherols, and lipoproteins in preeclamptic and normotensive pregnant Zimbabwean women. Am J Hypertens. 2003;16:665–72.
44. Jauniaux E, Poston L, Burton GJ. Placental-related diseases of pregnancy: involvement of oxidative stress and implications in human evolution. Hum Reprod Update. 2006;12:747–55.
45. Mikhail MS, Anyaegbunam A, Garfinkel D, Palan PR, Basu J, Romney SL. Preeclampsia and antioxidant nutrients: decreased plasma levels of reduced ascorbic acid, alpha-tocopherol, and beta-carotene in women with preeclampsia. Am J Obstet Gynecol. 1994;171:150–7.
46. Agarwal A, Gupta S, Sekhon L, Shah R. Redox considerations in female reproductive function and assisted reproduction: from molecular mechanisms to health implications. Antioxid Redox Signal. 2008;10:1375–403.
47. Ziari SA, Mireles VL, Cantu CG, Cervantes III M, Idrisa A, Bobsom D, Tsin AT, Glew RH. Serum vitamin A, vitamin E, and beta-carotene levels in preeclamptic women in northern Nigeria. Am J Perinatol. 1996;13:287–91.
48. Zhang C, Williams MA, Sanchez SE, King IB, Ware-Jauregui S, Larrabure G, Bazul V, Leisenring WM. Plasma concentrations of carotenoids, retinol, and tocopherols in preeclamptic and normotensive pregnant women. Am J Epidemiol. 2001;153:572–80.
49. Sharma JB, Kumar A, Malhotra M, Arora R, Prasad S, Batra S. Effect of lycopene on pre-eclampsia and intrauterine growth retardation in primigravidas. Int J Gynaecol Obstet. 2003;81:257–62.
50. Azar M, Basu A, Jenkins AJ, Nankervis AJ, Hanssen KF, Scholz H, Henriksen T, Garg SK, Hammad SM, Scardo JA, Aston CE, Lyons TJ. Serum carotenoids and fat-soluble vitamins in women with type 1 diabetes and preeclampsia: a longitudinal study. Diabetes Care. 2011;34:1258–64.
51. Banerjee S, Jeyaseelan S, Guleria R. Trial of lycopene to prevent pre-eclampsia in healthy primigravidas: results show some adverse effects. J Obstet Gynaecol Res. 2009;35:477–82.
52. Ortega-Senovilla H, Alvino G, Taricco E, Cetin I, Herrera E. Enhanced circulating retinol and non-esterified fatty acids in pregnancies complicated with intrauterine growth restriction. Clin Sci (Lond). 2010;118:351–8.
53. Kim YK, Wassef L, Chung S, Jiang H, Wyss A, Blaner WS, Quadro L. beta-Carotene and its cleavage enzyme beta-carotene-15,15′-oxygenase (CMOI) affect retinoid metabolism in developing tissues. FASEB J. 2011;25:1641–52.
54. Lampert JM, Holzschuh J, Hessel S, Driever W, Vogt K, von Lintig J. Provitamin A conversion to retinal via the beta, beta-carotene-15,15′-oxygenase (bcox) is essential for pattern formation and differentiation during zebrafish embryogenesis. Development. 2003;130:2173–86.
55. Duester G. Retinoic acid synthesis and signaling during early organogenesis. Cell. 2008;134:921–31.
56. Ross SA, McCaffery PJ, Drager UC, De Luca LM. Retinoids in embryonal development. Physiol Rev. 2000;80:1021–54.
57. Maden M, Gale E, Kostetskii I, Zile M. Vitamin A-deficient quail embryos have half a hindbrain and other neural defects. Curr Biol. 1996;6:417–26.
58. Spiegler E, Kim YK, Wassef L, Shete V, Quadro L. Maternal-fetal transfer and metabolism of vitamin A and its precursor beta-carotene in the developing tissues. Biochim Biophys Acta. 2012;1821:88–98.
59. Yeum KJ, Ferland G, Patry J, Russell RM. Relationship of plasma carotenoids, retinol and tocopherols in mothers and newborn infants. J Am Coll Nutr. 1998;17:442–7.
60. Rubin LP, Chan GM, Barrett-Reis BM, Fulton AB, Hansen RM, Ashmeade TL, Oliver JS, Mackey AD, Dimmit RA, Hartmann EE, Adamkin DH. Effect of carotenoid supplementation on plasma carotenoids, inflammation and visual development in preterm infants. J Perinatol. 2012;32(6):418–24.
61. de Barros Silva SS, Rondo PH, Erzinger GS. Beta-carotene concentrations in maternal and cord blood of smokers and non-smokers. Early Hum Dev. 2005;81:313–7.
62. Dijkhuizen MA, Wieringa FT, West CE, Muhilal. Zinc plus beta-carotene supplementation of pregnant women is superior to beta-carotene supplementation alone in improving vitamin A status in both mothers and infants. Am J Clin Nutr. 2004;80:1299–307.
63. Imdad A, Yakoob MY, Sudfeld C, Haider BA, Black RE, Bhutta ZA. Impact of vitamin A supplementation on infant and childhood mortality. BMC Public Health. 2011;11 Suppl 3:S20.
64. Mayo-Wilson E, Imdad A, Herzer K, Yakoob MY, Bhutta ZA. Vitamin A supplements for preventing mortality, illness, and blindness in children aged under 5: systematic review and meta-analysis. BMJ. 2011;343:d5094.
65. Malpel S, Mendelsohn C, Cardoso WV. Regulation of retinoic acid signaling during lung morphogenesis. Development. 2000;127:3057–67.
66. Biesalski HK. The significance of vitamin A for the development and function of the lung. Forum Nutr. 2003;56:37–40.
67. Zachman RD. Role of vitamin A in lung development. J Nutr. 1995;125:1634S–8.

68. Biesalski HK, Nohr D. Importance of vitamin-A for lung function and development. Mol Aspects Med. 2003;24:431–40.
69. Zachman RD. Vitamin A supplementation for extremely-low-birth-weight infants. J Pediatr. 2000;136:124–5.
70. Maden M, Hind M. Retinoic acid in alveolar development, maintenance and regeneration. Philos Trans R Soc Lond B Biol Sci. 2004;359:799–808.
71. Cho SJ, George CL, Snyder JM, Acarregui MJ. Retinoic acid and erythropoietin maintain alveolar development in mice treated with an angiogenesis inhibitor. Am J Respir Cell Mol Biol. 2005;33:622–8.
72. Massaro GD, Massaro D. Postnatal treatment with retinoic acid increases the number of pulmonary alveoli in rats. Am J Physiol. 1996;270:L305–10.
73. Massaro GD, Massaro D, Chan WY, Clerch LB, Ghyselinck N, Chambon P, Chandraratna RA. Retinoic acid receptor-beta: an endogenous inhibitor of the perinatal formation of pulmonary alveoli. Physiol Genomics. 2000;4:51–7.
74. Massaro D, Massaro GD. Dexamethasone accelerates postnatal alveolar wall thinning and alters wall composition. Am J Physiol. 1986;251:R218–24.
75. Zachman RD, Kakkad B, Chytil F. Perinatal rat lung retinol (vitamin A) and retinyl palmitate. Pediatr Res. 1984;18:1297–9.
76. Dirami G, Massaro GD, Clerch LB, Ryan US, Reczek PR, Massaro D. Lung retinol storing cells synthesize and secrete retinoic acid, an inducer of alveolus formation. Am J Physiol Lung Cell Mol Physiol. 2004;286:L249–56.
77. Shmarakov I, Fleshman MK, D'Ambrosio DN, Piantedosi R, Riedl KM, Schwartz SJ, Curley Jr RW, von Lintig J, Rubin LP, Harrison EH, Blaner WS. Hepatic stellate cells are an important cellular site for beta-carotene conversion to retinoid. Arch Biochem Biophys. 2010;504:3–10.
78. Pinto Mde L, Rodrigues P, Coelho AC, Pires Mdos A, dos Santos DL, Goncalves C, Bairos VA. Prenatal administration of vitamin A alters pulmonary and plasma levels of vascular endothelial growth factor in the developing mouse. Int J Exp Pathol. 2007;88:393–401.
79. Wei H, Huang HM, Li TY, Qu P, Liu YX, Chen J. Marginal vitamin A deficiency affects lung maturation in rats from prenatal to adult stage. J Nutr Sci Vitaminol (Tokyo). 2009;55:208–14.
80. Northway Jr WH, Rosan RC, Porter DY. Pulmonary disease following respirator therapy of hyaline-membrane disease. Bronchopulmonary dysplasia. N Engl J Med. 1967;276:357–68.
81. Shenai JP, Kennedy KA, Chytil F, Stahlman MT. Clinical trial of vitamin A supplementation in infants susceptible to bronchopulmonary dysplasia. J Pediatr. 1987;111:269–77.
82. Papagaroufalis C, Megreli C, Hagjigeorgi C, Xanthou M. A trial of vitamin A supplementation for the prevention of intraventricular hemorrhage in very low birth weight neonates. J Perinat Med. 1991;19 Suppl 1:382–7.
83. Sommer A. Vitamin A deficiency and clinical disease: an historical overview. J Nutr. 2008;138:1835–9.
84. Stephensen CB. Vitamin A, infection, and immune function. Annu Rev Nutr. 2001;21:167–92.
85. Biesalski HK, Nohr D. New aspects in vitamin A metabolism: the role of retinyl esters as systemic and local sources for retinol in mucous epithelia. J Nutr. 2004;134:3453S–7.
86. Cerwenka A, Bakker AB, McClanahan T, Wagner J, Wu J, Phillips JH, Lanier LL. Retinoic acid early inducible genes define a ligand family for the activating NKG2D receptor in mice. Immunity. 2000;12:721–7.
87. Kuwata T, Wang IM, Tamura T, Ponnamperuma RM, Levine R, Holmes KL, Morse HC, De Luca LM, Ozato K. Vitamin A deficiency in mice causes a systemic expansion of myeloid cells. Blood. 2000;95:3349–56.
88. Zhao Z, Ross AC. Retinoic acid repletion restores the number of leukocytes and their subsets and stimulates natural cytotoxicity in vitamin A-deficient rats. J Nutr. 1995;125:2064–73.
89. Smeland EB, Rusten L, Jacobsen SE, Skrede B, Blomhoff R, Wang MY, Funderud S, Kvalheim G, Blomhoff HK. All-*trans* retinoic acid directly inhibits granulocyte colony-stimulating factor-induced proliferation of CD34+ human hematopoietic progenitor cells. Blood. 1994;84:2940–5.
90. Chen X, Welner RS, Kincade PW. A possible contribution of retinoids to regulation of fetal B lymphopoiesis. Eur J Immunol. 2009;39:2515–24.
91. Fahlman C, Jacobsen SE, Smeland EB, Lomo J, Naess CE, Funderud S, Blomhoff HK. All-*trans*- and 9-*cis*-retinoic acid inhibit growth of normal human and murine B cell precursors. J Immunol. 1995;155:58–65.
92. Chen X, Esplin BL, Garrett KP, Welner RS, Webb CF, Kincade PW. Retinoids accelerate B lineage lymphoid differentiation. J Immunol. 2008;180:138–45.
93. Sen J. Signal transduction in thymus development. Cell Mol Biol (Noisy-le-Grand). 2001;47:197–215.
94. Reifen R. Vitamin A as an anti-inflammatory agent. Proc Nutr Soc. 2002;61:397–400.
95. Semba RD. Vitamin A, immunity, and infection. Clin Infect Dis. 1994;19:489–99.
96. West Jr KP, Howard GR, Sommer A. Vitamin A and infection: public health implications. Annu Rev Nutr. 1989;9:63–86.
97. Makori N, Peterson PE, Lantz K, Hendrickx AG. Exposure of cynomolgus monkey embryos to retinoic acid causes thymic defects: effects on peripheral lymphoid organ development. J Med Primatol. 2002;31:91–7.
98. Kiss I, Ruhl R, Szegezdi E, Fritzsche B, Toth B, Pongracz J, Perlmann T, Fesus L, Szondy Z. Retinoid receptor-activating ligands are produced within the mouse thymus during postnatal development. Eur J Immunol. 2008;38:147–55.

99. Wang W, Ballow M. The effects of retinoic acid on *in vitro* immunoglobulin synthesis by cord blood and adult peripheral blood mononuclear cells. Cell Immunol. 1993;148:291–300.
100. Ballow M, Wang W, Xiang S. Modulation of B-cell immunoglobulin synthesis by retinoic acid. Clin Immunol Immunopathol. 1996;80:S73–81.
101. Ballow M, Xiang S, Wang W, Brodsky L. The effects of retinoic acid on immunoglobulin synthesis: role of interleukin 6. J Clin Immunol. 1996;16:171–9.
102. Garcia AL, Ruhl R, Herz U, Koebnick C, Schweigert FJ, Worm M. Retinoid- and carotenoid-enriched diets influence the ontogenesis of the immune system in mice. Immunology. 2003;110:180–7.
103. Guzman JJ, Caren LD. Effects of prenatal and postnatal exposure to vitamin A on the development of the murine immune system. Life Sci. 1991;49:1455–62.
104. Gossage C, Deyhim M, Moser-Veillon PB, Douglas LW, Kramer TR. Effect of beta-carotene supplementation and lactation on carotenoid metabolism and mitogenic T lymphocyte proliferation. Am J Clin Nutr. 2000;71:950–5.
105. Ruhl R, Hanel A, Garcia AL, Dahten A, Herz U, Schweigert FJ, Worm M. Role of vitamin A elimination or supplementation diets during postnatal development on the allergic sensitisation in mice. Mol Nutr Food Res. 2007;51:1173–81.
106. Lee CM, Boileau AC, Boileau TW, Williams AW, Swanson KS, Heintz KA, Erdman Jr JW. Review of animal models in carotenoid research. J Nutr. 1999;129:2271–7.
107. Kawashima T. A marine carotenoid, fucoxanthin, induces regulatory T cells and inhibits Th17 cell differentiation *in vitro*. Biosci Biotechnol Biochem. 2011;75:2066–9.
108. Garey LJ. Structural development of the visual system of man. Hum Neurobiol. 1984;3:75–80.
109. Packer O, Hartmann EE, Teller DY. Infant color vision: the effect of test field size on Rayleigh discriminations. Vision Res. 1984;24:1247–60.
110. Yuodelis C, Hendrickson A. A qualitative and quantitative analysis of the human fovea during development. Vision Res. 1986;26:847–55.
111. Bone RA, Landrum JT, Fernandez L, Tarsis SL. Analysis of the macular pigment by HPLC: retinal distribution and age study. Invest Ophthalmol Vis Sci. 1988;29:843–9.
112. Bone RA, Landrum JT, Friedes LM, Gomez CM, Kilburn MD, Menendez E, Vidal I, Wang W. Distribution of lutein and zeaxanthin stereoisomers in the human retina. Exp Eye Res. 1997;64:211–8.
113. Malinow MR, Feeney-Burns L, Peterson LH, Klein ML, Neuringer M. Diet-related macular anomalies in monkeys. Invest Ophthalmol Vis Sci. 1980;19:857–63.
114. Feeney-Burns L, Neuringer M, Gao CL. Macular pathology in monkeys fed semipurified diets. Prog Clin Biol Res. 1989;314:601–22.
115. Snodderly DM. Evidence for protection against age-related macular degeneration by carotenoids and antioxidant vitamins. Am J Clin Nutr. 1995;62:1448S–61.
116. Leung IY, Sandstrom MM, Zucker CL, Neuringer M, Snodderly DM. Nutritional manipulation of primate retinas, II: effects of age, n-3 fatty acids, lutein, and zeaxanthin on retinal pigment epithelium. Invest Ophthalmol Vis Sci. 2004;45:3244–56.
117. Bettler J, Zimmer JP, Neuringer M, DeRusso PA. Serum lutein concentrations in healthy term infants fed human milk or infant formula with lutein. Eur J Nutr. 2010;49:45–51.
118. Hardy P, Dumont I, Bhattacharya M, Hou X, Lachapelle P, Varma DR, Chemtob S. Oxidants, nitric oxide and prostanoids in the developing ocular vasculature: a basis for ischemic retinopathy. Cardiovasc Res. 2000;47:489–509.
119. Choi JS, Kim D, Hong YM, Mizuno S, Joo CK. Inhibition of nNOS and COX-2 expression by lutein in acute retinal ischemia. Nutrition. 2006;22:668–71.
120. Kowluru RA, Menon B, Gierhart DL. Beneficial effect of zeaxanthin on retinal metabolic abnormalities in diabetic rats. Invest Ophthalmol Vis Sci. 2008;49:1645–51.
121. Wing GL, Blanchard GC, Weiter JJ. The topography and age relationship of lipofuscin concentration in the retinal pigment epithelium. Invest Ophthalmol Vis Sci. 1978;17:601–7.
122. Feeney-Burns L, Hilderbrand ES, Eldridge S. Aging human RPE: morphometric analysis of macular, equatorial, and peripheral cells. Invest Ophthalmol Vis Sci. 1984;25:195–200.
123. Dillon J, Zheng L, Merriam JC, Gaillard ER. Transmission of light to the aging human retina: possible implications for age related macular degeneration. Exp Eye Res. 2004;79:753–9.
124. Hammond Jr BR, Wenzel AJ, Luther MS, Rivera RO, King SJ, Choate ML. Scotopic sensitivity: relation to age, dietary patterns, and smoking status. Optom Vis Sci. 1998;75:867–72.
125. Romagnoli C, Giannantonio C, Cota F, Papacci P, Vento G, Valente E, Purcaro V, Costa S. A prospective, randomized, double blind study comparing lutein to placebo for reducing occurrence and severity of retinopathy of prematurity. J Matern Fetal Neonatal Med. 2011;24 Suppl 1:147–50.
126. Dani C, Lori I, Favelli F, Frosini S, Messner H, Wanker P, De Marini S, Oretti C, Boldrini A, Massimiliano C, Bragetti P, Germini C. Lutein and zeaxanthin supplementation in preterm infants to prevent retinopathy of prematurity: a randomized controlled study. J Matern Fetal Neonatal Med. 2012;25(5):523–7.

Chapter 11
Provitamin A Carotenoids and Cancer Prevention

Benchun Miao and Xiang-Dong Wang

Key Points

- Clinical intervention trials conducted to determine the chemoprotective effect of large doses of β-carotene as a potential chemopreventive agent on the incidence of lung cancer in smokers found either no protective effect or a harmful effect. However, evidence for a protective role of whole fruits and vegetables rich in provitamin A carotenoids (β-carotene, α-carotene, and β-cryptoxanthin) in the prevention of certain cancers and other chronic diseases (e.g., atherosclerosis, diabetics, age-related macular degeneration, UV damage in skin) continues to be reported in human epidemiological studies and small intervention trials, as well as in mechanistic studies using cell culture and animal models.
- These findings have led to an increased effort to better understand the role of carotenoids and their derivatives in the process of these chronic diseases, with special attention to their metabolism and biological actions, dose effects, organ-specific effects, and the oxidative environment especially in smokers and alcohol drinkers.
- Greater knowledge has been gained in the biological effects of provitamin A carotenoid derivatives on the potential for beneficial effects of small quantities or harmful effects of large quantities of the resulting metabolic products. Provitamin A carotenoids may have certain unique beneficial effects against cancer risks.
- The molecular biological properties of provitamin A carotenoids, such as β-cryptoxanthin, and their metabolites remain to be determined through further more detailed research.

Keywords Provitamin A carotenoids • Metabolism • Molecular mechanisms • Cancer prevention

B. Miao, Ph.D. • X.-D. Wang, M.D., Ph.D. (✉)
Nutrition and Cancer Biology Laboratory, Jean Mayer USDA Human Nutrition Research Center on Aging at Tufts University, 711 Washington Street, Boston, MA 02111, USA
e-mail: xiang-dong.wang@tufts.edu

S.A. Tanumihardjo (ed.), *Carotenoids and Human Health*, Nutrition and Health,
DOI 10.1007/978-1-62703-203-2_11, © Springer Science+Business Media New York 2013

Introduction

More than 700 carotenoids have been identified but only 40–50 of them are present in the typical human diet and can be absorbed, metabolized, and utilized by the body [1]. All carotenoids possess a polyisoprenoid structure, a long conjugated chain of double bonds with a near bilateral symmetry around the central double bond [2]. The conjugated double bond makes carotenoids susceptible to oxidative cleavage and geometric (*trans/cis*) conversion. Some carotenoids such as α-carotene, β-carotene, and β-cryptoxanthin can be cleaved to form vitamin A; therefore, they are called provitamin A carotenoids (Fig. 11.1). Provitamin A carotenoids have at least one β-ionone ring. β-Carotene, a strongly colored red-orange pigment, is one of the most well-known and well-studied provitamin A carotenoids. Much research on carotenoids to date has concentrated on β-carotene. β-Cryptoxanthin is another provitamin A carotenoid which has drawn more attention of researchers in recent years. Some carotenoids such as lutein, zeaxanthin, and lycopene cannot form vitamin A, so they are called non-provitamin A carotenoids.

The richest dietary sources of β-carotene are yellow, orange, and leafy green fruits and vegetables, such as carrots, spinach, sweet potatoes, and cantaloupe. β-Cryptoxanthin is closely related to β-carotene in structure, with only the addition of a hydroxyl group. It is a member of the class of carotenoids known as xanthophylls. In a pure form, cryptoxanthin is a red crystalline solid with a metallic luster. β-Cryptoxanthin is mainly derived from orange fruits like tangerine and papaya. α-Carotene is a form of carotene with a β-ring at one end and an ε-ring at the other. It is the second most common form of carotene. The following vegetables are rich in α-carotene: carrots, sweet potatoes, pumpkin, winter squash, and broccoli.

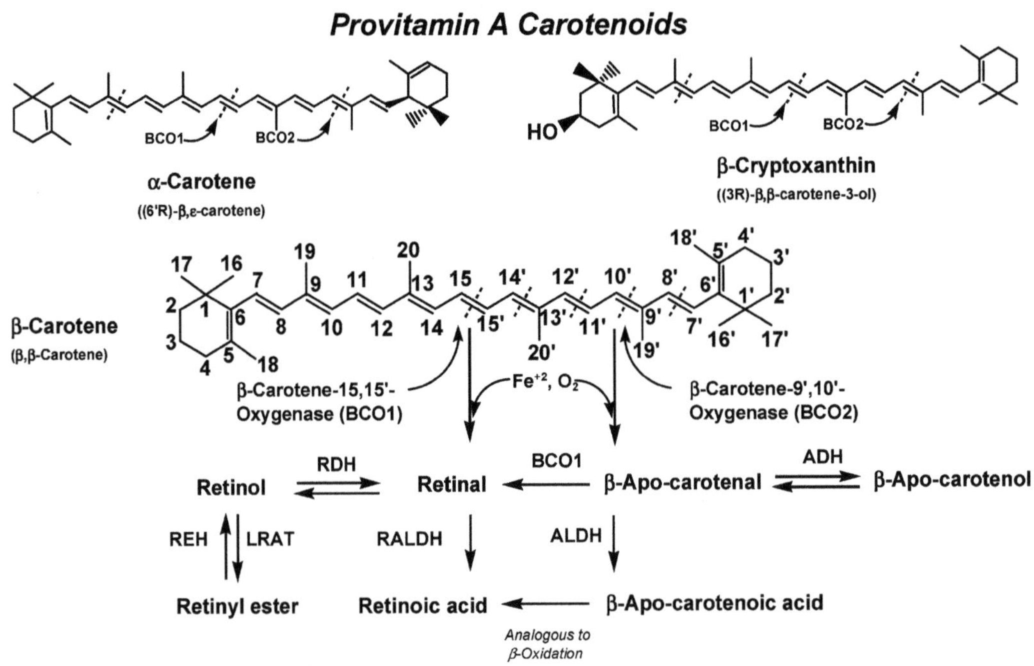

Fig. 11.1 Chemical structures of provitamin A carotenoids (β-carotene, α-carotene, and β-cryptoxanthin) and metabolic pathway of β-carotene. Figure adapted from Mernitz H, Wang XD. The bioconversion of carotenoids into retinoids: implications for cancer prevention. In: Vitamin A: New Research, editors, Loessing: KARGER press; 2007. p. 39–57

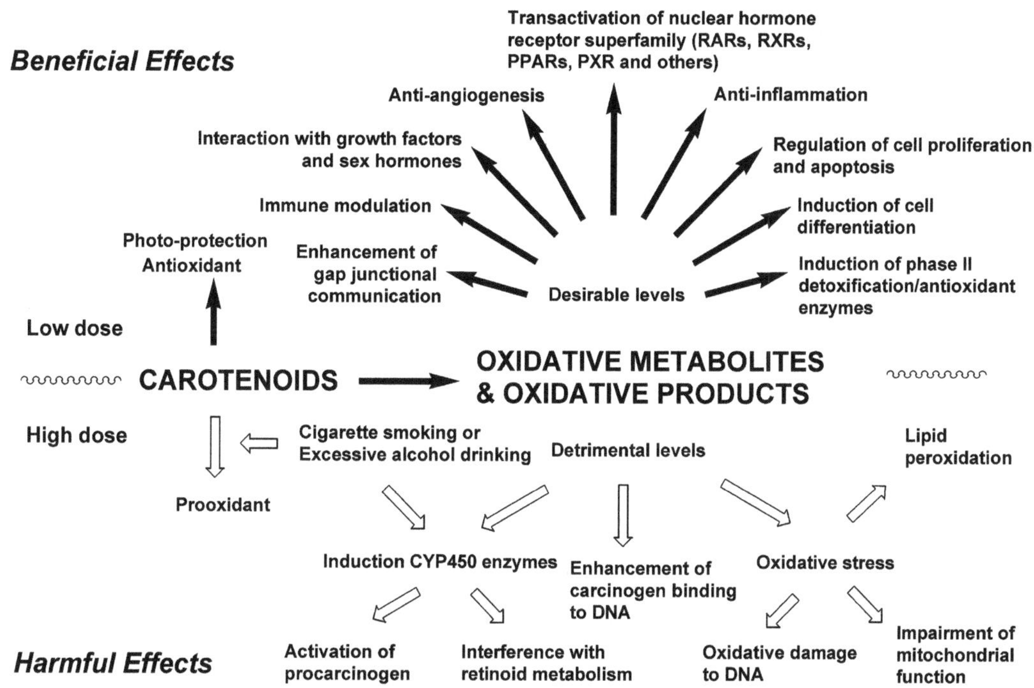

Fig. 11.2 Schematic illustration of beneficial and harmful effects of carotenoids on human health, including possible mechanisms related to carotenoid dose and oxidative metabolite formation. The biological activities of carotenoids could be related to the function of intact carotenoids or their metabolic products, which can possess either more or less activity than their parent compounds, or have entirely different functions. It appears that while small quantities of carotenoids can offer protection against certain cancers and chronic diseases related to free radical oxidation, larger amounts of carotenoid metabolites may actually be harmful, especially when coupled with a highly oxidative environment, such as the lungs of a cigarette smoker or liver of an excessive alcohol drinker. Oxidative destruction of β-carotene results in the formation of metabolites that may facilitate the carcinogenic process. Strong interactions among β-carotene, vitamin E, and vitamin C, and the capability of these compounds to "recycle" each other or antioxidant "network," regenerating efficient antioxidants from their radical cations, have led researchers to speculate about the potential utility of combined antioxidant therapy *in vivo*. It is possible that this additional protection against oxidative degradation may increase the utility of nutritional interventions targeting lung cancer in smoke-exposed models, surpassing effects seen in single-agent intervention studies. The combination of carotenoids and other antioxidants, such as vitamins E and C, which provide complementary or synergistic protective effects, would be a valuable strategy against cancer risk. Figure adapted from Wang XD. Carotenoid oxidative/degradative products and their biological activities. In: Krinsky NI, Mayne ST, Sies H, editors. Carotenoids in health and disease. New York: Marcel Dekker, Inc. press. 2004. p. 313–335

Epidemiological studies show that a high dietary intake of carotenoids may offer protective effects against the development of certain cancers [3]. However, other reports show that β-carotene alone or in combination with vitamin A could increase the risk of lung cancer in smokers [4, 5]. These observations have led to extensive research efforts to better understand the mechanisms involved in the action of carotenoids on carcinogenic processes. This chapter will focus on the roles of β-carotene specifically and other provitamin A carotenoids, especially β-cryptoxanthin, in cancer prevention as well as illustrate the potential mechanisms (Fig. 11.2).

Bioavailability and Metabolism of Provitamin A Carotenoids

The bioavailability of β-carotene from vegetables and fruits is generally not high [6] and is covered extensively in Section I of this book. The half-life of plasma carotenoids is 12 days and under for β-carotene, α-carotene, and β-cryptoxanthin. Food processing and cooking cause breakdown of the food matrix and release of embedded carotenoids increasing absorption and bioavailability [7, 8]. After release from the food matrix, ingested carotenoids must be emulsified and solubilized into micelles before they are absorbed into the intestinal mucosa. The efficiency of absorption of a moderate dose of β-carotene in oil is about 9–22%, so dietary fat promotes β-carotene absorption [9]. Both the cellular uptake and secretion of β-carotene are saturable, concentration-dependent processes. After β-carotene is taken up by the mucosa of the small intestine, it is either cleaved by β-carotene 15,15′-monooxygenase (CMO1 or BCO1) or β-carotene 9′,10′-monooxygenase (CMO2 or BCO1) into vitamin A and other metabolites, or packaged into chylomicrons and secreted into the lymphatic system for transport to the liver and other peripheral tissues.

The two metabolic pathways for β-carotene to convert to vitamin A include central and excentric cleavage (Fig. 11.1). For provitamin A carotenoids, central cleavage is the main pathway to form vitamin A. β-Carotene, α-carotene, and β-cryptoxanthin are cleaved symmetrically at their central double bond by CMO1. The excentric cleavage pathway [10, 11] was confirmed by the molecular identification of an excentric cleavage enzyme, CMO2, in mice, humans, zebrafish, and ferrets [12, 13]. CMO2 has been demonstrated to have the ability to catalyze the asymmetric cleavage of β-carotene to produce β-*apo*-10′-carotenal and β-ionone [12]. Although the contribution of CMO2 in vitamin A biosynthesis remains controversial, a quantitative trait locus associated with yellow adipose and milk color was identified to contain a premature stop codon mutation in the bovine CMO2 gene. This results in increased adipose, serum, and milk β-carotene concentrations and decreased liver retinol compared to wild types, yet no developmental or physiologic abnormalities in CMO2 mutants were observed [14]. β-*Apo*-carotenals can be cleaved further by CMO1 to produce retinol and retinoic acid [15], or oxidized to their corresponding *apo*-β-carotenoic acids. β-*Apo*-carotenoic acids may then undergo a process similar to β-oxidation of fatty acids, until further oxidation is blocked by the methyl group at the C13 position [16]. Recently, utilizing HPLC, LC-MS, and GC-MS, we have identified both volatile and non-volatile *apo*-carotenoid products including 3-OH-β-ionone, β-ionone, 3-OH-β-*apo*-10′-carotenal, and β-*apo*-10′-carotenal, indicating cleavage at both the 9,10 and 9′,10′ carbon–carbon double bond of β-cryptoxanthin [17]. Furthermore, in the presence of NAD^+, *in vitro* incubation of 3-OH-β-*apo*-10′-carotenal with ferret hepatic homogenates resulted in dose-dependent formation of 3-OH-β-*apo*-10′-carotenoic acid. Since *apo*-carotenoids serve as important signaling molecules in a variety of biological processes, enzymatic cleavage of β-cryptoxanthin by mammalian CMO2 represents a new avenue of research regarding vertebrate provitamin A carotenoid metabolism and biological function.

Biological Activity of β-Carotene on Cancer

Beneficial Effects and Potential Mechanisms

Regulation of Transcriptional Receptors

Provitamin A carotenoids can produce all-*trans*-retinoic acid and 9-*cis*-retinoic acid [18], the ligands for retinoic acid receptors (RARs) and retinoid X receptors (RXRs), respectively. β-Carotene and its oxidative metabolite, *apo*-14′-carotenoic acid, can reverse the downregulation of RARβ by smoke-borne carcinogens in normal bronchial epithelial cells [19], and the transactivation of the RARβ2 promoter induced by β-*apo*-14′-carotenoic acid is through its metabolism to all-*trans*-retinoic acid [19]. So the bioactivities of β-carotene may be mediated through transcriptional activation of a series of genes associated with antiproliferative or proapoptotic activities.

Antioxidant Function

In the early 1980s, two key publications [20, 21] revealed that β-carotene could be an antioxidant and anti-cancer agent. This greatly stimulated the field of carotenoid research. Cancer development has been linked to DNA damage, which could result from an increased level of oxidative stress. Provitamin A carotenoids are scavengers of singlet oxygen and other reactive oxygen species [22]. Therefore the antioxidant activities of provitamin A carotenoids may be one mechanism underlying their beneficial effects against carcinogenesis. β-Carotene is able to neutralize singlet oxygen ($^1O_2$) and interrupt lipid peroxidation chain reactions (see Chap. 4). Based on that activity, β-carotene can reduce the harmful effects of solar radiation on photosensitive individuals [23], decrease DNA oxidative damage in lymphocytes [24], and reduce the MDA level in human plasma [25]. In rats, β-carotene also exhibited antioxidant and anti-apoptotic properties to prevent ethanol-induced cytotoxicity in isolated hepatocytes by decreasing oxidative stress and inhibiting caspase-9 and caspase-3 expression [26].

β-Carotene and Antioxidant Combinations

The interactions among β-carotene, α-tocopherol (vitamin E), and ascorbic acid and the capability of these compounds to "recycle" each other, led researchers to characterize their combined antioxidant activities. α-Tocopherol enhances lymphatic transport of β-carotene and central cleavage of β-carotene to form vitamin A (rather than oxidative by-products) *in vivo* [27]. Further, α-tocopherol and ascorbic acid were able to decrease the production of undesirable oxidative metabolites and increase the formation of retinoids from β-carotene in lung tissues of smoke-exposed ferrets *in vitro* [28]. The formation of excentric cleavage products in ferret lung post-nuclear fractions after incubation with β-carotene was greatly increased while the formation of retinoic acid was decreased in animals that had been exposed to cigarette smoke. Retinoic acid reduction was reversed by addition of α-tocopherol or ascorbic acid both *in vitro* [29] and *in vivo* [30]. These studies suggest that α-tocopherol and ascorbic acid act synergistically to prevent the oxidative excentric cleavage of β-carotene induced by exposure to cigarette smoke and enhance vitamin A formation.

Combined antioxidant (i.e., β-carotene, α-tocopherol, and ascorbic acid) supplementation reversed smoke-induced changes of lung protein levels related to cellular proliferation and apoptosis [30, 31] and reversed the increased labeling of proliferating cellular nuclear antigen observed in smoke-exposed, carcinogen-injected ferrets. Supplementation also reversed smoke- and carcinogen-induced phosphorylation of mitogen-activated protein kinase (MAPK), c-jun N-terminal kinase (JNK), and extracellular signal-regulated kinase (ERK), which subsequently induced phosphorylation of p53 tumor suppressor protein and activated its downstream apoptotic protein Bax. In addition, the combined antioxidants also suppressed smoke-induced oxidative stress [31]. A human study showed that the beneficial effects of combined β-carotene, vitamin E, and selenium supplementation on mortality were still evident up to 10 years after the cessation of supplementation [32]. These data provide *in vivo* evidence of the utility of combined nutrients as a chemopreventive strategy to reduce the risk of lung cancer in smokers.

Inhibition of Proliferation and Induction of Apoptosis

β-Carotene was able to inhibit the activation of MAPK pathways, cell proliferation, and phosphorylation of p53 [31]. β-Carotene suppressed proliferation of some cancer cells, such as human squamous cells (SK-MES lung carcinoma or Scc-25 oral carcinoma) [33], and this inhibitory effect was accompanied by a rapid appearance of a unique 70 kDa protein, analogue to heat shock proteins. Moreover, β-carotene suppressed the growth of prostate tumor cells xenografted in nude mice [34]. β-Carotene inhibited cyclin D1-associated cdk4 kinase activity, along with a decrease in the levels of the hyperphosphorylated form of retinoblastoma protein in human fibroblasts [35], which may partially explain the inhibitory effect of β-carotene on cancer cell proliferation.

Genetic loss or functional aberration of cellular control mechanisms of apoptosis is considered to be a critical event in the initiation, promotion, or progression of cancer [36]. Apoptosis represents a protective mechanism against neoplastic transformation and development of tumors by eliminating genetically damaged cells or cells that may have been inappropriately induced to divide by mitogenic and proliferative stimuli. β-Carotene exhibits potential roles in the induction of apoptosis of human cervical cancer cells [37], colon adenocarcinoma [38, 39], gastric cancer cells [40], and leukemic cells [41]. One possible underlying mechanism for the proapoptotic effect of β-carotene could be its potential regulation on caspase cascade activation in tumor cells. For example, β-carotene induced apoptosis by the activation of caspase-8, caspase-9, and caspase-3 via cytochrome c release from mitochondria. Concomitantly, a dose-dependent decrease of B-cell lymphoma 2 and increase of BID protein cleavage were also observed [42].

Inhibition of Malignant Transformation

The potential tumor preventive effects of provitamin A carotenoids might associate with the inhibition of malignant transformation. For example, β-carotene can inhibit malignant transformation induced by 3-methylcholanthrene or X-ray treatment in a fibroblast cell line [43]. All-*trans*-β-carotene is consistently more active in suppressing neoplastic transformation in both murine and human keratinocytes as compared with 9-*cis*-β-carotene [44].

Harmful Effects and Potential Mechanisms

During 1994–1996, the human trials with β-carotene concluded no evidence of beneficial effect and actually showed an increased risk of lung cancer in heavy smokers and asbestos workers [4, 5, 18, 45]. These unexpected findings brought carotenoid researchers back to experimental research in animal and cell culture models in an attempt to find insight into this contradiction. The effects of dose responses, the antioxidant/pro-oxidant effect, and the coexistence of the central and excentric cleavage pathways reveal the complexity of carotenoid metabolism in organisms and raise questions regarding the potential effects of interaction between exogenous factors (e.g., tobacco smoking and chronic alcohol consumption) with carotenoids and their metabolites (Fig. 11.2) [46].

Dosage

Small quantities of β-carotene can offer protection against certain cancers related to free radical oxidation, while larger amounts might be harmful, especially when coupled with a highly oxidative environment. The dosages of β-carotene used in two human intervention studies mentioned above were 20–30 mg per day for 2–8 years. This is tenfold higher than the intake of β-carotene in the typical American diet (~2 mg per day) and resulted in accumulation of relatively high levels of β-carotene and its oxidative excentric cleavage metabolites in lung tissue. Research in animal and cell culture models suggest that β-carotene is unstable in the free radical-rich environment of lungs exposed to cigarette smoke, which will alter β-carotene metabolism to produce undesirable excentric cleavage metabolites (Fig. 11.2). These metabolites facilitate a number of changes associated with the carcinogenic process, including induction of carcinogen-activating enzymes, binding of carcinogen metabolites to DNA, interference with vitamin A metabolism, downregulation of tumor suppressor genes, upregulation of oncogenes, induction of oxidative stress, and enhanced induction of cell transformation by carcinogens [46]. Given that β-carotene in the diet is less bioavailable than supplemental β-carotene, no harmful effects have been associated with high levels of dietary β-carotene from natural food sources, aside from the occasional appearance of carotenodermia.

Pro-oxidant Effect

Some evidence indicates that carotenoids might behave as pro-oxidants in certain circumstances. At higher oxygen concentrations, carotenoid peroxy radicals such as Car-OO• or ROO-Car-OO• could be formed, which could act as pro-oxidants, promote hydrogen abstraction and oxidation of unsaturated lipids, and hence exacerbate membrane damage. β-Carotene at a concentration of 0.2 μM augmented UVA-induced heme oxygenase-1 expression [47]. In another study, β-carotene at a concentration of 10 μM increased the production of reactive oxygen species and the levels of cellular oxidized glutathione in leukemia and colon adenocarcinoma cell lines *in vitro* [48]. Lowe et al. demonstrated that β-carotene can protect HT29 cells against oxidative DNA damage at relatively low concentrations (1–3 μM), but lose this capacity at higher concentrations (4–10 μM) [49]. Based on the evidence obtained from the clinical trials of β-carotene supplementation in lung cancer, it appears that β-carotene may act as a protective antioxidant against cancer at physiological levels, but may lose its effectiveness or even exert pro-oxidant effects at pharmacological levels, especially in highly oxidative compartments of the body. The interactions among β-carotene, α-tocopherol, and ascorbic acid *in vitro* and their potential capability to transform each other, led researchers to their combination studies to eliminate potential pro-oxidant effects by a single agent. In animal studies, α-tocopherol and ascorbic acid decreased the production of undesirable oxidative metabolites and increased the formation of retinoids from β-carotene in lung tissue of smoke-exposed ferrets *in vitro* and *in vivo*.

Induction of Phase I Enzymes

In laboratory studies, tobacco smoking and chronic, excessive alcohol consumption, especially when coupled with a high dose of carotenoids, induced the expression of cytochrome P450 enzymes [29, 50]. These enzymes may activate procarcinogens present in alcoholic beverages, tobacco smoke, and diet, leading to increased formation of carcinogen-DNA adducts. If not repaired or repaired incorrectly, these adducts may eventually lead to mutations and ultimately cancer, especially, if the adducts are located in tumor suppressor genes. In addition, these same cytochrome P450 enzymes can break down retinoic acid and lead to significantly decreased tissue retinoic acid levels [29]. These studies provide possible mechanistic explanations for the discordance between the results of observational epidemiological studies and intervention trials using carotenoids as a potential beneficial agent.

Other Provitamin A Carotenoids and Their Cancer-Preventive Effects

β-Cryptoxanthin

Recently, several epidemiological studies have brought attention to β-cryptoxanthin for its potential benefits against lung cancer [51–53]. In two cohort studies involving Chinese populations, among all carotenoids examined, only serum levels of β-cryptoxanthin or the dietary intake of β-cryptoxanthin were significantly associated with a reduced risk of lung cancer [51, 52]. Similarly, in a pooled analysis of data from seven large cohorts in North America and Europe involving 3,155 incident cases of lung cancer, β-cryptoxanthin was the only dietary carotenoid significantly associated with a reduction of lung cancer risk (RR=0.76; 95% confidence interval, 0.67–0.86; highest versus lowest quintile) [53]. Data from our lab showed that β-cryptoxanthin inhibited the proliferation of premalignant human bronchial epithelial cells, which was associated with a decrease of cells in S phase, lowered protein levels of cyclin D and E, and increased levels of the cell cycle inhibitor p21, without inducing apoptosis [54]. β-Cryptoxanthin significantly increased RARβ mRNA in these cells. The effect of β-cryptoxanthin is, in part, due to the transactivation of RARs, supported by further observation that β-cryptoxanthin dramatically increased RARE-dependent promoter activity in cells co-transfected with RAR expression vector [54].

Recently, studies indicated that β-cryptoxanthin provides a beneficial effect against cigarette smoke-induced inflammation, oxidative DNA damage, and squamous metaplasia in the lungs of ferrets [55]. The effects of β-cryptoxanthin supplementation were evaluated on cigarette smoke-induced squamous metaplasia, inflammation, and changes in protein levels of pro-inflammatory cytokine tumor necrosis factor alpha (TNFα) and transcription factors nuclear factor kappa B (NF-κ B) and activator protein-1 (AP-1), as well as on smoke-induced oxidative DNA damage [8-hydroxy-2′-deoxyguanosine (8-OHdG)] in the lung tissue of ferrets. β-Cryptoxanthin supplementation dose-dependently increased plasma and lung β-cryptoxanthin levels. Both low-dose (7.5 μg/kg body weight per day) and high-dose (37.5 μg/kg body weight per day) β-cryptoxanthin lowered cigarette smoke-induced lung squamous metaplasia in ferrets. Lung squamous metaplastic lesions were observed in all ferrets in the smoke-exposed group, but only in two of the six ferrets in the low-dose β-cryptoxanthin group with smoke exposure and only in one of the six ferrets in the high-dose β-cryptoxanthin group with smoke exposure. No lung squamous metaplasia was found in the control group, the low-dose or high-dose β-cryptoxanthin alone groups. Cigarette smoke significantly increased inflammation in ferret lungs with the median grade of 3, and both low- and high-dose β-cryptoxanthin significantly lowered smoke-induced inflammation with the median grade of 2 (range: from 1 to 3). β-Cryptoxanthin substantially reduced smoke-elevated TNFα levels in alveolar, bronchial, bronchiolar, and bronchial serous/mucous gland epithelial cells and in lung macrophages. Moreover, β-cryptoxanthin decreased smoke-induced activation of NF-κB, expression of AP-1, c-Jun, and c-Fos, and levels of 8-OHdG in the same epithelial cells. The beneficial effects of β-cryptoxanthin were stronger by high-dose β-cryptoxanthin than those by low-dose β-cryptoxanthin [55].

Recent studies demonstrated that cancer-preventive effects of β-cryptoxanthin may depend on the enhancement of DNA repair as well as antioxidant protection against damage [56]. At low concentrations, close to those found in plasma, β-cryptoxanthin protects transformed human cells (HeLa and Caco-2) from damage induced by H_2O_2 or by visible light in the presence of a photosensitizer. In addition, it has a striking effect on two kinds of DNA repair—SB rejoining and excision repair of oxidized bases [56].

Several recent studies indicate that β-cryptoxanthin could suppress α7-nicotinic acetylcholine receptor (α7-nAChR) expression and its mediated PI3K signaling pathways in human immortalized lung cells and lung cancer cells [57]. The nicotinic acetylcholine receptors (nAChRs) were initially believed to exist only in the nervous system. However, emerging studies showed that nAChRs, their physiological agonist acetylcholine, and its synthesizing enzyme choline acetyltransferase are widely expressed in mammalian cells, including cancer cells [58–60]. Some tobacco components like nicotine and nicotine-derived nitrosamino ketone (NNK) are high-affinity nAChR agonists. The α7-nAChR is the main subunit of nAChRs in lung cancer cells, and numerous studies have reported that α7-nAChR plays critical roles in lung carcinogenesis and lung cancer development by regulation of multiple cellular signaling pathways [60, 61]. Nicotine and NNK can enhance lung cancer cell proliferation and motility through stimulation of α7-nAChR as well as upregulation of α7-nAChR expression [61, 62]. Therefore, α7-nAChR represents a valuable molecular target for prevention or therapy of tobacco-related lung cancers [60, 63]. The suppression of α7-nAChR expression and its downstream signaling, especially PI3K signaling pathways, by β-cryptoxanthin might provide mechanical explanation to the inhibitory effect of β-cryptoxanthin on lung cancer cell proliferation and survival *in vitro*, and the chemopreventive effects of β-cryptoxanthin among current smokers in human epidemiologic studies. Moreover, we found that β-cryptoxanthin is effective at inhibiting migration and invasion of α7-nAChR positive lung cancer cells by suppressing actin remodeling, ruffling/lamellipodia formation, but not in α7-nAChR negative cells. In addition, β-cryptoxanthin could suppress angiogenesis through inhibiting endothelial cell migration, invasion, tube formation, and microvessel outgrowth in aortic ring sprouting experiments. These results provided additional mechanical support for the anti-proliferation and anti-motility activities of β-cryptoxanthin.

α-Carotene

Several studies showed that α-carotene possesses higher activity than β-carotene to suppress tumorigenesis in skin, lung, liver, and colon [64, 65]. In the skin tumorigenesis experiment [64], the percentage of tumor-bearing mice in the control group was 69%, whereas the percentages of tumor-bearing mice in the groups treated with α- and β-carotene were 25% and 31%, respectively. The average number of tumors per mouse in the control group was 3.7, whereas the α-carotene-treated group had 0.3 tumors per mouse ($p<0.01$). β-Carotene treatment also decreased the average number of tumors per mouse (2.9 tumors per mouse), but the difference from the control group was not significant. The higher potency of α-carotene than β-carotene in the suppression of tumor promotion was further confirmed in this study. For example, in a 4-nitroquinoline 1-oxide (4NQO)-initiated and glycerol-promoted mouse lung carcinogenesis model, the average number of tumors per mouse in the control group was 4.1, whereas the α-carotene-treated group had 1.3 tumors per mouse ($p<0.001$). β-Carotene treatment did not show any suppressive effect on the average number of tumors per mouse, but rather induced a slight increase (4.9 tumors per mouse). In a liver carcinogenesis experiment [64], C3H/He mice, which have a high incidence of spontaneous liver tumor development, were treated for 40 weeks with α- and β-carotene with a 0.05% emulsion in drinking water or vehicle control. The mean number of hepatomas was significantly decreased by α-carotene treatment as compared with that in the control group; the control group developed 6.3 tumors per mouse, whereas the α-carotene-treated group had 3.0 tumors per mouse ($p<0.001$). On the other hand, the β-carotene-treated group only showed a tendency toward a decrease of tumors, as compared with the control group [64].

Conclusion and Future Directions

Many epidemiological studies show the benefit of provitamin A carotenoid-rich fruits and vegetables on the risk of chronic diseases; however, clinical supplementation trials have returned null findings or evidence of harm in certain populations. Based on these results, high-dose carotenoid supplementation is not recommended for the general population, and smokers and consumers of alcohol are warned to avoid high-dose carotenoid supplements. However, the metabolism and molecular biological properties of many carotenoids remain to be determined through further research. Recent studies indicated that provitamin A carotenoids other than β-carotene may be active in several important cellular signaling pathways in lung carcinogenesis, and excentric cleavage carotenoid metabolites could have greater biological roles than their parent compounds in several molecular targets. In particular, studies from seven large well-implemented cohort studies consistently show that among all of the specific carotenoids examined, increased dietary intake or elevated blood levels of β-cryptoxanthin is strongly associated with a reduced risk of lung cancer. The experimental evidence shows that β-cryptoxanthin inhibits the growth of both premalignant and malignant lung cell lines, and decreased dose-dependently the tobacco smoke-induced lung inflammation, TNFα levels, and squamous metaplasia in animal studies. These studies indicate that each of the provitamin A carotenoids has certain unique beneficial effects against cancer risks. In particular, whether there are great differences between β-carotene and β-cryptoxanthin in their biological activities and whether β-cryptoxanthin is a potentially effective chemopreventive agent against the development of lung cancer need further studies.

References

1. Rao AV, Rao LG. Carotenoids and human health. Pharmacol Res. 2007;55:207–16.
2. Britton G. Structure and properties of carotenoids in relation to function. FASEBJ. 1995;9:1551–8.
3. van Poppel G, Goldbohm RA. Epidemiologic evidence for beta-carotene and cancer prevention. Am J Clin Nutr. 1995;62:1393S–402.
4. Albanes D, Heinonen OP, Taylor PR, et al. Alpha-tocopherol and beta-carotene supplements and lung cancer incidence in the alpha-tocopherol, beta-carotene cancer prevention study: effects of base-line characteristics and study compliance. J Natl Cancer Inst. 1996;88:1560–70.
5. Omenn GS, Goodman GE, Thornquist MD, et al. Effects of a combination of beta carotene and vitamin A on lung cancer and cardiovascular disease. N Engl J Med. 1996;334:1150–5.
6. Castenmiller JJ, Lauridsen ST, Dragsted LO, et al. beta-Carotene does not change markers of enzymatic and nonenzymatic antioxidant activity in human blood. J Nutr. 1999;129:2162–9.
7. Parker RS. Absorption, metabolism, and transport of carotenoids. FASEB J. 1996;10:542–51.
8. Parker RS. Bioavailability of carotenoids. Eur J Clin Nutr. 1997;51 Suppl 1:S86–90.
9. Wang XD. Review: absorption and metabolism of beta-carotene. J Am Coll Nutr. 1994;13:314–25.
10. Wang XD, Tang GW, Fox JG, et al. Enzymatic conversion of beta-carotene into beta-*apo*-carotenals and retinoids by human, monkey, ferret, and rat tissues. Arch Biochem Biophys. 1991;285:8–16.
11. Wang XD, Krinsky NI, Tang GW, et al. Retinoic acid can be produced from excentric cleavage of beta-carotene in human intestinal mucosa. Arch Biochem Biophys. 1992;293:298–304.
12. Kiefer C, Hessel S, Lampert JM, et al. Identification and characterization of a mammalian enzyme catalyzing the asymmetric oxidative cleavage of provitamin A. J Biol Chem. 2001;276:14110–6.
13. Hu KQ, Liu C, Ernst H, et al. The biochemical characterization of ferret carotene-9′,10′-monooxygenase catalyzing cleavage of carotenoids *in vitro* and *in vivo*. J Biol Chem. 2006;281:19327–38.
14. Hessel S, Eichinger A, Isken A, et al. CMO1 deficiency abolishes vitamin A production from beta-carotene and alters lipid metabolism in mice. J Biol Chem. 2007;282:33553–61.
15. Lakshmanan MR, Pope JL, Olson JA. The specificity of a partially purified carotenoid cleavage enzyme of rabbit intestine. Biochem Biophys Res Commun. 1968;33:347–52.
16. Wang XD, Russell RM, Liu C, et al. Beta-oxidation in rabbit liver *in vitro* and in the perfused ferret liver contributes to retinoic acid biosynthesis from beta-apocarotenoic acids. J Biol Chem. 1996;271:26490–8.

17. Mein JR, Dolnikowski GG, Ernst H, et al. Enzymatic formation of *apo*-carotenoids from the xanthophyll carotenoids lutein, zeaxanthin and beta-cryptoxanthin by ferret carotene-9′,10′-monooxygenase. Arch Biochem Biophys. 2011;506:109–21.
18. Lee IM, Cook NR, Manson JE, et al. Beta-carotene supplementation and incidence of cancer and cardiovascular disease: the Women's Health Study. J Natl Cancer Inst. 1999;91:2102–6.
19. Prakash P, Liu C, Hu KQ, et al. Beta-carotene and beta-*apo*-14′-carotenoic acid prevent the reduction of retinoic acid receptor beta in benzo[a]pyrene-treated normal human bronchial epithelial cells. J Nutr. 2004;134:667–73.
20. Peto R, Doll R, Buckley JD, et al. Can dietary beta-carotene materially reduce human cancer rates? Nature. 1981;290:201–8.
21. Burton GW, Ingold KU. beta-Carotene: an unusual type of lipid antioxidant. Science. 1984;224:569–73.
22. Krinsky NI. The antioxidant and biological properties of the carotenoids. Ann N Y Acad Sci. 1998;854:443–7.
23. Krinsky NI. Effects of carotenoids in cellular and animal systems. Am J Clin Nutr. 1991;53:238S–46.
24. Fabiani R, De Bartolomeo A, Rosignoli P, et al. Antioxidants prevent the lymphocyte DNA damage induced by PMA-stimulated monocytes. Nutr Cancer. 2001;39:284–91.
25. Meraji S, Ziouzenkova O, Resch U, et al. Enhanced plasma level of lipid peroxidation in Iranians could be improved by antioxidants supplementation. Eur J Clin Nutr. 1997;51:318–25.
26. Peng HC, Chen JR, Chen YL, et al. beta-Carotene exhibits antioxidant and anti-apoptotic properties to prevent ethanol-induced cytotoxicity in isolated rat hepatocytes. Phytother Res. 2010;24 Suppl 2:S183–9.
27. Wang XD, Marini RP, Hebuterne X, et al. Vitamin E enhances the lymphatic transport of beta-carotene and its conversion to vitamin A in the ferret. Gastroenterology. 1995;108:719–26.
28. Liu C, Lian F, Smith DE, et al. Lycopene supplementation inhibits lung squamous metaplasia and induces apoptosis via up-regulating insulin-like growth factor-binding protein 3 in cigarette smoke-exposed ferrets. Cancer Res. 2003;63:3138–44.
29. Liu C, Russell RM, Wang XD. Exposing ferrets to cigarette smoke and a pharmacological dose of beta-carotene supplementation enhance *in vitro* retinoic acid catabolism in lungs via induction of cytochrome P450 enzymes. J Nutr. 2003;133:173–9.
30. Kim Y, Chongviriyaphan N, Liu C, et al. Combined antioxidant (beta-carotene, alpha-tocopherol and ascorbic acid) supplementation increases the levels of lung retinoic acid and inhibits the activation of mitogen-activated protein kinase in the ferret lung cancer model. Carcinogenesis. 2006;27:1410–9.
31. Kim Y, Lian F, Yeum KJ, et al. The effects of combined antioxidant (beta-carotene, alpha-tocopherol and ascorbic acid) supplementation on antioxidant capacity, DNA single-strand breaks and levels of insulin-like growth factor-1/IGF-binding protein 3 in the ferret model of lung cancer. Int J Cancer. 2007;120:1847–54.
32. Qiao YL, Dawsey SM, Kamangar F, et al. Total and cancer mortality after supplementation with vitamins and minerals: follow-up of the Linxian General Population Nutrition Intervention Trial. J Natl Cancer Inst. 2009;101:507–18.
33. Schwartz JL, Singh RP, Teicher B, et al. Induction of a 70 kD protein associated with the selective cytotoxicity of beta-carotene in human epidermal carcinoma. Biochem Biophys Res Commun. 1990;169:941–6.
34. Yang CM, Yen YT, Huang CS, et al. Growth inhibitory efficacy of lycopene and beta-carotene against androgen-independent prostate tumor cells xenografted in nude mice. Mol Nutr Food Res. 2011;55:606–12.
35. Stivala LA, Savio M, Quarta S, et al. The antiproliferative effect of beta-carotene requires p21waf1/cip1 in normal human fibroblasts. Eur J Biochem. 2000;267:2290–6.
36. Thompson CB. Apoptosis in the pathogenesis and treatment of disease. Science. 1995;267:1456 62.
37. Muto Y, Fujii J, Shidoji Y, et al. Growth retardation in human cervical dysplasia-derived cell lines by beta-carotene through down-regulation of epidermal growth factor receptor. Am J Clin Nutr. 1995;62:1535S–40.
38. Palozza P, Calviello G, Serini S, et al. beta-Carotene at high concentrations induces apoptosis by enhancing oxy-radical production in human adenocarcinoma cells. Free Radic Biol Med. 2001;30:1000–7.
39. Palozza P, Serini S, Maggiano N, et al. Induction of cell cycle arrest and apoptosis in human colon adenocarcinoma cell lines by beta-carotene through down-regulation of cyclin A and Bcl-2 family proteins. Carcinogenesis. 2002;23:11–8.
40. Jang SH, Lim JW, Kim H. Mechanism of beta-carotene-induced apoptosis of gastric cancer cells: involvement of ataxia-telangiectasia-mutated. Ann N Y Acad Sci. 2009;1171:156–62.
41. Palozza P, Serini S, Torsello A, et al. Regulation of cell cycle progression and apoptosis by beta-carotene in undifferentiated and differentiated HL-60 leukemia cells: possible involvement of a redox mechanism. Int J Cancer. 2002;97:593–600.
42. Palozza P, Serini S, Torsello A, et al. Mechanism of activation of caspase cascade during beta-carotene-induced apoptosis in human tumor cells. Nutr Cancer. 2003;47:76–87.
43. Merriman RL, Bertram JS. Reversible inhibition by retinoids of 3-methylcholanthrene-induced neoplastic transformation in C3H/10T1/2 clone 8 cells. Cancer Res. 1979;39:1661–6.
44. Hieber AD, King TJ, Morioka S, et al. Comparative effects of all-*trans* β-carotene vs. 9-*cis* beta-carotene on carcinogen-induced neoplastic transformation and connexin 43 expression in murine 10T1/2 cells and on the differentiation of human keratinocytes. Nutr Cancer. 2000;37:234–44.

45. Hennekens CH, Buring JE, Manson JE, et al. Lack of effect of long-term supplementation with beta carotene on the incidence of malignant neoplasms and cardiovascular disease. N Engl J Med. 1996;334:1145–9.
46. Wang XD. Carotenoid oxidative/degradative products and their biological activities. In: Krinsky NI, Mayne ST, Sies H, editors. Carotenoids in health and disease. New York: Marcel Dekker; 2004. p. 313–35.
47. Obermuller-Jevic UC, Francz PI, Frank J, et al. Enhancement of the UVA induction of haem oxygenase-1 expression by beta-carotene in human skin fibroblasts. FEBS Lett. 1999;460:212–6.
48. Palozza P, Serini S, Torsello A, et al. Beta-carotene regulates NF-kappaB DNA-binding activity by a redox mechanism in human leukemia and colon adenocarcinoma cells. J Nutr. 2003;133:381–8.
49. Lowe GM, Booth LA, Young AJ, et al. Lycopene and beta-carotene protect against oxidative damage in HT29 cells at low concentrations but rapidly lose this capacity at higher doses. Free Radic Res. 1999;30:141–51.
50. Veeramachaneni S, Ausman LM, Choi SW, et al. High dose lycopene supplementation increases hepatic cytochrome P4502E1 protein and inflammation in alcohol-fed rats. J Nutr. 2008;138:1329–35.
51. Yuan JM, Ross RK, Chu XD, et al. Prediagnostic levels of serum beta-cryptoxanthin and retinol predict smoking-related lung cancer risk in Shanghai, China. Cancer Epidemiol Biomarkers Prev. 2001;10:767–73.
52. Yuan JM, Stram DO, Arakawa K, et al. Dietary cryptoxanthin and reduced risk of lung cancer: the Singapore Chinese Health Study. Cancer Epidemiol Biomarkers Prev. 2003;12:890–8.
53. Mannisto S, Smith-Warner SA, Spiegelman D, et al. Dietary carotenoids and risk of lung cancer in a pooled analysis of seven cohort studies. Cancer Epidemiol Biomarkers Prev. 2004;13:40–8.
54. Lian F, Hu KQ, Russell RM, et al. Beta-cryptoxanthin suppresses the growth of immortalized human bronchial epithelial cells and non-small-cell lung cancer cells and up-regulates retinoic acid receptor beta expression. Int J Cancer. 2006;119:2084–9.
55. Liu C, Bronson RT, Russell RM, et al. Beta-cryptoxanthin supplementation prevents cigarette smoke-induced lung inflammation, oxidative damage and squamous metaplasia in ferrets. Cancer Prev Res (Phila). 2011;4(8): 1255–66.
56. Lorenzo Y, Azqueta A, Luna L, et al. The carotenoid beta-cryptoxanthin stimulates the repair of DNA oxidation damage in addition to acting as an antioxidant in human cells. Carcinogenesis. 2009;30:308–14.
57. Miao B, Iskandar A, Wang XD. Beta-cryptoxanthin inhibits phosphoinositide 3-kinase (PI3K) signaling and lung cancer cell motility. Submitted to Cancer Prev Res (the abstract was presented on AACR annual meeting 2011).
58. Schuller HM. Is cancer triggered by altered signalling of nicotinic acetylcholine receptors? Nat Rev Cancer. 2009;9:195–205.
59. Wessler I, Kirkpatrick CJ. Acetylcholine beyond neurons: the non-neuronal cholinergic system in humans. Br J Pharmacol. 2008;154:1558–71.
60. Egleton RD, Brown KC, Dasgupta P. Nicotinic acetylcholine receptors in cancer: multiple roles in proliferation and inhibition of apoptosis. Trends Pharmacol Sci. 2008;29:151–8.
61. Plummer III HK, Dhar M, Schuller HM. Expression of the alpha7 nicotinic acetylcholine receptor in human lung cells. Respir Res. 2005;6:29.
62. Catassi A, Servent D, Paleari L, et al. Multiple roles of nicotine on cell proliferation and inhibition of apoptosis: implications on lung carcinogenesis. Mutat Res. 2008;659:221–31.
63. Trombino S, Cesario A, Margaritora S, et al. Alpha7-nicotinic acetylcholine receptors affect growth regulation of human mesothelioma cells: role of mitogen-activated protein kinase pathway. Cancer Res. 2004;64:135–45.
64. Murakoshi M, Nishino H, Satomi Y, et al. Potent preventive action of alpha-carotene against carcinogenesis: spontaneous liver carcinogenesis and promoting stage of lung and skin carcinogenesis in mice are suppressed more effectively by alpha-carotene than by beta-carotene. Cancer Res. 1992;52:6583–7.
65. Narisawa T, Fukaura Y, Hasebe M, et al. Inhibitory effects of natural carotenoids, alpha-carotene, beta-carotene, lycopene and lutein, on colonic aberrant crypt foci formation in rats. Cancer Lett. 1996;107:137–42.

Chapter 12
Lycopene and Cancer

Nikki Ford and John W. Erdman Jr.

Key Points

- Epidemiological and human clinical trials suggest that dietary intake of tomatoes or lycopene protects against cancers of the prostate, breast, cervix, ovary, endometrium, lung, bladder, oral cavity, esophagus, stomach, colon, and pancreas.
- Tomatoes contain numerous bioactives that may work additively or synergistically to reduce cancer risk.
- The effects of lycopene cannot easily be distinguished from the effects of tomato products on cancer risk in epidemiological or human clinical trials.
- Lycopene or tomato intake may reduce cancer risk through modulation of growth factors, increased apoptosis and cell–cell communication, and reduction in cell proliferation, angiogenesis, and cell migration.
- More than ten independent epidemiological or clinical studies have examined the chemopreventative effects of lycopene on cancers of the prostate, breast, lung, and stomach.

Keywords Cancer • Lycopene • Tomato • Carotenoid • Growth factor • Apoptosis • Proliferation • Angiogenesis

Introduction

The red pigment lycopene is the most abundant carotenoid in tomatoes. Lycopene can also be found in lesser amounts in guava, pink grapefruit, papaya, and watermelon. Upon consumption, lycopene accumulates predominantly in the liver, adrenals, testes, and prostate [1]. Comprised of 40 carbons, lycopene is an acyclic, open chain polyisoprenoid carotenoid with 11 conjugated double bonds [2].

N. Ford, Ph.D. (✉)
Department of Nutritional Sciences, University of Texas at Austin,
1400 Barbara Jordan Blvd, Austin, TX 73723, USA
e-mail: nikkiannford@gmail.com

J.W. Erdman Jr., Ph.D.
Department of Nutritional Sciences, University of Illinois at Urbana-Champaign,
905 Goodwin Ave, 455 Bevier Hall, Urbana, IL 61801, USA

S.A. Tanumihardjo (ed.), *Carotenoids and Human Health*, Nutrition and Health,
DOI 10.1007/978-1-62703-203-2_12, © Springer Science+Business Media New York 2013

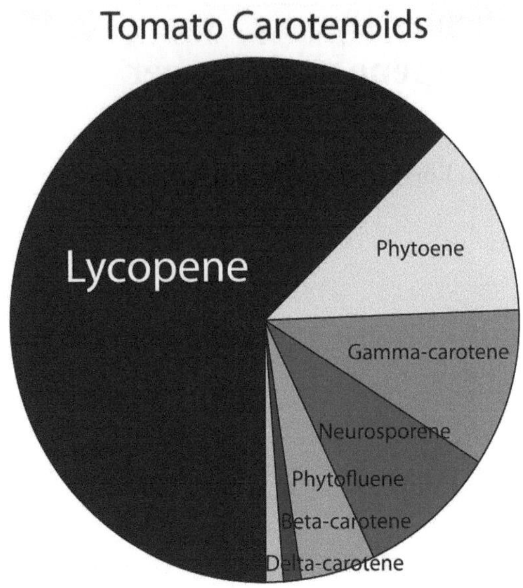

Fig. 12.1 Tomato carotenoid content (modified from previous publication [78])

Two primary forms of lycopene exist: the linear all-*trans* form and a variety of chain kinked *cis*-isomer forms. All-*trans* lycopene is the predominant isomer found in plants, but *cis* isomers are the form most commonly found in human tissues suggesting preferential absorption of *cis* isomers [3].

Tomatoes also contain a variety of carotenoids in addition to lycopene. While lycopene comprises approximately 60% of the total carotenoids found in red tomato products; phytoene, phytofluene, neurosporene, and γ-carotene are the next most abundant carotenoids (Fig. 12.1). The concentration of lycopene in tomatoes or tomato products also varies widely depending upon variety, ripeness of the fruit, and processing methods [4].

Dietary intake of tomatoes is inversely associated with numerous chronic diseases including cardiovascular disease and cancer. Both diseases share some common attributes including increased inflammation and oxidation and altered metabolism. Most research has been dedicated to investigating the effects of only lycopene on chronic disease risk. This review will focus on cancer risk and also will suggest that lycopene may not be wholly responsible for the anti-carcinogenic properties of tomato products.

Lycopene Modulates Cancer Pathways

Cells must be self-sufficient and versatile to withstand endogenous and exogenous stresses. The body comprises many autonomous controls to replace cells damaged by typical human exposures such as UV light, toxins, and stomach acid. These controls place each cell at risk for corruption of pathways which inevitably can lead to carcinogenesis. Mutations in DNA, genes, or cellular pathways can modify growth and differentiation, recruitment of nutrients, and migration or metastasis of cells. Lycopene has been reported to modulate many of these pathways resulting in reduced cellular carcinogenic properties (Fig. 12.2).

Balancing oxidants and antioxidants within the cellular environment is essential for optimal cell health. While necessary for energy production, cellular metabolism also produces reactive oxygen species (ROS) and reactive nitrogen species (RNS) that can damage lipids, proteins, and DNA. In properly maintained systems, our bodies counteract excess ROS or RNS through an antioxidant network thereby

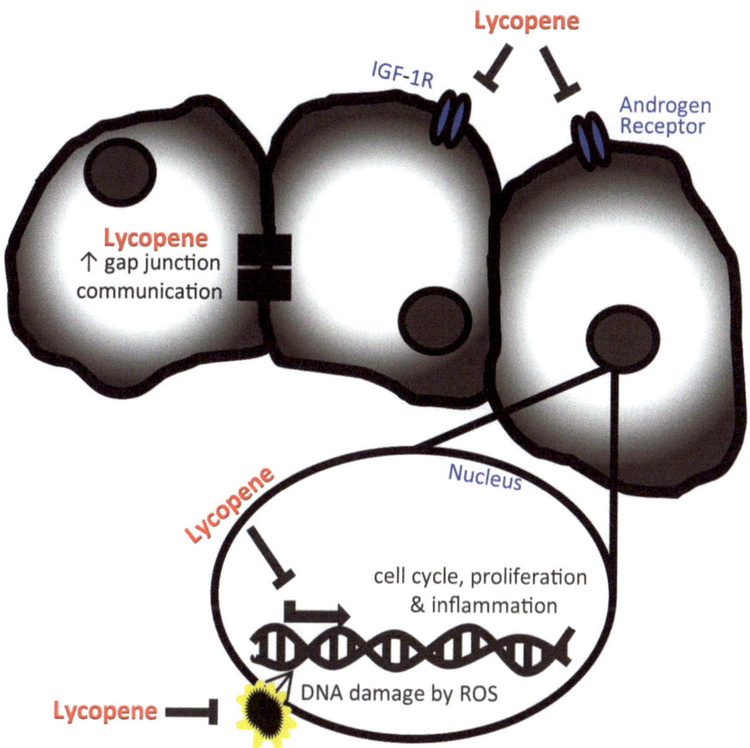

Fig. 12.2 Lycopene alters cancer pathways (for review see [6]). *Abbreviations*: *IGF-1R* insulin-like growth factor 1 receptor, *ROS* radical oxygen species

protecting us from an imbalance of excess oxidants. Early studies suggested that the antioxidant effect of lycopene may reduce chronic diseases such as cancer. *In vitro*, lycopene is the most proficient carotenoid singlet oxygen quencher in nature [5]. However, it is questionable whether lycopene is an important *in vivo* antioxidant because this fat-soluble compound circulates in the body in very low concentrations compared to other antioxidants, such as vitamin E [6]. Additionally, due to the physical nature of the molecule, lycopene may not be able to access the sites of highest ROS production. Lastly, little *in vivo* evidence supports the idea that lycopene works primarily through an antioxidant mechanism [6]. So, although lycopene is a potent antioxidant, it is unlikely that lycopene reduces cancer risk through a direct antioxidant mechanism.

Growth factors are key regulators of cell growth. Through target-specific receptors, cells receive extracellular signals such as hormones and cytokines which regulate their growth or differentiation. Studies demonstrate that lycopene plays a role in controlling proliferation pathways. Numerous studies suggest that lycopene decreases cell proliferation [7]. More specifically, animal and clinical studies show that lycopene inhibits the expression of insulin-like growth factor (IGF-1) or its receptor or increases IGF-1 binding proteins [8–13]. IGF-1 mimics many of the physiological traits of insulin to regulate growth and metabolism. Epidemiological studies indicate that circulating IGF-1 is related to increased risk for several types of cancers [14]. Lycopene also positively modulates inflammatory cytokine-driven pathways [12, 15–18], although lycopene may not be able to overcome the effects of certain stressors, such as obesity [19].

Some cancers strongly depend on sex steroids to promote growth and differentiation. For example, circulating androgens are tightly correlated with prostate cancer risk. Lycopene reduces testosterone, regulates androgen metabolizing pathways [8, 20], reduces serum estrogen and estrogenic activity [21–23]. Circulating estrogens are positively correlated with breast and other female reproductive cancers [24].

Another hallmark of cancer is the loss of intracellular signaling between cells. Cell growth is balanced through cell–cell communication through an intracellular exchange of small circulating signaling molecules. On the cell wall, gap junction proteins form channels between neighboring cells within a tissue. Some evidence suggests that lycopene enhances the expression of these gap junction proteins [25, 26], although we recently report no effect in a rodent model and *in vitro* [7]. Proper cell–cell communication allows cells to sense neighboring cells and possibly prevent uncontrolled cellular growth.

Cancer prevention therapies often target two common mechanisms, the normal cell cycle and apoptosis. Evidence suggests that lycopene may regulate cell growth by direct control of the cell cycle [27, 28]. By controlling a cell's progression through the cell cycle, lycopene can inhibit cell division and replication. To avoid replication of damaged cells which could promote carcinogenesis, the cells induce apoptosis which is a process whereby a cell undergoes morphological changes resulting in controlled cell death. This process allows for macrophages and other surrounding cells to remove cell debris without damaging neighboring tissues. Studies in humans and animals suggest that lycopene induces apoptosis [9, 28–36]. By inducing apoptosis in tissues, lycopene may modify risk for cancer by removing damaged cells from the DNA pool.

An essential component of tumor growth is recruitment and development of capillary networks to provide energy to the tumor cells. In 2008, Huang first reported that lycopene supplementation significantly reduced the expression of a key protein (VEGF) in angiogenesis [37]. Since that time, two more studies demonstrated that lycopene inhibits angiogenesis [38, 39]. A small body of evidence suggests that lycopene reduces cancer progression by limiting nutrient delivery through increased tumor capillary networks. In contrast, lycopene supplementation increased VEGF expression in mice that were exposed to smoke [40]. Again, this study suggests that the beneficial effects of lycopene may not overcome certain environmental or physiological stressors.

Primary tumors can metastasize to form proliferating colonies in distal tissues. Treatment is often more difficult after tumor metastasis and therefore preventing migration of tumor cells through the body improves an individual's cancer treatment success. In separate studies, lycopene treatment significantly reduced cell migration in hepatoma cells, hepatocarcinoma cells, and fibroblasts [41–44]. Future epidemiological studies of secondary tumor incidence in relation to lycopene intake could better identify whether reduced *in vitro* cell migration translates to fewer metastases of human cancers.

Cancers

Prostate Cancer

As a component of the male reproductive system, the prostate is a small walnut-shaped gland responsible for producing some of the fluid components of sperm. According to the National Cancer Institute, more than 215,000 new cases of prostate cancer were diagnosed and 32,050 men died from the disease in 2010 in the USA [45]. Prostate cancer typically occurs in older men and afflicts African-American men more than men of other races [45].

As men age, the prostate often swells to constrict the urethra. Although the swelling, also known as benign prostatic hyperplasia (BPH), is not cancerous it can cause inflammation that may promote prostate cancer if left untreated [46]. Prostate cancer is usually diagnosed by a digital rectal exam or by changes in blood prostate specific antigen (PSA) over time.

Surgery, radiation therapy, and active surveillance are the most common prostate cancer therapeutics. Active surveillance is defined as close monitoring to identify changes or growth of the cancer. Nutritionists have used the period of active surveillance to investigate the effects of dietary modifications on cancer progression. Additionally, there is generally a small window of time before clinical treatment (elective prostate removal), which provides nutritionists the opportunity to further investigate dietary modulations on prostate cancer progression.

A small clinical trial by Kucuk and colleagues opted to give men with newly diagnosed, but clinically localized, prostate cancer either a 15 mg lycopene supplement twice daily or no supplement for 3 weeks prior to prostatectomy [47]. The lycopene treatment significantly reduced the aggressiveness of the cancer as determined by reduced involvement of surgical margins and reduction in the areas determined to be high grade prostatic intraepithelial neoplasia (PIN). The lycopene treatment also reduced the inflammatory marker, IGF-1, which has been linked to prostate cancer incidence. Not only has lycopene shown promising results to reduce the progression of prostate cancer but also large epidemiological studies suggest that consumption of tomatoes, or blood lycopene levels, is inversely associated with prostate cancer incidence. A study published from the Harvard School of Public Health first drew attention to this relationship [48]. Using data from the Health Professionals Follow-up Study in 1986, Giovannucci and colleagues report that of the 46 vegetables and fruits investigated, only four were significantly associated with a reduced risk of prostate cancer: tomato sauce, tomatoes, pizza, and strawberries. Three of those foods (not strawberries) contain lycopene. The risk of prostate cancer was reduced by 21% on average in men with high intakes of lycopene-containing foods compared to low consumers of lycopene. Twenty-six clinical or epidemiological studies have investigated the relationship between tomato or lycopene intake and prostate cancer risk. No studies report an increased risk with consumption, but ten studies suggest a protective effect. A meta-analysis [49] analyzing published studies up to 2003 reported a 10–20% reduction in prostate cancer risk with high tomato or lycopene intake. In conclusion, a large body of human data suggests that tomatoes or lycopene-containing foods reduce prostate cancer risk.

Breast Cancer

Almost 210,000 new cases of breast cancer with nearly 40,000 deaths occurred in the USA in 2010 [45]. Breast cancer normally develops in the ducts and lobules in breast tissue of both men and women, although male breast cancer is uncommon. Primary breast tumors are detected using mammography or magnetic resonance imagining (MRI). If a tumor is detected, further diagnosis is required because there are currently five recognized subtypes of breast cancer with different molecular profiles that differentiate treatment. Common therapies include mastectomy, hormone therapy, radiation therapy, and chemotherapy. Prevention of breast cancer by tomatoes or lycopene was investigated in 24 studies; 18 found no effect and 6 reported a protective effect of lycopene or tomato dietary intake (see Table 12.1 for review). Due to lack of knowledge at the time, older human studies often failed to account for important mitigating factors that may have washed out further positive effects including: menopause status, breast tumor subtype, and race. For example, one recent study suggests that African-American women with a low intake of lycopene have a greater risk of developing cancer of the breast compared to Caucasian women with low intakes [50]. Future epidemiological and clinical trials will be better equipped to model and interpret dietary influences on breast cancer risk. Additionally, lycopene's mechanism of preventative action within each breast cancer subtype should be identified.

Cancers of the Female Reproductive Tract

As a less common cancer of the female reproductive tract, only 12,000 new cases of cervical cancer were diagnosed in 2010 according to the National Cancer Institute. Regular screening by a Papanicolaou (Pap) Test reduces cervical cancer mortality by at least 80%. Additionally, although cervical cancer is generally a slower growing cancer, more than one-third of women diagnosed with cervical cancer die from the disease because of late diagnosis suggesting that proper screening is not done in many women [45].

Table 12.1 Results of epidemiological trials investigating the relative risk of dietary intake of tomato or lycopene or blood lycopene levels on cancer risk by cancer site

Cancer site	References	Country	No. of cases	Assessment	Relative risk (95% CI)
Prostate	Mills [79]	USA	180 (7th DA)	Tomato intake by diet history (quartiles)	0.60 (0.37–0.97)
	Giovannucci [80]	USA	773	Tomato intake by FFQ (quintiles)	0.65 (0.44–0.95)
	Schuman [81]	USA	223	Tomato intake by diet history (quartiles)	0.70 (NA)
	Cerhan [82]	USA	101	Tomato intake by diet history (quintiles)	0.50 (0.30–0.90)
	Salem [83]	Iran	194	Tomato intake by FFQ (tertiles)	0.33 (0.16–0.65)
	Darlington [84]	Canada	752	Tomato intake by FFQ (quartiles)	1.2 (0.9–1.6)
	Stram [85]	USA	3,922	Tomato intake by FFQ (quintiles)	1.02 (0.92–1.14)
	Norrish [86]	New Zealand	318	Tomato product intake by FFQ (quartiles)	0.82 (0.53–1.26)
	Gallus [87]	Italy	1,294	Pizza intake by diet history (median)	1.04 (0.88–1.23)
	Gann [88]	USA	581	Blood lycopene (quintiles)	0.56 (0.34–0.91)
	Jian [89]	China	130	Lycopene intake by diet history (quartiles)	0.18 (0.08–0.39)
	Vogt [90]	USA	483	Blood lycopene (quartiles)	0.65 (NA)
	Lu [91]	USA	65	Blood lycopene (tertiles)	0.24 (0.06–0.90)
	McCann [92]	USA	433	Lycopene intake by FFQ (quartiles)	0.62 (0.42–0.92)
	Hsing [93]	USA	103 (7th DA)	Blood lycopene (quartiles)	0.50 (0.20–1.29)
	Key [94]	UK	328	Blood lycopene (quartiles)	0.99 (0.68–1.45)
	Nomura [95]	USA	142	Blood lycopene (quartiles)	1.10 (0.50–2.20)
	Norrish [86]	New Zealand	317	Lycopene intake by FFQ (quartiles)	0.76 (0.50–1.17)
	Gann [88]	USA	578	Blood lycopene (quintiles)	0.75 (0.54–1.06)
	Kirsh [96]	USA	1,338	Lycopene intake by FFQ (quintiles)	0.95 (0.79, 1.13)
	Pourmand [97]	Iran	130	Lycopene intake by diet history (quartiles)	0.45 (0.09–2.12)
	Bosetti [98]	Italy	1294	Lycopene intake by FFQ (quintiles)	0.94 (0.72–1.23)
	Wu [99]	USA	450	Lycopene intake by FFQ (quintiles)	0.66 (0.38–1.13)
	Huang [100]	USA	182	(CLUE I Blood lycopene (quintiles)	0.83 (0.46–1.48)
		USA	142	(CLUE II Blood lycopene (quintiles)	0.79 (0.41–1.54)
	Schuurman [101]	Netherlands	642	Lycopene intake by FFQ (quintiles)	0.98 (0.71–1.34)
	Le Marchand [102]	USA	452	Lycopene intake by diet history (quartiles)	0.9 (NA)
Breast	Do [103]	Korea	359	Tomato intake by FFQ (quartiles)	0.59 (0.38–0.89)
	Gallus [87]	Italy	2,569	Pizza intake by diet history (median)	0.97 (0.86–1.10)
	Ewertz [104]	Denmark	1,486	Tomato intake by FFQ (quartiles)	1.04 (0.79–1.31)
	Levi [105]	Switzerland	107	Tomato intake by diet history (tertiles)	0.9 (NA)
	Levi [105]	Switzerland	289	Lycopene intake by FFQ (tertiles)	0.43 (0.35–0.71)
	Zhang [106]	USA	46	Breast adipose lycopene	0.32 (0.11–0.94)
	Dorjgochoo [107]	China	365	Blood lycopene (quartiles)	0.56 (0.32–0.97)

(continued)

Table 12.1 (continued)

Cancer site	References	Country	No. of cases	Assessment	Relative risk (95% CI)
	Huang [108]	China	122	Lycopene intake by diet history (quartiles)	0.38 (0.21–0.71)
	Gaudet [23]	USA	770 (post) 367 (pre)	Lycopene intake by FFQ (quintiles)	0.66 (0.48–0.90) 1.53 (0.92–2.52)
	Tamimi [109]	USA	604	Blood lycopene (quintiles)	1.0 (0.7–1.4)
	Kabat [110]	USA	190	Blood lycopene (tertiles)	1.47 (0.98–2.22)
	Freudenheim [111]	USA	297	Lycopene intake by diet history (quartiles)	0.87 (0.55–1.39)
	Wang [112]	USA	157	Lycopene intake by diet history (quartiles)	0.90 (0.74–1.11)
	Cui [21]	USA	462	Lycopene intake by FFQ (quintiles)	0.85 (0.73–1.00)
	Sesso [113]	USA	1,076	Blood lycopene (quartiles)	0.93 (0.56–1.52)
	Tamimi [114]	USA	969	Blood lycopene (quintiles)	1.01 (0.73–1.39)
	Terry [115]	Canada	1,452	Lycopene intake by FFQ (quintiles)	1.01 (0.8, 1.22)
	Sato [116]	USA	295	Blood lycopene (quintiles)	0.55 (0.29–1.06)
	Hulten [117]	Sweden	201	Blood lycopene (quartiles)	1.0 (0.60–1.80)
	La Vecchia [118]	Italy	1,953	Lycopene intake by FFQ (quintiles)	1.2 (1.0–1.4)
	Potischman [119]	USA	83	Blood lycopene (quartiles)	0.62 (0.19–2.0)
	London [120]	USA	377	Blood lycopene (quintiles)	1.0 (0.70–1.70)
	Dorgan [121]	USA	105	Blood lycopene (quartiles)	0.5 (0.20–1.20)
Cervix	VanEenwyk [122]	USA	102	Blood lycopene (quartiles)	0.26 (0.08–0.9)
	VanEenwyk [122]	USA	102	Lycopene intake by diet history (quartiles)	0.19 (0.04–0.77)
	Batieha [123]	USA	50	Blood lycopene (tertiles)	0.40 (0.15–1.04)
	Potischman [124]	Latin America	387	Blood lycopene (quartiles)	1.14 (0.8–2.1)
	Kanetsky [125]	USA	32 (Black F)	Blood lycopene (tertiles)	0.32 (0.8–1.3)
	Goodman [126]	USA	147	Blood lycopene (quartiles)	0.60 (0.20–1.40)
	Nagata [127]	Japan	152	Lycopene intake by diet history (quartiles)	0.28 (0.08–1.01)
	Schiff [128]	USA	81 (Am Ind)	Blood lycopene (tertiles)	0.80 (0.40–1.90)
Ovary	Cramer [53]	USA	549	Lycopene intake by diet history (quintiles)	0.53 (0.35–0.82)
	Jeong [52]	Korea	45	Blood lycopene (tertiles)	0.09 (0.03–0.32)
	Zhang [129]	China	254	Lycopene intake by FFQ (quartiles)	1.01 (0.62–1.64)
	Koushik [130]	Many	2,012	Lycopene intake by FFQ	1.01 (0.97–1.05)
	La Vecchia [118]	Italy	1,030	Lycopene intake by FFQ (quintiles)	1.1 (0.9–1.5)
	Helzlsouer [131]	USA	35	Blood lycopene (tertiles)	1.36 (0.4–4.3)

(continued)

Table 12.1 (continued)

Cancer site	References	Country	No. of cases	Assessment	Relative risk (95% CI)
Endometrium	Jeong [52]	Korea	28	Blood lycopene (tertiles)	0.85 (0.04–0.61)
	Jain [132]	Canada	221	Lycopene intake by diet history (quartiles)	0.63 (0.43–0.94)
	Pelucchi [133]	Italy	454	Lycopene intake by FFQ (quartiles)	0.95 (0.68–1.34)
	McCann [54]	USA	232	Lycopene intake by diet (quartiles)	0.6 (0.4–1.0)
Lung	Agudo [134]	Spain	103	Tomato intake by FFQ (tertiles)	0.45 (0.22–0.91)
	Brennan [135]	EU	506	Tomato intake by FFQ (tertiles)	0.5 (0.4–0.6)
	Darby [136]	UK	982	Tomato intake by FFQ (quartiles)	0.74 (0.57–0.96)
	Forman [137]	China	183 (TM)	Tomato intake by FFQ (quartiles)	0.42 (NA)
	Goodman [138]	USA	463 (M) 212 (F)	Tomato intake by diet history (quartiles)	0.77 (NA) M 0.50 (NA) F
	Le Marchand [139]	USA	597 (M) 268 (F)	Tomato intake by diet history (quartiles)	0.63 (NA) M 0.42 (NA) F
	Ziegler [140]	USA	11,084	Tomato intake by FFQ (quartiles)	0.93 (0.58–1.49)
	Garcia-Closas [141]	Spain	103	Tomato intake by FFQ (tertiles)	0.56 (0.26–1.24)
	Smith-Warner [57]	EU & NA	3,206	Tomato intake (quartiles) meta-analysis	0.83 (0.74–1.02)
	Fraser [142]	USA	61 (7th DA)	Tomato intake by FFQ (median)	1.24 (0.51–2.99)
	Knekt [143]	Finland	138	Tomato intake by diet history (median)	1.00 (0.67–1.50)
	Mayne [144]	USA	413	Tomato intake by FFQ (quartiles)	0.79 (NA)
	Kvale [145]	Norway	168	Tomato intake by diet history (median)	0.87 (NA)
	Axelsson [146]	Sweden	308	Tomato intake by FFQ (tertiles)	0.67 (0.43–1.05)
	Bond [147]	USA	308	Tomato intake by FFQ (median)	0.42 (0.14–1.33)
	De Stefani [148]	Uruguay	541	Tomato intake by FFQ (tertiles)	0.76 (0.49–1.16)
	Muscat [149]	USA	94	Tomato intake by FFQ (quartiles)	0.40 (0.2–1.9)
	Mannisto [58]	EU & NA	3,155	Lycopene intake (quintiles) meta-analysis	0.77 (0.68–0.88)
	Yuan [150]	China	209	Blood lycopene (quintiles)	0.46 (0.27–0.79)
	Holick [151]	Finland	1,644	Lycopene intake by FFQ (quintiles)	0.72 (0.61–0.84)
	Michaud [152]	USA	519	Lycopene intake by FFQ (quintiles)	0.8 (0.64–0.99)
	Le Marchand [153]	USA	230 (M) 102 (F)	Lycopene intake by diet history (quartiles)	0.67 (NA) M 0.77 (NA) F
	Speizer [154]	USA	593 (F)	Lycopene intake by FFQ (quintiles)	0.80 (0.60–1.10)
	Voorrips [155]	Netherlands	939 (M)	Lycopene intake by FFQ (quintiles)	1.05 (0.75–1.46)
	Wright [156]	USA	587	Lycopene intake by FFQ (quartiles)	0.73 (0.48–1.1)
	Ito [157]	Japan	147	Blood lycopene (quartiles)	0.46 (0.21–1.04)

(continued)

Table 12.1 (continued)

Cancer site	References	Country	No. of cases	Assessment	Relative risk (95% CI)
	Yuan [158]	Singapore	482	Blood lycopene (quintiles)	0.89 (0.65–1.21)
	Rohan [159]	Canada	155	Lycopene intake by FFQ (quartiles)	1.04 (0.61–1.76)
	Steinmetz [160]	USA	138	Lycopene intake by FFQ (quintiles)	1.21 (0.69–2.10)
	Candelora [161]	USA	124 (F)	Lycopene intake by FFQ (quartiles)	0.60 (0.30–1.20)
	Comstock [162]	USA	258	Blood lycopene (quintiles)	1.01 (NA)
Bladder	Castelao [61]	USA	771	Tomato intake by diet history (quintiles)	0.73 (0.57–0.93)
	Bruemmer [163]	USA	262	Tomato intake by diet history (median)	0.71 (0.39–1.29)
	Helzlsouer [164]	USA	135	Blood lycopene (tertiles)	0.5 (NA)
	Nomura [165]	USA	195 (M) 66 (F)	Lycopene intake by diet history (quintiles)	0.7 (NA) M 0.9 (NA) F
	Hung [166]	USA	84	Blood lycopene (quartiles)	0.90 (0.81–1.00)
	Nomura [167]	USA	111 (Japan)	Blood lycopene (quartiles)	0.60 (0.28–1.29)
	Michaud [168]	Finland	344	Lycopene intake by FFQ (quintiles)	1.32 (0.95–1.83)
	Zeegers [169]	Netherlands	569	Lycopene intake by FFQ (quintiles)	1.08 (0.77–1.51)
Oral	Franceschi [170]	Italy	314	Tomato intake by diet history (quartiles)	0.5 (NA)
	Zheng [171]	China	404	Tomato intake by diet history (median)	0.49 (0.26–0.94)
	Zheng [172]	China	177 (M) 24 (F)	Tomato intake by diet history (tertiles)	1.2 (NA) M 1.1 (0.4–3.1) F
	Sapkota [173]	Europe	378	Tomato intake by diet history (tertiles)	0.70 (0.31–1.58)
	La Vecchia [118]	Italy	754	Lycopene intake by FFQ (quintiles)	0.9 (0.8–1.0)
Esophagus	Cook-Mozaffari [174]	Iran	217 (M) 127 (F)	Tomato intake by diet history (median)	0.61 (0.43–0.86) M 1.08 (0.69–1.67) F
	Lagiou [175]	Europe	2,304	Fresh tomato intake by FFQ (tertiles)	0.84 (0.77–0.91)
	Sapkota [173]	Europe	187	Tomato intake by diet history (tertiles)	0.42 (0.18–0.95)
	Brown [176]	USA	207 (M)	Tomato intake by FFQ (quartiles)	0.70 (0.4–1.4)
	De Stefani [177]	Uruguay	234	Lycopene intake by diet history (quartiles)	0.70 (0.6–0.9)
	La Vecchia [118]	Italy	304	Lycopene intake by FFQ (quintiles)	0.80 (0.7–1.0)

(continued)

Table 12.1 (continued)

Cancer site	References	Country	No. of cases	Assessment	Relative risk (95% CI)
Stomach	Haenszel [178]	USA	223 (Japan)	Tomato intake by FFQ (tertiles)	0.39 (NA)
	Modan [179]	Israel	406	Tomato intake by diet history (median)	0.55 (NA)
	Correa [180]	USA	391	Tomato intake by diet history (median)	0.56 (0.34–0.90)
	Tuyns [181]	Belgium	449	Tomato intake by diet history (median)	0.12 (NA)
	Franceschi [170]	Italy	723	Tomato intake by FFQ (quartile)	0.43 (0.33–0.55)
	Buiatti [65]	Italy	1,016	Tomato intake by diet history (tertiles)	0.70 (NA)
	Boeing [182]	Poland	741	Tomato intake by FFQ (tertile)	0.77 (NA)
	Ramon [64]	Spain	177	Tomato intake by diet history (tertiles)	1.03 (NA)
	Gonzalez [183]	Spain	354	Tomato intake by diet history (quartiles)	0.90 (0.50–1.50)
	Tajima [184]	Japan	93	Tomato intake by diet history (tertiles)	1.24 (NA)
	Ekstrom [185]	Sweden	74	Tomato intake by diet history (tertiles)	0.60 (0.30–1.10)
	Pelucchi [186]	Italy	230	Tomato intake by FFQ (quartiles)	0.70 (0.41–1.17)
	De Stefani [187]	Uruguay	120	Lycopene intake by diet history (tertiles)	0.37 (0.19–0.73)
	Nouraie [188]	Finland	126	Lycopene intake by FFQ (quartiles)	0.67 (0.47–0.95)
	Lissowska [189]	Poland	274	Lycopene intake by diet history (quartiles)	1.19 (0.77–1.82)
	Garcia-Closas [190]	Spain	354	Lycopene intake by FFQ (quartiles)	1.55 (0.91–2.64)
	Yuan [191]	China	191	Blood lycopene (quartiles)	0.63 (0.34–1.15)
	Jenab [192]	Europe	244	Blood lycopene (quartiles)	0.63 (0.36–1.09)
	Botterweck [193]	Netherlands	282	Lycopene intake by FFQ (quartiles)	1.0 (0.7–1.5)
	Larsson [194]	Sweden	139	Lycopene intake by FFQ (quartiles)	0.92 (0.53–1.58)
Colon	Franceschi [170]	Italy	955	Tomato intake by FFQ (quartiles)	0.39 (0.31–0.49)
	Hu [67]	China	111	Tomato intake by diet history (tertiles)	0.4 (0.17–0.94) M 0.26 (0.12–0.55) F
	Malila [195]	Finland	184	Tomato intake by FFQ (quartiles)	1.06 (0.68–1.66)
	Centonze [196]	Italy	132	Pizza intake by FFQ (median)	0.89 (0.51–1.53)
	Tuyns [197]	Belgium	453	Tomato intake by diet history (median)	1.15 (NA)
	La Vecchia [118]	Italy	1,953	Lycopene intake by FFQ (quintiles)	1.0 (0.80–1.2)
	Mannisto [198]	Numerous	7,885	Tomato intake by FFQ (quintiles)	1.02 (0.93–1.11)

(continued)

Table 12.1 (continued)

Cancer site	References	Country	No. of cases	Assessment	Relative risk (95% CI)
Pancreas	Mesquita [199]	Netherlands	164	Tomato intake by diet history (quintiles)	0.23 (NA)
	Nkondjock [200]	Canada	462	Tomato intake by FFQ (quartiles)	0.69 (0.46–0.96)
	Nothlings [201]	USA	429	Tomato intake by FFQ (quintiles)	0.83 (0.62–1.10)
	Burney [202]	USA	22	Lycopene intake by diet history (tertiles)	0.16 (0.04–0.57)

Abbreviations: *7th DA* 7th Day Adventists, *FFQ* food frequency questionnaire, *NA* not available, *CI* confidence intervals, *pre* pre-menopausal, *post* post-menopausal, *EU & NA* Europe and North America, *Japan* Japanese Americans, *Black F* African-American females, *Am Ind* American Indian, *TM* tin miners, *F* female, *M* male

The standard treatments for cancer of the cervix include radiation therapy, surgery, and chemotherapy. Like many other cancers, dietary and lifestyle modifications may prevent cervical cancer [51]. Specifically, in relation to this chapter, eight studies have investigated the relationship between tomato or lycopene dietary intake and cervical cancer. Two studies reported a protective effect of lycopene and six studies demonstrated no effect on cervical cancer incidence (see Table 12.1 for review). Currently, there are no reports of the effects of dietary tomato intake on cervical cancer risk. Because cervical cancer is most commonly caused by human papillomavirus (HPV) infection, adopting lifestyle modifications to prevent infection would most reduce incidence of cervical cancer [45].

Cancer of the ovary claimed almost 14,000 lives in 2010 with an average annual diagnosis rate of nearly 22,000 new cases in the USA [45]. There are two primary ovarian cancer types; epithelial carcinomas and malignant germ cell tumors. The three current screening tests are pelvic exam, transvaginal ultrasound, and serum protein levels (CA-125). Once diagnosed, patients have three primary therapy options: surgery, radiation therapy, and chemotherapy [45]. Evidence suggests that dietary factors, including high fruit, vegetable, and antioxidant intake, reduce risk of gynecological cancers including ovarian cancer [51]. Six epidemiological or clinical trials report the relationship between lycopene intake or blood levels on ovarian cancer risk (see Table 12.1 for review). Two of these studies report a protective effect, although one study [52] only included 45 Korean subjects which may not demonstrate a true effect at the US population level. A study by Cramer and colleagues reported that serum lycopene levels most predicted ovarian cancer risk in pre-menopausal women suggesting that lycopene may modulate estrogen levels [53]. Additionally, they hypothesized that lycopene may reduce circulating IGF-1 levels, which ultimately results in reduced ovarian gonadotropin production.

Very few epidemiological or clinical trials investigated the effects of dietary tomato or lycopene intake on endometrial cancer. Two of four total studies suggest that dietary lycopene reduces endometrial cancer risk (see Table 12.1 for review). Additionally, a study by McCann and colleagues found that relative risk of endometrial cancer was reduced to 0.6, but the 95% confidence intervals (0.4–1.0) do not consider this to be a significant effect [54]. Early research appears promising, but further studies should investigate the relationship between lycopene intake and cancer of the endometrium with emphasis on mechanisms of action.

Lung Cancer

The two main types of lung cancer are small cell and non-small cell which are distinguished morphologically under a microscope. More than 220,000 new cases of lung cancer were diagnosed and nearly

160,000 individuals died from the disease in the USA in 2010 [45]. The overall 5-year relative survival from the 1999–2006 Surveillance Epidemiology and End Results (SEER) data was only 15.8% [55]. There is currently no regular screening for lung cancer, although once symptoms are detected it can be diagnosed by chest X-ray or sputum cytology. Although nine types of standard treatment are used to combat lung cancer, prognosis remains poor [45].

Lung cancer is strongly impacted by lifestyle. Cigarette smoking is the primary risk factor for development of lung carcinoma. Therefore, many dietary trials are conducted in populations of smokers. Six out of 31 epidemiological or clinical trials report that dietary intake of tomatoes or lycopene reduces incidence of lung cancer (see Table 12.1 for review). Although very high intakes of supplemental β-carotene may increase risk in smokers (for further discussion, see [56]), no studies suggest that dietary lycopene increases lung cancer risk.

Two meta-analyses conducted with subjects from the European Union and North America also examined the relationship between lycopene or tomato intake with lung cancer. The analysis by Smith-Warner and colleagues suggests that tomato intake is not significantly associated with lung cancer incidence in a population of 3,206 individuals [57]. In contrast, the analysis by Mannisto and colleagues suggests that increased dietary lycopene reduced lung cancer risk in a population of 3,155 individuals [58]. It is possible that due to the radical and sometimes irreversible changes caused by smoking, dietary modification may not significantly improve health outcomes in populations of smokers. In a recent review, Drs. Lian and Wang suggest that studying the metabolism and mechanistic basis of lycopene chemoprevention will help to elucidate optimal dosing, the production of bioactive metabolites, and possible interactions with other dietary components *in vivo* [59].

Bladder Cancer

Bladder cancer is the third most prevalent cancer in the USA and, one of the most expensive cancers to treat due to long courses of treatment and frequent follow-up surveillance [60]. There is currently no standard or routine screening for bladder cancer but instead discovery relies upon symptoms including blood in the urine and pain during urination. Once diagnosed, treatment options include surgery, radiation therapy, and chemotherapy [45]. Dietary components may reduce the incidence of bladder cancer including carrots, selenium, cruciferous vegetables, and fruits [60]. The relationship between tomato or lycopene intake with bladder cancer incidence has also been investigated. Eight studies investigated this relationship and three report an inverse association suggesting that dietary tomatoes or lycopene reduces incidence of bladder cancer (see Table 12.1 for review). Individuals with high exposures to environmental arylamines often arising from industrial dyes are at an increased risk of developing bladder cancer [61]. The case–control study by Castelao and colleagues reports that lycopene intake increased arylamine detoxification [61]. Studies in high risk populations are necessary to elucidate a clear relationship between dietary lycopene and bladder cancer [62].

Cancers of the Digestive Tract

Food is passed from the oral cavity through the esophagus to the stomach. According to the National Cancer Institute, more than 36,000 new cases of oral cancer, 16,000 new cases of esophageal, and 21,000 new cases of stomach cancer were diagnosed in 2010 [45]. There is no standard screening method for any of these cancer types. Once diagnosed, patients have the option of surgery or radiation therapy. Additionally, for esophageal cancer patients, chemotherapy, laser therapy, and electrocoagulation are accepted therapies. Stomach cancer patients may also receive chemoradiation therapy.

Smoke and tobacco use is the primary risk factor for oral–esophageal cancers [45]. Incidence of oral, esophageal, and stomach cancer is highest in Asia and linked to nutritional deficiencies and contaminated food and water [63]. It appears diet and lifestyle modifications strongly modulate risk for these cancers. In relation to this chapter, epidemiological and clinical studies examined the relationship between dietary intake of tomatoes or lycopene and cancers of the digestive tract. Five studies investigated the relationship with oral cancer, 6 with esophageal, and 20 studies examined stomach cancer. Two studies reported that intake of tomatoes reduced oral cancer risk, four reported that dietary tomatoes or lycopene reduced esophageal cancer risk, and eight studies reported that dietary tomatoes or lycopene provided protection against stomach cancer (see Table 12.1 for review). Stomach cancer risk is strongly associated with increased consumption of smoked meats due to the nitrosation process. Two of the stomach cancer studies hypothesized that tomato or lycopene intake inhibits intragastric formation of nitrosamines [64, 65].

In 2010, nearly 103,000 new colon cancer cases were diagnosed thanks to numerous screening techniques including: fecal occult blood test, sigmoidoscopy, barium enema, colonoscopy, and digital rectal exam [45]. Once diagnosed with colon cancer, a patient has the option of surgery, chemotherapy, radiation, or targeted therapies. Prevention of the disease may include dietary and lifestyle modifications. Calorie restriction, increased intake of omega-3 fatty acids, sulforaphane from broccoli, fiber, folate, calcium, vitamin D, and curcumin from the spice turmeric were reported to reduce colon cancer risk [59, 66]. Additionally, case–control studies have reported a reduced risk of colon cancer with increased intake of fruits and vegetables [59]. Seven studies explored a relationship between dietary tomatoes or lycopene and colon cancer risk. Two reports suggest that increased tomato intake reduces colon cancer risk (see Table 12.1 for review). One of these studies examined males and females separately and reported that although both sexes benefit from tomato intake, females received the greatest benefit from tomato consumption [67]. *In vitro* and *in vivo* animal studies attribute lycopene's antioxidant properties, enhancement of cell–cell communication, modification of IGF-1 signaling, and induction of detoxification enzymes to reduce colon cancer risk (for further review, see [59]) although thorough understanding of lycopene's mechanisms of action needs to be elucidated.

The pancreas is an organ of the digestive tract that connects to the small intestine through the common bile duct. The pancreas is responsible for making digestive enzymes and hormones, including insulin. There are currently no common screening methods for pancreatic cancer, even though more than 43,000 new cases were diagnosed in 2010 [45]. For those unfortunate enough to develop pancreatic cancer, the 5-year survival rate is around 5% with surgery, radiation, and chemotherapy as the currently accepted therapies [55]. Because of the rapid mortality, data are limited regarding diet and lifestyle as modifiers of pancreatic cancer risk. Four epidemiological or clinical trials examined the relationship between dietary intake of tomatoes or lycopene and pancreatic cancer risk (see Table 12.1 for review). Three of those studies found that intake of tomatoes or lycopene resulted in reduced incidence of pancreatic cancer. Although ¾ of the studies support lycopene as a chemopreventative, more studies are required in high risk populations to clarify this relationship and define the mechanisms by which lycopene might modify pancreatic cancer risk.

Lycopene Versus Tomato

Epidemiological evidence provides data sets which are used to define associations between food intake and disease. Because of the broad nature of data collection such as food frequency questionnaires or serum analysis, epidemiological data often cannot distinguish between the protective effects of foods versus food bioactive components. In these large studies, serum lycopene can only be used as a biomarker of tomato intake, but its effects on disease cannot be distinguished from those of tomatoes. As discussed earlier, serum lycopene or consumption of tomato products is associated with reduced risk of many cancers. These data may suggest that lycopene is responsible, but only supplementation trials, animal work, or *in vitro* studies can demonstrate a cause and effect relationship.

Lycopene, at high concentrations *in vitro*, reduces cancer growth and modulates associated biomarkers [7]. Few *in vitro* or animal studies demonstrate that lower levels of lycopene intake, closer to what could be physiologically attained through the diet, significantly reduce cancer progression [68, 69]. This suggests that lycopene is bioactive, but may not be consumed in high enough concentrations in the diet to have a significant physiological effect suggesting that other components of tomatoes may affect cancer risk.

Tomato products are good sources of vitamins A, C, E, potassium, and folate [70]. Tomatoes also contain other phytochemicals including the carotenoids, β-carotene, phytoene, and phytofluene [70]. Additionally, the skin of the tomato contains the flavonols, quercetin, and kaempferol. Animal studies from our laboratory comparing the effects of diets containing lycopene or dried tomato powder suggest that the whole food more effectively reduces prostate tumor growth than lycopene alone [31, 71]. Animal and *in vitro* studies also suggest that combinations of lycopene with other tomato components modulate cancer biomarkers more effectively than lycopene alone [72–76]. Together these data suggest that bioactive components of tomatoes, including lycopene, work additively or synergistically to reduce growth of cancer cells. Incorporating tomato products into the diet ensures consumption of multiple cancer fighting phytochemicals in one food.

Conclusion

No reports suggest that lycopene or tomato products increase cancer risk in any cancer type while a number show significant reduction in a variety of cancers (Fig. 12.3). Epidemiological and clinical trials indicate that dietary intake of tomatoes or lycopene protects against cancers of the prostate, breast, cervix, ovary, endometrium, lung, bladder, oral cavity, esophagus, stomach, colon, and pancreas. More than ten independent epidemiological or clinical studies have examined the chemopreventative effects of lycopene on cancers of the prostate, breast, lung, and stomach.

Numerous mechanisms of action have been proposed for lycopene's effect on cancer risk including modulation of growth factors and sex steroids, inhibition of normal cell proliferation, and antioxidant effects (see Fig. 12.2). Animal and *in vitro* studies suggest that lycopene is bioactive in high concentrations, but requires additive or synergistic effects of other tomato bioactive components to reduce prostate cancer [6, 77]. Because tomatoes contain other important vitamins and minerals, consumption of tomato products, as opposed to lycopene alone, is likely to reduce cancer risk as indicated by epidemiological and clinical trials of tomato intake.

Future Directions

As the scientific community better defines cancer subtypes and their risk factors, human trials can be designed to obtain the maximum benefits from dietary and lifestyle modifications. With the emergence of epigenetics and personalized medicine, specific dietary components may modulate cancer risk of subsets of the human population. Future studies should focus on the variance within population-based studies to define mitigating factors that influence the chemopreventative effects of tomatoes or lycopene.

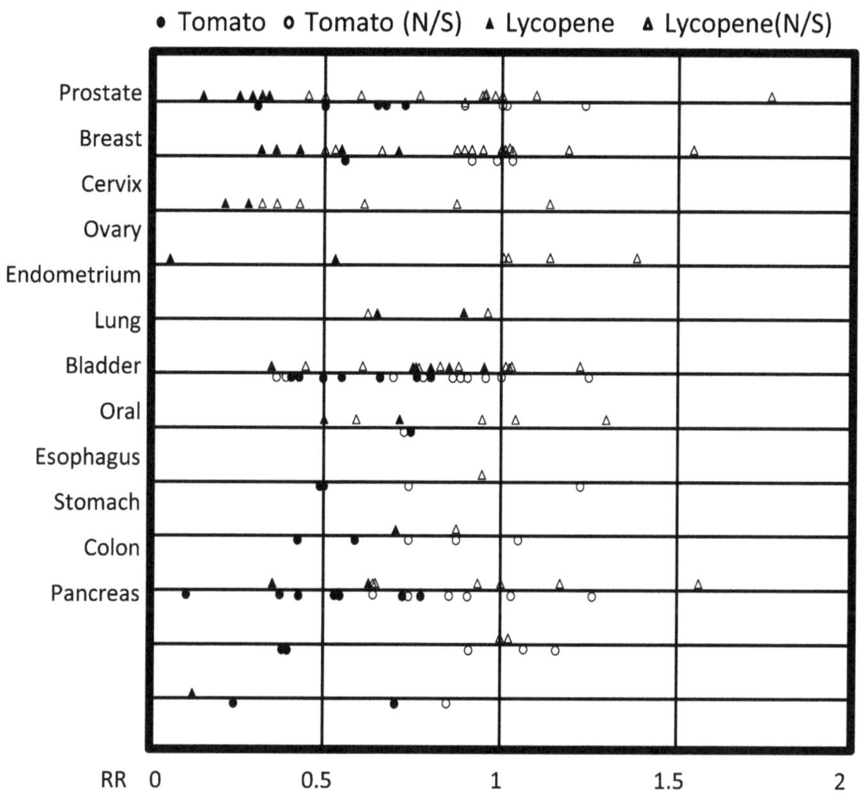

Fig. 12.3 Tomato intake or lycopene levels in relation to relative risk (RR) of cancer by site. *Closed shapes* represent studies with statistically significant outcomes; *open center shapes* represent studies with non-significant outcomes. See Table 12.1 for references

References

1. Wertz K, Siler U, Goralczyk R. Lycopene: modes of action to promote prostate health. Arch Biochem Biophys. 2004;430(1):127–34.
2. Hadley CW, Miller EC, Schwartz SJ, Clinton SK. Tomatoes, lycopene, and prostate cancer: progress and promise. Exp Biol Med. 2002;227(10):869–80.
3. Erdman Jr JW. How do nutritional and hormonal status modify the bioavailability, uptake, and distribution of different isomers of lycopene? J Nutr. 2005;135(8):2046S–7.
4. Rubio-Diaz DE, Santos A, Francis DM, Rodriguez-Saona LE. Carotenoid stability during production and storage of tomato juice made from tomatoes with diverse pigment profiles measured by infrared spectroscopy. J Agric Food Chem. 2010;58(15):8692–8.
5. Di Mascio P, Kaiser S, Sies H. Lycopene as the most efficient biological carotenoid singlet oxygen quencher. Arch Biochem Biophys. 1989;274(2):532–8.
6. Erdman Jr JW, Ford NA, Lindshield BL. Are the health attributes of lycopene related to its antioxidant function? Arch Biochem Biophys. 2009;483(2):229–35.
7. Ford NA, Elsen AC, Zuniga K, Lindshield BL, Erdman Jr. JW. Lycopene and *apo*-12′-lycopenal reduce cell proliferation and alter cell cycle progression in human prostate cancer cells. Nutr Cancer. 2011;63(2):256–63.
8. Siler U, Barella L, Spitzer V, et al. Lycopene and vitamin E interfere with autocrine/paracrine loops in the Dunning prostate cancer model. FASEB J. 2004;18(9):1019–21.
9. Liu C, Lian F, Smith DE, Russell RM, Wang XD. Lycopene supplementation inhibits lung squamous metaplasia and induces apoptosis via up-regulating insulin-like growth factor-binding protein 3 in cigarette smoke-exposed ferrets. Cancer Res. 2003;63(12):3138–44.

10. Walfisch S, Walfisch Y, Kirilov E, et al. Tomato lycopene extract supplementation decreases insulin-like growth factor-I levels in colon cancer patients. Eur J Cancer Prev. 2007;16(4):298–303.
11. Riso P, Brusamolino A, Martinetti A, Porrini M. Effect of a tomato drink intervention on insulin-like growth factor (IGF)-1 serum levels in healthy subjects. Nutr Cancer. 2006;55(2):157–62.
12. Herzog A, Siler U, Spitzer V, et al. Lycopene reduced gene expression of steroid targets and inflammatory markers in normal rat prostate. FASEB J. 2005;19(2):272–4.
13. Voskuil DW, Vrieling A, Korse CM, et al. Effects of lycopene on the insulin-like growth factor (IGF) system in premenopausal breast cancer survivors and women at high familial breast cancer risk. Nutr Cancer. 2008;60(3):342–53.
14. Hursting SD, Berger NA. Energy balance, host-related factors, and cancer progression. J Clin Oncol. 2010;28(26):4058–65.
15. Yamaguchi M, Hasegawa I, Yahagi N, Ishigaki Y, Takano F, Ohta T. Carotenoids modulate cytokine production in Peyer's patch cells *ex vivo*. J Agric Food Chem. 2010;58(15):8566–72.
16. Palozza P, Simone R, Catalano A, et al. Lycopene prevention of oxysterol-induced proinflammatory cytokine cascade in human macrophages: inhibition of NF-kappaB nuclear binding and increase in PPARgamma expression. J Nutr Biochem. 2011;22(3):259–68.
17. Feng D, Ling WH, Duan RD. Lycopene suppresses LPS-induced NO and IL-6 production by inhibiting the activation of ERK, p38MAPK, and NF-kappaB in macrophages. Inflamm Res. 2010;59(2):115–21.
18. Saedisomeolia A, Wood LG, Garg ML, Gibson PG, Wark PA. Lycopene enrichment of cultured airway epithelial cells decreases the inflammation induced by rhinovirus infection and lipopolysaccharide. J Nutr Biochem. 2009;20(8):577–85.
19. Markovits N, Ben Amotz A, Levy Y. The effect of tomato-derived lycopene on low carotenoids and enhanced systemic inflammation and oxidation in severe obesity. Isr Med Assoc J. 2009;11(10):598–601.
20. Campbell JK, Stroud CK, Nakamura MT, Lila MA, Erdman Jr JW. Serum testosterone is reduced following short-term phytofluene, lycopene, or tomato powder consumption in F344 rats. J Nutr. 2006;136(11):2813–9.
21. Cui Y, Shikany JM, Liu S, Shagufta Y, Rohan TE. Selected antioxidants and risk of hormone receptor-defined invasive breast cancers among postmenopausal women in the Women's Health Initiative Observational Study. Am J Clin Nutr. 2008;87(4):1009–18.
22. Murtaugh MA, Ma KN, Benson J, Curtin K, Caan B, Slattery ML. Antioxidants, carotenoids, and risk of rectal cancer. Am J Epidemiol. 2004;159(1):32–41.
23. Gaudet MM, Britton JA, Kabat GC, et al. Fruits, vegetables, and micronutrients in relation to breast cancer modified by menopause and hormone receptor status. Cancer Epidemiol Biomarkers Prev. 2004;13(9):1485–94.
24. AICR. Food, nutrition, physical activity, and the prevention of cancer: a global perspective. Washington DC: AICR; 2007.
25. Krutovskikh V, Asamoto M, Takasuka N, Murakoshi M, Nishino H, Tsuda H. Differential dose-dependent effects of alpha-, beta-carotenes and lycopene on gap-junctional intercellular communication in rat liver *in vivo*. Jpn J Cancer Res. 1997;88(12):1121–4.
26. Kucuk O, Sarkar FH, Djuric Z, et al. Effects of lycopene supplementation in patients with localized prostate cancer. Exp Biol Med. 2002;227(10):881–5.
27. Cheng HC, Chien H, Liao CH, Yang YY, Huang SY. Carotenoids suppress proliferating cell nuclear antigen and cyclin D1 expression in oral carcinogenic models. J Nutr Biochem. 2007;18(10):667–75.
28. Tang L, Jin T, Zeng X, Wang JS. Lycopene inhibits the growth of human androgen-independent prostate cancer cells *in vitro* and in BALB/c nude mice. J Nutr. 2005;135(2):287–90.
29. Kim HS, Bowen P, Chen L, et al. Effects of tomato sauce consumption on apoptotic cell death in prostate benign hyperplasia and carcinoma. Nutr Cancer. 2003;47(1):40–7.
30. Bowen P, Chen L, Stacewicz-Sapuntzakis M, et al. Tomato sauce supplementation and prostate cancer: lycopene accumulation and modulation of biomarkers of carcinogenesis. Exp Biol Med. 2002;227(10):886–93.
31. Canene-Adams K, Lindshield BL, Wang S, Jeffery EH, Clinton SK, Erdman Jr JW. Combinations of tomato and broccoli enhance antitumor activity in Dunning R3327-H prostate adenocarcinomas. Cancer Res. 2007;67(2):836–43.
32. Liu C, Russell RM, Wang XD. Lycopene supplementation prevents smoke-induced changes in p53, p53 phosphorylation, cell proliferation, and apoptosis in the gastric mucosa of ferrets. J Nutr. 2006;136(1):106–11.
33. Sengupta A, Ghosh S, Das S. Tomato and garlic can modulate azoxymethane-induced colon carcinogenesis in rats. Eur J Cancer Prev. 2003;12(3):195–200.
34. Dias MC, Vieiralves NF, Gomes MI, Salvadori DM, Rodrigues MA, Barbisan LF. Effects of lycopene, synbiotic and their association on early biomarkers of rat colon carcinogenesis. Food Chem Toxicol. 2010;48(3):772–80.
35. Velmurugan B, Mani A, Nagini S. Combination of S-allylcysteine and lycopene induces apoptosis by modulating Bcl-2, Bax, Bim and caspases during experimental gastric carcinogenesis. Eur J Cancer Prev. 2005;14(4):387–93.
36. Kurcer MA, Kurcer Z, Koksal M, et al. Effect of lycopene on caspase-3 enzyme activation in liver of methanol-intoxicated rats: comparison with fomepizole. J Med Food. 2010;13(4):985–91.

37. Huang CS, Liao JW, Hu ML. Lycopene inhibits experimental metastasis of human hepatoma SK-Hep-1 cells in athymic nude mice. J Nutr. 2008;138(3):538–43.
38. Yang CM, Yen YT, Huang CS, Hu ML. Growth inhibitory efficacy of lycopene and beta-carotene against androgen-independent prostate tumor cells xenografted in nude mice. Mol Nutr Food Res. 2010;55(4):606–12.
39. Moselhy SS, Al mslmani MA. Chemopreventive effect of lycopene alone or with melatonin against the genesis of oxidative stress and mammary tumors induced by 7,12 dimethyl(a)benzanthracene in Sprague Dawley female rats. Mol Cell Biochem. 2008;319(1–2):175–80.
40. Kasagi S, Seyama K, Mori H, et al. Tomato juice prevents senescence-accelerated mouse P1 strain from developing emphysema induced by chronic exposure to tobacco smoke. Am J Physiol Lung Cell Mol Physiol. 2006;290(2):L396–404.
41. Hwang ES, Lee HJ. Inhibitory effects of lycopene on the adhesion, invasion, and migration of SK-Hep1 human hepatoma cells. Exp Biol Med (Maywood). 2006;231(3):322–7.
42. Chiang HS, Wu WB, Fang JY, et al. Lycopene inhibits PDGF-BB-induced signaling and migration in human dermal fibroblasts through interaction with PDGF-BB. Life Sci. 2007;81(21–22):1509–17.
43. Wu WB, Chiang HS, Fang JY, Hung CF. Inhibitory effect of lycopene on PDGF-BB-induced signalling and migration in human dermal fibroblasts: a possible target for cancer. Biochem Soc Trans. 2007;35(Pt 5):1377–8.
44. Huang CS, Shih MK, Chuang CH, Hu ML. Lycopene inhibits cell migration and invasion and upregulates Nm23-H1 in a highly invasive hepatocarcinoma, SK-Hep-1 cells. J Nutr. 2005;135(9):2119–23.
45. National Cancer Institute. 2011. http://www.cancer.gov/cancertopics/types. http://www.cancer.gov/cancertopics/types/prostate. Accessed 14 Mar.
46. Djavan B. The correlation between inflammation, BPH, and prostate cancer. Eur Urol Suppl. 2009;8(13):863–4.
47. Kucuk O, Sarkar FH, Sakr W, et al. Phase II randomized clinical trial of lycopene supplementation before radical prostatectomy. Cancer Epidemiol Biomarkers Prev. 2001;10(8):861–8.
48. Giovannucci E, Ascherio A, Rimm EB, Stampfer MJ, Colditz GA, Willett WC. Intake of carotenoids and retinol in relation to risk of prostate cancer. J Natl Cancer Inst. 1995;87(23):1767–76.
49. Etminan M, Takkouche B, Caamano-Isorna F. The role of tomato products and lycopene in the prevention of prostate cancer: a meta-analysis of observational studies. Cancer Epidemiol Biomarkers Prev. 2004;13(3):340–5.
50. Simon MS, Djuric Z, Dunn B, Stephens D, Lababidi S, Heilbrun LK. An evaluation of plasma antioxidant levels and the risk of breast cancer: a pilot case control study. Breast J. 2000;6(6):388–95.
51. Rieck G, Fiander A. The effect of lifestyle factors on gynaecological cancer. Best Pract Res Clin Obstet Gynaecol. 2006;20(2):227–51.
52. Jeong NH, Song ES, Lee JM, et al. Plasma carotenoids, retinol and tocopherol levels and the risk of ovarian cancer. Acta Obstet Gynecol Scand. 2009;88(4):457–62.
53. Cramer DW, Kuper H, Harlow BL, Titus-Ernstoff L. Carotenoids, antioxidants and ovarian cancer risk in pre- and postmenopausal women. Int J Cancer. 2001;94(1):128–34.
54. McCann SE, Freudenheim JL, Marshall JR, Brasure JR, Swanson MK, Graham S. Diet in the epidemiology of endometrial cancer in western New York (United States). Cancer Causes Control. 2000;11(10):965–74.
55. Horner MJ, Ries LAG, Krapcho M, et al. SEER cancer statistics review, 1975–2006. Bethesda, MD: National Cancer Institute; 2009. http://seer.cancer.gov/csr/1975_2006/, based on November 2008 SEER data submission, posted to the SEER web site.
56. Goodman GE, Thornquist MD, Balmes J, et al. The beta-carotene and retinol efficacy trial: incidence of lung cancer and cardiovascular disease mortality during 6-year follow-up after stopping beta-carotene and retinol supplements. J Natl Cancer Inst. 2004;96(23):1743–50.
57. Smith-Warner SA, Spiegelman D, Yaun SS, et al. Fruits, vegetables and lung cancer: a pooled analysis of cohort studies. Int J Cancer. 2003;107(6):1001–11.
58. Mannisto S, Smith-Warner SA, Spiegelman D, et al. Dietary carotenoids and risk of lung cancer in a pooled analysis of seven cohort studies. Cancer Epidemiol Biomarkers Prev. 2004;13(1):40–8.
59. Preedy VR, Watson RR, editors. Lycopene: nutritional medicinal and therapeutic properties. Enfield, NH: Science Publishers; 2008.
60. Busby JE, Kamat AM. Chemoprevention for bladder cancer. J Urol. 2006;176(5):1914–20.
61. Castelao JE, Yuan JM, Gago-Dominguez M, et al. Carotenoids/vitamin C and smoking-related bladder cancer. Int J Cancer. 2004;110(3):417–23.
62. Sasaki T, Horikawa M, Orikasa K, et al. Possible relationship between the risk of Japanese bladder cancer cases and the CYP4B1 genotype. Jpn J Clin Oncol. 2008;38(9):634–40.
63. Lambert R, Hainaut P. The multidisciplinary management of gastrointestinal cancer. Epidemiology of oesophagogastric cancer. Best Pract Res Clin Gastroenterol. 2007;21(6):921–45.
64. Ramon JM, Serra L, Cerdo C, Oromi J. Dietary factors and gastric cancer risk. A case-control study in Spain. Cancer. 1993;71(5):1731–5.
65. Buiatti E, Palli D, Decarli A, et al. A case-control study of gastric cancer and diet in Italy: II. Association with nutrients. Int J Cancer. 1990;45(5):896–901.

66. Tammariello AE, Milner JA. Mouse models for unraveling the importance of diet in colon cancer prevention. J Nutr Biochem. 2010;21(2):77–88.
67. Hu JF, Liu YY, Yu YK, Zhao TZ, Liu SD, Wang QQ. Diet and cancer of the colon and rectum: a case-control study in China. Int J Epidemiol. 1991;20(2):362–7.
68. Burgess LC, Rice E, Fischer T, et al. Lycopene has limited effect on cell proliferation in only two of seven human cell lines (both cancerous and noncancerous) in an in vitro system with doses across the physiological range. Toxicol In Vitro. 2008;22(5):1297–300.
69. Hantz HL, Young LF, Martin KR. Physiologically attainable concentrations of lycopene induce mitochondrial apoptosis in LNCaP human prostate cancer cells. Exp Biol Med. 2005;230(3):171–9.
70. Canene-Adams K, Campbell JK, Zaripheh S, Jeffery EH, Erdman Jr JW. The tomato as a functional food. J Nutr. 2005;135(5):1226–30.
71. Boileau TW, Liao Z, Kim S, Lemeshow S, Erdman Jr JW, Clinton SK. Prostate carcinogenesis in N-methyl-N-nitrosourea (NMU)-testosterone-treated rats fed tomato powder, lycopene, or energy-restricted diets. J Natl Cancer Inst. 2003;95(21):1578–86.
72. Balestrieri ML, De Prisco R, Nicolaus B, et al. Lycopene in association with alpha-tocopherol or tomato lipophilic extracts enhances acyl-platelet-activating factor biosynthesis in endothelial cells during oxidative stress. Free Radic Biol Med. 2004;36(8):1058–67.
73. Nara E, Hayashi H, Kotake M, Miyashita K, Nagao A. Acyclic carotenoids and their oxidation mixtures inhibit the growth of HL-60 human promyelocytic leukemia cells. Nutr Cancer. 2001;39(2):273–83.
74. Pastori M, Pfander H, Boscoboinik D, Azzi A. Lycopene in association with alpha-tocopherol inhibits at physiological concentrations proliferation of prostate carcinoma cells. Biochem Biophys Res Commun. 1998;250(3): 582–5.
75. Bureyko T, Hurdle H, Metcalfe JB, Clandinin MT, Mazurak VC. Reduced growth and integrin expression of prostate cells cultured with lycopene, vitamin E and fish oil in vitro. Br J Nutr. 2009;101(7):990–7.
76. Richards LR, Benghuzzi H, Tucci M, Hughes J. The synergistic effect of conventional and sustained delivery of antioxidants on LNCaP prostate cancer cell line. Biomed Sci Instrum. 2003;39:402–7.
77. Basu A, Imrhan V. Tomatoes versus lycopene in oxidative stress and carcinogenesis: conclusions from clinical trials. Eur J Clin Nutr. 2007;61(3):295–303.
78. Clinton SK. Lycopene: chemistry, biology, and implications for human health and disease. Nutr Rev. 1998;56 (2 Pt 1):35–51.
79. Mills PK, Beeson WL, Phillips RL, Fraser GE. Cohort study of diet, lifestyle, and prostate cancer in Adventist men. Cancer. 1989;64(3):598–604.
80. Giovannucci E. Tomato products, lycopene, and prostate cancer: a review of the epidemiological literature. J Nutr. 2005;135(8):2030S–1.
81. Schuman LM, Mandel JS, Radke A, Seal U, Halberg F. Some selected features of the epidemiology of prostatic cancer: Minneapolis-St. Paul, Minnesota case-control study, 1976–1979. In: Magnus K, editor. Trends in cancer incidence; causes and practical implications. Washington, DC: Hemisphere; 1982. p. 345–54.
82. Cerhan JR, Cantor KP, Williamson K, Lynch CF, Torner JC, Burmeister LF. Cancer mortality among Iowa farmers: recent results, time trends, and lifestyle factors (United States). Cancer Causes Control. 1998;9(3):311–9.
83. Salem S, Salahi M, Mohseni M, et al. Major dietary factors and prostate cancer risk: a prospective multicenter case-control study. Nutr Cancer. 2011;63(1):21–7.
84. Darlington GA, Kreiger N, Lightfoot N, Purdham J, Sass-Kortsak A. Prostate cancer risk and diet, recreational physical activity and cigarette smoking. Chronic Dis Can. 2007;27(4):145–53.
85. Stram DO, Hankin JH, Wilkens LR, et al. Prostate cancer incidence and intake of fruits, vegetables and related micronutrients: the multiethnic cohort study* (United States). Cancer Causes Control. 2006;17(9):1193–207.
86. Norrish AE, Jackson RT, Sharpe SJ, Skeaff CM. Prostate cancer and dietary carotenoids. Am J Epidemiol. 2000;151(2):119–23.
87. Gallus S, Talamini R, Bosetti C, et al. Pizza consumption and the risk of breast, ovarian and prostate cancer. Eur J Cancer Prev. 2006;15(1):74–6.
88. Gann PH, Ma J, Giovannucci E, et al. Lower prostate cancer risk in men with elevated plasma lycopene levels: results of a prospective analysis. Cancer Res. 1999;59(6):1225–30.
89. Jian L, Lee AH, Binns CW. Tea and lycopene protect against prostate cancer. Asia Pac J Clin Nutr. 2007;16 Suppl 1:453–7.
90. Vogt TM, Mayne ST, Graubard BI, et al. Serum lycopene, other serum carotenoids, and risk of prostate cancer in US Blacks and Whites. Am J Epidemiol. 2002;155(11):1023–32.
91. Heber D, Lu QY. Overview of mechanisms of action of lycopene. Exp Biol Med. 2002;227(10):920–3.
92. McCann SE, Ambrosone CB, Moysich KB, et al. Intakes of selected nutrients, foods, and phytochemicals and prostate cancer risk in western New York. Nutr Cancer. 2005;53(1):33–41.
93. Hsing AW, Comstock GW, Abbey H, Polk BF. Serologic precursors of cancer. Retinol, carotenoids, and tocopherol and risk of prostate cancer. J Natl Cancer Inst. 1990;82(11):941–6.

94. Key TJ, Silcocks PB, Davey GK, Appleby PN, Bishop DT. A case-control study of diet and prostate cancer. Br J Cancer. 1997;76(5):678–87.
95. Nomura AM, Stemmermann GN, Lee J, Craft NE. Serum micronutrients and prostate cancer in Japanese Americans in Hawaii. Cancer Epidemiol Biomarkers Prev. 1997;6(7):487–91.
96. Kirsh VA, Mayne ST, Peters U, et al. A prospective study of lycopene and tomato product intake and risk of prostate cancer. Cancer Epidemiol Biomarkers Prev. 2006;15(1):92–8.
97. Pourmand G, Salem S, Mehrsai A, et al. The risk factors of prostate cancer: a multicentric case-control study in Iran. Asian Pac J Cancer Prev. 2007;8(3):422–8.
98. Bosetti C, Talamini R, Montella M, et al. Retinol, carotenoids and the risk of prostate cancer: a case-control study from Italy. Int J Cancer. 2004;112(4):689–92.
99. Wu K, Erdman Jr JW, Schwartz SJ, et al. Plasma and dietary carotenoids, and the risk of prostate cancer: a nested case-control study. Cancer Epidemiol Biomarkers Prev. 2004;13(2):260–9.
100. Huang HY, Alberg AJ, Norkus EP, Hoffman SC, Comstock GW, Helzlsouer KJ. Prospective study of antioxidant micronutrients in the blood and the risk of developing prostate cancer. Am J Epidemiol. 2003;157(4):335–44.
101. Schuurman AG, Goldbohm RA, Brants HA, van den Brandt PA. A prospective cohort study on intake of retinol, vitamins C and E, and carotenoids and prostate cancer risk (Netherlands). Cancer Causes Control. 2002;13(6): 573–82.
102. Le Marchand L, Hankin JH, Kolonel LN, Wilkens LR. Vegetable and fruit consumption in relation to prostate cancer risk in Hawaii: a reevaluation of the effect of dietary beta-carotene. Am J Epidemiol. 1991;133(3):215–9.
103. Do MH, Lee SS, Kim JY, Jung PJ, Lee MH. Fruits, vegetables, soy foods and breast cancer in pre- and postmenopausal Korean women: a case-control study. Int J Vitam Nutr Res. 2007;77(2):130–41.
104. Ewertz M, Gill C. Dietary factors and breast-cancer risk in Denmark. Int J Cancer. 1990;46(5):779–84.
105. Levi F, Pasche C, Lucchini F, La Vecchia C. Dietary intake of selected micronutrients and breast-cancer risk. Int J Cancer. 2001;91(2):260–3.
106. Zhang S, Tang G, Russell RM, et al. Measurement of retinoids and carotenoids in breast adipose tissue and a comparison of concentrations in breast cancer cases and control subjects. Am J Clin Nutr. 1997;66(3):626–32.
107. Dorjgochoo T, Gao YT, Chow WH, et al. Plasma carotenoids, tocopherols, retinol and breast cancer risk: results from the Shanghai Women Health Study (SWHS). Breast Cancer Res Treat. 2009;117(2):381–9.
108. Huang JP, Zhang M, Holman CD, Xie X. Dietary carotenoids and risk of breast cancer in Chinese women. Asia Pac J Clin Nutr. 2007;16 Suppl 1:437–42.
109. Tamimi RM, Colditz GA, Hankinson SE. Circulating carotenoids, mammographic density, and subsequent risk of breast cancer. Cancer Res. 2009;69(24):9323–9.
110. Kabat GC, Kim M, Adams-Campbell LL, et al. Longitudinal study of serum carotenoid, retinol, and tocopherol concentrations in relation to breast cancer risk among postmenopausal women. Am J Clin Nutr. 2009;90(1):162–9.
111. Freudenheim JL, Marshall JR, Vena JE, et al. Premenopausal breast cancer risk and intake of vegetables, fruits, and related nutrients. J Natl Cancer Inst. 1996;88(6):340–8.
112. Wang C, Baumgartner RN, Yang D, et al. No evidence of association between breast cancer risk and dietary carotenoids, retinols, vitamin C and tocopherols in Southwestern Hispanic and non-Hispanic White women. Breast Cancer Res Treat. 2009;114(1):137–45.
113. Sesso HD, Buring JE, Norkus EP, Gaziano JM. Plasma lycopene, other carotenoids, and retinol and the risk of cardiovascular disease in men. Am J Clin Nutr. 2005;81(5):990–7.
114. Tamimi RM, Hankinson SE, Campos H, et al. Plasma carotenoids, retinol, and tocopherols and risk of breast cancer. Am J Epidemiol. 2005;161(2):153–60.
115. Terry P, Jain M, Miller AB, Howe GR, Rohan TE. Dietary carotenoids and risk of breast cancer. Am J Clin Nutr. 2002;76(4):883–8.
116. Sato R, Helzlsouer KJ, Alberg AJ, Hoffman SC, Norkus EP, Comstock GW. Prospective study of carotenoids, tocopherols, and retinoid concentrations and the risk of breast cancer. Cancer Epidemiol Biomarkers Prev. 2002;11(5):451–7.
117. Hulten K, Van Kappel AL, Winkvist A, et al. Carotenoids, alpha-tocopherols, and retinol in plasma and breast cancer risk in northern Sweden. Cancer Causes Control. 2001;12(6):529–37.
118. La Vecchia C. Tomatoes, lycopene intake, and digestive tract and female hormone-related neoplasms. Exp Biol Med (Maywood). 2002;227(10):860–3.
119. Potischman N, McCulloch CE, Byers T, et al. Breast cancer and dietary and plasma concentrations of carotenoids and vitamin A. Am J Clin Nutr. 1990;52(5):909–15.
120. London SJ, Stein EA, Henderson IC, et al. Carotenoids, retinol, and vitamin E and risk of proliferative benign breast disease and breast cancer. Cancer Causes Control. 1992;3(6):503–12.
121. Dorgan JF, Sowell A, Swanson CA, et al. Relationships of serum carotenoids, retinol, alpha-tocopherol, and selenium with breast cancer risk: results from a prospective study in Columbia, Missouri (United States). Cancer Causes Control. 1998;9(1):89–97.

122. VanEenwyk J, Davis FG, Bowen PE. Dietary and serum carotenoids and cervical intraepithelial neoplasia. Int J Cancer. 1991;48(1):34–8.
123. Batieha AM, Armenian HK, Norkus EP, Morris JS, Spate VE, Comstock GW. Serum micronutrients and the subsequent risk of cervical cancer in a population-based nested case-control study. Cancer Epidemiol Biomarkers Prev. 1993;2(4):335–9.
124. Potischman N, Herrero R, Brinton LA, et al. A case-control study of nutrient status and invasive cervical cancer. II. Serologic indicators. Am J Epidemiol. 1991;134(11):1347–55.
125. Kanetsky PA, Gammon MD, Mandelblatt J, et al. Dietary intake and blood levels of lycopene: association with cervical dysplasia among non-Hispanic, black women. Nutr Cancer. 1998;31(1):31–40.
126. Goodman MT, Kiviat N, McDuffie K, et al. The association of plasma micronutrients with the risk of cervical dysplasia in Hawaii. Cancer Epidemiol Biomarkers Prev. 1998;7(6):537–44.
127. Nagata C, Shimizu H, Yoshikawa H, et al. Serum carotenoids and vitamins and risk of cervical dysplasia from a case-control study in Japan. Br J Cancer. 1999;81(7):1234–7.
128. Schiff MA, Patterson RE, Baumgartner RN, et al. Serum carotenoids and risk of cervical intraepithelial neoplasia in Southwestern American Indian women. Cancer Epidemiol Biomarkers Prev. 2001;10(11):1219–22.
129. Zhang M, Holman CD, Binns CW. Intake of specific carotenoids and the risk of epithelial ovarian cancer. Br J Nutr. 2007;98(1):187–93.
130. Koushik A, Hunter DJ, Spiegelman D, et al. Intake of the major carotenoids and the risk of epithelial ovarian cancer in a pooled analysis of 10 cohort studies. Int J Cancer. 2006;119(9):2148–54.
131. Helzlsouer KJ, Alberg AJ, Norkus EP, Morris JS, Hoffman SC, Comstock GW. Prospective study of serum micronutrients and ovarian cancer. J Natl Cancer Inst. 1996;88(1):32–7.
132. Jain MG, Rohan TE, Howe GR, Miller AB. A cohort study of nutritional factors and endometrial cancer. Eur J Epidemiol. 2000;16(10):899–905.
133. Pelucchi C, Dal Maso L, Montella M, et al. Dietary intake of carotenoids and retinol and endometrial cancer risk in an Italian case-control study. Cancer Causes Control. 2008;19(10):1209–15.
134. Agudo A, Esteve MG, Pallares C, et al. Vegetable and fruit intake and the risk of lung cancer in women in Barcelona, Spain. Eur J Cancer. 1997;33(8):1256–61.
135. Brennan P, Butler J, Agudo A, et al. Joint effect of diet and environmental tobacco smoke on risk of lung cancer among nonsmokers. J Natl Cancer Inst. 2000;92(5):426–7.
136. Darby S, Whitley E, Doll R, Key T, Silcocks P. Diet, smoking and lung cancer: a case-control study of 1000 cases and 1500 controls in South-West England. Br J Cancer. 2001;84(5):728–35.
137. Forman MR, Yao SX, Graubard BI, et al. The effect of dietary intake of fruits and vegetables on the odds ratio of lung cancer among Yunnan tin miners. Int J Epidemiol. 1992;21(3):437–41.
138. Goodman MT, Kolonel LN, Wilkens LR, Yoshizawa CN, Le Marchand L, Hankin JH. Dietary factors in lung cancer prognosis. Eur J Cancer. 1992;28(2–3):495–501.
139. Le Marchand L, Yoshizawa CN, Kolonel LN, Hankin JH, Goodman MT. Vegetable consumption and lung cancer risk: a population-based case-control study in Hawaii. J Natl Cancer Inst. 1989;81(15):1158–64.
140. Ziegler RG, Mayne ST, Swanson CA. Nutrition and lung cancer. Cancer Causes Control. 1996;7(1):157–77.
141. Garcia-Closas R, Agudo A, Gonzalez CA, Riboli E. Intake of specific carotenoids and flavonoids and the risk of lung cancer in women in Barcelona, Spain. Nutr Cancer. 1998;32(3):154–8.
142. Fraser GE, Beeson WL, Phillips RL. Diet and lung cancer in California Seventh-day Adventists. Am J Epidemiol. 1991;133(7):683–93.
143. Knekt P, Jarvinen R, Teppo L, Aromaa A, Seppanen R. Role of various carotenoids in lung cancer prevention. J Natl Cancer Inst. 1999;91(2):182–4.
144. Mayne ST, Janerich DT, Greenwald P, et al. Dietary beta carotene and lung cancer risk in U.S. nonsmokers. J Natl Cancer Inst. 1994;86(1):33–8.
145. Kvale G, Bjelke E, Gart JJ. Dietary habits and lung cancer risk. Int J Cancer. 1983;31(4):397–405.
146. Axelsson G, Liljeqvist T, Andersson L, Bergman B, Rylander R. Dietary factors and lung cancer among men in west Sweden. Int J Epidemiol. 1996;25(1):32–9.
147. Bond GG, Thompson FE, Cook RR. Dietary vitamin A and lung cancer: results of a case-control study among chemical workers. Nutr Cancer. 1987;9(2–3):109–21.
148. De Stefani E, Brennan P, Boffetta P, et al. Diet and adenocarcinoma of the lung: a case-control study in Uruguay. Lung Cancer. 2002;35(1):43–51.
149. Muscat JE, Huncharek M. Dietary intake and the risk of malignant mesothelioma. Br J Cancer. 1996;73(9):1122–5.
150. Yuan JM, Ross RK, Chu XD, Gao YT, Yu MC. Prediagnostic levels of serum beta-cryptoxanthin and retinol predict smoking-related lung cancer risk in Shanghai, China. Cancer Epidemiol Biomarkers Prev. 2001;10(7):767–73.
151. Holick CN, Michaud DS, Stolzenberg-Solomon R, et al. Dietary carotenoids, serum beta-carotene, and retinol and risk of lung cancer in the alpha-tocopherol, beta-carotene cohort study. Am J Epidemiol. 2002;156(6):536–47.

152. Michaud DS, Feskanich D, Rimm EB, et al. Intake of specific carotenoids and risk of lung cancer in 2 prospective US cohorts. Am J Clin Nutr. 2000;72(4):990–7.
153. Le Marchand L, Hankin JH, Kolonel LN, Beecher GR, Wilkens LR, Zhao LP. Intake of specific carotenoids and lung cancer risk. Cancer Epidemiol Biomarkers Prev. 1993;2(3):183–7.
154. Speizer FE, Colditz GA, Hunter DJ, Rosner B, Hennekens C. Prospective study of smoking, antioxidant intake, and lung cancer in middle-aged women (USA). Cancer Causes Control. 1999;10(5):475–82.
155. Voorrips LE, Goldbohm RA, Brants HA, et al. A prospective cohort study on antioxidant and folate intake and male lung cancer risk. Cancer Epidemiol Biomarkers Prev. 2000;9(4):357–65.
156. Wright ME, Mayne ST, Swanson CA, Sinha R, Alavanja MC. Dietary carotenoids, vegetables, and lung cancer risk in women: the Missouri women's health study (United States). Cancer Causes Control. 2003;14(1):85–96.
157. Ito Y, Wakai K, Suzuki K, et al. Serum carotenoids and mortality from lung cancer: a case-control study nested in the Japan Collaborative Cohort (JACC) study. Cancer Sci. 2003;94(1):57–63.
158. Yuan JM, Stram DO, Arakawa K, Lee HP, Yu MC. Dietary cryptoxanthin and reduced risk of lung cancer: the Singapore Chinese Health Study. Cancer Epidemiol Biomarkers Prev. 2003;12(9):890–8.
159. Rohan TE, Jain M, Howe GR, Miller AB. A cohort study of dietary carotenoids and lung cancer risk in women (Canada). Cancer Causes Control. 2002;13(3):231–7.
160. Steinmetz KA, Potter JD, Folsom AR. Vegetables, fruit, and lung cancer in the Iowa Women's Health Study. Cancer Res. 1993;53(3):536–43.
161. Candelora EC, Stockwell HG, Armstrong AW, Pinkham PA. Dietary intake and risk of lung cancer in women who never smoked. Nutr Cancer. 1992;17(3):263–70.
162. Comstock GW, Alberg AJ, Huang HY, et al. The risk of developing lung cancer associated with antioxidants in the blood: ascorbic acid, carotenoids, alpha-tocopherol, selenium, and total peroxyl radical absorbing capacity. Cancer Epidemiol Biomarkers Prev. 1997;6(11):907–16.
163. Bruemmer B, White E, Vaughan TL, Cheney CL. Nutrient intake in relation to bladder cancer among middle-aged men and women. Am J Epidemiol. 1996;144(5):485–95.
164. Helzlsouer KJ, Comstock GW, Morris JS. Selenium, lycopene, alpha-tocopherol, beta-carotene, retinol, and subsequent bladder cancer. Cancer Res. 1989;49(21):6144–8.
165. Nomura AM, Kolonel LN, Hankin JH, Yoshizawa CN. Dietary factors in cancer of the lower urinary tract. Int J Cancer. 1991;48(2):199–205.
166. Hung RJ, Zhang ZF, Rao JY, et al. Protective effects of plasma carotenoids on the risk of bladder cancer. J Urol. 2006;176(3):1192–7.
167. Nomura AM, Lee J, Stemmermann GN, Franke AA. Serum vitamins and the subsequent risk of bladder cancer. J Urol. 2003;170(4 Pt 1):1146–50.
168. Michaud DS, Pietinen P, Taylor PR, Virtanen M, Virtamo J, Albanes D. Intakes of fruits and vegetables, carotenoids and vitamins A, E, C in relation to the risk of bladder cancer in the ATBC cohort study. Br J Cancer. 2002;87(9):960–5.
169. Zeegers MP, Goldbohm RA, van den Brandt PA. Are retinol, vitamin C, vitamin E, folate and carotenoids intake associated with bladder cancer risk? Results from the Netherlands Cohort Study. Br J Cancer. 2001;85(7):977–83.
170. Franceschi S, Bidoli E, La Vecchia C, Talamini R, D'Avanzo B, Negri E. Tomatoes and risk of digestive-tract cancers. Int J Cancer. 1994;59(2):181–4.
171. Zheng W, Blot WJ, Diamond EL, et al. Serum micronutrients and the subsequent risk of oral and pharyngeal cancer. Cancer Res. 1993;53(4):795–8.
172. Zheng W, Blot WJ, Shu XO, et al. Risk factors for oral and pharyngeal cancer in Shanghai, with emphasis on diet. Cancer Epidemiol Biomarkers Prev. 1992;1(6):441–8.
173. Sapkota A, Hsu CC, Zaridze D, et al. Dietary risk factors for squamous cell carcinoma of the upper aerodigestive tract in central and eastern Europe. Cancer Causes Control. 2008;19(10):1161–70.
174. Cook-Mozaffari PJ, Azordegan F, Day NE, Ressicaud A, Sabai C, Aramesh B. Oesophageal cancer studies in the Caspian Littoral of Iran: results of a case-control study. Br J Cancer. 1979;39(3):293–309.
175. Lagiou P, Talamini R, Samoli E, et al. Diet and upper-aerodigestive tract cancer in Europe: the ARCAGE study. Int J Cancer. 2009;124(11):2671–6.
176. Brown LM, Blot WJ, Schuman SH, et al. Environmental factors and high risk of esophageal cancer among men in coastal South Carolina. J Natl Cancer Inst. 1988;80(20):1620–5.
177. De Stefani E, Ronco AL, Boffetta P, et al. Nutrient intake and risk of squamous cell carcinoma of the esophagus: a case-control study in Uruguay. Nutr Cancer. 2006;56(2):149–57.
178. Haenszel W, Kurihara M, Segi M, Lee RK. Stomach cancer among Japanese in Hawaii. J Natl Cancer Inst. 1972;49(4):969–88.
179. Modan B, Cuckle H, Lubin F. A note on the role of dietary retinol and carotene in human gastro-intestinal cancer. Int J Cancer. 1981;28(4):421–4.

180. Correa P, Fontham E, Pickle LW, Chen V, Lin YP, Haenszel W. Dietary determinants of gastric cancer in south Louisiana inhabitants. J Natl Cancer Inst. 1985;75(4):645–54.
181. Tuyns AJ, Kaaks R, Haelterman M, Riboli E. Diet and gastric cancer. A case-control study in Belgium. Int J Cancer. 1992;51(1):1–6.
182. Boeing H, Jedrychowski W, Wahrendorf J, Popiela T, Tobiasz-Adamczyk B, Kulig A. Dietary risk factors in intestinal and diffuse types of stomach cancer: a multicenter case-control study in Poland. Cancer Causes Control. 1991;2(4):227–33.
183. Gonzalez CA, Sanz JM, Marcos G, et al. Dietary factors and stomach cancer in Spain: a multi-centre case-control study. Int J Cancer. 1991;49(4):513–9.
184. Tajima K, Tominaga S. Dietary habits and gastro-intestinal cancers: a comparative case-control study of stomach and large intestinal cancers in Nagoya, Japan. Jpn J Cancer Res. 1985;76(8):705–16.
185. Ekstrom AM, Serafini M, Nyren O, Hansson LE, Ye W, Wolk A. Dietary antioxidant intake and the risk of cardia cancer and noncardia cancer of the intestinal and diffuse types: a population-based case-control study in Sweden. Int J Cancer. 2000;87(1):133–40.
186. Pelucchi C, Tramacere I, Bertuccio P, Tavani A, Negri E, La Vecchia C. Dietary intake of selected micronutrients and gastric cancer risk: an Italian case-control study. Ann Oncol. 2009;20(1):160–5.
187. De Stefani E, Boffetta P, Brennan P, et al. Dietary carotenoids and risk of gastric cancer: a case-control study in Uruguay. Eur J Cancer Prev. 2000;9(5):329–34.
188. Nouraie M, Pietinen P, Kamangar F, et al. Fruits, vegetables, and antioxidants and risk of gastric cancer among male smokers. Cancer Epidemiol Biomarkers Prev. 2005;14(9):2087–92.
189. Lissowska J, Gail MH, Pee D, et al. Diet and stomach cancer risk in Warsaw, Poland. Nutr Cancer. 2004;48(2):149–59.
190. Garcia-Closas R, Gonzalez CA, Agudo A, Riboli E. Intake of specific carotenoids and flavonoids and the risk of gastric cancer in Spain. Cancer Causes Control. 1999;10(1):71–5.
191. Yuan JM, Ross RK, Gao YT, Qu YH, Chu XD, Yu MC. Prediagnostic levels of serum micronutrients in relation to risk of gastric cancer in Shanghai, China. Cancer Epidemiol Biomarkers Prev. 2004;13(11 Pt 1):1772–80.
192. Jenab M, Riboli E, Ferrari P, et al. Plasma and dietary carotenoid, retinol and tocopherol levels and the risk of gastric adenocarcinomas in the European prospective investigation into cancer and nutrition. Br J Cancer. 2006;95(3):406–15.
193. Botterweck AA, van den Brandt PA, Goldbohm RA. Vitamins, carotenoids, dietary fiber, and the risk of gastric carcinoma: results from a prospective study after 6.3 years of follow-up. Cancer. 2000;88(4):737–48.
194. Larsson SC, Bergkvist L, Naslund I, Rutegard J, Wolk A. Vitamin A, retinol, and carotenoids and the risk of gastric cancer: a prospective cohort study. Am J Clin Nutr. 2007;85(2):497–503.
195. Malila N, Hakulinen T. Epidemiological trends of colorectal cancer in the Nordic countries. Scand J Surg. 2003;92(1):5–9.
196. Centonze S, Boeing H, Leoci C, Guerra V, Misciagna G. Dietary habits and colorectal cancer in a low-risk area. Results from a population-based case-control study in southern Italy. Nutr Cancer. 1994;21(3):233–46.
197. Tuyns AJ, Kaaks R, Haelterman M. Colorectal cancer and the consumption of foods: a case-control study in Belgium. Nutr Cancer. 1988;11(3):189–204.
198. Mannisto S, Yaun SS, Hunter DJ, et al. Dietary carotenoids and risk of colorectal cancer in a pooled analysis of 11 cohort studies. Am J Epidemiol. 2007;165(3):246–55.
199. Bueno de Mesquita HB, Maisonneuve P, Runia S, Moerman CJ. Intake of foods and nutrients and cancer of the exocrine pancreas: a population-based case-control study in The Netherlands. Int J Cancer. 1991;48(4):540–9.
200. Nkondjock A, Ghadirian P, Johnson KC, Krewski D. Dietary intake of lycopene is associated with reduced pancreatic cancer risk. J Nutr. 2005;135(3):592–7.
201. Nothlings U, Wilkens LR, Murphy SP, Hankin JH, Henderson BE, Kolonel LN. Vegetable intake and pancreatic cancer risk: the multiethnic cohort study. Am J Epidemiol. 2007;165(2):138–47.
202. Burney PG, Comstock GW, Morris JS. Serologic precursors of cancer: serum micronutrients and the subsequent risk of pancreatic cancer. Am J Clin Nutr. 1989;49(5):895–900.

Chapter 13
Lutein and Zeaxanthin and Eye Disease

Rohini Vishwanathan and Elizabeth J. Johnson

Key Points

- The xanthophylls lutein and zeaxanthin are oxygenated carotenoids that preferentially accumulate in the macular region of the retina. Lutein, zeaxanthin, and *meso*-zeaxanthin (a conversion product of lutein formed in the macula) are referred to as macular pigment. Lutein and zeaxanthin are also present in all other ocular structures except the vitreous, cornea, and sclera; although, their concentrations are much lower than in the macular region. Lutein and zeaxanthin protect the ocular tissues by their ability to filter damaging blue light and their antioxidant potential.
- Eye diseases that have been associated with low lutein and zeaxanthin include age-related macular degeneration (AMD)—due to the exclusive location of lutein and zeaxanthin in the macula, which is the sight of AMD insult; cataract—due to the presence of lutein and zeaxanthin in the lens, which is constantly exposed to light and oxygen; and retinitis pigmentosa—due to the presence of lutein and zeaxanthin in the rod outer segments and in the macula.
- The etiology of each eye disease will be discussed briefly followed by a review of epidemiological evidence and findings from intervention studies with lutein and zeaxanthin, alone and in combination with other nutrients.
- The role of lutein and zeaxanthin in improving visual function will also be examined.
- The chapter will close with a brief summary of conclusions and future directions.

Keywords Lutein • Zeaxanthin • Macular pigment • Eye disease • Age-related macular degeneration • Cataract • Retinitis pigmentosa • Visual function

R. Vishwanathan, Ph.D. • E.J. Johnson, Ph.D. (✉)
Carotenoids and Health Laboratory, Jean Mayer USDA Human Nutrition Research Center on Aging at Tufts University, 711 Washington St., Boston, MA 02111, USA
e-mail: rohini.vishwanathan@tufts.edu; elizabeth.johnson@tufts.edu

S.A. Tanumihardjo (ed.), *Carotenoids and Human Health*, Nutrition and Health,
DOI 10.1007/978-1-62703-203-2_13, © Springer Science+Business Media New York 2013

Introduction

Structure and Tissue Distribution of Lutein and Zeaxanthin

Lutein and zeaxanthin are known as oxygenated carotenoids or xanthophylls due to the presence of two hydroxyl groups, one on each of the two ionone rings (Fig. 13.1). They are 40 carbon polyisoprenoid compounds with nine conjugated double bonds in the polyene chain [1]. Lutein and zeaxanthin are stereoisomers of one another but are not interchangeable wherever they have a functional role [2]. Lutein has both β and ε type ionone rings, while zeaxanthin has two β type ionone rings [2]. The hydroxyl groups make lutein and zeaxanthin more polar in nature compared with lycopene, α-carotene, and β-carotene, which are pure hydrocarbons. The relative orientation of the hydroxyl groups dictates the observed specificity in tissue accumulation and orientation within the cell membranes. The structure is also important in the specific recognition of lutein and zeaxanthin by binding proteins [3].

Of the 700 carotenoids identified in nature, only 13 carotenoids and their 12 isomers are found in the serum and only two, lutein and zeaxanthin, exclusively accumulate in the macula of the human eye. The macula lutea is a yellowish region 5–6 mm in diameter in the posterior pole of the human retina responsible for the central 15–20° of vision [4, 5]. Lutein, zeaxanthin, and *meso*-zeaxanthin, a conversion product of lutein formed in the macula [6], are collectively referred to as macular pigment (MP). The macular region has a central depression, a region called the fovea (Fig. 13.2), an area so rich in cone receptors that permits maximal visual acuity [2]. The concentration of xanthophylls in the central macula is about 1 mM, which corresponds to more than 3 orders of their concentration in normal serum [7, 8]. However, in regions just a few millimeters from the central fovea the concentration of xanthophylls drops more than 100-fold [5]. The ratio of lutein to zeaxanthin increases from about 1:2.4 in the central 0–0.25 mm of the macula to greater than 2:1 in the periphery, distances exceeding 6 mm from the fovea [7, 9, 10]. *Meso*-zeaxanthin was shown to be present in the macular

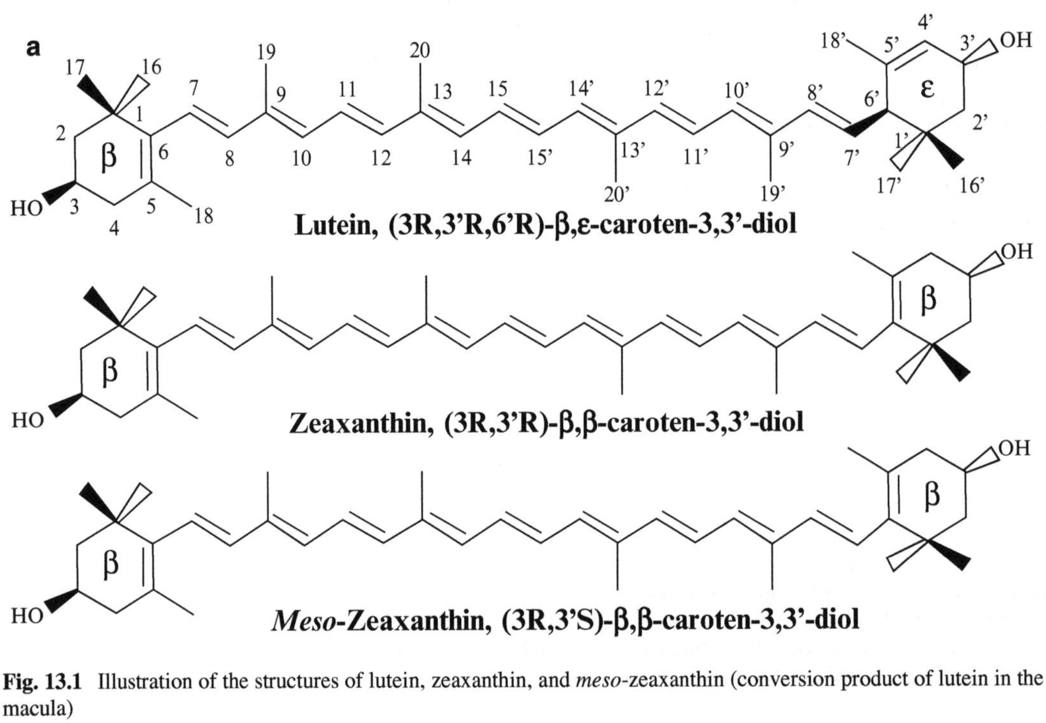

Fig. 13.1 Illustration of the structures of lutein, zeaxanthin, and *meso*-zeaxanthin (conversion product of lutein in the macula)

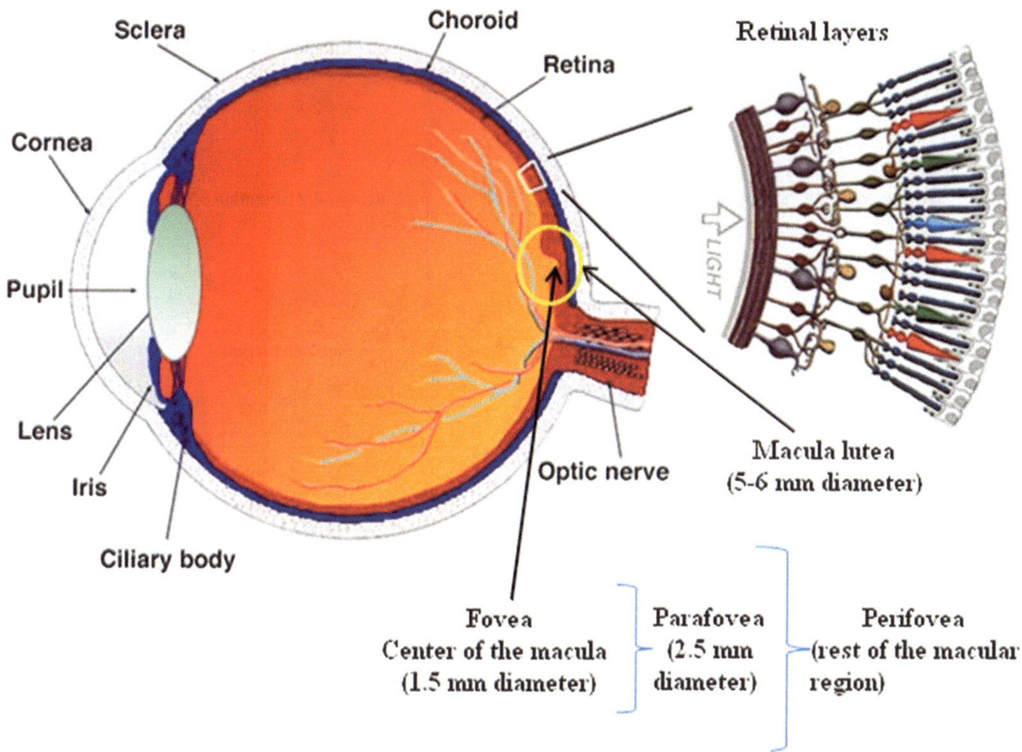

Fig. 13.2 An illustration of the structure of the eye showing the different regions including the macular regions where lutein and zeaxanthin exclusively accumulate. Credit for the eye image: Webvision (http://webvision.med.utah.edu/sretina.html), with permission

region (not 8 mm and peripheral retina) of xanthophyll-free rhesus monkeys that were fed a pure lutein diet and not those that were fed a pure zeaxanthin diet demonstrating that lutein isomerizes to *meso*-zeaxanthin via migration of a double bond [6]. This partially explains the disparity between the 3:1 ratio of lutein to zeaxanthin in the blood and the 1:2 in the macula and also the lower lutein to zeaxanthin ratio in the fovea compared to the periphery [5]. The lutein:zeaxanthin:*meso*-zeaxanthin ratio in the macula is 1:1:1 [6, 7].

Knowing that these xanthophylls are present in the fovea and peripheral regions of the retina, the question arises to their precise location within the cellular and subcellular structures. Lutein and zeaxanthin are said to be asymmetrically distributed across the depth of the retina (Fig. 13.3), with highest concentrations in the inner retinal layers [7, 11, 12]. In 1984, Snodderly et al. described MP distribution patterns that hypothesized the cone axons (outer plexiform layer) to contain the highest densities of MP due to the high density of cone photoreceptors in the fovea [12]. Others have also shown the majority of the pigments to be concentrated in the outer plexiform layers of the fovea as well as the outer and inner plexiform layers of the adjacent areas [7, 12–14]. There is strong evidence showing the presence of lutein and zeaxanthin in the photoreceptor rod outer segments (ROS), where they were shown to represent 10–15% and 25% of total retinal lutein and zeaxanthin in two separate studies [15, 16]. Within the ROS, the highest density of lutein and zeaxanthin exists in the perifoveal region (Fig. 13.2), where the concentration of pigments was 2.5-times greater than in the peripheral regions of the retina [15]. Lutein and zeaxanthin were also detected in the retinal pigment epithelium (RPE), but their concentrations were less than half of that found in ROS [15]. The high selectivity and distribution of lutein and zeaxanthin in these retinal layers suggests the presence of specific binding proteins. Bernstein et al. have shown the presence of carotenoid binding proteins in the retina, which specifically bind lutein and zeaxanthin.

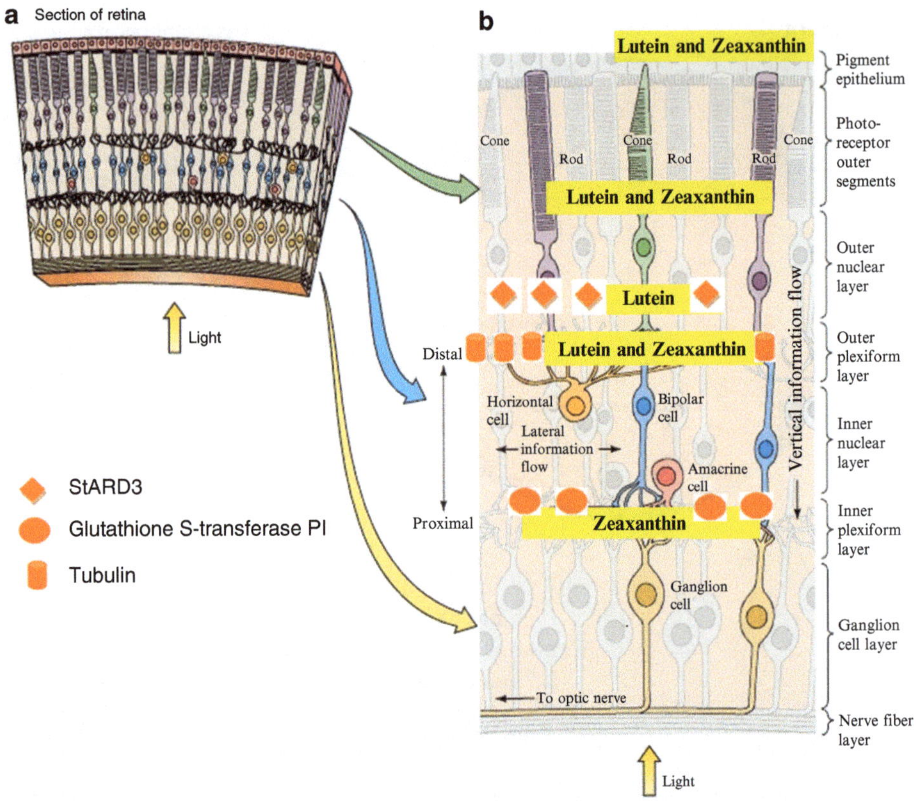

Fig. 13.3 (**a**) Cross section of the retina showing the different neuronal cells. (**b**) Distribution of lutein and zeaxanthin within the cellular structures and the associated specific carotenoid binding proteins that have been detected in these regions. Credit for cross section of the retina: Purves D, Augustine GJ, Fitzpatrick D et al., editors. The retina. Neuroscience. 2nd ed. Sunderland (MA): Sinauer Associates, 2001, with permission

Tubulin was shown to bind lutein and zeaxanthin in the photoreceptor axon layer, glutathione *S*-transferase P1 (GSTP1) concentrated in the outer and inner plexiform layers of the fovea and in the photoreceptor inner segment ellipsoid region specifically bound to zeaxanthin, and the steroidogenic acute regulatory domain protein 3 (StARD3) specifically bound to lutein (Fig. 13.3) [3, 17].

Lutein and zeaxanthin are present in all other ocular structures with the exception of the vitreous, cornea, and sclera [5]. Approximately 30% of the ocular lutein and zeaxanthin are present in the uveal structures (i.e., iris, ciliary body, and RPE/choroid) [5]. Long-term supplementation with high doses of lutein can increase lutein concentration in ocular tissues such as the lens and peripheral retina that generally contain low levels of lutein and zeaxanthin [18]. In the lens, 75% of the lutein and zeaxanthin are present in the epithelium and cortex [19]. Other than the ocular tissues, lutein and zeaxanthin are found in the adipose tissue, ovaries, testes, liver, skin, human milk, and more recently have been detected in the brain [20–25].

Role of Lutein and Zeaxanthin in the Eye

Unlike α-carotene, β-carotene, and β-cryptoxanthin, lutein and zeaxanthin do not have provitamin A activity [26]. The presence of hydroxyl groups in the ionone rings prevents enzymatic cleavage at the 15-15′ bond which is involved in the formation of vitamin A aldehyde [27].

Lutein and zeaxanthin are believed to function in ocular health through their ability to absorb damaging blue radiation of light and their strong antioxidant potential. The cornea and lens filter UV radiation of light allowing visible blue light to reach the retina. MP has an absorption maximum of about 450 nm and acts as an effective filter diminishing the intensity of blue light reaching the photoreceptors [28]. Lutein and zeaxanthin as MP attenuate as much as 40% of the blue light from reaching the retina [29]. Lutein has a greater filtering efficiency compared to zeaxanthin [28] due to the difference in position of the double bond within the ionone ring. Lutein is able to orient itself both parallel and perpendicular to the plane of the membrane, while zeaxanthin can only lie perpendicular to the membrane [28, 30]. The two orientations of the lutein molecule allow for blue light absorption from all directions, which is not the case with zeaxanthin [5]. Even though β-carotene and lycopene have absorption maxima around 450 nm, the absence of hydrophilic groups causes them to remain within the hydrophobic core of the membrane making them unable to efficiently filter blue light [1]. Furthermore, these carotenes are not present in significant concentrations in ocular tissue [31]. Evidence for MP providing protection from light damage comes from observations in older adults in whom an increased loss of sensitivity of the short wavelength-sensitive-cones (S-cone) was observed across the retina compared to younger adults, with more loss of sensitivity at the nonfoveal locations compared to the fovea, an area where MP is at its peak [32].

Because of their slightly hydrophilic nature, lutein and zeaxanthin are able to quench singlet oxygen more effectively in the water phase compared to the completely hydrophobic hydrocarbon carotenoids [33]. Lutein and zeaxanthin have the ability to scavenge reactive oxygen species and limit peroxidation of membrane phospholipids. Under conditions of prolonged UV exposure, zeaxanthin is more effective than lutein in diminishing UV-induced lipid oxidation [30]. The retina is particularly susceptible to oxidative damage because of its high consumption of oxygen, its high concentration of polyunsaturated fatty acids, such as docosahexaenoic acid (DHA), and its exposure to visible light [34]. The photoreceptor cells are constantly exposed to light which could lead to generation of electrically excited species. These could react with molecular oxygen to produce reactive oxygen species and cause lipid peroxidation and cellular damage [5]. Furthermore, the presence of oxidative metabolites of lutein and zeaxanthin in the retina, such as 3-hydroxy-beta, epsilon-caroten-3′-one, and 3′-epilutein, which are not of dietary origin, is evidence for the antioxidative role of lutein and zeaxanthin in the retina [31].

In the iris, lutein and zeaxanthin most likely act as blue light filters, while in the ciliary body, an area of high metabolic activity, they most likely act as antioxidants [35]. In the lens as well, lutein and zeaxanthin most likely have an antioxidant function, with the constant exposure to oxygen and UV radiation. Due to their presence in the eye, lutein and zeaxanthin have been extensively researched in the prevention and treatment of eye diseases. The focus of this chapter is to discuss the most current findings on lutein and zeaxanthin in the treatment and prevention of age-related macular degeneration, cataract, and retinitis pigmentosa. The role of these macular carotenoids in visual function will also be discussed.

Eye Diseases

Age-Related Macular Degeneration

Age-related macular degeneration (AMD) is the leading cause of blindness in adults aged 60 years and over in industrialized countries. The prevalence of AMD increases dramatically with age. Nearly 30% of Americans >75 years have early signs of AMD and 7% have advanced AMD, whereas the respective prevalence is 8% and 0.1% in adults aged 43–54 years [36]. None of the current treatment options can reverse the damage caused by AMD.

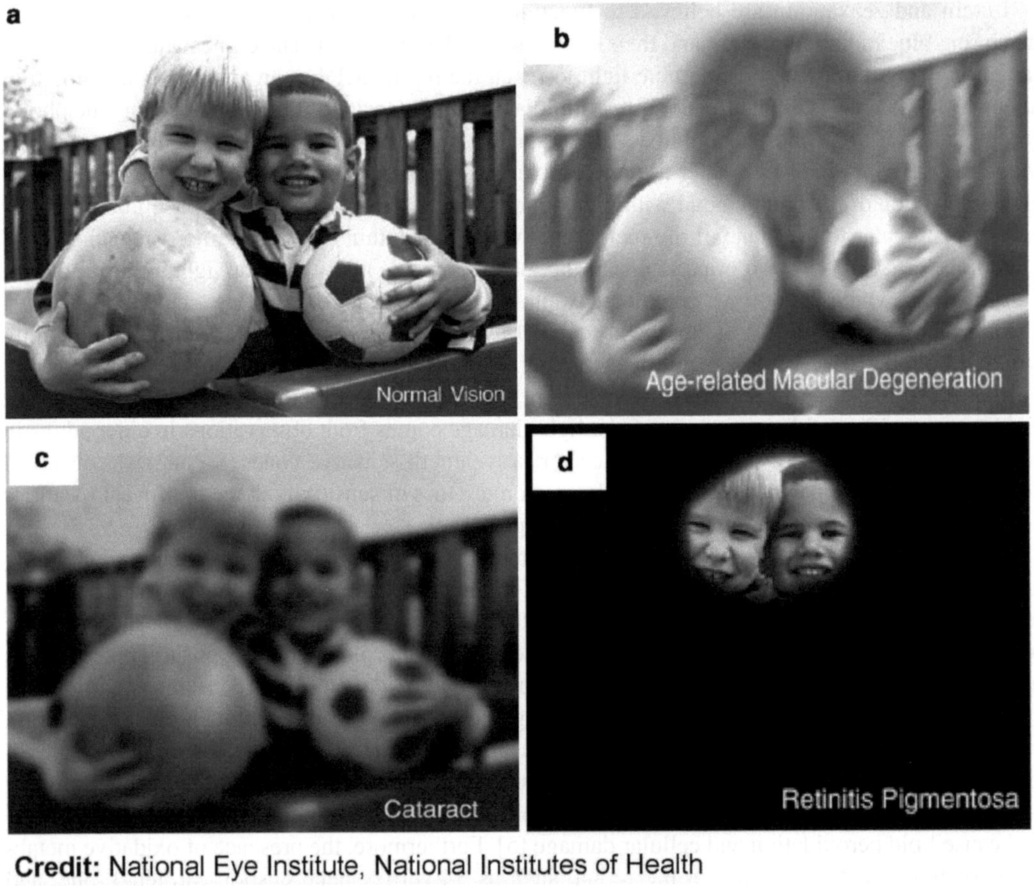

Fig. 13.4 A scene viewed by a person with (**a**) normal vision, (**b**) age-related macular degeneration, (**c**) cataract, and (**d**) retinitis pigmentosa. Credit: National Eye Institute, National Institutes of Health

AMD is a disease that affects the macular region of the retina causing loss of central vision (Fig. 13.4) and as the disease advances can lead to complete blindness. Posterior to the photoreceptors lies the RPE, part of the blood-ocular barrier, which has several functions including phagocytosis of the photoreceptors [37]. The clinical hallmark and usually the first clinical signs of AMD is the presence of drusen. Drusen are extracellular deposits that accumulate between the RPE and inner layer of the Bruch's membrane and appear as pale yellow spots on the retina [38]. They are formed due to inability of the RPE to adequately perform its function of phagocytosis. Drusen can also be present in the normal aging eye. AMD can be classified into the following types based on the Age-Related Eye Disease Study (AREDS) classification system: (1) Early AMD—presence of few (<20) medium-sized drusen or retinal pigmentary abnormalities, (2) Intermediate AMD—presence of at least one large drusen, numerous medium-sized drusen, or geographic atrophy that does not extend to the center of the macula, (3) Advanced or late AMD—can either be neovascular (wet, exudative) or non-neovascular (dry, atrophic, non-exudative) [39]. Neovascular non-exudative is characterized by drusen and geographic atrophy that extends to the macula [37]. Neovascular exudative is characterized by the growth of new blood vessels under the RPE and sometimes into the sub-retinal space. The early stages of AMD are generally asymptomatic. In the later stages there may be distortion of vision or complete loss of visual function, especially central vision [40]. The pathogenesis of AMD is complex; however, the mechanisms of importance are chemical and light-induced oxidative stress, blue light induced damage to the RPE and photoreceptor rod cells, RPE dysfunction, hemodynamic processes, and also genetic factors. Age, family history, race, and female gender are considered to be non-modifiable risk factors of AMD. The modifiable risk factors include smoking, hypertension, raised serum cholesterol, excessive alcohol consumption, lifetime exposure to visible blue light, low MP levels, and possibly low intake of vitamins, minerals, and carotenoids in the diet [34, 41, 42].

Macular Pigment

Lutein and zeaxanthin are uniquely located in the fovea, which is the site of AMD insult. The association of MP density with AMD is biologically plausible given the ability of lutein and zeaxanthin to filter blue light and act as antioxidants protecting the retina from oxidative stress. Evidence shows that MP density decreases with AMD. Concentrations of lutein and zeaxanthin in the retinas from AMD donors were lower than in controls suggesting that low MP density could be a risk factor for AMD [43]. Subjects with advanced AMD in one eye had significantly lower MP density in the other eye compared to healthy eyes of subjects without AMD [44]. MP density was found to be 32% lower in the eyes of AMD patients compared to normal disease-free eyes [45]. However, in a cross-sectional study of women participating in the Carotenoids in Age-related Eye Disease Study (CAREDS) MP density was not related to intermediate AMD. After an exploratory analysis, the authors suggested that the observations may have been biased in older women, whose diets improved with age. The authors also suggested the possibility that low MP density could be the result, rather than the cause, of damage to the retina with AMD [46]. A similar observation was reported in a subset of the Rotterdam Eye Study, another cross-sectional study that examined MP density in subjects ≥55 years with or without AMD [47]. The reason for these conflicting observations may be the cross-sectional nature of the studies, as data from a prospective study found MP density to be reduced in subjects with late AMD [48]. Evidence that MP density is reduced in AMD suggests that higher dietary intake of lutein and zeaxanthin could increase their accumulation in the macula and thus protect against AMD.

Epidemiological Evidence

A number of studies have looked at the relationship between dietary intake of lutein and zeaxanthin and the risk of AMD. Three case–control studies showed high dietary intakes or plasma levels of lutein and zeaxanthin were related to reduced risk of advanced neovascular AMD [49–51]. In the Eye Disease Case–Control Study, subjects in the highest quintile of spinach consumption, a rich source of lutein and zeaxanthin had 86% lower odds of advanced AMD [50]. Case–control analysis of the AREDS population found that subjects in the highest quintile of lutein and zeaxanthin intake had lower odds of neovascular AMD and large or extensive intermediate drusen compared to the lowest quintile. Cross-sectional data from CAREDS showed that high lutein and zeaxanthin intakes (~3 mg/day) were related to a decreased risk of intermediate AMD compared to low intakes (792 μg/day) in women <75 years, who are at risk of diet changes, but not in women ≥75 years [52]. In this population of women <75 years of age, a strong inverse relationship was observed between prevalence of intermediate AMD and high intake of green vegetables (12 servings/day of cooked greens, lettuce, spinach salad, broccoli, peas, and zucchini squash). Prospective data from the Blue Mountains Eye Study (BMES) showed that high intake of lutein/zeaxanthin (>942 μg/day) reduced the risk of incident neovascular AMD and subjects with above median intakes (>743 μg/day) had a reduced risk of indistinct soft or reticular drusen during a 5–10-year follow-up [42]. Again, subjects in the highest quintile of vegetable intake in the BMES also had reduced odds of developing any AMD. However, the observations reported by Robman et al. were exactly the opposite. In this study, higher dietary intakes of lutein and zeaxanthin were related to increased rate of progression of AMD [53]. The study included subjects who had either participated in the Melbourne Visual Impairment Project (MVIP), a population-based study that evaluated the association of cataract and dietary intake of lutein and zeaxanthin or in the Vitamin E, Cataract, and Age-related Macular Degeneration Trial (VECAT), a randomized controlled trial that showed no effect of intake of 500 IU/day of vitamin E for 4 years on cataract. One of the possible reasons for greater AMD risk could be that these subjects started eating a diet high in lutein and zeaxanthin based on the knowledge of the beneficial effects of these xanthophylls gained by participating in the MVIP and VECAT. Also, high intake may not translate to higher retinal uptake as these AMD- and cataract-affected eyes may have impaired uptake mechanisms. Intake levels of 0.88–1 mg/day of lutein and zeaxanthin combined were associated with higher odds of AMD. In other studies, the levels of 1–3 mg/day of lutein alone or up to 6 mg/day of lutein and zeaxanthin combined were associated with reduced risk of AMD. Thus, it appears that the levels may have been too low to see a beneficial effect in eyes already affected with AMD and cataract.

In a case–control study in China, serum lutein and zeaxanthin concentrations were lower in subjects with exudative AMD compared to controls [54]. In a cross-sectional study, Gale et al. found that subjects with the lowest plasma zeaxanthin concentration (<0.03 μM), not plasma lutein or lutein plus zeaxanthin, had a twofold greater risk of AMD compared to subjects with high plasma zeaxanthin (>0.05 μM) [55]. Cross-sectional examination of the baseline data from the POLA study revealed similar associations of high plasma zeaxanthin concentrations (>0.09 μM) with reduced risk of AMD compared to low plasma zeaxanthin (<0.04 μM). They also reported an association with plasma lutein and zeaxanthin combined [56]. However, in the POLA study population, the high plasma zeaxanthin concentrations were much greater than in the Gale et al. study. The authors attributed this to a higher dietary intake of these xanthophylls. Contrary to these protective inverse associations, a nested case–control study of the Beaver Dam Eye Study cohort found no difference in serum lutein and zeaxanthin concentrations between early AMD and age, sex, and smoking matched controls [57]. Serum concentrations, unlike tissue concentration, are not a good measure of long-term dietary intake, which may have caused the null findings. Indeed, high retinal levels of lutein and zeaxanthin were associated with an 82% lower risk of AMD compared with low levels [43].

Intervention Studies

Epidemiological evidence listed earlier suggests that low MP density could increase the risk of AMD. The most apparent prevention and treatment strategy would thus be to increase MP density via increasing lutein and zeaxanthin intake in the diet through foods and/or supplements. Consumption of lutein- and zeaxanthin-rich foods such as spinach, corn, and eggs for periods ranging from 5 to 15 weeks has significantly increased MP density in a population aged 24–60 years and also in a population >60 years, who are at an increased risk of AMD [58–60]. However, in an ancillary study of the Women's Health Initiative, a low-fat, high fruit and vegetable diet for about 8 years did not alter MP density in postmenopausal women [61]. The increase in fruit and vegetable intake (approximately 1.5 servings/day) was possibly of insufficient magnitude to raise MP density. Additionally, subjects in the intervention group also appeared to have similar lutein and zeaxanthin intake (2.5 mg/day) as the comparison group (2 mg/day), indicating that the increase in consumption of fruits and vegetables was not necessarily from lutein- and zeaxanthin-rich foods [61].

In addition, MP density has been shown to significantly increase through intake of supplements containing lutein and zeaxanthin in adults without and with AMD [8, 62–69]. Bone et al. were the first to show that *meso*-zeaxanthin is absorbed by the body. They observed increases in serum *meso*-zeaxanthin and also MP density following 120 days of supplementation with 15 mg *meso*-zeaxanthin, 5.5 mg lutein, and 1.4 mg zeaxanthin [70]. Following this, in a recent exploratory study, improvements in MP density and MP spatial profile were reported after 2 weeks of supplementation with a formulation containing 3.7 mg lutein, 0.8 mg zeaxanthin, and 7.3 mg *meso*-zeaxanthin [71].

Change in MP density post-supplementation appears to be related to baseline MP density levels with supplementation being most beneficial in a population with low baseline MP density [59, 60, 72]. Zeimer et al. suggested that long-term supplementation with high doses of lutein may be necessary to cause a significant improvement in MP density, but lutein and zeaxanthin levels in foods are sufficient to maintain high MP density [63]. MP enrichment can also be achieved through intake of foods that are rich in lutein and zeaxanthin, such as spinach, corn, and eggs [58–60]. All studies listed above, with the exception of one, evaluated high doses of lutein supplementation (6, 10, 12, 20, or 30 mg/day), while zeaxanthin doses were lower (1–3 mg/day). The Lutein Xanthophyll Eye Accumulation Study (LUXEA) evaluated the effects of supplementation with lutein (11 mg/day) or zeaxanthin (13 mg/day) for 6 months on MP density. Increases in MP density in the fovea were similar to the parafovea for the zeaxanthin-supplemented group. This confounded MP density measurements because parafoveal measures are used as a reference measure. Therefore, a correction was needed to determine MP increases with zeaxanthin supplementation. This was not the case with lutein supplementation, which caused MP density increase in the fovea only [67]. These findings suggest zeaxanthin is deposited more widely in the retina during supplementation, while lutein accumulates more in the fovea. Normal distribution in unsupplemented individuals is the reverse, zeaxanthin is dominant in the fovea and lutein in the periphery [9]. The authors speculated that higher amounts of zeaxanthin in the fovea compared to lutein at baseline possibly caused greater zeaxanthin deposition in the parafoveal regions during supplementation. Similarly, the normally high lutein levels in the peripheral regions of the retina compared to zeaxanthin possibly caused greater deposition of lutein in the fovea during lutein supplementation.

Supplementation with lutein and zeaxanthin as well as *meso*-zeaxanthin can significantly improve MP density in populations without and with AMD. The ability of supplementation with these xanthophylls to slow the progression of AMD and/or influence other visual function parameters will now be discussed. In the Lutein Antioxidant Supplementation Trial (LAST), a double-blinded, placebo-controlled, randomized trial, 10 mg/day lutein alone or in combination with antioxidants, vitamins, and minerals for 1 year improved visual function and subjective results of Amsler grid testing in patients with atrophic AMD [66]. Improvements were also reported in glare recovery and contrast sensitivity in this study. In the Age-related Maculopathy Italian Study, nonadvanced AMD patients supplemented with 10 mg lutein, 1 mg zeaxanthin, and 4 mg astaxanthin together with vitamins C and E, zinc, and copper daily for 12 months showed improvements in a selective dysfunction that affects the central retina (0°–5°) but no functional changes were reported in the more peripheral (5°–20°) regions of the retina [73]. However, supplementation with 6 mg lutein in combination with vitamins C and E, retinol, zinc, and copper for 9 months did not affect contrast sensitivity in atrophic AMD patients when compared to controls [74]. The 6 mg lutein used in this study was in an ester form, which would be equivalent to only about 3 mg of lutein [75]. Also, the authors suggested that the change in contrast sensitivity was clinically important. The authors provided plausible explanations for their counterintuitive results, which include genetic factors that affect lutein binding proteins in the retina, lower dosage of lutein, and bioavailability of lutein esters. However, free lutein and lutein esters had comparable bioavailability [75]. Supplementation with 12 mg lutein and 1 mg zeaxanthin together with vitamins C and E, zinc, and selenium for 6 months significantly increased MP density in an older adult population, 90% of whom exhibited some clinical features of AMD [76]. The AREDS intervention of vitamin C (500 mg), vitamin E (400 IU), β-carotene (15 mg), zinc (as zinc oxide, 80 mg), and copper (as copper oxide, 2 mg), but not lutein or zeaxanthin, was found to lower the risk of AMD by 25% in individuals who had intermediate or advanced AMD in one eye but not the other eye [77]. The ongoing AREDS 2 intervention is evaluating the effect of lutein, zeaxanthin, and omega-3 fatty acids on progression to advanced AMD [78].

On a slightly different note, cataract surgery, where the natural crystalline lens is replaced with a clear artificial intraocular lens, is an independent risk factor of AMD [79, 80]. There is increased transmission of short wavelength light to the retina after cataract surgery and an induced intraocular inflammatory response; either or both of these could enhance AMD risk [81, 82]. Interestingly, implantation of a blue light filtering intraocular lens, not a standard intraocular lens, during cataract surgery increased MP density 3 months post-surgery in the absence of raised serum lutein and zeaxanthin concentrations [83]. The authors did not hypothesize an increase in MP density with blue light filtering lens, but only a stabilization of MP density. They speculate that there is enhanced retinal capture of lutein and zeaxanthin following cataract surgery to offset the increased photo-oxidative damage from the increased visible light irradiation of the retina, but the photo-oxidative damage does not occur with blue light filtering lens causing an increase in MP density.

Cataract

Age-related cataract is one of the major causes of visual impairment and blindness in the aging US population. Approximately 50% of the 30–50 million cases of worldwide blindness result from unoperated cataract [84, 85]. A clinically significant cataract is present in about 5% of Caucasian Americans aged 52–64 years and rises to 46% in those aged 75–85 years [36]. In the USA, cataract extraction accompanied by ocular lens implant is the most common surgical procedure of the eye [86]. Lens implantation enables many to have reduced dependence on glasses. However, the procedure is costly, accounting for 12% of the Medicare budget and more than $3 billion in annual health expenditures [86, 87]. For these reasons, the prevention of cataract is a preferred alternative to surgery.

Three types of cataract are defined by their location in the lens. Nuclear cataract occurs in the center or nucleus of the lens and is the most common type [36], which interferes with a person's ability to see distant objects and is usually the result of advancing age. Cortical cataract begins at the outer rim of the lens (the cortex) and progresses towards the center, and is most common in diabetics. Posterior subcapsular cataract (PSC) occurs in the central posterior cortex, just under the posterior capsule, the membrane that envelops the lens. PSC can occur in younger individuals progressing rapidly and resulting in glare and blurriness [88]. This type of cataract is usually seen in patients who use steroids, are diabetic, or have extreme nearsightedness. Figure 13.4 shows a scene viewed by a person affected with cataract.

Various factors are involved in the development of cataracts, such as long-term light exposure, diabetes, smoking, alcohol use, and advancing age [88]. Such factors can lead to aggregation of the lens proteins and osmotic damage resulting in increased scattering of light and loss of lens transparency. Protein aggregation mainly occurs in the lens nucleus and osmotic damage occurs in the lens cortex [89]. Free radicals are generated in the lens during normal metabolic activities and as a result of photo-oxidative reactions due to increased UVB exposure (related to cortical and PSC). These free radicals can also cause electrolyte imbalance and protein aggregation. Lutein and zeaxanthin are ideally located in the lens to provide protection against free radical damage. Other innate antioxidant defense mechanisms, which include enzymes such as superoxide dismutase and glutathione and non-enzymatic molecules such as vitamins C and E also protect the lens from oxidative stress.

Epidemiological Studies

A number of studies have investigated the relationship between dietary intake of lutein and zeaxanthin and the incidence of cataract. In prospective data from the Nurses' Health Study population, a significant reduction in the incidence of cataract extraction was observed with high dietary intake of dark green vegetables such as spinach, which are rich in lutein, but not with vegetables such as carrots, sweet potatoes, and squash, which are rich in carotenes [90]. The risk of cataract extraction was 19% lower in the US male health professionals who had the highest lutein and zeaxanthin intake compared to those with the lowest intake [91]. Again, broccoli and spinach were more consistently associated with reduced risk compared to iceberg and romaine lettuce and corn indicating a protective effect of lutein-rich foods. A similar inverse association was observed in a case–control study conducted in Northern Italy. In this study, reduced odds of cataract extraction were reported in subjects with the highest intake of cruciferous vegetables and spinach [92]. The evidence of a beneficial association between lutein and zeaxanthin intake and nuclear cataract seems promising. Higher dietary intake of lutein and zeaxanthin was associated with a reduced risk of nuclear cataract compared to low intakes [93, 94]. When examining specific foods, Christen et al. found a borderline significant inverse relation with green leafy vegetables and raw spinach. The MVIP found an inverse association between high dietary intake of lutein and zeaxanthin and prevalence of nuclear cataract, but not cortical and PSC in an Australian population aged 40 years and older [95]. Also, CAREDS found that women in the highest quintile of dietary intake or serum lutein and zeaxanthin were 32% less likely to have nuclear cataract compared to those in the lowest quintile [96]. In the prospective POLA study, plasma zeaxanthin, and not lutein, was associated with a 75% reduced risk of nuclear cataract in residents of Southern France [56]. Similarly, high zeaxanthin intake was protective against cataract in institutionalized men aged 65 years and older [97]. In the same study, men and women who consumed >3.29 mg/day of lutein were less likely to have cataracts than those whose consumption was <0.26 mg/day. Neither dietary intake nor plasma lutein and zeaxanthin were found to be related to cortical cataract risk [98–100]. Risk of PSC was 50% lower in women with the highest vs. lowest lutein/zeaxanthin intake and also in individuals with high plasma lutein/zeaxanthin concentrations [99, 101]. Among the epidemiological studies mentioned above, lutein and zeaxanthin intake in only one study included intake from both diet and supplements [98]; in the other studies, dietary intake represents lutein and zeaxanthin from food sources alone. Unlike the protective effects reported by other studies, the Beaver Dam Eye study reported an increased risk of nuclear cataract in women with high serum lutein levels [102]. This inconsistent finding may be due to the cross-sectional nature of the study or the fact that serum lutein may not reflect lutein levels in the lens [103].

Intervention Studies

Two intervention studies to date have evaluated the effect of lutein supplementation on subjects diagnosed with cataract. In these two separate long-term intervention studies, supplementation with 7 mg/day of lutein (equivalent to lutein in ~100 g of spinach [104]) and 12 mg of lutein three times a week was shown to improve visual acuity and glare sensitivity in cataract patients [105, 106]. Several randomized controlled trials have evaluated a combination of vitamins and micronutrients; the most frequently studied were vitamins C and E and β-carotene. The AREDS, the Antioxidants in the Prevention of Cataract (APC) study done in southern India, the Roche European American Cataract Trial (REACT), and the Alpha-tocopherol Beta-carotene (ATBC) study did not demonstrate beneficial effects of supplementation [107–110]. Reduction in lens opacity or nuclear cataract incidence with supplementation was observed in the US population of the REACT study, the Linxian study done in rural China, and the Italian Clinical Trial of Nutritional Supplements and Age-related cataract study [109, 111, 112]. However, the interventions used in these studies were a combination of multivitamins and minerals, which included β-carotene but not lutein and zeaxanthin. The ability of lutein and zeaxanthin to retard the development or progression of cataract or lens opacity has not been evaluated.

In conclusion, epidemiological studies provide strong evidence to suggest that long-term intake of dietary lutein and zeaxanthin may provide protection against the incidence of nuclear cataract, to a lesser extent PSC, but not cortical cataract. Most noteworthy is the fact that pharmacological doses are not necessary, because an adequate amount is found in foods such as spinach, kale, and broccoli.

Retinitis Pigmentosa

Retinitis pigmentosa (RP) is the leading cause of inherited blindness in the developed world, affecting 50,000–100,000 people in the USA and an estimated 1.5 million people worldwide [113, 114]. RP refers to a group of inherited retinal disorders that result in the degeneration of rod and cone photoreceptors [115]. Clinically, rod cell death translates to night blindness which generally precedes defects in peripheral visual field, i.e., tunnel vision (Fig. 13.4), by years or even decades. Cones are seldom directly affected by identified mutations. They degenerate secondarily to the rods as the disease progresses, which results in loss of central vision and complete blindness [113]. Many individuals with RP are not legally blind until their 40s or 50s and some RP patients even retain partial sight throughout life. On the other hand, some RP patients go completely blind during childhood.

RP can be inherited as an autosomal-dominant (30–40% of cases), autosomal-recessive (50–60%), or X-linked (5–15%) trait [115]. Mutations in the rhodopsin gene account for ~25% of dominant RP. Mutations in the USH2A gene may be the cause of ~20% of the recessive RP [116]. The USH2A gene encodes for the protein usherin and may be important for retinal development and maintaining homeostasis. Mutations in the GTPase regulator gene may account for ~70% of X-linked RP [115]. These mutations cause ~30% of all cases of RP. Mutations identified in other genes include: enzymes of the phototransduction cascade [transducin α-subunit, guanylate cyclase, cGMP-dependent phosphodiesterase, and arrestin]; structural or trafficking proteins [peripherin/RD, ABCR]; more rarely genes encoding proteins involved in vitamin A metabolism [CRALBP, RPE 65] and phagocytosis of photoreceptor outer segments [117–125]. Mutations affecting proteins involved in specific biochemical pathways that transduce light can cause hyperpolarization and apoptosis of the rod photoreceptor cells.

The high concentration of lutein and zeaxanthin in the ROS and also in the macula warrants their investigation in the treatment of RP. In a small, uncontrolled study of 13 RP patients and 3 patients with other retinal diseases, supplementation with 40 mg lutein/day for 9 weeks improved visual acuity and visual field area [126]. Lutein supplementation (10 mg/day for 12 weeks followed by 30 mg/day for 12 weeks) also improved central visual field in 34 RP patients in a randomized, cross-over, placebo-controlled, double-blinded study [127]. In another double-blinded, randomized control trial (RCT), nonsmoking RP patients supplemented with 12 mg/day of lutein along with 15,000 IU/day of vitamin A for 4 years had a slower decline in midperipheral visual field sensitivity compared to controls who were taking 15,000 IU/day of vitamin A [128]. Maximum slowing of midperipheral sensitivity also occurred among those with the highest serum lutein concentration and greatest increase in MP density and was not limited to those with milder disease. Unlike the previous two studies, no significant effect of this intervention was observed on central field sensitivity. The detectable benefit of lutein supplementation in preserving midperipheral function but not central function may reflect an increased requirement for antioxidants in the photoreceptor outer segments, where cells are most impaired. No toxic effects of lutein supplementation were observed in this study. No beneficial effect on central vision was observed in a small group of patients ($n=23$) with RP and Usher's syndrome who were supplemented with 20 mg lutein/day for 6 months [129]. MP density profile was not significantly different between controls and RP patients. MP density was related to foveal structure in RP patients compared with controls. MP density was lower in patients with reduced inner retinal thickness, suggesting that loss of inner retinal tissue is known to occur with outer retinal degenerations. Similar observations were made in a cross-sectional study that showed decreased MP density in eyes with more photoreceptor cell loss and in eyes with cystoid macular edema, which occurs in more than 25% of RP patients [130]. MP density increased in only half the subjects post-lutein supplementation of 20 mg/day for 6 months despite increases in serum lutein concentration [129]. The nonresponse in MP density may have been due to loss of photoreceptor cells or disruption of lutein uptake mechanisms in the macula [130]. Supplementation may have also caused increases in lutein levels in peripheral regions of the retina, which cannot be detected by heterochromatic flicker photometry. This is a noninvasive, psychophysical technique that can measure pigment density in the macular region only.

The evidence to date indicates that short-term lutein supplementation at doses of ≥30 mg/day or long-term supplementation at doses of 10–20 mg/day in combination with 15,000 IU/day of vitamin A may benefit central or midperipheral visual fields, respectively. Larger-scale placebo-controlled dose–response clinical studies are needed to derive more conclusive evidence of the benefits of lutein supplementation in specific types of RP. Preservation of central vision is necessary for preventing complete blindness in RP patients. Vitamins A and E and omega-3 fatty acids benefit RP patients [131–136]. More studies are needed to determine if lutein in combination with vitamin A and omega-3 fatty acids can help preserve central vision and also improve peripheral vision in RP patients.

Visual Function

The role of lutein and zeaxanthin as MP and also their importance in the retina and lens is now well-established. Data are also accumulating that suggest lutein and zeaxanthin as MP can improve visual function. There are two hypotheses that explain the mechanism by which MP improves visual function [137]. The acuity hypothesis states that MP reduces the effect of chromatic aberration. The visibility hypothesis states that MP may improve vision through the atmosphere by preferentially absorbing blue haze (short-wave dominant air light that produces a veiling luminance when viewing objects at a distance). MP may improve glare disability and photostress recovery because of its light filtering properties [138]. Some biological mechanisms, such as improvement in neuronal signaling efficiency in the eye, have also been suggested by which lutein and zeaxanthin may improve visual function [139].

High lutein and zeaxanthin intake improves MP density; therefore, it may improve visual function measures. Subjects from the LUXEA study, described in the AMD section, showed improved contrast acuity thresholds at high mesopic levels, which means better visual performance when ambient illumination is low [140]. Although increases in MP density were not related to contrast acuity thresholds, the results of this study suggest that lutein and zeaxanthin supplementation may benefit activities such as driving at night. Six months of supplementation with 12 mg/day of lutein was shown to increase MP density in healthy subjects with a mean age of 23 years and improve visual performance in glare function tests [141]. Lutein has been reported to protect against the detrimental effects of long-term computer display light exposure in healthy subjects aged 22–30 years of age [142]. In this study, 12 weeks of supplementation with 12 mg/day of lutein also improved contrast sensitivity. Lutein supplementation (5 mg) in combination with zeaxanthin (1 mg) and blackcurrant extract (200 mg) was also shown to reduce symptoms of visual fatigue associated with visual proof-reading tasks in healthy subjects aged 22–45 years [143].

The effect of lutein supplementation on visual performance was evaluated in patients with eye disease. In a double-blind, placebo-controlled study involving cataract patients ($n = 17$), supplementation with 15 mg lutein three times a week resulted in improved visual acuity and glare sensitivity [105]. In patients with retinal degeneration, lutein supplementation (20–40 mg/day, 26 weeks) improved visual acuity and mean visual field area, which began 2–4 weeks after the intervention but plateaued at 6–14 weeks [126]. RCTs involving AMD patients have shown that lutein supplementation, ranging in dose from 8 to 15 mg, improved dark adaptation, visual acuity, foveal sensitivity, contrast sensitivity, and glare recovery [66, 144, 145]. Evidence suggests that high MP density can improve visual function measures.

Conclusions

Epidemiological evidence suggests that high dietary intake of lutein and zeaxanthin is related to reduced risk of AMD. The majority of these studies evaluated neovascular or advanced AMD risk. Lower AMD risk was associated with higher consumption of lutein-rich dark green vegetables, such as spinach, broccoli, and lettuce, indicating supraphysiological doses may not be necessary for prevention. The lutein amounts in the high intake groups of epidemiological studies were 1–3 mg/day, while the lutein and zeaxanthin combined amount was ~6 mg/day. MP density can be augmented by consumption of lutein- and zeaxanthin-rich foods, such as spinach, eggs, and corn. Also, intake of high doses of lutein and *meso*-zeaxanthin supplements increases MP density. High dose zeaxanthin supplementation, however, may increase pigment levels in the peripheral regions of the retina and not necessarily in the macular region. Evidence suggests that increased MP density can be maintained by consumption of lutein- and zeaxanthin-rich foods. MP density can also be increased in AMD affected eyes. Long-term lutein supplementation at doses of 10 mg/day with or without supplementation with other antioxidants may improve visual function measures in AMD patients. Lutein and zeaxanthin have potential impact in the prevention and treatment of AMD.

Despite the limitations associated with evaluating dietary intakes, epidemiological studies have consistently shown high dietary intake of lutein and zeaxanthin to be protective against the incidence of nuclear cataract and cataract extraction. The most noteworthy is that among the different food groups evaluated, high intake of lutein-rich dark green vegetables, such as spinach and broccoli, was related to decreased cataract risk [90–94]. In the reviewed studies, high lutein and zeaxanthin amounts were 6 mg/day [91, 94], >3.2 mg/day [96, 97], and >1 mg/day [93, 95] and the corresponding low doses were 1 mg/day and 250–600 μg/day. The evidence of a beneficial effect of high lutein and zeaxanthin intake on PSC is very scarce and no associations have been observed with cortical cataract. More lutein and zeaxanthin intervention studies are necessary to provide convincing evidence that lutein and zeaxanthin can improve visual function in cataract patients.

Supplementation with high doses of lutein preserved central visual acuity in small RCTs on RP patients. Lutein in combination with 15,000 IU/day of vitamin A preserved midperipheral visual function. Both these findings indicate that lutein may play a role in preventing complete blindness in RP patients.

In 2006, the Food and Drug Administration reviewed all the epidemiological and clinical intervention studies on AMD and cataract and concluded that there is no credible evidence for a health claim about the intake of lutein or zeaxanthin (or both) on the risk of AMD and cataract [146]. In observational studies, lutein and zeaxanthin intake was calculated using food frequency questionnaires, diet recalls, or diet records, in which the type and amount of foods consumed was recorded. Lutein and zeaxanthin intake was then estimated from the USDA's database on carotenoid composition of foods. The limitations of these dietary assessment tools include subject's poor memory, overestimation or underestimation of portion sizes, the variation in lutein and zeaxanthin levels in the foods, the effect of consumption method (i.e., cooked vs. raw), type and amount of fat or fiber consumed with the lutein and zeaxanthin source, and other factors that affect bioavailability. Dietary assessments do not allow nutrients or food components to be studied in isolation, which may not yield the same findings. Thus, the findings of observational studies presented in this chapter must be interpreted with caution.

Future Directions

The evidence to date suggests that lutein and zeaxanthin can have a significant impact on AMD and cataract risk. Of note is that these are the only two carotenoids that are preferentially taken up into the retina and the lens. More randomized, controlled clinical trials are necessary to determine the dosage at which lutein and zeaxanthin interventions are most effective. In the case of AMD, it is evident that low MP density is one of the modifiable pre-disposing risk factors. MP density can be measured with ease using techniques such as heterochromatic flicker photometry, motion detection photometry, fundus reflectance spectroscopy, Raman spectrometry, and autofluorescence spectrometry [147].

Clinical models of these MP measurement devices are now available that could be potentially used by ophthalmologists to assess an individual's MP density as part of a routine eye examination. If low MP density is detected early in life, consumption of lutein- and zeaxanthin-rich foods can increase pigment levels and possibly prevent AMD development later in life. Future studies should focus on standardizing the clinical devices used for MP assessment and comparing measurements to other established techniques. Thus, there is scope of prevention of AMD through early identification of depleted MP levels in the retina. The majority of studies have focused on effects of lutein supplementation on MP enrichment. Supplementation with lutein or zeaxanthin alone seems to increase pigment density in different regions of the macula. One study showed supplementation with a high dose of zeaxanthin increased pigment levels more in the peripheral regions, which normally contain higher lutein levels. Future studies need to delve deeper into the differential effects of lutein and zeaxanthin supplementation on pigment enrichment and also functional effects. Studies should also be designed to evaluate different doses of lutein and zeaxanthin and also the impact of supplementation on different stages of AMD.

There is an urgent need to evaluate the effect of lutein and zeaxanthin intervention on progression of cataract, especially because epidemiological evidence showed a positive effect of high lutein and zeaxanthin intake on nuclear cataract. Nuclear cataract is the result of advancing age; thus, consuming a lutein- and zeaxanthin-rich diet early in life may possibly prevent incidence. Large-scale studies are required to evaluate the effect of lutein intervention in the preservation of vision in RP patients to prevent the incidence of blindness.

Other than their role in eye disease prevention and visual function, lutein and zeaxanthin may influence neural functions within the retina and enhance gap junctional communication, which in the retina is crucial for light processing and may be important for the development of neural circuitry within the visual system [148]. High MP density has been associated with improved visual processing speed, which is measured as critical flicker fusion threshold [149, 150]. MP density was shown to be inversely related to scotopic noise; lutein and zeaxanthin may thus improve efficiency of rod cell functioning [151, 152]. The exclusive accumulation of lutein and zeaxanthin in the neural retina warrants further investigation of their role in modifying neural functions.

References

1. Britton G. Structure and properties of carotenoids in relation to function. FASEB J. 1995;9(15):1551–8.
2. Krinsky NI, Landrum JT, Bone RA. Biologic mechanism of the protective role of lutein and zeaxanthin in the eye. Annu Rev Nutr. 2003;23:171–201.
3. Li B, Vachali P, Bernstein PS. Human ocular carotenoid-binding proteins. Photochem Photobiol Sci. 2010;9(11): 1418–25.
4. Frederick K. Distribution and metabolism of dietary carotenoids in humans as a criterion for development of nutritional supplements. Pure Appl Chem. 2006;78(8):7.
5. Ahmed SS, Lott MN, Marcus DM. The macular xanthophylls. Surv Ophthalmol. 2005;50(2):183–93.
6. Johnson EJ, Neuringer M, Russell RM, Schalch W, Snodderly DM. Nutritional manipulation of primate retinas. III: Effects of lutein or zeaxanthin supplementation on adipose tissue and retina of xanthophyll-free monkeys. Invest Ophthalmol Vis Sci. 2005;46(2):692–702.
7. Bone RA, Landrum JT, Friedes LM, et al. Distribution of lutein and zeaxanthin stereoisomers in the human retina. Exp Eye Res. 1997;64(2):211–8.
8. Landrum JT, Bone RA, Sprague K, Moore L. A one-year study of supplementation with lutein on the macular pigment. Exp Eye Res. 1997;65:57–62.

9. Bone RA, Landrum JT, Fernandez L, Tarsis SL. Analysis of the macular pigment by HPLC: retinal distribution and age study. Invest Ophthalmol Vis Sci. 1988;29:843–9.
10. Handelman GJ, Dratz EA, Reay CC, van Kuijk JG. Carotenoids in the human macula and whole retina. Invest Ophthalmol Vis Sci. 1988;29(6):850–5.
11. Algvere PV, Marshall J, Seregard S. Age-related maculopathy and the impact of blue light hazard. Acta Ophthalmol Scand. 2006;84(1):4–15.
12. Snodderly DM, Auran JD, Delori FC. The macular pigment. II. Spatial distribution in primate retinas. Invest Ophthalmol Vis Sci. 1984;25:12.
13. Landrum JT, Bone RA. Lutein, zeaxanthin, and the macular pigment. Arch Biochem Biophys. 2001; 385(1):28–40.
14. Bone RA, Landrum JT. Macular pigment in henle fiber membranes: a model for Haidinger's brushes. Vision Res. 1984;24(2):103–8.
15. Rapp LM, Maple SS, Choi JH. Lutein and zeaxanthin concentrations in rod outer segment membranes from perifoveal and peripheral human retina. Invest Ophthalmol Vis Sci. 2000;41(5):1200–9.
16. Sommerburg LG, Siems WG, Hurst JS, Lewis JW, van Kuijk FJGM. Lutein and zeaxanthin are associated with photoreceptors in the human retina. Curr Eye Res. 1999;19:491–5.
17. Li B, Vachali P, Frederick JM, Bernstein PS. Identification of StARD3 as a lutein-binding protein in the macula of the primate retina. Biochemistry. 2011;50(13):2541–9.
18. Bhosale P, Zhao DY, Bernstein PS. HPLC measurement of ocular carotenoid levels in human donor eyes in the lutein supplementation era. Invest Ophthalmol Vis Sci. 2007;48(2):543–9.
19. Yeum K-J, Shang F, Schalch W, Russell RM, Taylor A. Fat-soluble nutrient concentrations in different layers of human cataractous lens. Curr Eye Res. 1999;19(6):502–5.
20. Yeum KJ, Ahn SH, Rupp de Paiva SA, Lee Kim YC, Krinsky NI, Russell RM. Correlation between carotenoid concentrations in serum and normal breast adipose tissue of women with benign breast tumor or cancer. J Nutr. 1998;128:1920–6.
21. Khachik F, Spangler CJ, Smith Jr JC, Canfield LM, Steck A, Pfander H. Identification, quantificantion, and relative concentrations of carotenoids and their metabolites in human milk and serum. Anal Chem. 1997;69(10):7.
22. Leo MA, Ahmed S, Aleynik SI, Siegel JH, Kasmin F, Lieber CS. Carotenoids and tocopherols in various hepatobiliary conditions. J Hepatol. 1995;23(5):550–6.
23. Peng YM, Peng YS, Lin Y. A nonsaponification method for the determination of carotenoids, retinoids, and tocopherols in solid human tissues. Cancer Epidemiol Biomarkers Prev. 1993;2(2):6.
24. Furr HC, Clark RM. Intestinal absorption and tissue distribution of carotenoids. J Nutr Biochem. 1997;8(7):364–77.
25. Craft NE, Haitema TB, Garnett KM, Fitch KA, Dorey CK. Carotenoid, tocopherol, and retinol concentrations in elderly human brain. J Nutr Health Aging. 2004;8:156–62.
26. Demmig-Adams B, Adams WW. Antioxidants in photosynthesis and human nutrition. Science. 2002;298(5601): 2149–53.
27. Kim Y-S, Oh D-K. Biotransformation of carotenoids to retinal by carotenoid 15,15′-oxygenase. Appl Microbiol Biotechnol. 2010;88(4):807–16.
28. Junghans A, Sies H, Stahl W. Macular pigments lutein and zeaxanthin as blue light filters studied in liposomes. Arch Biochem Biophys. 2001;391:160–4.
29. Snodderly DM, Auran JD, Delori FC. The macular pigment. II. Spatial distribution in primate retinas. Invest Ophthalmol Vis Sci. 1984;25(6):674–85.
30. Sujak A, Gabrielska J, Grudzinski W, Borc R, Mazurek P, Gruszecki WI. Lutein and zeaxanthin as protectors of lipid membranes against oxidative damage: the structual evidence. Arch Biochem Biophys. 1999;371(2):301–7.
31. Khachik F, Bernstein PS, Garland DL. Identification of lutein and zeaxanthin oxidation products in human and monkey retinas. Invest Ophthalmol Vis Sci. 1997;38(9):1802–11.
32. Haegerstrom-Portney G. Short-wavelength-sensitive-cone sensitivity loss with aging: a protective role for macular pigment? J Opt Soc Am A. 1988;5:2140–4.
33. Ojima F, Sakamoto H, Ishiguro Y, Terao J. Consumption of carotenoids in photosensitized oxidation of human plasma and plasma low-density lipoprotein. Free Radic Biol Med. 1993;15(4):377–84.
34. Nolan J, O'Donovan O, Beatty S. The role of macular pigment in the defence against AMD. AMD. 2003;39–41.
35. Bernstein PS, Khachik F, Carvalho LS, et al. Identification and quantitation of carotenoids and their metabolites in the tissues of the human eye. Exp Eye Res. 2001;72:215–23.
36. Congdon N, O'Colmain B, Klaver CCW, et al. Causes and prevalence of visual impairment among adults in the United States. Arch Ophthalmol. 2004;122(4):477–85.
37. Jager RD, Mieler WF, Miller JW. Age-related macular degeneration. N Engl J Med. 2008;358(24):2606–17.
38. Abdelsalam A, Del Priore L, Zarbin MA. Drusen in age-related macular degeneration: pathogenesis, natural course, and laser photocoagulation-induced regression. Surv Ophthalmol. 1999;44(1):1–29.

39. Age-related Eye Disease Study Research Group. A simplified severity scale for age-related macular degeneration. AREDS report No. 18. Arch Ophthalmol. 2005;123(11):5.
40. Snodderly DM. Evidence for protection against age-related macular degeneration by carotenoids and antioxidant vitamins. Am J Clin Nutr. 1995;62(6 Suppl):1448S–61.
41. Ambati J, Ambati BK, Yoo SH, Ianchulev S, Adamis AP. Age-related macular degeneration: etiology, pathogenesis, and therapeutic strategies. Surv Ophthalmol. 2003;48(3):257–93.
42. Tan JSL, Wang JJ, Flood V, Rochtchina E, Smith W, Mitchell P. Dietary antioxidants and the long-term incidence of age-related macular degeneration: the Blue Mountains Eye Study. Ophthalmology. 2008;115(2):334–41.
43. Bone RA, Landrum JT, Mayne ST, Gomez CM, Tibor SE, Twaroska EE. Macular pigment in donor eyes with and without AMD: a case-control study. Invest Ophthalmol Vis Sci. 2001;42(1):235–40 [Erratum appears in Invest Ophthalmol Vis Sci 2001 Mar;42(3):548].
44. Beatty S, Murray IJ, Henson DB, Carden D, Koh H, Boulton ME. Macular pigment and risk for age-related macular degeneration in subjects from a Northern European population. Invest Ophthalmol Vis Sci. 2001; 42(2):439–46.
45. Bernstein PS, Shao D-Y, Wintch SW. Resonance Raman measurement of macular carotenoids in normal subjects and in age-related macular degeneration patients. Ophthalmology. 2002;109:1780–7.
46. LaRowe TL, Mares JA, Snodderly DM, et al. Macular pigment density and age-related maculopathy in the Carotenoids in Age-Related Eye Disease Study. An ancillary study of the women's health initiative. Ophthalmology. 2008;115(5):876–83. e871.
47. Berendschot TTJM, Willemse-Assink JJM, Bastiaanse M, de Jong PTVM, van Norren D. Macular pigment and melanin in age-related maculopathy in a general population. Invest Ophthalmol Vis Sci. 2002;43(6):1928–32.
48. Schweitzer D, Lang GE, Remsch H, et al. Age-related maculopathy. Comparative studies of patients, their children and healthy controls. (German). Ophthalmologe. 2000;97:84–90.
49. Eye Disease Case-Control Study Group (EDCCSG). Antioxidant status and neovascular age-related macular degeneration. Arch Ophthalmol. 1993;111:104–9.
50. Seddon JM, Ajani UA, Sperduto RD, et al. Dietary carotenoids, vitamins A, C, and E, and advanced age-related macular degeneration. Eye Disease Case-Control Study Group. JAMA. 1994;272(18):1413–20.
51. Snellen EL, Verbeek AL, Van Den Hoogen GW, Cruysberg JR, Hoyng CB. Neovascular age-related macular degeneration and its relationship to antioxidant intake. Acta Ophthalmol Scand. 2002;80(4):368–71.
52. Moeller SM, Parekh N, Tinker L, et al. Associations between intermediate age-related macular degeneration and lutein and zeaxanthin in the Carotenoids in Age-related Eye Disease Study (CAREDS): ancillary study of the Women's Health Initiative. Arch Ophthalmol. 2006;124(8):1151–62.
53. Robman L, Vu H, Hodge A, et al. Dietary lutein, zeaxanthin, and fats and the progression of age-related macular degeneration. Can J Ophthalmol. 2007;42(5):7.
54. Zhou H, Zhao X, Johnson EJ, et al. Serum carotenoids and risk of age-related macular degeneration in a Chinese population sample. Invest Ophthalmol Vis Sci. 2011;52:4338–44.
55. Gale CR, Hall NF, Phillips DIK, Martyn CN. Lutein and zeaxanthin status and risk of age-related macular degeneration. Invest Ophthalmol Vis Sci. 2003;44:2461–5.
56. Delcourt C, Carrière I, Delage M, Barberger-Gateau P, Schalch W, POLA Study Group. Plasma lutein and zeaxanthin and other carotenoids as modifiable risk factors for age-related maculopathy and cataract: the POLA study. Invest Ophthalmol Vis Sci. 2006;47(6):2329–35.
57. Mares-Perlman JA, Brady WE, Klein R, et al. Serum antioxidants and age-related macular degeneration in a population-based case-control study. Arch Ophthalmol. 1995;113(12):1518–23.
58. Hammond Jr BR, Johnson EJ, Russell RM, et al. Dietary modification of human macular pigment density. Invest Ophthalmol Vis Sci. 1997;38:1795–801.
59. Wenzel AJ, Gerweck C, Barbato D, Nicolosi RJ, Handelman GJ, Curran-Celentano J. A 12-wk egg intervention increases serum zeaxanthin and macular pigment optical density in women. J Nutr. 2006;136(10):2568–73.
60. Vishwanathan R, Goodrow-Kotyla EF, Wooten BR, Wilson TA, Nicolosi RJ. Consumption of 2 and 4 egg yolks/d for 5 wk increases macular pigment concentrations in older adults with low macular pigment taking cholesterol-lowering statins. Am J Clin Nutr. 2009;90(5):1272–9.
61. Moeller SM, Voland R, Sarto GE, Gobel VL, Streicher SL, Mares JA. Women's health initiative diet intervention did not increase macular pigment optical density in an ancillary study of a subsample of the women's health initiative. J Nutr. 2009;139(9):1692–9.
62. Bone RA, Landrum JT. Dose-dependent response of serum lutein and macular pigment optical density to supplementation with lutein esters. Arch Biochem Biophys. 2010;504(1):50–5.
63. Zeimer M, Hense HW, Heimes B, Austermann U, Fobker M, Pauleikhoff D. The macular pigment: short- and intermediate-term changes of macular pigment optical density following supplementation with lutein and zeaxanthin and co-antioxidants. The LUNA Study. Ophthalmologe. 2009;106(1):29–36.
64. Johnson EJ, Chung H-Y, Caldarella SM, Snodderly DM. The influence of supplemental lutein and docosahexaenoic acid on serum, lipoproteins, and macular pigmentation. Am J Clin Nutr. 2008;87(5):1521–9.

65. Wenzel AJ, Sheehan JP, Gerweck C, Stringham JM, Fuld K, Curran-Celentano J. Macular pigment optical density at four retinal loci during 120 days of lutein supplementation. Ophthalmic Physiol Opt. 2007;27(4):329–35.
66. Richer S, Stiles W, Statkute L, et al. Double masked, placebo-controlled, randomized trial of lutein and antioxidant supplementation in the intervention of atrophic age-related macular degeneration: the Veteran's LAST study (Lutein Antioxidant Supplementation Trial). Optometry. 2004;75:216–30.
67. Schalch W, Cohn W, Barker FM, et al. Xanthophyll accumulation in the human retina during supplementation with lutein or zeaxanthin—the LUXEA (LUtein Xanthophyll Eye Accumulation) study. Arch Biochem Biophys. 2007;458:128–35.
68. Koh H-H, Murray IJ, Nolan D, Carden D, Feather J, Beatty S. Plasma and macular responses to lutein supplement in subjects with and without age-related maculopathy: a pilot study. Exp Eye Res. 2004;79(1):21–7.
69. Bone RA, Landrum JT, Guerra LH, Ruiz CA. Lutein and zeaxanthin dietary supplements raise macular pigment density and serum concentrations of these carotenoids in humans. J Nutr. 2003;133:992–8.
70. Bone RA, Landrum JT, Cao Y, Howard AN, Alvarez-Calderon F. Macular pigment response to a supplement containing *meso*-zeaxanthin, lutein and zeaxanthin. Nutr Metab (Lond). 2007;4:12.
71. Connolly EE, Beatty S, Thurnham DI, et al. Augmentation of macular pigment following supplementation with all three macular carotenoids: an exploratory study. Curr Eye Res. 2010;35(4):335–51.
72. Richer S, Devenport J, Lang JC. LAST II: differential temporal responses of macular pigment optical density in patients with atrophic age-related macular degeneration to dietary supplementation with xanthophylls. Optometry. 2007;78(5):213–9.
73. Parisi V, Tedeschi M, Gallinaro G, Varano M, Saviano S, Piermarocchi S. Carotenoids and antioxidants in age-related maculopathy Italian study: multifocal electroretinogram modifications after 1 year. Ophthalmology. 2008;115(2):324–33. e322.
74. Bartlett HE, Eperjesi F. Effect of lutein and antioxidant dietary supplementation on contrast sensitivity in age-related macular disease: a randomized controlled trial. Eur J Clin Nutr. 2007;61(9):1121–7.
75. Chung H-Y, Rasmussen HM, Johnson EJ. Lutein bioavailability is higher from lutein-enriched eggs than from supplements and spinach in men. J Nutr. 2004;134(8):1887–93.
76. Trieschmann M, Beatty S, Nolan JM, et al. Changes in macular pigment optical density and serum concentrations of its constituent carotenoids following supplemental lutein and zeaxanthin: The LUNA study. Exp Eye Res. 2007;84(4):718–28.
77. Age-Related Eye Disease Study Research Group. A randomized, placebo-controlled, clinical trial of high-dose supplementation with vitamins C and E, beta carotene, and zinc for age-related macular degeneration and vision loss: AREDS report no. 8. Arch Ophthalmol. 2001;119(10):1417–36 [Erratum appears in Arch Ophthalmol. 2008;126(9):1251].
78. Age-related Eye Disease Study. AREDS 2. www.areds2.org. Accessed 10 June 2011.
79. Cugati S, Mitchell P, Rochtchina E, Tan AG, Smith W, Wang JJ. Cataract surgery and the 10-year incidence of age-related maculopathy: the Blue Mountains Eye study. Ophthalmology. 2006;113(11):2020–5.
80. Wang JJ, Klein R, Smith W, Klein BEK, Tomany S, Mitchell P. Cataract surgery and the 5-year incidence of late-stage age-related maculopathy: pooled findings from the Beaver Dam and Blue Mountains Eye Studies. Ophthalmology. 2003;110(10):1960–7.
81. Brockmann C, Schulz M, Laube T. Transmittance characteristics of ultraviolet and blue-light-filtering intraocular lenses. J Cataract Refract Surg. 2008;34(7):1161–6.
82. Gaillard ER, Zheng L, Merriam JC, Dillon J. Age-related changes in the absorption characteristics of the primate lens. Invest Ophthalmol Vis Sci. 2000;41(6):1454–9.
83. Nolan JM, O'Reilly P, Loughman J, et al. Augmentation of macular pigment following implantation of blue light-filtering intraocular lenses at the time of cataract surgery. Invest Ophthalmol Vis Sci. 2009;50(10):4777–85.
84. World Health Organization. Use of intraocular lenses in cataract surgery in developing countries. Bull World Health Organ. 1991;69:657–66.
85. Thylefors B, Negrel AD, Pararajasegaram R, Dadzie KY. Global data on blindness. Bull World Health Organ. 1995;69:115–21.
86. Javitt JC. Who does cataract surgery in the United States? Arch Ophthalmol. 1993;111:1329.
87. Steinberg EP, Javitt JC, Sharkey PD, et al. The content and cost of cataract surgery. Arch Ophthalmol. 1993;111:1041–9.
88. Asbell PA, Dualan I, Mindel J, Brocks D, Ahmad M, Epstein S. Age-related cataract. Lancet. 2005;365(9459):599–609.
89. Bunce GE, Kinoshita J, Horwitz J. Nutritional factors in cataract. Annu Rev Nutr. 1990;10(1):233–54.
90. Hankinson SE, Stampfer MJ, Seddon JM, et al. Nutrient intake and cataract extraction in women: a prospective study. BMJ. 1992;305:244–51.
91. Brown L, Rimm EB, Seddon JM, et al. A prospective study of carotenoid intake and risk of cataract extraction in US men. Am J Clin Nutr. 1999;70:517–24.
92. Tavani A, Negri E, LaVeccia C. Food and nutrient intake and risk of cataract. Ann Epidemiol. 1996;6:41–6.

93. Lyle B, Mares-Perlman JA, Klein BEK, Klein R, Gregor JL. Antioxidant intake and risk of incident of age-related nuclear cataracts in the Beaver Dam Eye Study. Am J Epidemiol. 1999;149:801–9.
94. Christen WG, Liu S, Glynn RJ, Gaziano JM, Buring JE. Dietary carotenoids, vitamins C and E, and risk of cataract in women: a prospective study. Arch Ophthalmol. 2008;126(1):102–9.
95. Vu HTV, Robman L, Hodge A, McCarty CA, Taylor HR. Lutein and zeaxanthin and the risk of cataract: the Melbourne visual impairment project. Invest Ophthalmol Vis Sci. 2006;47(9):3783–6.
96. Moeller SM, Voland R, Tinker L, et al. Associations between age-related nuclear cataract and lutein and zeaxanthin in the diet and serum in the carotenoids in the age-related eye disease study (CAREDS), an ancillary study of the women's health initiative. Arch Ophthalmol. 2008;126(3):354–64.
97. Rodriguez RE, Ortega RM, Lopez-Sobaler AM, Aparicio A, Bermejo LM, Marin-Arias LI. The relationship between antioxidant nutrient intake and cataracts in older people. Int J Vitam Nutr Res. 2006;76(6):8.
98. Taylor A, Jacques PF, Chylack Jr LT, et al. Long-term intake of vitamins and carotenoids and odds of early age-related cortical and posterior subcapsular lens opacities. Am J Clin Nutr. 2002;75(3):540–9.
99. Gale CR, Hall NF, Phillips DIK, Martyn CN. Plasma antioxidant vitamins and carotenoids and age-related cataract. Ophthalmology. 2001;108:1992–8.
100. Vitale S, West S, Hallfrisch J, et al. Plasma antioxidants and risk of cortical and nuclear cataract. Epidemiology. 1993;4:195–203.
101. Chasen-Taber L, Willett WC, Seddon JM, et al. A prospective study of carotenoid and vitamin A intakes and risk of cataract extraction in US women. Am J Clin Nutr. 1999;70:517–24.
102. Mares-Perlman JA, Brady WE, Klein BE, et al. Serum carotenoids and tocopherols and severity of nuclear and cortical opacities. Invest Ophthalmol Vis Sci. 1995;36:276–88.
103. Moeller SM, Jacques PF, Blumberg JB. The potential role of dietary xanthophylls in cataract and age-related macular degeneration. J Am Coll Nutr. 2000;19(5 Suppl):522S–7.
104. USDA, ARS. National Nutrient Database for Standard Reference, Release 19. Nutrient Data Laboratory Home Page. 2006.
105. Olmedilla B, Granado F, Blanco I, Vaquero M. Lutein, but not alpha-tocopherol, supplementation improves visual function in patients with age-related cataracts: a 2-y double-blind, placebo-controlled pilot study. Nutrition. 2003;19(1):21–4.
106. Olmedilla B, Granado F, Blanco I, Vaquero M, Cajigal C. Lutein in patients with cataracts and age-related macular degeneration: a long-term supplementation study. J Sci Food Agric. 2001;81:904–9.
107. Age-Related Eye Disease Study Research Group. A randomized, placebo-controlled, clinical trial of high-dose supplementation with vitamins C and E and beta carotene for age-related cataract and vision loss: AREDS report no. 9. Arch Ophthalmol. 2001;119(10):1439–52 [Erratum appears in Arch Ophthalmol. 2008 Sep;126(9):1251].
108. Gritz DC, Srinivasan M, Smith SD, et al. The antioxidants in prevention of cataracts study: effects of antioxidant supplements on cataract progression in south India. Br J Ophthalmol. 2006;90(7):847–51.
109. Chylack LTJ, Brown NB, Bron A, et al. The Roche European American Cataract Trial (REACT): a randomized clinical trial to investigate the efficiency of a antioxidant micronutrient mixture to slow progression of age-related cataract. Ophthalmic Epidemiol. 2002;9:49–80.
110. Teikari JM, Virtamo J, Rautalahti M, Palmgren J, Liesto K, Heinonen OP. Long-term supplementation with alpha-tocopherol and beta-carotene and age-related cataract. Acta Ophthalmol Scand. 1997;75(6):634–40.
111. Sperduto RD, Hu TS, Milton RC, et al. The Linxian cataract studies. Two nutrition intervention trials. Arch Ophthalmol. 1993;111(9):1246–53.
112. Clinical Trial of Nutritional Supplements and Age-Related Cataract Study Group, Maraini G, Sperduto RD, et al. A randomized, double-masked, placebo-controlled clinical trial of multivitamin supplementation for age-related lens opacities. Clinical trial of nutritional supplements and age-related cataract report no. 3. Ophthalmology. 2008;115(4):599–607. e591.
113. Delyfer M-N, Léveillard T, Mohand-Saïd S, Hicks D, Picaud S, Sahel J-A. Inherited retinal degenerations: therapeutic prospects. Biol Cell. 2004;96(4):261–9.
114. Berson EL. Nutrition and retinal degenerations. Int Ophthalmol Clin. 2000;40(4):93–111.
115. Hartong DT, Berson EL, Dryja TP. Retinitis pigmentosa. Lancet. 2006;368:1795–809.
116. Liu X, Bulgakov OV, Darrow KN, et al. Usherin is required for maintenance of retinal photoreceptors and normal development of cochlear hair cells. Proc Natl Acad Sci U S A. 2007;104(11):4413–8.
117. Dryja TP, Hahn LB, Reboul T, Arnaud B. Missense mutation in the gene encoding the alpha subunit of rod transducin in the Nougaret form of congenital stationary night blindness. Nat Genet. 1996;13(3):358–60.
118. Perrault I, Rozet JM, Calvas P, et al. Retinal-specific guanylate cyclase gene mutations in Leber's congenital amaurosis. Nat Genet. 1996;14(4):461–4.
119. McLaughlin ME, Sandberg MA, Berson EL, Dryja TP. Recessive mutations in the gene encoding the beta-subunit of rod phosphodiesterase in patients with retinitis pigmentosa. Nat Genet. 1993;4(2):130–4.

120. Fuchs S, Nakazawa M, Maw M, Tamai M, Oguchi Y, Gal A. A homozygous 1-base pair deletion in the arrestin gene is a frequent cause of Oguchi disease in Japanese. Nat Genet. 1995;10(3):360–2.
121. Dryja TP, Hahn LB, Kajiwara K, Berson EL. Dominant and digenic mutations in the peripherin/RDS and ROM1 genes in retinitis pigmentosa. Invest Ophthalmol Vis Sci. 1997;38(10):1972–82.
122. Allikmets R. Simple and complex ABCR: Genetic predisposition to retinal disease. Am J Hum Genet. 2000;67(4):793–9.
123. Maw MA, Kennedy B, Knight A, et al. Mutation of the gene encoding cellular retinaldehyde-binding protein in autosomal recessive retinitis pigmentosa. Nat Genet. 1997;17(2):198–200.
124. Marlhens F, Bareil C, Griffoin JM, et al. Mutations in RPE65 cause Leber's congenital amaurosis. Nat Genet. 1997;17(2):139–41.
125. D'Cruz PM, Yasumura D, Weir J, et al. Mutation of the receptor tyrosine kinase gene Mertk in the retinal dystrophic RCS rat. Hum Mol Genet. 2000;9(4):645–51.
126. Dagnelie G, Zorge IS, McDonald TM. Lutein improves visual function in some patients with retinal regeneration: a pilot study via the internet. Optom Vis Sci. 2000;71:147–64.
127. Bahrami H, Melia M, Dagnelie G. Lutein supplementation in retinitis pigmentosa: PC-based vision assessment in a randomized double-masked placebo-controlled clinical trial [NCT00029289]. BMC Ophthalmol. 2006;6(1):23.
128. Berson EL, Rosner B, Sandberg MA, et al. Clinical trial of lutein in patients with retinitis pigmentosa receiving vitamin A. Arch Ophthalmol. 2010;128(4):403–11.
129. Aleman TS, Duncan JL, Bieber ML, et al. Macular pigment and lutein supplementation in retinitis pigmentosa and usher syndrome. Invest Ophthalmol Vis Sci. 2001;42(8):1873–81.
130. Sandberg MA, Johnson EJ, Berson EL. The relationship of macular pigment optical density to serum lutein in retinitis pigmentosa. Invest Ophthalmol Vis Sci. 2010;51(2):1086–91.
131. Berson EL, Rosner B, Sandberg MA, et al. A randomized trial of vitamin A and vitamin E supplementation for retinitis pigmentosa. Arch Ophthalmol. 1993;111(6):761–72.
132. Berson EL, Rosner B, Sandberg MA, et al. Vitamin A supplementation for retinitis pigmentosa. Arch Ophthalmol. 1993;111(11):1456–9.
133. Bishara S, Merin S, Cooper M, Azizi E, Delpre G, Deckelbaum RJ. Combined vitamin A and E therapy prevents retinal electrophysiological deterioration in abetalipoproteinaemia. Br J Ophthalmol. 1982;66(12):767–70.
134. Yokota T, Shiojiri T, Gotoda T, Arai H. Retinitis pigmentosa and ataxia caused by a mutation in the gene for the α-tocopherol-transfer protein. N Engl J Med. 1996;335(23):1770–1.
135. Berson EL, Rosner B, Sandberg MA, et al. Clinical trial of docosahexaenoic acid in patients with retinitis pigmentosa receiving vitamin A treatment. Arch Ophthalmol. 2004;122(9):1297–305.
136. Berson EL, Rosner B, Sandberg MA, et al. Further evaluation of docosahexaenoic acid in patients with retinitis pigmentosa receiving vitamin A treatment: subgroup analyses. Arch Ophthalmol. 2004;122(9):1306–14.
137. Wooten BR, Hammond BR. Macular pigment: influences on visual acuity and visibility. Prog Retin Eye Res. 2002;21(2):225–40.
138. Stringham JM, Hammond BR. The glare hypothesis for macular pigment function. Optom Vis Sci. 2007;84(9):859–64.
139. Stringham JM, Hammond Jr BR. Dietary lutein and zeaxanthin: possible effects on visual function. Nutr Rev. 2005;63(2):59–64.
140. Kvansakul J, Rodriguex-Carmona M, Edgar D, Barker FM, Kopcke W, Barbur JL. Supplementation with the carotenoids lutein or zeaxanthin improves human visual performance. Ophthalmic Physiol Opt. 2006;26:362–71.
141. Stringham JM, Hammond BR. Macular pigment and visual performance under glare conditions. Optom Vis Sci. 2008;85:82–8.
142. Ma L, Lin X-M, Zou Z-Y, Xu X-R, Li Y, Xu R. A 12-week lutein supplementation improves visual function in Chinese people with long-term computer display light exposure. Br J Nutr. 2009;102(2):186–90.
143. Yagi A, Fujimoto K, Michihiro K, Goh B, Tsi D, Nagai H. The effect of lutein supplementation on visual fatigue: a psychophysiological analysis. Appl Ergon. 2009;40:1047–54.
144. Falsini B, Piccardi M, Iarossi G, Fadda A, Merendino E, Valentini P. Influence of short-term antioxidant supplementation on macular function in age-related maculopathy: a pilot study including electrophysiologic assessment. Ophthalmology. 2003;110(1):51–60. discussion 61.
145. Cangemi FE. TOZAL study: an open case-control study of an oral antioxidant and omega-3 supplement for dry AMD. BMC Ophthalmol. 2007;7:3.
146. Trumbo PR, Ellwood KC. Lutein and zeaxanthin intakes and risk of age-related macular degeneration and cataracts: an evaluation using the Food and Drug Administration's evidence-based review system for health claims. Am J Clin Nutr. 2006;84(5):971–4.
147. Leung IYF. Macular pigment: new clinical methods of detection and the role of carotenoids in age-related macular degeneration. Optometry. 2008;79(5):266–72.

148. Stahl W, Seis H. Effects of carotenoids and retinoids on gap junctional communication. Biofactors. 2001;15:95–8.
149. Hammond BR, Wooten BR. CFF thresholds: relation to macular pigment optical density. Ophthalmic Physiol Opt. 2005;25(4):315–9.
150. Renzi LM, Hammond BR. The relation between the macular carotenoids, lutein and zeaxanthin, and temporal vision. Ophthalmic Physiol Opt. 2010;30(4):351–7.
151. Zimmer JP, Hammond BR. Possible influences of lutein and zeaxanthin on the developing retina. Clin Ophthalmol. 2007;1(1):11.
152. Gutherie AH, Hammond BR. Macular pigment and scotopic noise. ARVO Abstracts [abstract]. Invest Ophthalmol Vis Sci. 2005;E1784.

Chapter 14
Carotenoids and Bone Health

Sherry A. Tanumihardjo and Neil Binkley

Key Points

- The role of vitamin A in bone health remains controversial. Some human studies associate higher concentrations of specific carotenoids with improved bone health.
- *In vitro* and animal studies suggest that carotenoids, in particular β-cryptoxanthin, have favorable effects on bone remodeling parameters.
- Population-based studies associate high dietary intake of preformed vitamin A with greater osteoporosis and hip fracture risk.
- Practitioners need to be aware of the regulatory mechanisms controlling provitamin A carotenoid bioconversion to retinol to alleviate concern in regard to seemingly "high" dietary vitamin A intakes that are associated with healthy diets at recommended fruit and vegetable intakes.
- Future studies are needed to clarify the associations between specific carotenoids, total body stores of vitamin A, and bone health.
- This chapter reviews the associations of various carotenoids with beneficial and adverse bone health consequences and suggests future work that should be accomplished to clarify the role of carotenoids in bone.

Keywords Bone Health • Osteoporosis • β-Cryptoxanthin • Provitamin A

Introduction

Osteoporosis is a common disease characterized by low bone mass and deterioration of bone microarchitecture leading to an increased risk of fragility fracture. Approximately 40–50 % of postmenopausal women and ~25 % of older men sustain osteoporosis-related fractures in their lifetime [1, 2]. These fractures reduce quality and quantity of life and cause major healthcare costs [3, 4]. Given

S.A. Tanumihardjo, M.S., Ph.D. (✉)
Department of Nutritional Sciences, University of Wisconsin-Madison,
1415 Linden Dr., Madison, WI 53706, USA
e-mail: sherry@nutrisci.wisc.edu

N. Binkley, M.D.
School of Medicine & Public Health, University of Wisconsin-Madison,
2870 University Avenue, Madison, WI 53705, USA

S.A. Tanumihardjo (ed.), *Carotenoids and Human Health*, Nutrition and Health,
DOI 10.1007/978-1-62703-203-2_14, © Springer Science+Business Media New York 2013

current population demographics [5], the number of osteoporosis-related fractures will increase for the foreseeable future. Nutritional deficiencies, or excesses, may be causally related to bone loss with advancing age. As such, determining optimal nutritional approaches to reduce the impact of this devastating disease is an active area of research.

Ultimately, osteoporosis results from disordered bone remodeling in which osteoclastic bone resorption exceeds osteoblastic bone formation. One consequence of such unbalanced bone remodeling is a reduction in bone mass. As such, measurement of bone mineral density (BMD) by dual-energy X-ray absorptiometry (DXA) is commonly used as part of the fragility fracture risk assessment process [6]. In fact, the World Health Organization [7] identified criteria for bone health classification (i.e., osteoporosis/osteopenia/normal) based on BMD measurement (Table 14.1).

Bone remodeling is a normal physiologic process in which a quantum of bone is removed by osteoclasts and, ideally, an equal amount is replaced by osteoblasts. The control of bone remodeling is extremely complex, but a central role for nuclear factor-κB (NF-κB) in osteoclastogenesis and osteoclast activity has recently been appreciated [8]. Briefly, osteoblasts produce the receptor activator of NF-κB ligand (RANKL), which, upon binding to its receptor (RANK), stimulates both development of new osteoclasts and activity of mature osteoclasts [9]. Importantly, RANKL is upregulated upon estrogen withdrawal, which occurs during menopause, leading to rapid transmenopausal bone loss. RANKL is naturally regulated by a decoy receptor called osteoprotegerin [10], which is overwhelmed at menopause leading to increased osteoclast number/activity and thus, to rapid bone loss.

The process of bone remodeling is essential in maintaining bone strength, in part by repair of microfractures. A number of markers have been identified to assist in assessing bone remodeling [6]. Examples of commonly utilized bone turnover markers include serum or urine N-Telopeptide of type 1 collagen (NTX), serum bone specific alkaline phosphatase (BSAP), serum C-Telopeptide (CTX), osteocalcin, and serum procollagen type 1 N-terminal propeptide (P1NP). These serum and/or urinary measures are commonly quantified in studies of bone health and increasingly being utilized in clinical care. These markers, among others, have been reviewed in Brown et al. [6].

Some literature suggests that carotenoids are important in bone remodeling regulation (Fig. 14.1). It is possible that carotenoids might reduce fragility fracture risk either by reducing osteoclastic bone resorption or by enhancing osteoblastic bone formation. Dietary interventions that could slow or halt bone loss are obviously appealing in that low cost, population-based preventive approaches would be feasible. Moreover, such a diet-based approach would likely be embraced by those people who do not like to utilize prescription drugs to maintain their health. This chapter reviews the associations of carotenoids to various indices of bone health, discusses hypervitaminosis A, and suggests future work that should be accomplished to clarify the role of carotenoids in bone health.

Table 14.1 World Health Organization criteria for diagnosing osteopenia and osteoporosis[a]

Category	Criteria based on bone mineral density (BMD)
Normal	BMD within 1 SD[b] of the young adult mean
Low bone mass (osteopenia)	BMD between 1 and 2.5 SD below the young adult mean
Osteoporosis	BMD ≥2.5 SD below the young adult mean
Severe osteoporosis	Fragility fractures plus BMD ≥2.5 SD below the young adult mean

[a]Adapted from [7]. This classification applies only to BMD as measured by dual-energy X-ray absorptiometry at the lumbar spine, femoral neck, total proximal femur, and one-third radius sites

[b]Standard deviation (SD)

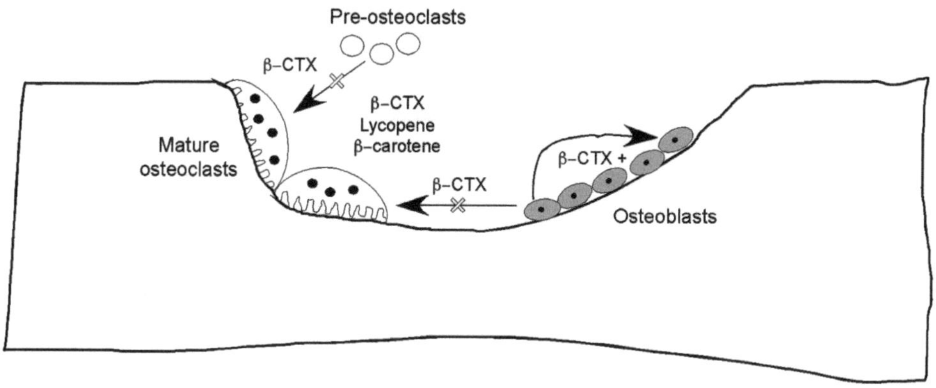

Fig. 14.1 Speculative roles of carotenoids in bone remodeling. The regulation of bone remodeling is extremely complex. Some of the factors affecting this process include sex steroids (e.g., estrogen/testosterone), cytokines (e.g., IL-1, IL-6, RANK/RANKL), growth factors (e.g., IGF-1), mechanical loading, toxins (e.g., chemotherapeutic agents, glucocorticoids, alcohol, tobacco), and nutrition (e.g., calcium, vitamin D, carotenoids). Carotenoids may favorably or adversely affect the bone remodeling cycle as indicated here. Specifically, β-cryptoxanthin (β-CTX) may inhibit both differentiation of pre-osteoclasts to osteoclasts and also inhibit mature osteoclast activity. Lycopene and β-carotene may inhibit function of mature osteoclasts, whereas retinol may stimulate their activity. β-CTX may blunt the osteoblast-induced activation of osteoclasts and also stimulate osteoblastic activity

Potential Mechanisms of Carotenoids in Osteoporosis

It is possible that carotenoids might produce a beneficial bone benefit via their antioxidant properties, which are discussed in Chap. 4. Increases in oxidative stress caused by reactive oxygen species may be involved in bone resorption [11, 12] and also adversely modulate osteoblastic differentiation [13]. Either of these effects could negatively impact bone balance at the remodeling site, thereby ultimately adversely affecting bone mass. An increased presence of free radicals activates the oxidative stress-responsive transcription factor, NF-κB [14, 15]. Carotenoids as antioxidants [16] can quench singlet oxygen and trap peroxyl radicals [17], thus potentially reducing bone resorption. Consistent with this, in epidemiologic studies, high antioxidant intake is associated with lower fracture risk. For example, a population-based study in which β-carotene intake was assessed by food frequency questionnaire and included supplement usage found an odds ratio of 0.39 for β-carotene intake in relation to hip fracture risk in past and present smokers for the extreme quintiles of intake [18]. Cigarette smoke contains many prooxidants. Moreover, a similar association was not found among those who had never smoked.

In Italian women with osteoporosis, lower plasma levels of zeaxanthin, β-cryptoxanthin, lycopene, and α- and β-carotene were found [19]. A similar finding was noted in US women in regards to lycopene and β-cryptoxanthin serum concentrations [20]. Both of these cohorts also reported lower serum vitamin A concentrations in women with osteoporosis [21, 22]. These results are somewhat counter-intuitive because supplementation or fortification with preformed vitamin A is associated with greater age-related bone loss [23–25]. It is plausible that plant sources of vitamin A are protective to bone or alternatively that the carotenoids are acting as biomarkers for other phytochemicals in fruits and vegetables that protect bone [26], or that high vitamin A intake is a marker of a generally healthy lifestyle.

Of the major carotenoids found in human serum, lycopene has the greatest antioxidant potential with twice the activity of β-carotene for quenching singlet oxygen [27]. Higher dietary lycopene intake alone has been associated with lower hip fracture risk. In the Framingham Osteoporosis Study, the relative risk for an osteoporotic fracture was 0.66 for the highest versus lowest lycopene intake tertile as assessed by food frequency questionnaire [28]. The protective effect was most pronounced when lycopene-containing foods exceeded 4.4 servings/week. Furthermore, higher lycopene intake was associated with less bone loss over time at the lumbar spine in women and the trochanter in men [29].

Supplementing postmenopausal women with lycopene derived from tomato products decreased the bone resorption serum marker NTX [30]. Restricting dietary lycopene in a small number of postmenopausal women resulted in a significant increase in serum NTX [31], leading the authors to conclude that lycopene is important in maintaining bone health. As discussed in Section I of this book, dietary lycopene is predominantly in tomatoes and readily available in a variety of processed forms throughout the world. Future studies need to tease out whether the beneficial bone effects are truly associated with isolated lycopene or products from the whole tomato.

In addition to the human *in vivo* studies noted above, *in vitro* studies found effects of carotenoids on bone. For example, in tissue culture, β-cryptoxanthin has a direct stimulatory effect on bone formation and an inhibitory effect on bone resorption [32–35]. Specifically, β-cryptoxanthin inhibits osteoclast-like cell formation induced by RANKL *in vitro* [32]. In this mouse marrow culture model, the effect of β-cryptoxanthin to inhibit osteoclast formation was blocked by protein synthesis inhibition. This led the authors to speculate that the inhibitory action of β-cryptoxanthin may involve a protein component related to RANKL stimulation of osteoclastogenesis [32]. Furthermore, in this *in vitro* system, β-cryptoxanthin inhibition of osteoclast-like cell formation was equal to that produced by estradiol [32]. Supporting a role of this carotenoid in postmenopausal women, β-cryptoxanthin was lower in women with osteoporosis than those without [20].

In addition to an anti-resorptive effect, potentially mediated via RANKL inhibition, *in vitro* work suggests that β-cryptoxanthin may have direct effects to stimulate osteoblastic bone formation. For example, β-cryptoxanthin stimulates osteoblast-like cell proliferation and increases insulin-like growth factor-1 mRNA [33]. Additionally, β-cryptoxanthin enhanced mineralization in osteoblast-like cell culture [33]. Consistent with this, increased calcium content has been observed in cultured rat femur tissue cultures exposed to β-cryptoxanthin [34, 35]. Thus, *in vitro* work suggests that β-cryptoxanthin may possess bone formation stimulating effects.

Limited *in vivo* work supports the *in vitro* studies noted above. For example, β-cryptoxanthin increased bone calcium content in young [36] and old [37] rats. Moreover, β-cryptoxanthin reduced bone loss induced by ovariectomy in rats [38]. Small studies of men and women receiving juice fortified with β-cryptoxanthin appear to be consistent with the *in vitro* and animal data with increases in markers of bone formation and reduction in bone resorption markers reported [39–41]. However, existing human data are quite limited due to small study size and inclusion of both men and women across a wide age range. In summary, *in vitro*, animal, and limited human data suggest that β-cryptoxanthin has potential to stimulate bone formation and inhibit bone resorption [42]. These observations with β-cryptoxanthin are of direct clinical relevance given the projected increase in osteoporotic fractures in the foreseeable future. Further investigations are needed to elucidate the action of β-cryptoxanthin on bone health. Dietary sources of β-cryptoxanthin are limited but do include citrus fruits, which are quite popular and have wide-reaching global distribution.

Most of the evidence for beneficial effects of carotenoids on bone health has been associated with the hydrocarbon carotenes and β-cryptoxanthin. In addition, lutein and zeaxanthin intakes were positively correlated with bone mass in Australian premenopausal women [43] and a 4-year change in BMD measured by DXA in US men [29].

Other Bone-Related Associations

In US case–control studies, higher circulating concentrations of lutein and β-cryptoxanthin have been associated with lower risk of knee osteoarthritis [44]. Another study implicated a beneficial effect of fruit intake on factors associated with the pathogenesis of knee osteoarthritis and the number of bone marrow lesions as assessed by magnetic resonance imaging [45]. This conclusion was based on a food frequency questionnaire that showed a positive association of the carotenoids lutein, zeaxanthin, and β-cryptoxanthin to healthy knee structure [45]. In contrast, no association was found with any carotenoid and knee osteoarthritis in a cohort of Japanese subjects [46]. Thus, although a link of fruit or other dietary factors with osteoarthritis may exist, such a relationship requires further evaluation and benefits may not result from a single carotenoid.

Osteoarthritis, with its commonly observed osteophyte (i.e., bone spur) formation, is a common accompaniment of advancing age. Although higher serum concentrations for many carotenoids were associated with a lower incidence of lumbar spine osteophytes, only lower serum β-carotene was associated with a higher incidence of bone spurs in a group of Japanese volunteers after multivariate analysis [47]. As osteoarthritis is virtually ubiquitous in older adults, randomized controlled trials are needed to determine if dietary modification or β-carotene supplementation may reduce the overall risk of developing this common disease.

Hypervitaminosis A

Provitamin A carotenoids are converted by the human body to vitamin A; however, this process is highly regulated as discussed in Chap. 3. Considering current dietary intakes and regulation, it seems unlikely that hypervitaminosis A can occur from provitamin A carotenoid intake alone [48]. Nonetheless, as dietary recommendations to increase fruit and vegetable intake are promoted, calculated vitamin A intakes could increase if humans ate the recommended 4.5 cups/day of fruit and vegetables for the typical 2,000-cal eating plan [49]. For example, if a person ate a combination of 1 cup raw carrots, 1 cup cooked spinach, and 1/2 cup raw tomatoes for their 2.5 cups recommended vegetables in 1 day and entered these amounts into the USDA nutrient database [50], a value of 2,050 μg retinol activity equivalents (RAE) would be obtained. This is about three times the vitamin A recommended intake for a 19–30-year-old women, which is 700 μg RAE [51], which may cause concern to the consumer. However, it is unlikely that the person would make this amount of vitamin A from this continued level of provitamin A intake due to the many factors that affect carotenoid bioavailability and bioconversion [48, 52]. Nonetheless, considering the widespread use of preformed vitamin A supplements and fortified foods, the topic of excessive dietary vitamin A and bone health will be reviewed here briefly.

Excessive dietary preformed vitamin A leading to hypervitaminosis A is associated with osteoporosis [53] and fragility fractures [54]. Association studies relate chronic high preformed vitamin A intake with low bone mass, potentially leading to osteoporosis [23–25, 55, 56]. However, this does not seem to be the case for the dietary provitamin A carotenoids [21]. Considering that most people in developed countries get more vitamin A than recommended [57] and most studies that have been done are observational, more questions are currently raised than answered in regard to the association of preformed vitamin A to bone health. Interpretation of epidemiological studies must be done with caution until these associations are further evaluated by research that links actual vitamin A status measured by total body stores with bone mass and fracture incidence. Reflecting this current uncertainty, the Expert Group on Vitamins and Minerals concluded that the risk of hip fracture is a continuous graded response that includes exposure levels within dietary vitamin A intakes, and thus, a Safe Upper Limit could not be established because of overlap with reasonable dietary intakes [58].

Historically, hypervitaminosis A has been associated with bone alterations in human remains [59, 60], reports of toxicity in Arctic people [61], and in children with excessive vitamin A intakes [62–67]. Case studies linking abnormal bone parameters and excessive vitamin A intake continue to appear in the literature [68]. The hypothesis that skeletal toxicities may occur with retinoid use is supported by observations of myalgias, arthralgias, decreases in BMD, and hyperostoses (e.g., bone spurs) with systemic retinoid treatment for acne [69]. However to date, no population studies directly linking excessive or hypervitaminotic vitamin A status to bone health at the population level using sensitive biomarkers of vitamin A status have been performed [70]. Moreover, in captive nonhuman primates with long-term hypervitaminosis A, bone health appeared to be normal [71, 72].

Prospective, observational studies conducted in countries where the incidence of osteoporosis is high [5], found associations between preformed vitamin A intake and hip fracture or osteoporosis [24, 25, 55, 56]. The amount of dietary vitamin A associated with this effect was approximately two times the RDA at 1,500 μg retinol equivalents. In comparison, the Tolerable Upper Intake Level is 3,000 μg preformed vitamin A, which is the highest level thought to pose no risk of adverse health effects in the general population [51]. Other studies reviewed in Myhre et al. [73] have not linked vitamin A intake to osteoporosis. In summary, associational studies suggest that high dietary intake of preformed vitamin A may have adverse bone consequences including bone loss and fracture. However, it is axiomatic that association does not prove causation and randomized controlled trials of retinol supplementation and/or retinoid treatment are necessary to further evaluate the effect on bone health.

Other Things in Fruits and Vegetables

While this chapter reviews the association of carotenoids and vitamin A with bone health, both beneficial and adverse, it is possible that such reported associations simply reflect carotenoids acting as a biomarker for other components in fruit and vegetables that affect skeletal status. For example, calcium from vegetable intake was positively associated with BMD in Korean women [26]. Furthermore in the same study, potassium, vitamins C and E, and β-carotene were positively associated with BMD. Additionally, vegetables are an important source of dietary potassium, which is associated with higher bone density. However, adjusting a large data set for potassium intake did not change the beneficial association of carotenoid intake and hip fracture [29] suggesting that carotenoids do play a beneficial role in optimal bone health. Moreover, other dietary minerals (e.g., magnesium, strontium, selenium) may have skeletal effects.

Fruits also contain other phytochemicals, in addition to carotenoids, which may explain improved bone health. For example in citrus fruits, a natural occurring flavonoid called naringin was found to perturb osteoclast formation and bone resorption [74]. Furthermore, other plant-derived flavonoids are associated with bone-building properties [75]. Eating whole foods, especially fruits and vegetables, seems to promote optimal health rather than any one single component serving as the "magic bullet." Studies of whole foods must appreciate and acknowledge the complexity of these diet/bone interactions rather than assuming that the single nutrient being studied is causally related to the outcome observed.

Conclusions

The beneficial associations reported between carotenoids and bone health, notably for β-cryptoxanthin, could be causally related, or alternatively, merely be an indicator for the intake of other antioxidants, other nutrients and minerals, or potentially reflect an overall healthy lifestyle that is more common in people with high dietary intakes of carotenoids, i.e., fruits and vegetables. Further research is essential to clarify whether the currently observed associations are causally related to bone health, perhaps with foods that have enhanced concentrations of β-cryptoxanthin or other carotenoids. If beneficial bone effects are confirmed, such nutritional approaches could potentially offer safe, inexpensive approaches to reduce bone loss with advancing age with resultant reduction in fragility fracture risk and consequently major beneficial personal and societal benefits. Conversely, the potential negative impact of preformed vitamin A on bone needs to be further investigated to determine if vitamin A status per se or other synergistic nutritional or non-nutritional interactions negatively impact bone health.

References

1. Chrischilles EA, Butler CD, Davis CS, Wallace RB. A model of lifetime osteoporosis impact. Arch Intern Med. 1990;151:2026–32.
2. Nguyen TV, Eisman JA, Kelly PJ, Sambrook PN. Risk factors for osteoporotic fractures in elderly men. Am J Epidemiol. 1996;144:255–63.
3. Pande I, Scott DL, O'Neill TW, Pritchard C, Woolf AD, Davis MJ. Quality of life, morbidity and mortality after low trauma hip fracture in men. Ann Rheum Dis. 2006;65:87–92.
4. Johnell O, Kanis JA, Oden A, Sernbo I, Redlund-Johnell I, Petterson C, De Laet C, Jönsson B. Mortality after osteoporotic fractures. Osteoporos Int. 2004;15:38–42.
5. Lips P. Epidemiology and predictors of fractures associated with osteoporosis. Am J Med. 1997;103:3S–8.
6. Brown JP, Albert C, Nassar BA, Adachi JD, Cole D, Davison KS, Dooley KC, Don-Wauchope A, Douville P, Hanley DA, Jamal SA, Josse R, Kaiser S, Krahn J, Krause R, Kremer R, Lepage R, Letendre E, Morin S, Ooi DS, Papaioaonnou A, Ste-Marie L-G. Bone turnover markers in the management of postmenopausal osteoporosis. Clin Biochem. 2009;42:929–42.
7. Report of WHO Study Group. Assessment of fracture risk and its application to screening for postmenopausal osteoporosis. WHO reference number: WHO/TSR/843. 1994.
8. Kearns AE, Khosla S, Kosternuik PJ. Receptor activator of nuclear factor κB ligand and osteoprotegerin regulation of bone remodeling in health and disease. Endocr Rev. 2008;29:155–92.
9. Boyce BF, Xing L. Functions of RANKL/RANK/OPG in bone modeling and remodeling. Arch Biochem Biophys. 2008;473:139–46.
10. Gallagher JC. Advances in bone biology and new treatments for bone loss. Maturitas. 2008;60:65–9.
11. Garrett IR, Boyce BF, Oreffo RO, Bonewald L, Poser J, Mundy GR. Oxygen-derived free radicals stimulate osteoclastic bone resorption in rodent bone *in vitro* and *in vivo*. J Clin Invest. 1990;85:632–9.
12. Basu S, Michaelsson K, Olofsson H, Johansson S, Melhus H. Association between oxidative stress and bone mineral density. Biochem Biophys Res Commun. 2001;288:275–9.
13. Mody N, Parhami F, Sarafian TA, Demer LL. Oxidative stress modulates osteoblastic differentiation of vascular and bone cells. Free Radic Biol Med. 2001;31:509–16.
14. Schreck R, Albermann K, Baeuerle PA. Nuclear factor κB: an oxidative stress-responsive transcription factor of eukaryotic cells. Free Radic Res Commun. 1992;17:221–7.
15. Schreck R, Rieber P, Baeuerle PA. Reactive oxygen intermediates as apparently widely used messengers in the activation of the NF-κB transcription factor and HIV-1. EMBO J. 1991;10:2247–58.
16. Rock CL. Carotenoids: biology and treatment. Pharmacol Ther. 1997;75:185–97.
17. Terao J. Astaxanthin as a chain-breaking antioxidant in phospholipid peroxidation. In: Yagi K, Kondo M, Niki E, Yoshikawa T, editors. Oxygen radicals. New York: Elsevier Science Publishers; 1992. p. 657–60.
18. Zhang J, Munger RG, West NA, Cutler DR, Wengreen HJ, Corcoran CD. Antioxidant intake and risk of osteoporotic hip fracture in Utah: an effect modified by smoking status. Am J Epidemiol. 2006;163:9–17.
19. Maggio D, Barabani M, Pierandrei M, Polidori MC, Catani M, Mecocci P, Senin U, Pacifici R, Cherubini A. Marked decrease in plasma antioxidants in aged osteoporotic women: results of a cross-sectional study. J Clin Endocrinol Metab. 2003;88:1523–7.
20. Yang Z, Zhang Z, Penniston KL, Binkley N, Tanumihardjo SA. Serum carotenoid concentrations in postmenopausal women from the US with and without osteoporosis. Int J Vitam Nutr Res. 2008;78:105–11.
21. Maggio D, Polidori MC, Barabani M, Tufi A, Ruggiero C, Cecchetti R, Aisa MC, Stahl W, Cherubini A. Low levels of carotenoids and retinol in involutional osteoporosis. Bone. 2006;38:244–8.
22. Penniston KL, Weng N, Binkley N, Tanumihardjo SA. Serum retinyl esters are not elevated in postmenopausal women with and without osteoporosis whose preformed vitamin A intakes are high. Am J Clin Nutr. 2006;84:1350–6.
23. Melhus H, Michaelsson K, Kindmark A, Bergström R, Holmberg L, Mallmin H, Wolk A, Ljunghall S. Excessive dietary intake of vitamin A is associated with reduced bone mineral density and increased risk for hip fracture. Ann Intern Med. 1998;129:770–8.
24. Promislow JHE, Goodman-Gruen D, Slymen DJ, Barrett-Connor E. Retinol intake and bone mineral density in the elderly: the Rancho Bernardo study. J Bone Miner Res. 2002;17:1349–58.
25. Feskanich D, Singh V, Willett WC, Colditz GA. Vitamin A intake and hip fractures among postmenopausal women. JAMA. 2002;287:47–54.
26. Park H-M, Heo J, Park Y. Calcium from plant sources is beneficial to lowering the risk of osteoporosis in postmenopausal Korean women. Nutr Res. 2011;31:27–31.
27. DiMascio P, Kaiser S, Sies H. Lycopene as the most efficient biological carotenoid singlet oxygen quencher. Arch Biochem Biophys. 1989;274:532–8.

28. Sahni S, Hannan MT, Blumberg J, Cupples LA, Kiel DP, Tucker KL. Protective effect of total carotenoid and lycopene intake on the risk of hip fracture: a 17-year follow-up from the Framingham Osteoporosis Study. J Bone Miner Res. 2009;24:1086–94.
29. Sahni S, Hannan MT, Blumberg J, Cupples LA, Kiel DP, Tucker KL. Inverse association of carotenoid intakes with 4-y change in bone mineral density in elderly men and women: the Framingham Osteoporosis Study. Am J Clin Nutr. 2009;89:416–24.
30. Mackinnon ES, Rao AV, Josse RG, Rao LG. Supplementation with the antioxidant lycopene significantly decreases oxidative stress parameters and the bone resorption marker N-telopeptide of type I collagen in postmenopausal women. Osteoporos Int. 2011;22:1091–101.
31. Mackinnon ES, Rao AV, Rao LG. Dietary restriction of lycopene for a period of one month resulted in significantly increased biomarkers of oxidative stress and bone resorption in postmenopausal women. J Nutr Health Aging. 2011;15:133–8.
32. Uchiyama S, Yamaguchi M. Inhibitory effect of β-cryptoxanthin on osteoclast-like cell formation in mouse marrow cultures. Biochem Pharmacol. 2004;67:1297–305.
33. Uchiyama S, Yamaguchi M. β-Cryptoxanthin stimulates cell proliferation and transcriptional activity in osteoblastic MC3T3-E1 cells. Int J Mol Med. 2005;15:675–81.
34. Yamaguchi M, Uchiyama S. Effect of carotenoid on calcium content and alkaline phosphatase activity in rat femoral tissues *in vitro*: the unique anabolic effect of β-cryptoxanthin. Biol Pharm Bull. 2003;26:1188–91.
35. Yamaguchi M, Uchiyama S. β-Cryptoxanthin stimulates bone formation and inhibits bone resorption in tissue culture *in vitro*. Mol Cell Biochem. 2004;258:137–44.
36. Uchiyama S, Sumida T, Yamaguchi M. Oral administration of β-cryptoxanthin induces anabolic effects on bone components in the femoral tissues of rats *in vivo*. Biol Pharm Bull. 2004;27:232–5.
37. Uchiyama S, Sumida T, Yamaguchi M. Anabolic effect of β-cryptoxanthin on bone components in the femoral tissues of aged rats *in vivo* and *in vitro*. J Health Sci. 2004;50:491–6.
38. Uchiyama S, Yamaguchi M. Oral administration of β-cryptoxanthin prevents bone loss in ovariectomized rats. Int J Mol Med. 2006;17:15–20.
39. Yamaguchi M, Igarashi A, Uchiyama S, Morita S, Sugawara K, Sumida T. Prolonged intake of juice (*Citrus unshiu*) reinforced with β-cryptoxanthin has an effect on circulating bone biochemical markers in normal individuals. J Health Sci. 2004;50:619–24.
40. Yamaguchi M, Igarashi A, Morita S, Sumida T, Sugawara K. Relationship between serum β-cryptoxanthin and circulating bone metabolic markers in healthy individuals with the intake of juice (*Citrus unshiu*) containing β-cryptoxanthin. J Health Sci. 2005;51:738–43.
41. Yamaguchi M, Igarashi A, Uchiyama S, Sugawara K, Sumida T, Morita S, Ogawa H, Nishitani M, Kajimoto Y. Effect of β-cryptoxanthin on circulating bone metabolic markers: intake of juice (*Citrus unshiu*) supplemented with β-cryptoxanthin has an effect in menopausal women. J Health Sci. 2006;52:758–68.
42. Uchiyama S. β-Cryptoxanthin and bone metabolism: the preventive role in osteoporosis. J Health Sci. 2008;54:356–69.
43. Wattanapenpaiboon N, Lukito W, Wahlqvist ML, Strauss BJ. Dietary carotenoid intake as a predictor of bone mineral density. Asia Pac J Clin Nutr. 2003;12:467–73.
44. De Roos AJ, Arab L, Renner JB, Craft N, Luta G, Helmick CG, Hochberg MC, Jordan JM. Serum carotenoids and radiographic knee osteoarthritis: the Johnston County Osteoarthritis Project. Public Health Nutr. 2001;4:935–42.
45. Wang Y, Hodge AM, Wluka AE, English DR, Giles GG, O'Sullivan R, Forbes A, Cicuttini FM. Effect of antioxidants on knee cartilage and bone in healthy, middle-aged subjects: a cross-sectional study. Arthritis Res Ther. 2007;9:R66.
46. Seki T, Hasegawa Y, Yamaguchi J, Kanoh T, Ishiguro N, Tsuboi M, Ito Y, Hamajima N, Suzuki K. Association of serum carotenoids, retinol, and tocopherols with radiographic knee osteoarthritis: possible risk factors in rural Japanese inhabitants. J Orthop Sci. 2010;15:477–84.
47. Imagama S, Hasegawa Y, Seki T, Matsuyama Y, Sakai Y, Ito Z, Ishiguro N, Ito Y, Hamajima N, Suzuki K. The effect of β-carotene on lumbar osteophyte formation. Spine (Phila Pa 1976). 2011;36(26):2293–8.
48. Tanumihardjo SA. Food-based approaches for ensuring adequate vitamin A nutrition. Compr Rev Food Sci Food Saf. 2008;7:373–81.
49. U.S. Department of Agriculture and U.S. Department of Health and Human Services. Dietary guidelines for Americans, 2010. 7th ed. Washington, DC: U.S. Government Printing Office; December 2010.
50. USDA National Nutrient Database for Standard Reference, Release 21. Composition of foods raw, processed, prepared. 2008. Available from: http://www.nal.usda.gov/fnic/foodcomp/search/. Accessed Nov 2011.
51. Institute of Medicine, Food and Nutrition Board. Dietary reference intakes for vitamin A, vitamin K, arsenic, boron, chromium, copper, iodine, iron, molybdenum, nickel, silicon, vanadium, and zinc. Washington, DC: National Academy Press; 2001. p. 65–126.
52. Tanumihardjo SA, Palacios N, Pixley KV. Provitamin A carotenoid bioavailability: what really matters? Int J Vitam Nutr Res. 2010;80:336–50.

53. Penniston KL, Tanumihardjo SA. The acute and chronic toxic effects of vitamin A. Am J Clin Nutr. 2006;83:191–201.
54. Binkley N, Krueger D. Hypervitaminosis A and bone. Nutr Rev. 2000;58:138–44.
55. Lim LS, Harnack LJ, Lazovich D, Folsom AR. Vitamin A intake and the risk of hip fracture in postmenopausal women: the Iowa Women's Health Study. Osteoporos Int. 2004;15:552–9.
56. Michaelsson K, Lithell H, Vessby B, Melhus H. Serum retinol levels and the risk of fracture. N Engl J Med. 2003;348:287–94.
57. Penniston KL, Tanumihardjo SA. Vitamin A in dietary supplements and fortified foods: too much of a good thing? J Am Diet Assoc. 2003;103:1185–7.
58. Expert Group on Vitamins and Minerals. Risk assessment: vitamin A (retinol). In: Safe upper levels for vitamins and minerals. May 2003. p. 110–26. Internet: http://www.food.gov.uk/multimedia/pdfs/vitmin2003.pdf. Accessed 1 Dec 2011.
59. Walker A, Zimmerman MR, Leakey REF. A possible case of hypervitaminosis A in *Homo erectus*. Nature. 1982;296:248–50.
60. Zimmerman MR. The paleopathology of the liver. Ann Clin Lab Sci. 1990;20:301–6.
61. Landy D. Pibloktoq (hysteria) and Inuit nutrition: possible implication of hypervitaminosis A. Soc Sci Med. 1985;21:173–85.
62. Frame B, Jackson CE, Reynolds WA, Umphrey JE. Hypercalcemia and skeletal effects in chronic hypervitaminosis A. Ann Intern Med. 1974;80:44–8.
63. Coghlan D, Cranswick NE. Complementary medicine and vitamin A toxicity in children. Med J Aust. 2001;175:223–4.
64. Gamble JG, Ip SC. Hypervitaminosis A in a child from megadosing. J Pediatr Orthop. 1985;5:219–21.
65. Bush ME, Dahms BB. Fatal hypervitaminosis A in a neonate. Arch Pathol Lab Med. 1984;108:838–42.
66. Scherl S, Goldberg NS, Volpe L, Juster F. Overdosage of vitamin A supplements in a child. Cutis. 1992;50:209–10.
67. Grissom LE, Griffin GC, Mandell GA. Hypervitaminosis A as a complication of treatment for neuroblastoma. Pediatr Radiol. 1996;26:200–2.
68. Saltzman MD, King EC. Central physeal arrests as a manifestation of hypervitaminosis A. J Pediatr Orthop. 2007;27:351–3.
69. Nesher G, Zuckner J. Rheumatologic complications of vitamin A and retinoids. Semin Arthritis Rheum. 1995;24:291–6.
70. Tanumihardjo SA. Vitamin A: biomarkers of nutrition for development. Am J Clin Nutr. 2011;94:658S–65.
71. Penniston KL, Tanumihardjo SA. Subtoxic hepatic vitamin A concentrations in captive rhesus monkeys *(Macaca mulatta)*. J Nutr. 2001;131:2904–9.
72. Escaron AL, Green MH, Howe JA, Tanumihardjo SA. Mathematical modeling of serum ^{13}C-retinol in captive rhesus monkeys provides new insights on hypervitaminosis A. J Nutr. 2009;139:2000–6.
73. Myhre AM, Carlsen MH, Bohn SK, Wold HL, Laake P, Blomhoff R. Water-miscible, emulsified, and solid forms of retinol supplements are more toxic than oil-based preparations. Am J Clin Nutr. 2003;78:1152–9.
74. Ang ES, Yang X, Chen H, Liu Q, Zheng MH, Xu J. Naringin abrogates osteoclastogenesis and bone resorption via the inhibition of RANKL-induced NF-κB and ERK activation. FEBS Lett. 2011;585:2755–62.
75. Horcajada MN, Offord E. Naturally plant-derived compounds: role in bone anabolism. Curr Mol Pharmacol. 2012;5(2):205–18.

Section III
International Perspectives

Chapter 15
Provitamin A Carotenoids as a Dietary Source of Vitamin A

Marjorie J. Haskell

Key Points

- Vitamin A deficiency (VAD) is an important public health problem that affects low-income populations in developing countries throughout the world.
- VAD tends to occur in populations with chronic low dietary intake of vitamin A and frequent infections and can have serious adverse effects on human health.
- Populations in developing countries rely on dietary provitamin A (PVA) carotenoids to a greater extent to meet their vitamin A needs. Nationally representative data on dietary intakes of preformed vitamin A and PVA carotenoids do not exist in most developing countries.
- Dietary surveys have been conducted in populations at risk of VAD, and insufficient dietary intake of vitamin A has been reported for women of reproductive age and for preschool-age children.
- Food-based interventions that aim to increase dietary intake of PVA carotenoids have been implemented to increase vitamin A status in populations at risk of deficiency.
- The vitamin A equivalency of PVA carotenoids from plant source foods is highly variable and can be affected by many factors, as discussed in previous chapters.
- This chapter is focused on the public health significance of VAD and the importance of PVA carotenoids as a dietary source of vitamin A. Evidence on the efficacy of dietary interventions for increasing vitamin A status in populations at risk of VAD is also discussed.

Keywords Provitamin A carotenoids • Vitamin A • Diet • Food supply

Introduction

Vitamin A deficiency (VAD) is an important public health problem that affects low-income populations in developing countries throughout the world. VAD tends to occur in populations with chronic low dietary intake of vitamin A and frequent infections and can have serious adverse effects on human health [1]. Intervention programs to increase vitamin A status in vulnerable populations exist in many countries.

M.J. Haskell, B.S., M.P.H., Ph.D. (✉)
Department of Nutrition, University of California, Davis, One Shields Avenue, Davis, CA 95616, USA
e-mail: mjhaskell@ucdavis.edu

S.A. Tanumihardjo (ed.), *Carotenoids and Human Health*, Nutrition and Health,
DOI 10.1007/978-1-62703-203-2_15, © Springer Science+Business Media New York 2013

The World Health Organization (WHO) recommends providing high-dose vitamin A capsules (200,000 IU) to children 6–59 months of age, every 4–6 months, and a single high-dose vitamin A capsule (200,000 IU) to women within the first 6 weeks of giving birth in areas where VAD is endemic [2]. Food-based interventions that aim to increase dietary intake of provitamin A carotenoids are also a strategy for increasing vitamin A status in populations at risk of deficiency. However, the vitamin A equivalency of provitamin A carotenoids from plant source foods is highly variable and can be affected by many factors, as discussed in Section I of this book. Thus, the potential of food-based interventions for increasing vitamin A status in populations at risk of VAD is not yet well-understood. This chapter is focused on the public health significance of VAD and the importance of provitamin A carotenoids as a dietary source of vitamin A. Evidence on the efficacy of dietary interventions for increasing vitamin A status in populations at risk of VAD is also discussed.

Public Health Importance of VAD

The global prevalence of VAD is based on estimates of the numbers of preschool-age children and pregnant women who have serum retinol concentrations <0.70 μmol/L or a history of night blindness, which is a functional indicator of VAD. The most recent estimates were reported by the World Health Organization in 2009 and are based on prevalence data on VAD in countries with a gross domestic product (GDP) of <US $15,000 in 2005; populations in countries with a GDP >US $15,000 in 2005 are not considered to be at risk of VAD [1]. For countries for which there are no survey data available, the prevalence of VAD in preschool-age children and pregnant women is estimated using regression equations that are based on indicators of population health status, such as the human development index, under 5 mortality, adult female mortality, stunting, wasting, and population growth rates [1]. It is currently estimated that 190 million preschool-age children and 19.1 million pregnant women have low serum retinol concentrations; this represents 33.3% of preschool-age children and 15.3% of pregnant women in populations that are considered to be at risk of VAD [1]. Approximately 5.2 million preschool-age children and 9.8 million pregnant women are affected by night blindness; this represents 0.9 and 7.8% of preschool-age children and pregnant women in populations that are considered to be at risk of VAD. The global prevalence of VAD is shown in Figs. 15.1, 15.2, 15.3, and 15.4. The greatest estimated numbers of children with low serum retinol concentration are in South and South East Asia (91.5 million) and Africa (56.4 million). The greatest numbers of pregnant women with low serum retinol are in South and South East Asia (6.7 million), the Western Pacific (4.9 million), and Africa (4.2 million) [1].

The main causes of VAD in low-income populations in developing countries are chronic low dietary vitamin A intake and frequent infections [1]. Populations at risk of deficiency tend to consume monotonous diets that consist mainly of staple crops, small amounts of vegetables and fruits, and occasionally animal source foods. Most of their dietary vitamin A is obtained from plant sources of provitamin A carotenoids, such as dark green leafy vegetables and orange vegetables and fruits. Animal sources of preformed vitamin A, such as dairy products, egg yolk, and animal liver, are relatively expensive and are often not available. Preschool-age children and pregnant and lactating women are particularly vulnerable to developing VAD because of their increased nutritional demands and because of frequent diarrheal and respiratory infections, which can adversely affect vitamin A status. Diarrheal infections can reduce intestinal absorption of vitamin A, and fever can result in increased utilization and excretion of vitamin A [3–5]. Food intake can also decline during infection because of poor appetite [1].

VAD can have serious health consequences for preschool-age children and pregnant women. VAD is the leading cause of childhood blindness and is associated with reduced immune function and

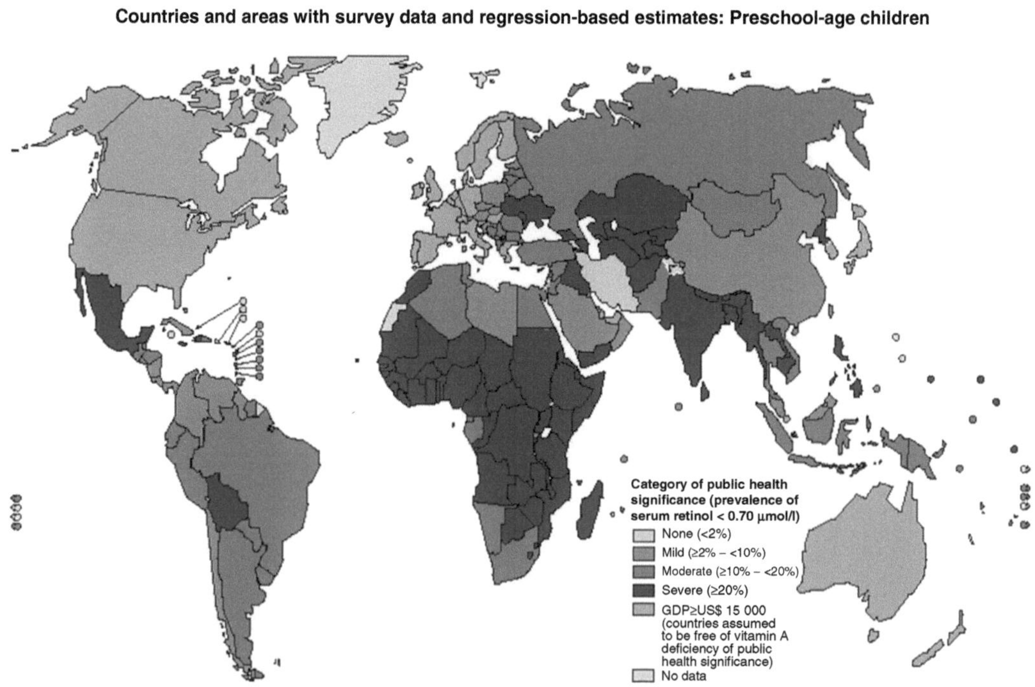

Fig. 15.1 Public health significance of vitamin A deficiency based on serum retinol <0.70 μmol/L in preschool-age children. *Source*: World Health Organization, 2009 [1], with permission

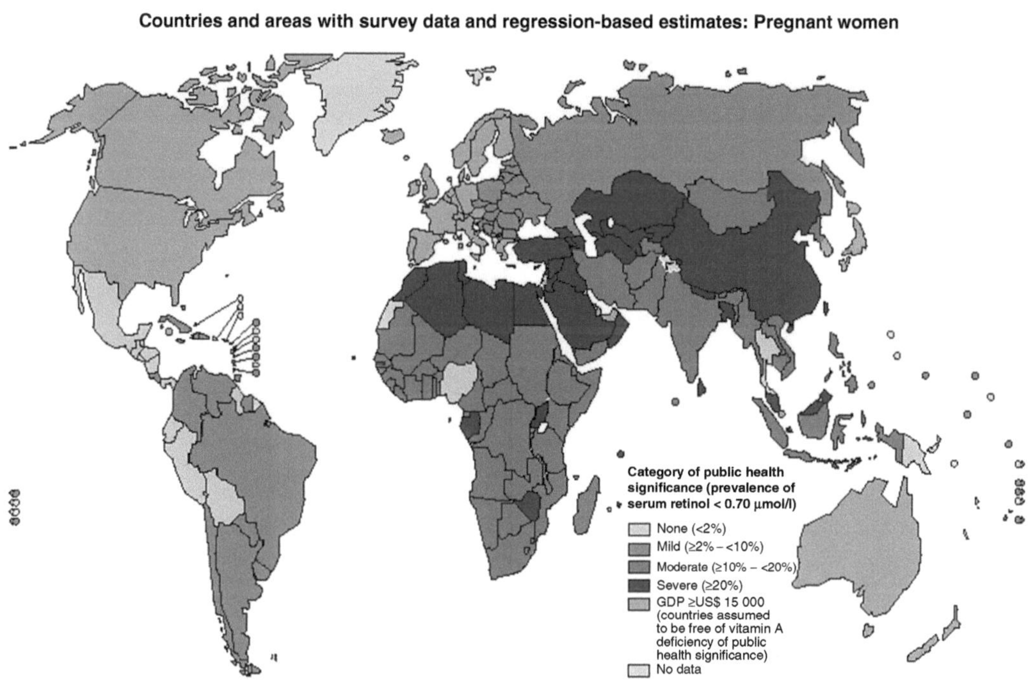

Fig. 15.2 Public health significance of vitamin A deficiency based on serum retinol <0.70 μmol/L in pregnant women. *Source*: World Health Organization, 2009 [1], with permission

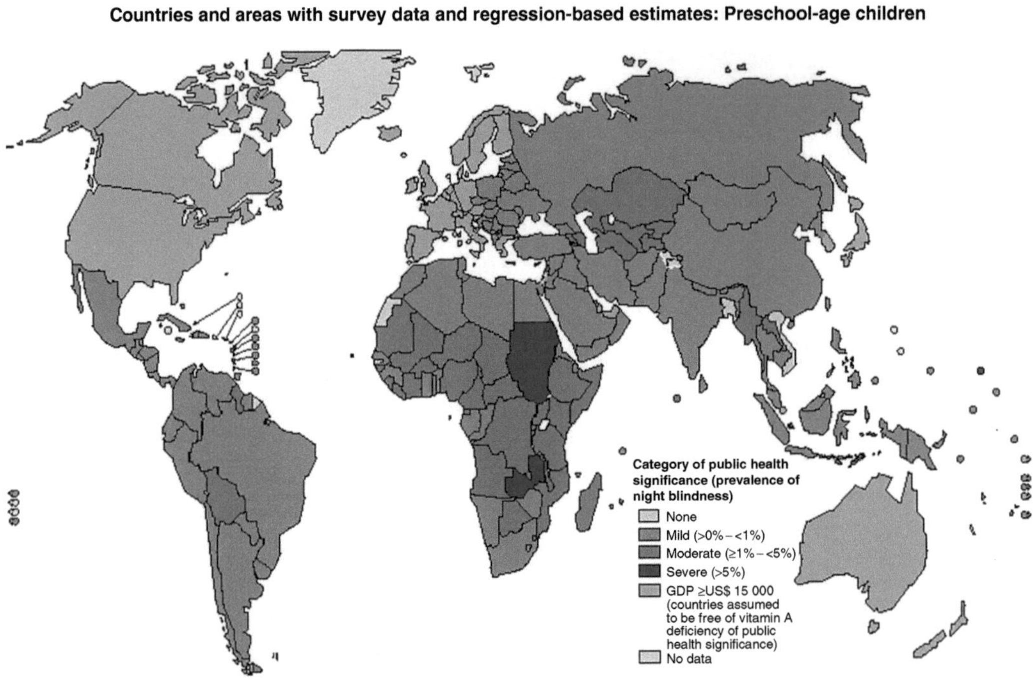

Fig. 15.3 Public health significance of vitamin A deficiency based on reported nightblindness in preschool-age children. *Source*: World Health Organization, 2009 [1], with permission

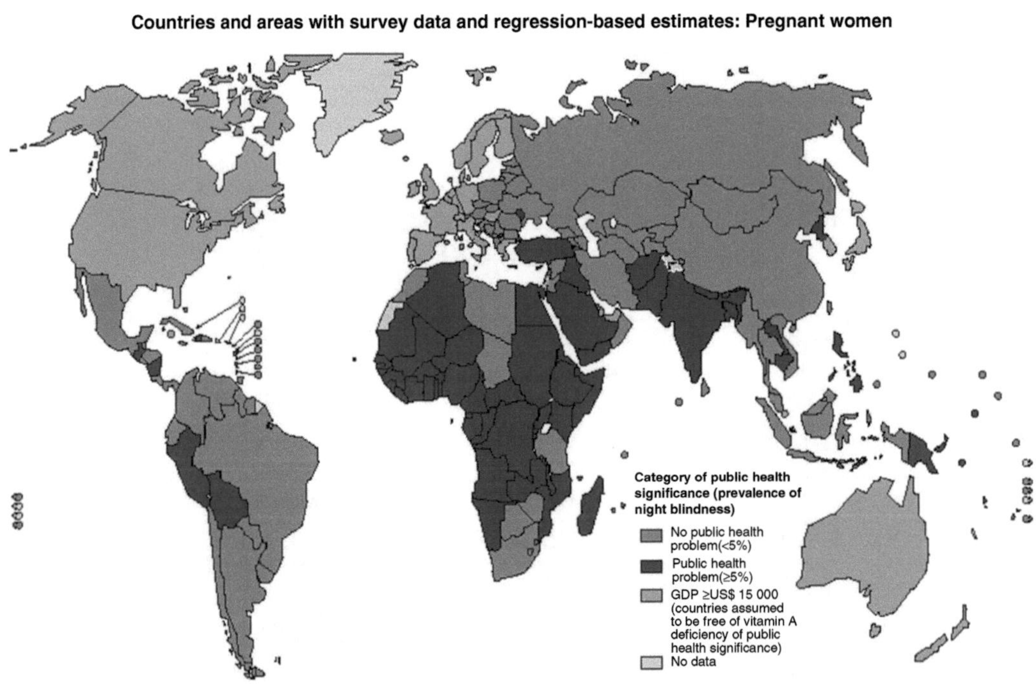

Fig. 15.4 Public health significance of vitamin A deficiency based on reported nightblindness in pregnant women. *Source*: World Health Organization, 2009 [1], with permission

increased risk of mortality from diarrheal diseases and measles in preschool-age children [1, 6]. Similarly, night blind pregnant women are five times more likely to die of infection during or shortly after pregnancy than non-night blind women [7].

Supplementation with vitamin A reduces childhood and maternal mortality. Supplementation of 6–59 month-old children with high-dose vitamin A capsules (200,000 IU) reduces childhood mortality by 23–30%, based on meta-analyses of randomized controlled intervention trials [6, 8]. Weekly supplementation of pregnant women with smaller doses of vitamin A or β-carotene (7 mg retinol equivalents (RE)/week) reduced maternal mortality by 44% in Nepal [9]. However, in a recent study, weekly vitamin A supplementation (25,000 IU/week) of pregnant Ghanaian women had no effect on maternal mortality [10]. These conflicting results may be related to differences in the vitamin A status of the Ghanaian and Nepali women. Night blindness was rare among the Ghanaian women, but was prevalent among the Nepali women, and the reduction in mortality in the Nepali women was greatest among night-blind women [11].

Importance of Provitamin A Carotenoids as a Dietary Source of Vitamin A

Provitamin A carotenoids are an important source of dietary vitamin A and are found in dark green leafy vegetables, such as spinach and kale, and in orange and yellow vegetables and fruits, such as carrot, mango, and papaya. β-Carotene, β-cryptoxanthin, and α-carotene are the provitamin A carotenoids that are commonly found in foods in human diets [12]. The vitamin A equivalency of provitamin A carotenoids is controversial and can be affected by many food and diet-related factors, as well as by health, nutritional, and genetic characteristics of human populations [12]. In the USA, a vitamin A equivalency ratio of 12:1, by weight, (12 μg β-carotene = 1 μg retinol = 1 retinol activity equivalent (RAE)) is recommended for β-carotene from mixed diets containing vegetables and fruits [13]. This is based on an absorption efficiency of ~16% for β-carotene from a mixed diet (6 μg plant β-carotene = 1 μg pure β-carotene) and an intestinal conversion ratio of 2:1, by weight, for pure β-carotene to vitamin A (2 μg β-carotene = 1 μg retinol). The other provitamin A carotenoids are assumed to have half the vitamin A activity of β-carotene based on differences in their chemical structures; thus, a vitamin A equivalency ratio of 24:1 is recommended for α-carotene and β-cryptoxanthin [13].

The vitamin A activities of α-carotene and β-cryptoxanthin have not been determined experimentally in humans. Recent data suggest that the vitamin A activity of β-cryptoxanthin may be greater than is currently assumed. In human volunteers who consumed similar amounts of α-carotene, β-cryptoxanthin, or β-carotene, plasma concentrations of α-carotene and β-cryptoxanthin were ~53% and ~725% higher, respectively, than plasma β-carotene concentrations, suggesting that α-carotene and β-cryptoxanthin may be more efficiently absorbed than β-carotene [14]. However, the greater apparent absorption of intact α-carotene and β-cryptoxanthin, compared to β-carotene, may be related to differences in intestinal conversion of these provitamin A carotenoids to vitamin A. The extent to which α-carotene and β-cryptoxanthin are converted to vitamin A in the human intestine is not known. In Mongolian gerbils that were fed pure α-carotene or β-carotene, 5.5 μg α-carotene was equivalent to 1 μg retinol, whereas 2.8 μg β-carotene was equivalent to 1 μg retinol; confirming that α-carotene has approximately half the vitamin A activity of β-carotene [15]. In contrast, in Mongolian gerbils that were fed pure β-cryptoxanthin or β-carotene, 2.7 μg β-cryptoxanthin was equivalent to 1 μg retinol, whereas 2.5 μg β-carotene was equivalent to 1 μg retinol, indicating that β-cryptoxanthin has ~92% of the vitamin A activity of β-carotene. As stated above, it is currently assumed that β-cryptoxanthin has ~50% of the vitamin A activity of β-carotene [16]. Thus, these data suggest that β-cryptoxanthin may have greater vitamin A activity and that food sources of β-cryptoxanthin such as citrus fruits, papaya, and yellow and orange maize may be better sources of dietary vitamin A than is currently assumed.

It is important to note that the vitamin A equivalency ratios for provitamin A carotenoids that are recommended by the Food and Agricultural Organization (FAO) and the World Health Organization (WHO) differ from those recommended by the Institute of Medicine in the USA. A vitamin A equivalency ratio of 6:1, by weight, for β-carotene from a mixed diet (6 μg β-carotene = 1 μg retinol = 1 retinol equivalent (RE)) is recommended by FAO/WHO, and a ratio of 12:1, by weight, is recommended for the other provitamin A carotenoids based on the assumption that their vitamin A activities are approximately half that of β-carotene because of differences in their chemical structures [17].

Safety of β-Carotene as a Dietary Source of Vitamin A

The safety of dietary provitamin A carotenoids as a vitamin A source is based on data for β-carotene. β-Carotene is considered a safe source of vitamin A because intestinal conversion of β-carotene to vitamin A decreases as an oral dose of β-carotene increases, which prevents formation of excessive vitamin A [18]. Also, expression of the BCMO1 gene is regulated by vitamin A status; thus, expression of the intestinal BCMO1 enzyme is upregulated in VAD, favoring greater intestinal conversion of β-carotene to vitamin A when vitamin A status is low, and downregulated when vitamin A status is adequate [19]. In contrast, preformed dietary vitamin A is easily absorbed from the diet [3] and has been associated with adverse health effects if consumed in excessive amounts. High intakes of preformed vitamin A (≥3,000 μg RE/day) were associated with an increased risk of hip fracture in postmenopausal women [20]. Also, because preformed vitamin A is potentially teratogenic, pregnant women are advised to avoid consuming large amounts of preformed vitamin A, and dietary β-carotene is considered to be a safer source of vitamin A during pregnancy [12].

However, there is concern that large doses of supplemental β-carotene may have adverse effects on human health. In early intervention trials, participants were supplemented with large doses of synthetic β-carotene (20 mg/day or 30 mg/day) to assess the effect of β-carotene on the incidence of lung cancer or cardiovascular disease. The results of these trials indicated that supplementation with large daily doses of β-carotene was not associated with a reduced risk of cancer or cardiovascular disease and may be harmful to smokers or to workers exposed to asbestos [21–23]. The amounts of supplemental β-carotene that were given to participants are much higher than the amounts that are commonly consumed in the diet. Dietary intake of β-carotene in the USA and UK is ~1–2 mg/day for most people and ~4–9 mg/day for vegans and vegetarians [12]. There are no known adverse health effects associated with usual dietary intakes of provitamin A carotenoids. However, in some individuals, chronic high intakes of carotenoids can result in a yellow discoloration of the skin, which is considered a benign condition [24].

Food Supply of Vitamin A

The global food supply of vitamin A is based on food balance sheets that are compiled by the FAO. As shown in Table 15.1, in Europe and The Americas, 37% of vitamin A in the food supply is provided by preformed vitamin A from animal sources, and 64% is provided by provitamin A carotenoids from plant sources. In contrast, in Africa and South and South East Asia, animal sources provide only 12% and 16% of preformed vitamin A in the food supply, respectively, and plant sources provide 84% and 88%, respectively. This is an important difference because preformed vitamin A from animal sources

Table 15.1 Available food supply of vitamin A, by WHO region

Region	Animal sources (μg RE/day)	Vegetable sources (μg RE/day)	Total (μg RE/day)
Africa	122 (16%)	654 (84%)	776
The Americas	295 (36%)	519 (64%)	814
South East Asia	53 (12%)	378 (88%)	431
Europe	271 (37%)	467 (63%)	738
Eastern Mediterranean	345 (37%)	591 (63%)	936
Western Pacific	216 (22%)	781 (78%)	997
Total	212 (27%)	565 (73%)	777

Numbers in parentheses indicate the percentage of total retinol equivalents (RE) from carotenoid food sources
WHO (2004), with permission

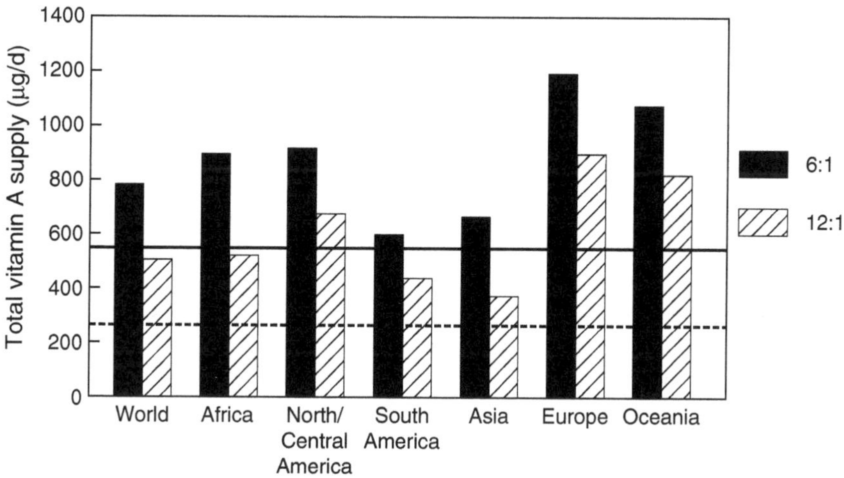

Fig. 15.5 Estimated global food supply of vitamin A based on the retinol equivalent (RE) or retinol activity equivalent (RAE). Based on data from West, 2002 (adapted). The *dashed line* represents the average vitamin A requirement for non-pregnant, non-lactating women of reproductive age (270 μg/day); the *solid line* represents the recommended safe level of intake of vitamin A for non-pregnant, non-lactating women of reproductive age (500 μg/day) (FAO/WHO, 2004). RE = 1 μg retinol = 6 μg β-carotene = 12 μg other PVA carotenoids; RAE = 1 μg retinol = 12 μg β-carotene = 24 μg other PVA carotenoids

is easily absorbed and utilized in the body, whereas provitamin A carotenoids are less well-absorbed and must be converted to vitamin A in intestinal cells.

Estimates of the global food supply of vitamin A are based on the retinol equivalent (RE); thus, a vitamin A equivalency ratio of 6:1 was used to estimate the vitamin A content of plant sources of β-carotene. Figure 15.5 compares estimates of the food supply of vitamin A based on the retinol equivalent (RE) and RAE, in relation to the FAO/WHO estimated vitamin A requirement and recommended safe intake of vitamin A for non-pregnant, non-lactating women [17, 25]. The adequacy of the global daily food supply of vitamin A is greatly affected by the vitamin A equivalency ratio that is used to estimate the vitamin A content of plant sources of vitamin A. Based on the RE (vitamin A equivalency ratio of 6:1), the per capita daily food supply of vitamin A exceeds the daily vitamin A requirement of non-pregnant, non-lactating women (270 μg/day) and recommended safe level of intake (500 μg/day). However, based on the RAE (vitamin A equivalency ratio of 12:1) the per capita daily food supply exceeds the daily vitamin A requirement of non-pregnant, non-lactating women, but falls short of the recommended daily safe intake in Africa, South America, and Asia. Because of the continuing controversy on the vitamin A equivalency of provitamin A carotenoids, it is difficult to estimate the vitamin A content of diets that consist primarily of plant sources of vitamin A.

Dietary Intake of Provitamin A Carotenoids as a Vitamin A Source

In the USA, the dietary reference intakes for vitamin A are for total dietary vitamin A; separate intakes are not specified for preformed vitamin A and provitamin A carotenoids (Table 15.2) [13]. It is assumed that vegetarians and vegans in the USA can meet their vitamin A requirements by carefully choosing foods that contain high amounts of provitamin A carotenoids [13]. Based on the US NHANES (National Health and Nutrition Examination Survey) data set for 2007–2008, mean dietary intakes of vitamin A were 654 RAE/day and 598 RAE/day for men (n=3,748) and women (n=3,958) 19–64 years of age, respectively [26]. These intakes exceed their estimated average vitamin A requirements (EAR) of 625 μg RAE/day (men) and 500 μg RAE/day (women) [13]. Of the provitamin A carotenoids, mean intakes of β-carotene were highest, 1,988 μg/day and 2,050 μg/day for men and women, respectively. Mean intakes of β-cryptoxanthin were 80 μg/day and 75 μg/day for men and women, respectively; and mean intakes of α-carotene were 386 μg/day and 402 μg/day, respectively. Provitamin A carotenoids provided ~28% and ~32% of mean vitamin A intakes for US men and women, respectively (based on vitamin A equivalency ratios of 12:1 for β-carotene and 24:1 for the other provitamin A carotenoids). In US children 3–4 years of age (n=677), mean dietary vitamin A intake was 594 μg RAE/day, which exceeds their EAR of 210 μg RAE/day (3 years of age) and 275 μg RAE/day (4 years of age) [13]. Mean intakes of β-carotene, β-cryptoxanthin, and α-carotene were 1,388 μg/day, 94 μg/day, and 346 μg/day, respectively, and provitamin A carotenoids provided ~49–64% of their mean vitamin A intake. The estimates of intakes for adults and children were based on 1–2 days of 24-h recall data.

The FAO/WHO recommended dietary intakes for vitamin A are commonly used in developing countries (Table 15.3) [17]. Populations in developing countries rely on dietary provitamin A carotenoids to a greater extent to meet their vitamin A needs. Nationally representative data on dietary intakes of vitamin A and provitamin A carotenoids do not exist in most developing countries. However, dietary surveys have been conducted in populations at risk of VAD, and insufficient dietary intake of

Table 15.2 US dietary reference intakes for vitamin A

Group	Adequate intake (μg RAE/day)	EAR (μg RAE/day)	RDA (μg RAE/day)
Infants			
0–6 months	400		
7–12 months	500		
Children			
1–3 years		210	300
4–8 years		275	400
Women			
19–30 years		500	700
Men			
19–30 years		625	900
Pregnant women		550	770
Lactating women		900	1,300

Adapted from Institute of Medicine (2001)
EAR estimated average requirement, *RDA* recommended daily allowance, *RAE* retinol activity equivalents

Table 15.3 FAO/WHO recommended dietary intakes for vitamin A

Group	Mean requirement (μg RE/day)	Recommended safe intake (μg RE/day)
Infants and children		
0–6 months	180	375
7–12 months	190	400
1–3 years	200	400
4–6 years	200	450
Women		
19–65 years	270	500
Men		
19–65 years	300	600
Pregnant women	370	800
Lactating women	450	850

Adapted from FAO/WHO (2004)
RE (retinol equivalent) = 1 μg retinol = 6 μg β-carotene = 12 μg other provitamin A carotenoids

vitamin A has been reported for women of reproductive age and for preschool-age children. A recent review examined reported micronutrient intakes of women living in resource-poor settings in Latin America, Africa, and Asia, and the data indicate that mean/median vitamin A intakes were below the FAO/WHO estimated mean requirement in ~29% of all studies examined; however, there were regional differences [27]. Vitamin A intakes were above the estimated mean requirement in Latin America and most African studies examined, but below the estimated mean requirement in 47% of studies that were conducted in Asia [27]. Information was not provided on intakes of provitamin A carotenoids. In urban women of reproductive age (n = 178) in Burkina Faso, 33% had inadequate vitamin A intakes in relation to the FAO/WHO estimated mean vitamin A requirement (270 μg RE/day), based on 3 days of quantitative 24-h recall data [17, 28]. The prevalence of inadequate intakes may be underestimated because a vitamin A equivalency ratio of 6:1 was used for β-carotene in the diet. Similarly, in urban women 15–45 years of age in Mali (n = 102), the median vitamin A intake was 245 μg RE/day based on two 24-h recalls, which is below the FAO/WHO estimated mean vitamin A requirement [29].

Low vitamin A intakes have also been reported for preschool-age children in developing countries. A recent study in 2–5 year old children in Kenya (n = 449) and Nigeria (n = 793) found that ~41% of Kenyan children and ~83% of Nigerian children had inadequate vitamin A intakes in relation to their recommended daily intakes (300 μg RAE/day for children 2–4 years of age or 400 μg RAE/day for children 4–5 years of age) [13, 30]. Data from a single 24-h recall in the Indian National Family Health Survey, 2005–2006, indicate that ~42% of children 12–35 months of age did not receive vitamin A-rich foods [31]. In Mozambiquean children 4–38 months of age (n = 234), median vitamin A intake was 56 μg RAE/day and median β-carotene intake was 62 μg/day, based on a 24-h recall. Collectively these data suggest that preschool-age children in low-income settings are at risk of inadequate intakes of preformed vitamin A and provitamin A carotenoids.

Effect of Dietary Provitamin A-Carotenoid Interventions on Vitamin A Status

Few controlled community-based intervention trials have been carried out to assess the effect of dietary provitamin A carotenoids on the vitamin A status of women of reproductive age or preschool-age children in populations at risk of VAD. The few trials that have been carried out in women have had mixed results. Feeding Indonesian lactating women 3.5 mg/day β-carotene as dark green leafy vegetables for 12 weeks had no effect on serum or milk retinol concentrations [32]. In contrast, feeding Vietnamese lactating women 4.8 mg/day or 5.6 mg/day β-carotene as dark green leafy vegetables or fruit, respectively, for 10 weeks, increased serum and milk retinol concentrations, compared to a negative control group [33]. Similarly, feeding Zimbabwean women 1.1 mg/day β-carotene for 60 days as pureed papaya or grated carrot increased serum retinol concentrations compared to a negative control group, and the proportion of women with inadequate liver stores of vitamin A decreased in the papaya group compared to the control group [34]. Feeding night-blind, pregnant Nepali women with 850 μg/day β-carotene for 6 weeks as dark green leafy vegetables or carrots normalized dark adaptation and increased plasma β-carotene concentrations, but had no effect on serum retinol concentrations [35].

There is also evidence that dietary interventions can increase vitamin A status in preschool-age and older children. In Gambian children, 2–7 years of age, feeding 1.8 mg/day of β-carotene as dried mango, for 4 months, increased serum retinol concentrations, compared to a negative control group [36]. In Mozambique, promotion of production and consumption of orange-fleshed sweet potatoes increased serum retinol concentrations in children 4–38 months of age in intervention villages compared to control villages, after 2 years [37]. In Chinese children, 5–6 years of age, feeding 4.6 mg/day of β-carotene, for 10 weeks, maintained total body vitamin A stores and prevented the decline in vitamin A stores of ~7.7 mg that was observed in the negative control group [38]. A few school-based intervention trials have been carried out in older children to assess the effect of feeding dietary provitamin A carotenoids on vitamin A status. In South African children, 5–10 years of age, feeding ~12.4 mg/day β-carotene as orange-fleshed sweet potatoes for 53 days improved liver vitamin A stores, compared with a negative control group [39]. In Indonesian children, 7–11 years of age, feeding 4.1 mg/day or 3.0 mg/day β-carotene as dark green leafy vegetables or fruit, respectively, for 9 weeks, increased serum retinol concentrations, compared with a negative control group [40]. Collectively, these intervention trials demonstrate that feeding dietary provitamin A carotenoids can increase vitamin A status in populations at risk of deficiency. However, in most cases, the magnitude of the increase in vitamin A status cannot be quantified because the biochemical indicators that were used to assess vitamin A status do not provide quantitative estimates of change in vitamin A stores in response to the intervention [41]. Information on the effect of dietary interventions on vitamin A-dependent physiologic functions, such as dark adaptation, in addition to information on changes in biochemical indicators of vitamin A status, would be useful for better interpreting the biological impact of food-based interventions.

Summary

VAD continues to be a serious public health problem in preschool-age children and women of reproductive age in developing countries. Plant sources of provitamin A carotenoids make a substantial contribution to the global food supply of vitamin A; however, the vitamin A equivalency of provitamin A carotenoids from plant sources remains controversial. Different vitamin A equivalency ratios are recommended for provitamin A carotenoids in the USA and by the FAO/WHO, and because of this, vitamin A intakes and the adequacy of intakes are difficult to interpret and compare across studies. Nevertheless, data from a few efficacy trials indicate that feeding plant sources of provitamin A carotenoids can increase vitamin A status in populations at risk of VAD. Further research is needed to better understand factors affecting bioavailability of provitamin A carotenoids and to better understand the biological impact of dietary interventions on the health and vitamin A status of populations.

References

1. World Health Organization. Global prevalence of vitamin A deficiency in populations at risk 1995–2005. WHO Global database on vitamin A deficiency. Geneva, Switzerland: WHO; 2009.
2. World Health Organization. Vitamin A supplements: a guide to their use in the treatment and prevention of vitamin A deficiency and xerophthalmia. Geneva, Switzerland: WHO; 1997. p. 9–18.
3. Sivakumar B, Reddy V. Absorption of labelled vitamin A in children during infection. Br J Nutr. 1972;27: 299–304.
4. Alvarez JO, Salazar-Lindo E, Kohatsu J, et al. Urinary excretion of retinol in children with acute diarrhea. Am J Clin Nutr. 1995;61:1273–6.
5. Stephensen CB, Alvarez JO, Kohatsu J, et al. Vitamin A is excreted in the urine during acute infection. Am J Clin Nutr. 1994;60:388–92.
6. Beaton GH, Martorell R, L'Abbe KA, et al. Effectiveness of vitamin A supplementation in the control of young child morbidity and mortality in developing countries. Nutrition Policy Discussion Paper No.13 ACC/SCN. 1993.
7. Christian P, West KP Jr, Khatry S, et al. Night blindness during pregnancy and subsequent mortality among women in Nepal: effects of vitamin A and β-carotene supplementation. Am J Epidemiol. 2000;152:542–7.
8. Glasziou P, Mackerras D. Vitamin A supplementation in infectious diseases: a meta-analysis. Br Med J. 1993;306:366–70.
9. West KP Jr, Katz J, Khatry S, et al. Double blind, cluster randomised trial of low dose supplementation with vitamin A or β-carotene on mortality related to pregnancy in Nepal. BMJ. 1999;318:570–5.
10. Kirkwood B, Hurt L, Amenga-Etego S, et al. Effect of vitamin A supplementation in women of reproductive age on maternal survival in Ghana (ObaapaVitA): a cluster-randomised, placebo-controlled trial. Lancet. 2010;375:1640–9.
11. West KP Jr, Christian P, Katz J, et al. Effect of vitamin A supplementation on maternal survival. Lancet. 2010; 376:873–4.
12. Grune T, Lietz G, Palou A, et al. β-carotene is an important vitamin A source for humans. J Nutr. 2010; 140:2268S–85.
13. Institute of Medicine. Dietary reference intakes: vitamin A, vitamin K, arsenic, boron, chromium, copper, iodine, iron, manganese, molybdenum, nickel, silicon, vanadium and zinc. Washington, DC: National Academy Press; 2001.
14. Burri B, Chang J, Neidlinger T. β-Cryptoxanthin and α-carotene rich foods have greater apparent bioavailability than β-carotene rich foods in Western diets. Br J Nutr. 2011;105:212–9.
15. Tanumihardjo S, Howe J. Twice the amount of alpha-carotene isolated from carrots is as effective as beta-carotene in maintaining the vitamin A status of Mongolian gerbils. J Nutr. 2005;135:2622–6.
16. Davis D, Jing H, Howe J, et al. Beta-cryptoxanthin from supplements or carotenoid-enhanced maize maintains liver vitamin A in Mongolian gerbils (*Meriones unguiculatus*) better than or equal to beta-carotene supplements. Br J Nutr. 2008;3:1–8.
17. Food and Agricultural Organization. Vitamin and mineral requirements in human nutrition. Report of joint FAO/WHO expert consultation. FAO, Rome: Bangkok, Thailand; 2004.
18. Novotny J, Harrison D, Pawlosky R, et al. β-Carotene conversion to vitamin A decreases as the dietary dose increases in humans. J Nutr. 2010;140:915–8.
19. Lietz G, Lange J, Rimbach G. Molecular and dietary regulation of β, β-carotene 15,15′-monooxygenase 1 (BCMO1). Arch Biochem Biophys. 2010;502:8–16.
20. Feskanich D, Singh V, Willett WC, et al. Vitamin A intake and hip fractures among postmenopausal women. JAMA. 2002;287:47–54.
21. Gaziano J, Hennekens C. The role of beta-carotene in the prevention of cardiovascular disease. Ann N Y Acad Sci. 1993;691:148–55.
22. The Alpha-Tocopherol β-Carotene Cancer Prevention Study Group. The effect of vitamin E and β-carotene on the incidence of lung cancer and other cancers in male smokers. N Engl J Med. 1994;330:1029–35.
23. Omenn G, Goodman GE, Thornquist MD, et al. Risk factors for lung cancer and for intervention effects in CARET, the beta-carotene and retinol efficacy trial. J Natl Cancer Inst. 1996;88:1550–9.
24. Vijayalakshmi A. Carotenodermia. Indian Pediatr. 2008;45:61.
25. West C, Eilander A, van Lieshout M. Consequences of revised estimates of carotenoid bioefficacy for dietary control of vitamin A deficiency in developing countries. J Nutr. 2002;132:2920S–6.
26. Centers for Disease Control and Prevention (CDC), National Center for Health Statistics (NCHS). National Health and Nutrition Examination Survey Data. Hyattsville, MD: U.S. Department of Health and Human Services, Centers for Disease Control and Prevention, 2007–2008; 2008.
27. Torheim L, Ferguson E, Penrose K, et al. Women in resource-poor settings are at risk of inadequate intakes of multiple micronutrients. J Nutr. 2010;140:2051S–8.

28. Becquey E, Martin-Prevel Y. Micronutrient adequacy of women's diet in urban Burkina Faso is low. J Nutr. 2010;140:2079S–85.
29. Kennedy G, Fanou-Fogny N, Seghieri C, et al. Food groups associated with a composite measure of probability of adequate intake of 11 micronutrients in the diets of women in urban Mali. J Nutr. 2010;140:2070S–80.
30. Gegios A, Amthor R, Maziya-Dixon B, et al. Children consuming cassava as a staple food are at risk for inadequate zinc, iron, and vitamin A intake. Plant Foods Hum Nutr. 2010;65:64–70.
31. Semba R, de Pee S, Sun K, et al. Low intake of vitamin A-rich foods among children, aged 12–35 months, in India: association with malnutrition, anemia, and missed child survival interventions. Nutr J. 2010;26:958–62.
32. de Pee S, West CE, Muhilal, et al. Lack of improvement in vitamin A status with increased consumption of dark-green leafy vegetables. Lancet. 1995;346:75–81.
33. Khan N, West CE, de Pee S, et al. The contribution of plant foods to the vitamin A supply of lactating women in Vietnam: a randomized controlled trial. Am J Clin Nutr. 2007;85:1112–20.
34. Ncube T, Greiner T, Malaba L, et al. Supplementing lactating women with pureed papaya and grated carrots improved vitamin A status in a placebo-controlled trial. J Nutr. 2001;131:1497–502.
35. Haskell M, Pandey P, Graham J, et al. Recovery from impaired dark adaptation does not differ among nightblind pregnant Nepali women who receive small daily doses of vitamin A as either liver, vitamin A-fortified Ultra-riceTM, green leafy vegetables, carrots, or vitamin A capsules. Am J Clin Nutr. 2005;81:461–71.
36. Drammeh B, Marquis G, Funkhouser E, et al. A randomized, 4-month mango and fat supplementation trial improved vitamin A status among young Gambian children. J Nutr. 2002;132:3693–9.
37. Low J, Arimond M, Osman N, et al. A food-based approach introducing orange-fleshed sweet potatoes increased vitamin A intake and serum retinol concentrations in young children in rural Mozambique. J Nutr. 2007;137:1320–7.
38. Tang G, Gu X, Hu S, et al. Green and yellow vegetables can maintain vitamin A body stores in Chinese children. Am J Clin Nutr. 1999;70:1069–76.
39. van Jaarsveld P, Faber M, Tanumihardjo S, Nestel P, Lombard C, Spinnler Benadé A. β-Carotene-rich orange-fleshed sweet potato improves the vitamin A status of primary school children assessed with the modified-relative-dose-response test. Am J Clin Nutr. 2005;81:1080–7.
40. de Pee S, West C, Permaesih D, et al. Orange fruit is more effective than are dark-green, leafy vegetables in increasing serum concentrations of retinol and β-carotene in schoolchildren in Indonesia. Am J Clin Nutr. 1998;68:1058–67.
41. Tanumihardjo SA. Vitamin A: biomarkers of nutrition for development. Am J Clin Nutr. 2011;94:658S–65.

Chapter 16
Provitamin A Carotenoids and Immune Function

Charles B. Stephensen

Key Points

- Vitamin A was called the anti-infective vitamin early in the twentieth century when vitamin A deficiency was shown to increase the severity of infections of experimental animals.
- Squamous metaplasia caused by vitamin A deficiency was known to disrupt the mucosal barrier to infection at that time but later insights into how vitamin A deficiency impaired immunity awaited the development of research methods in cellular immunology, and identification of retinoic acid as the key vitamin A metabolite active in the immune system, late in the twentieth century.
- It is now evident from studies in rodents that vitamin A deficiency impairs many aspects of both innate and adaptive immunity, but particularly development of antibody responses to T-cell-dependent antigens, secretory IgA responses at mucosal surfaces, development of T-helper cell subsets, and trafficking of lymphocytes to the intestinal tract.
- These defects are also presumed to occur in humans, although data are quite limited. Correcting such defects is presumably responsible for the ability of vitamin A supplementation to decrease the risk of mortality from some common infections of childhood (e.g., diarrhea and measles) in infants over 6 months of age in developing country settings where the risk of death from such infections is high.

Keywords Vitamin A • Retinol • Retinoic acid • Mortality • Immunity • Innate • Adaptive • Lymphocyte • Mucosal • Antibody

Introduction

The biological activities of vitamin A in promoting growth and sustaining vision were described nearly a century ago [1]. Within a few years vitamin A was additionally termed the "anti-infective vitamin" because deficient animals were found to develop symptomatic infections of mucosal surfaces at a much greater rate than non-deficient animals [2]. These infections were thought to result from compromised barrier defenses resulting from the patchy squamous metaplasia that was described at

C.B. Stephensen, Ph.D. (✉)
Immunity and Disease Prevention Research Unit, United States Department of Agriculture, Agricultural Research Service, Western Human Nutrition Research Center, University of California, 430 West Health Sciences Drive, Davis, CA 95616, USA
e-mail: Charles.Stephensen@ars.usda.gov

S.A. Tanumihardjo (ed.), *Carotenoids and Human Health*, Nutrition and Health,
DOI 10.1007/978-1-62703-203-2_16, © Springer Science+Business Media New York 2013

respiratory and intestinal epithelial surfaces. As a result of such observations, treatment studies were conducted into the 1940s to determine if vitamin A-rich preparations (e.g., cod liver oil) could be used to treat respiratory and enteric infections in humans. Some successes were reported but results were mixed overall [3]. Interest in such studies waned with the advent of antibiotics. The mechanisms underlying this increase in risk were not understood at that time, primarily because the science of immunology was only in its infancy [4]. In addition, the principal mechanism of action of vitamin A outside of the visual cycle was not defined until 1987 when retinoic acid was found to be the ligand for the retinoic acid receptor (RAR) [5]. This discovery showed that vitamin A could regulate gene expression and thus affect many cellular processes known to be responsive to vitamin A, such as cellular differentiation. This mechanism appears to account for the effects of vitamin A in the immune system. Other mechanisms may also be involved.

The major effect of provitamin A carotenoids on immunity occurs via production of vitamin A. However, carotenoids, apart from their provitamin A activity, can also affect immune function, primarily through their role as lipid-soluble antioxidants, as has been reviewed [6, 7]. While the focus of this chapter is on the role of vitamin A in immunity, the other activities of carotenoids will also be considered.

Vitamin A Deficiency and Childhood Mortality

Vitamin A deficiency is common in many developing countries in pregnant women and young children (Fig. 16.1). Worldwide, 190 million infants and young children have low serum retinol concentrations sometimes indicative of inadequate vitamin A stores (<0.70 μmol/l) with the majority living in South Asia and Africa. Controlled intervention trials conducted in the 1990s demonstrated that

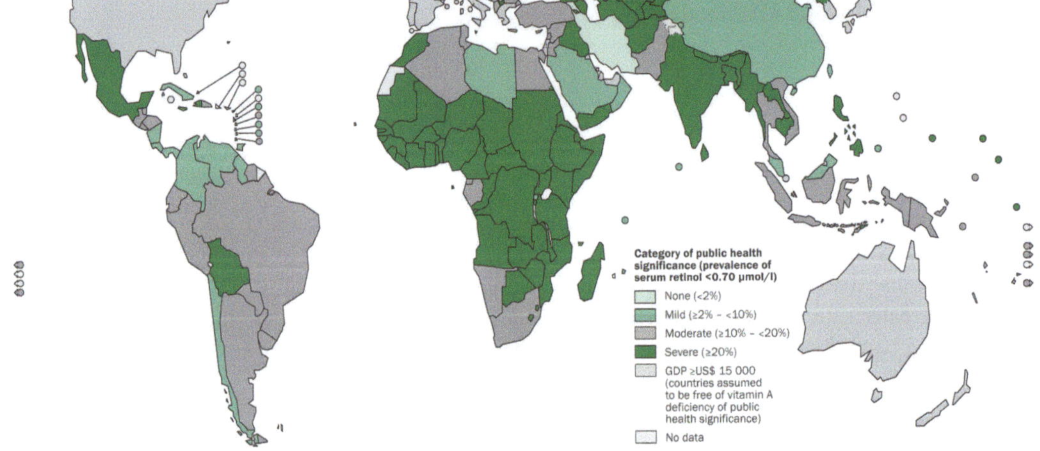

Fig. 16.1 Map of vitamin A deficiency in preschool children based on the prevalence of low serum retinol concentration. The map was provided with the permission from the World Health Organization (http://www.who.int/vmnis/vitamina/prevalence/vita_fig2b.pdf)

treatment of vitamin A deficiency in populations at risk of vitamin A deficiency in Africa and Asia decreases mortality from early childhood infections by ~24 % relative to subjects receiving placebo. In particular, diarrhea- and measles-related deaths were decreased by 28 % and 24 %, respectively. The risk of symptomatic measles infection was decreased by 50 %. These results come from a meta-analysis of many intervention trials in Asia and Africa [8]. Indicators of vitamin A deficiency also decreased dramatically in these studies: Night blindness decreased by 68 %, corneal signs of vitamin A deficiency (xerophthalmia) by 55 %, and deficiency as assessed by serum retinol by 29 %.

Based on these studies, vitamin A supplementation is currently recommended by the World Health Organization (WHO) for young children 6–59 months of age in populations where vitamin A deficiency is common [9]. (It should be noted that vitamin A supplementation to individuals with significant risk of deficiency is always recommended to improve vitamin A status, but WHO recommendations at the population level are strongly influenced by preventing mortality.) Providing vitamin A supplements to infants from 1 to 6 months of age has had mixed results in reducing mortality and is not currently recommended to decrease infant mortality [10]. Vitamin A supplementation in neonates, particularly within a day or 2 of birth, may also protect against death from infectious diseases but results vary by geographic region and sex of the infant [11]. When these studies are examined together there is not currently a sufficiently strong case to make an overall recommendation for supplementation [12]. While the specific biological mechanisms underlying the protective effect of vitamin A have not been clearly defined in human studies, it is likely that providing vitamin A supplements to deficient individuals restores impaired immune function thus improving recovery from infections and decreasing the risk of death. The impact in specific populations will also be influenced by the prevalence of various infectious diseases, the extent and duration of breastfeeding, and, of course, the underlying vitamin A status of infants and young children.

The Immune System

The principal function of the immune system is to protect us from death (and disability) caused by pathogenic parasites and microorganisms. Immunologists currently think of the immune system as having two components: "innate" and "adaptive" [13], although the two work together as an integrated whole. The innate system is evolutionarily older than the adaptive system and it is fully functional at birth. Innate immune cells (e.g., neutrophils, eosinophils, macrophages, and antigen presenting cells such as dendritic cells) use a diverse group of receptors (e.g., Toll-like receptors or TLRs) to recognize and respond to signature molecules from classes of microorganisms (e.g., flagella from some bacteria, cell-wall carbohydrate from yeast, RNA from viral genomes). These protective responses (e.g., phagocytosis, production of cytokines to promote inflammation) are essentially the same for all individuals within a species and do not vary after exposure to specific pathogens. Tissue damage from trauma, such as surgery, or physiologic damage, such as the development of lesions in the coronary arteries due to a poor diet, can also trigger the innate immune response. The adaptive immune system is different in that the host's response adapts to a specific pathogen (e.g., measles virus specifically and not RNA viruses in general) in order to develop "immunologic memory" that will respond more quickly and more efficiently the next time the same pathogen is encountered. This adaptation includes production of antigen-specific T and B lymphocytes, as well as antibodies. The innate immune system can help steer the development of the adaptive immune response by interacting with T and B lymphocytes, the principal cellular components of the adaptive immune system. Thus, individuals have different levels of adaptive immunity depending on their exposure history. Such an adaptive immune response occurs more rapidly after the second exposure to an antigen than it does after the first exposure. Thus the first encounter with a childhood pathogen (e.g., measles) can make a child quite ill, but subsequent infections will likely go unnoticed if an effective adaptive immune response has developed.

Vitamin A and Innate Immunity

Epithelial Surfaces

The first lines of defense against pathogens for any animal are its epithelial tissues, including the skin and mucosal epithelial surfaces of the respiratory, gastrointestinal, and urogenital tracts. The surface of the eye is also covered by epithelial cells that can play a defensive role. Vitamin A deficiency causes squamous metaplasia of mucosal epithelial surfaces. That is, the ciliated, columnar epithelial cells that help protect the respiratory tract from infection are replaced by squamous epithelium (which is normally limited to the skin) during vitamin A deficiency. This is most pronounced when these cells are challenged by external factors, including cigarette smoke or a respiratory tract infection. Squamous metaplasia is not limited to the respiratory tract and is seen at mucosal epithelial surfaces throughout the body, including the gastrointestinal tract and urinary bladder. Mucus-producing goblet cells are also lost from mucosal epithelial surfaces as a result of vitamin A deficiency. Squamous metaplasia and decreased mucus production can decrease protection of epithelial surfaces from bacterial pathogens. These changes may increase adherence of some pathogens, as can occur in the respiratory tract and urinary bladder, and can increase tissue damage by viral infection in the gut. These epithelial changes may increase the risk of invasive diseases, which could be life threatening [14].

Phagocytic Cells

Granulocytes are a group of white blood cells of the innate immune system that include neutrophils, eosinophils, basophils, and mast cells. These cells have a variety of responses to infection but primarily phagocytose and kill bacteria. They also secrete anti-microbial compounds to kill bacteria outside the cell. This killing process involves generation of reactive oxygen and nitrogen species that can cause oxidative damage to bystander cells. These cells also produce soluble mediators of inflammation (e.g., cytokines, chemokines, leukotrienes, prostaglandins) that regulate immune responses [13]. Neutrophils are a part of the initial response of the innate immune system to invasive infection that will result when microbial pathogens cross a mucosal barrier.

Retinoic acid is required for normal differentiation of neutrophils and dietary vitamin A deficiency impairs development of mature neutrophils in rodents and results in circulating neutrophils with significantly impaired ability to phagocytose and kill bacteria [14]. One study in vitamin A-deficient children reported improved neutrophil phagocytosis with vitamin A supplementation [15]. The mechanism of impaired granulopoesis in vitamin A deficiency is not well-described, although many genes involved in neutrophil development are responsive to retinoic acid. This impairment in neutrophil development implies that a reduced resistance to invasive bacterial disease may result from vitamin A deficiency. Consistent with this prediction, clearance of bacteria from the blood is impaired in vitamin A-deficient rats [16]. Increased or unchanged numbers of neutrophils have been reported from vitamin A-deficient rodents but neutrophil function was not examined in the studies describing neutrophilia [14]. In rats, a paradoxical increase in vitamin A levels is seen in the bone marrow during development of vitamin A deficiency [17], perhaps suggesting a compensatory response by the deficient animal to maintain normal development of neutrophils and other cells of the immune system in bone marrow. Thus vitamin A deficiency impairs neutrophil function although under some circumstances, the numbers of neutrophils are not depressed in the blood.

Since oxidative damage to healthy cells, including the phagocytic cells themselves, could have adverse effects for the host, deficiencies in antioxidant nutrients can affect phagocyte function and related tissue damage. Carotenoids are protective with regard to maintaining phagocyte function and minimizing collateral tissue damage [6, 7]. In human studies, elderly subjects are more likely to have poor antioxidant status and thus supplementation trials with antioxidants, such as vitamin E or carotenoids, are more effective in older rather than younger volunteers [18]. Interestingly, preventing such collateral damage via adequate carotenoid levels appears to be relevant to species other than humans who utilize carotenoid for pigments and also as antioxidants, including crustaceans [19] and avian species. In songbirds, carotenoids may enhance immune function and thus enhance fitness. This enhanced fitness may be evident to other birds of the same species thanks to the coloration resulting from high carotenoid intake. Such robust coloration may signal female finches that a particular male is better nourished and therefore a healthier potential mate [20, 21]. Thus carotenoids may play a dual role in enhancing survival of well-nourished finches (see Chap. 8).

Natural Killer Cells

Natural killer (NK) cells are cytotoxic lymphocytes that play an important role in the protection against viral infections before the development of an adaptive immune response [13]. Vitamin A-deficient animals have lower numbers of NK cells with a decreased ability to kill damaged or virus-infected cells. Treatment with retinoic acid restores the NK cell population and increases cytotoxic activity [22]. Thus vitamin A deficiency impairs NK cell function and this deficit may result in a decreased ability to clear infections once they occur.

Monocytes/Macrophages

Monocytes develop in the bone marrow and travel through the bloodstream to tissue sites, where they differentiate into macrophages. Some macrophages are found in healthy tissues and their numbers increase during most infections, particularly infection by viruses and other intracellular pathogens. Their preferred method of killing is through phagocytosis, as is seen with neutrophils. Macrophages also secrete many cytokines that act to promote inflammation by attracting other immune cells [13]. The number of macrophages in secondary lymphoid tissues may be increased by vitamin A deficiency in rodents. When such animals are treated with retinoic acid, the number of monocytes decreases [23]. This apparently paradoxical observation may result from increased production of some cytokines (e.g., interleukin [IL]-12 and interferon [IFN]-γ) in vitamin A deficiency that can promote macrophage-mediated inflammation, thus potentially increasing macrophage numbers in tissues. Vitamin A deficiency also impairs the ability of macrophages to ingest bacteria, which is enhanced with vitamin A supplementation [14]. Thus macrophage function is impaired by vitamin A deficiency but counter-balancing effects may minimize the impact on macrophage-mediated inflammation.

Vitamin A and Adaptive Immunity

Antigen Presenting Cells

Antigen presenting cells, such as dendritic cells, are found in peripheral tissues and in lymph nodes. When they encounter microbial products during an infection or immunization they are activated to take up and process antigen, produce specific cytokines (which may vary depending on the type of microbe encountered) and other signaling molecules (e.g., retinoic acid in some cases), and migrate to the draining lymph node. Activation will increase the expression of major histocompatibility complex (MHC) and costimulatory molecules on dendritic cells to enhance presentation of antigen and activation of antigen-specific T cells. The pattern of cytokines produced by the activated dendritic cells helps to regulate T-cell differentiation (e.g., IL-12 will promote Th1 cell development) [13].

Vitamin A has diverse effects on dendritic cell development but the most important feature of dendritic cells with regard to vitamin A biology is that they produce retinoic acid, the active metabolite of vitamin A, from retinol [24, 25]. Retinoic acid produced by dendritic cells can have autocrine effects on the dendritic cells themselves (e.g., to affect antigen presentation and dendritic cell migration to lymph nodes) but the most pronounced effects are on lymphocytes that interact with dendritic cells during antigen presentation to stimulate development of memory T and B lymphocytes during the initiation of an adaptive immune response. These effects are discussed below.

Dendritic cells presumably receive retinol via the retinol binding protein (RBP) complex from the liver. In the intestinal lymphoid tissue it is also possible that dietary vitamin A and provitamin A carotenoids could also be a more direct source of vitamin A or retinoic acid. Intestinal epithelial cells, which absorb vitamin A and provitamin A carotenoids from digested food, may contribute to local retinoic acid production in two ways. First, intestinal epithelial cells themselves produce retinoic acid from both dietary retinol [26–28] and dietary provitamin A carotenoids [29–31] and may thus contribute a source of retinoic acid in the intestinal lamina propria and draining lymph that could enhance mucosal immunity. In addition, rather than being transported via chylomicrons, some retinol is transported directly across intestinal cells [32] into hepatic portal blood and this retinol could also be a source of retinoic acid production in the gut [33].

Thymic Function

The thymus is an important organ of the immune system where T-cell development occurs. The rate of production of T cells by the thymus peaks within the first few months of life but does persist at a lower level into adulthood [13]. RARs are expressed in the thymus, and thymocyte development and survival are dependent on retinoic acid signaling during selection of mature T cells in the thymus. These data indicate that vitamin A is important for normal thymic development [34]. Impairment of thymic development by vitamin A deficiency in infancy could result in long-term loss of T-cell diversity and thus potentially diminish the efficacy of the adaptive immune response to infections later in life.

Peripheral T Cells

Following thymic development, retinoic acid is also required for normal proliferation and survival of T cells in response to antigenic stimulation in the periphery [34]. In addition, retinoic acid directly modulates development of T-cell differentiation following antigen exposure [14, 35, 36]. Naïve $CD4^+$ T-helper cells differentiate into many phenotypes based on the need to deal with different types of pathogens [13]. Current, well-established subsets of memory/effector T-helper (Th) cells include the following: Th1 cells produce the effector cytokine IFN-γ that activates macrophages to kill intracellular pathogens (e.g., *Mycobacterium tuberculosis* and some *Salmonella* species) and promote antiviral responses (e.g., development of cytotoxic $CD8^+$ T cells). Production of IL-27 and IL-12 by dendritic cells drives Th1 development (as well as production of IFN-γ itself by Th1 and other cell types). Th1 cell responses can be enhanced by vitamin A deficiency [37] perhaps primarily due to the ability of retinoic acid to decrease IFN-γ production, although this pattern is not unvarying and may depend on the patterns of cytokines produced in response to specific conditions (i.e., specific infections or types of vaccination). Th2 cells produce IL-4, IL-5, and IL-13 and promote "weep and sweep" responses in the gut and eosinophilic inflammation to expel metazoan parasites. Production of IL-4 by dendritic cells or other cell types drives Th2 development. Retinoic acid enhances Th2 development *ex vivo* in the presence of IL-4. Th17 cells produce the effector cytokines IL-17A and IL-22 which promote epithelial production of anti-bacterial peptides to kill extracellular bacteria and chemokines to attract neutrophils, which phagocytose and kill such bacteria. IL-17A also promotes neutrophil differentiation in the bone marrow. Th17 development is promoted by IL-6 from dendritic cells working together with TGF-β, which can be produced by many cell types, particularly in gut lymphoid tissue. Cytokines produced by Th17 cells, including IL-23, are also needed to sustain Th17 development. Inducible regulatory (iTreg) cells also develop in the periphery after encountering antigen (while natural Treg cells [nTreg] develop in the thymus in response to self-antigen) and act to inhibit rather than promote inflammation. This development of iTreg cells is an inherent regulatory component of adaptive immunity to control inflammation in order to prevent excessive pathology. TGF-β in the absence of inflammatory cytokines drives iTreg development but data also show that retinoic acid acts in concert with TGF-β to enhance iTreg development. Both TGF-β and retinoic acid [38] are produced by immune cells in the gut and mesenteric lymph nodes, which are key sites of Treg development [36].

During proliferation of T cells, antioxidant protection is also an important factor in ensuring cell survival. Signaling through the T-cell receptor involves significant involvement of membrane proteins and reorganization of regions of the membrane into lipid rafts. Cell-signaling events near the membrane also involve oxidation–reduction reactions during T-cell activation. Apart from vitamin A activity, carotenoids are also associated with enhanced proliferative responses of T cells presumably due to their role as membrane antioxidants [6, 7].

Vitamin A and Mucosal Targeting of Immune Cells

A final key, vitamin A-dependent aspect of maintenance of the mucosal immune system is the ability of lymphocytes first exposed to antigen at mucosal sites to return to mucosal sites as effector or memory cells [13]. The teleological explanation for this return is to allow these gut-derived lymphocytes to be present at sites where their cognate pathogens are likely to re-appear. Interestingly, retinoic acid produced by $CD103^+$ dendritic cells in the gut facilitates such return by inducing the expression of CC-chemokine receptor 9 (CCR9) and the $\alpha4\beta7$ integrin dimer on the surface of T and B lymphocytes undergoing differentiation in the gut. CCR9 responds to CC-chemokine ligand 25 (CCL25), which is constitutively expressed in the intestine, and $\alpha4\beta7$ integrin binds to mucosal addressin cell adhesion molecule-1 (MAdCAM-1), which is expressed on vascular endothelium associated with intestinal lymphoid tissue [39]. These two molecules combine to provide a gut-homing signature for lymphocytes. Acquisition of CCR9 and $\alpha4\beta7$ expression *in vitro* by T cells is blocked by inhibition of aldehyde dehydrogenase activity in dendritic cells, and by RAR-α antagonists and disruption of RAR-α in T cells, and can be induced by exogenous retinoic acid [40–42]. Dietary vitamin A deficiency decreases retinoic acid production by gut dendritic cells [41, 43] and inflammation may also have a similar effect [44]. In addition, development of mucosally targeted $CD103^+$ dendritic cells expressing retinaldehyde dehydrogenase occurs in the bone marrow and this development is also directed by production of retinoic acid, in this case by bone marrow cells [45].

B Cells and Antibody Responses

Naïve B cells develop into antibody-producing plasma cells and memory B cells following appropriate exposure to antigen. Thus B cells are responsible for development of the humoral immune response [13]. Some antibody responses develop without T-cell help (e.g., bacterial polysaccharides), and these are not impaired by vitamin A deficiency but many humoral responses require such help. Vitamin A deficiency generally impairs T-cell-mediated antibody responses, particularly Th2-dependent antibody responses, such as IgE and IgG1 responses [46, 47]. Antibody responses promoted by Th1 cells may not be affected or can be slightly increased by vitamin A deficiency in mice [14].

IgA antibody is secreted across mucosal surfaces to neutralize pathogens in the respiratory, urogenital, and intestinal tracts. It is a crucial element of the adaptive immune response protecting against such mucosal pathogens [13]. Vitamin A deficiency impairs the serum and secretory IgA response in the gut and respiratory tracts [14]. This phenomenon is partially explained by diminished Th2 development and mucosal targeting of lymphocytes but vitamin A also promotes IgA responses by enhancing class switching to IgA by plasma cells [48]. Thus, vitamin A deficiency impairs this crucial protective mechanism at mucosal surfaces.

Conclusions

Vitamin A deficiency in the developing world contributes significantly to the increased risk of death from infectious disease in infants and young children. Prevention of deficiency to decrease mortality is currently being attempted on a wide scale, via WHO recommendations implemented by national ministries of health. These programs rely on distribution of vitamin A capsules. Nutritionists usually think of supplementation programs as interim measures that, hopefully, will be supplanted with fortification and improved diets. Dietary improvements in the developing world could utilize provitamin A carotenoids both to improve stores and, perhaps, also to directly affect mucosal immune function via local production of vitamin A in the gut. While the effect of provitamin A carotenoids on mucosal immunity has not been evaluated in this manner, such research may offer a useful approach to evaluating the effectiveness of provitamin A carotenoids in improving health.

References

1. Wolf G. The discovery of the visual function of vitamin A. J Nutr. 2001;131:1647–50.
2. Green HN, Mellanby E. Vitamin A as an anti-infective agent. Br Med J. 1928;2:691–6.
3. Semba RD. Vitamin A as "anti-infective" therapy, 1920–1940. J Nutr. 1999;129:783–91.
4. Scrimshaw NS, Taylor CE, Gordon JE. Interactions of nutrition and infection. Geneva: World Health Organization; 1968.
5. Germain P, Chambon P, Eichele G, Evans RM, Lazar MA, Leid M, De Lera AR, Lotan R, Mangelsdorf DJ, Gronemeyer H. International Union of Pharmacology. LX. Retinoic acid receptors. Pharmacol Rev. 2006;58:712–25.
6. Chew BP, Park JS. Carotenoid action on the immune response. J Nutr. 2004;134:257S–61.
7. Hughes DA. Dietary carotenoids and human immune function. Nutrition. 2001;17:823–7.
8. Imdad A, Herzer K, Mayo-Wilson E, Yakoob MY, Bhutta ZA. Vitamin A supplementation for preventing morbidity and mortality in children from 6 months to 5 years of age. Cochrane Database Syst Rev. 2010;8:CD008524.
9. WHO. Guideline: vitamin A supplementation in infants and children 6–59 months of age. Geneva: World Health Organization; 2011.
10. WHO. Guideline: vitamin A supplementation in infants and children 1–5 months of age. Geneva: World Health Organization; 2011.

11. Kirkwood B, Humphrey J, Moulton L, Martines J. Neonatal vitamin A supplementation and infant survival. Lancet. 2010;376:1643–4.
12. WHO. Guideline: neonatal vitamin A supplementation. Geneva: World Health Organization; 2011.
13. Murphy KP, Travers P, Walport M, Janeway C. Janeway's immunobiology. New York: Garland Science; 2011.
14. Stephensen CB. Vitamin A infection, and immune function. Annu Rev Nutr. 2001;21:167–92.
15. Jimenez C, Leets I, Puche R, Anzola E, Montilla R, Parra C, Aguilera A, Garcia-Casal MN. A single dose of vitamin A improves haemoglobin concentration, retinol status and phagocytic function of neutrophils in preschool children. Br J Nutr. 2010;103:798–802.
16. Wiedermann U, Tarkowski A, Bremell T, Hanson LA, Kahu H, Dahlgren UI. Vitamin A deficiency predisposes to *Staphylococcus aureus* infection. Infect Immun. 1996;64:209–14.
17. Twining SS, Schulte DP, Wilson PM, Fish BL, Moulder JE. Retinol is sequestered in the bone marrow of vitamin A-deficient rats. J Nutr. 1996;126:1618–26.
18. Meydani SN, Wu D, Santos MS, Hayek MG. Antioxidants and immune response in aged persons: overview of present evidence. Am J Clin Nutr. 1995;62:1462S–76.
19. Cornet S, Biard C, Moret Y. Is there a role for antioxidant carotenoids in limiting self-harming immune response in invertebrates? Biol Lett. 2007;3:284–8.
20. Blount JD, Metcalfe NB, Birkhead TR, Surai PF. Carotenoid modulation of immune function and sexual attractiveness in zebra finches. Science. 2003;300:125–7.
21. Vinkler M, Albrecht T. Carotenoid maintenance handicap and the physiology of carotenoid-based signalisation of health. Naturwissenschaften. 2010;97:19–28.
22. Ross AC, Stephensen CB. Vitamin A and retinoids in antiviral responses. FASEB J. 1996;10:979–85.
23. Miller SC, Kearney SL. Effect of *in vivo* administration of all trans-retinoic acid on the hemopoietic cell populations of the spleen and bone marrow: profound strain differences between A/J and C57BL/6J mice. Lab Anim Sci. 1998;48:74–80.
24. Duriancik DM, Lackey DE, Hoag KA. Vitamin A as a regulator of antigen presenting cells. J Nutr. 2010;140:1395–9.
25. Manicassamy S, Pulendran B. Retinoic acid-dependent regulation of immune responses by dendritic cells and macrophages. Semin Immunol. 2009;21:22–7.
26. Lampen A, Meyer S, Arnhold T, Nau H. Metabolism of vitamin A and its active metabolite all-*trans*-retinoic acid in small intestinal enterocytes. J Pharmacol Exp Ther. 2000;295:979–85.
27. Arnhold T, Nau H, Meyer S, Rothkoetter HJ, Lampen AD. Porcine intestinal metabolism of excess vitamin A differs following vitamin A supplementation and liver consumption. J Nutr. 2002;132:197–203.
28. Thomas S, Prabhu R, Balasubramanian KA. Retinoid metabolism in the rat small intestine. Br J Nutr. 2005;93:59–63.
29. Wang XD, Russell RM, Marini RP, Tang G, Dolnikowski GG, Fox JG, Krinsky NI. Intestinal perfusion of beta-carotene in the ferret raises retinoic acid level in portal blood. Biochim Biophys Acta. 1993;1167:159–64.
30. Hebuterne X, Wang XD, Johnson EJ, Krinsky NI, Russell RM. Intestinal absorption and metabolism of 9-*cis*-beta-carotene in vivo: biosynthesis of 9-*cis*-retinoic acid. J Lipid Res. 1995;36:1264–73.
31. Crain FD, Lotspeich FJ, Krause RF. Biosynthesis of retinoic acid by intestinal enzymes of the rat. J Lipid Res. 1967;8:249–54.
32. During A, Harrison EH. Mechanisms of provitamin A (carotenoid) and vitamin A (retinol) transport into and out of intestinal Caco-2 cells. J Lipid Res. 2007;48:2283–94.
33. Harrison EH. Mechanisms of digestion and absorption of dietary vitamin A. Annu Rev Nutr. 2005;25:87–103.
34. Engedal N. Immune regulator vitamin A and T cell death. Vitam Horm. 2011;86:153–78.
35. Iwata M. The roles of retinoic acid in lymphocyte differentiation. Semin Immunol. 2009;21:1.
36. Mucida D, Park Y, Cheroutre H. From the diet to the nucleus: vitamin A and TGF-beta join efforts at the mucosal interface of the intestine. Semin Immunol. 2009;21:14–21.
37. Cantorna MT, Nashold FE, Hayes CE. In vitamin A deficiency multiple mechanisms establish a regulatory T helper cell imbalance with excess Th1 and insufficient Th2 function. J Immunol. 1994;152:1515–22.
38. Sun CM, Hall JA, Blank RB, Bouladoux N, Oukka M, Mora JR, Belkaid Y. Small intestine lamina propria dendritic cells promote de novo generation of Foxp3 T reg cells via retinoic acid. J Exp Med. 2007;204:1775–85.
39. Gorfu G, Rivera-Nieves J, Ley K. Role of beta7 integrins in intestinal lymphocyte homing and retention. Curr Mol Med. 2009;9:836–50.
40. Coombes JL, Siddiqui KR, Arancibia-Carcamo CV, Hall J, Sun CM, Belkaid Y, Powrie F. A functionally specialized population of mucosal CD103+ DCs induces Foxp3+ regulatory T cells via a TGF-beta and retinoic acid-dependent mechanism. J Exp Med. 2007;204:1757–64.
41. Molenaar R, Knippenberg M, Goverse G, Olivier BJ, de Vos AF, O'Toole T, Mebius RE. Expression of retinaldehyde dehydrogenase enzymes in mucosal dendritic cells and gut-draining lymph node stromal cells is controlled by dietary vitamin A. J Immunol. 2011;186:1934–42.
42. Iwata M, Yokota A. Retinoic acid production by intestinal dendritic cells. Vitam Horm. 2011;86:127–52.

43. Jaensson-Gyllenback E, Kotarsky K, Zapata F, Persson EK, Gundersen TE, Blomhoff R, Agace WW. Bile retinoids imprint intestinal CD103(+) dendritic cells with the ability to generate gut-tropic T cells. Mucosal Immunol. 2011;4:438–47.
44. Laffont S, Siddiqui KR, Powrie F. Intestinal inflammation abrogates the tolerogenic properties of MLN CD103+ dendritic cells. Eur J Immunol. 2010;40:1877–83.
45. Feng T, Cong Y, Qin H, Benveniste EN, Elson CO. Generation of mucosal dendritic cells from bone marrow reveals a critical role of retinoic acid. J Immunol. 2010;185:5915–25.
46. Ross AC, Chen Q, Ma Y. Augmentation of antibody responses by retinoic acid and costimulatory molecules. Semin Immunol. 2009;21:42–50.
47. Ertesvag A, Naderi S, Blomhoff HK. Regulation of B cell proliferation and differentiation by retinoic acid. Semin Immunol. 2009;21:36–41.
48. Watanabe K, Sugai M, Nambu Y, Osato M, Hayashi T, Kawaguchi M, Komori T, Ito Y, Shimizu A. Requirement for Runx proteins in IgA class switching acting downstream of TGF-beta 1 and retinoic acid signaling. J Immunol. 2010;184:2785–92.

Chapter 17
Biofortification of Maize with Provitamin A Carotenoids

Kevin Pixley, Natalia Palacios Rojas, Raman Babu, Raphael Mutale, Rebecca Surles, and Eliab Simpungwe

Key Points

- Biofortification, or the breeding of staple food crops to increase their micronutrient density, is widely viewed as a valuable strategy for sustainably improving the nutritional status of some malnourished populations.
- Successful biofortified varieties must be agronomically competitive with the best available local varieties, must be acceptable to consumers for all intended uses, including home consumption and marketing, and must be able to improve nutritional status of the target consumers.
- We describe the agricultural, nutrition, food technology, economic, and other multidisciplinary research that has resulted in provitamin A biofortified maize hybrids released for commercialization and consumption in Zambia in 2012.
- We conclude by describing elements of a demand-creation strategy, including advocacy and involvement of Zambian governmental, public, and private institutions; nutrition education; farmer-participatory evaluation of varieties; and marketing considerations.
- This chapter provides an overview of how basic and applied sciences are contributing to alleviate vitamin A deficiency in maize-consuming populations of Zambia and elsewhere.

Keywords Vitamin A • Maize • Corn • Biofortification • Provitamin A carotenoids • Vitamin A deficiency • Agriculture • Nutrition and health

K. Pixley, Ph.D. (✉)
Genetic Resources Program, International Maize and Wheat Improvement Center, CIMMYT, Km. 45 Carretera Mexico-Veracruz, El Batan, Texcoco 56130, Mexico

Department of Agronomy, University of Wisconsin, 1575 Linden Dr., Madison, WI
e-mail: k.pixley@cgiar.org

N.P. Rojas, Ph.D. • R. Babu, Ph.D. • R. Surles, Ph.D.
Global Maize Program, International Maize and Wheat Improvement Center, CIMMYT, Km. 45 Carretera Mexico-Veracruz, El Batan, Texcoco 56130, Mexico

R. Mutale, B.Sc.
HarvestPlus, Department of Crop Development, c/o World Fish Centre, Plot 4186 Addis Ababa Drive Long Acres, 51289, Lusaka 10101, Zambia

E. Simpungwe, Ph.D.
HarvestPlus, Zambia Country Program, c/o World Fish Centre,
Plot 4186 Addis Ababa Drive Long Acres, 51289, Ridgeway, Lusaka 10101, Zambia

S.A. Tanumihardjo (ed.), *Carotenoids and Human Health*, Nutrition and Health,
DOI 10.1007/978-1-62703-203-2_17, © Springer Science+Business Media New York 2013

Introduction

This book summarizes a wealth of research that has led to our collective, growing understanding about the crucial roles of carotenoids in human health. Chapter 15 informs us (citing WHO [1]) that despite all this knowledge, 190 million preschool-age children and 19 million pregnant women, mostly in Africa and South Asia, suffer from vitamin A deficiency (VAD) and increased morbidity and mortality. The reader and vitamin A researchers alike will be rightfully dissatisfied if opportunities to apply this knowledge are not created and availed to reduce the prevalence and consequences of VAD.

This chapter is about the food we eat, and especially about the food we eat when we cannot afford or chronically fail to access balanced, nutritious diets. Staple foods[1] are mainly rice in South Asia, wheat in Central Asia, and maize for most of sub-Saharan Africa. These are rich sources of energy, but they typically contain nutritionally inadequate quantities of micronutrients, including provitamin A carotenoids, iron, and zinc [2]. As food prices increase, over-reliance on these generally abundant, relatively inexpensive, widely traded, and easily stored staple grains often increases. Average per capita consumption of maize in Zambia, which will be the main case study for this chapter, is more than 130 kg per year (356 g per day), and maize provides more than half the calories and protein for most Zambians (FAOSTAT, as cited by 3), while providing only traces or no provitamin A [2].

Biofortification is the breeding of staple food crops to increase micronutrient density [4]. Graham et al. [5] suggested that because of the widespread consumption of staple crops, biofortification may be an effective and sustainable way of addressing micronutrient malnutrition. Hotz and McClafferty [6], however, highlighted the complex challenge of demonstrating the ability of biofortified crops to improve consumer health. Bouis and Welch [7] summarized the requirements for successful application of a biofortification strategy as: (1) developing a high yielding, profitable biofortified variety, (2) demonstrating its effectiveness at reducing malnutrition, and (3) ensuring that the biofortified crop is acceptable to farmers and consumers. Further, another crucial requirement is the creation of awareness and demand for the biofortified crop and its foods.

The proponents of biofortification include more than nutritionists and agriculturalists. From an economic point of view, investments in biofortification are justified as a complementary strategy to supplementation and fortification, particularly suited to rural or remote areas where other approaches may have incomplete coverage [8]. Strong endorsement of the concept of biofortification came from the 2008 Copenhagen Consensus [9], in which a panel of expert economists ranked biofortification (5th), micronutrient fortification (3rd), micronutrient supplements (1st), and community-based nutrition education (9th) among the best 30 ways of advancing global welfare [10].

Although conceptually simple—"make the most popular and affordable foods more nutritious"—implementing a biofortification strategy from its underlying sciences to achieving widespread impact on malnutrition is tremendously challenging. The objectives of this chapter are to describe elements of the ongoing HarvestPlus[2] project of provitamin A biofortified maize for Zambia to: (1) illustrate the science, methods, and progress towards developing biofortified maize at the International Maize and Wheat Improvement Center (CIMMYT)[3]; (2) describe a pathway towards achieving impact on malnutrition through biofortified maize; and (3) highlight some of the lessons, challenges, and opportunities for biofortified maize to address problems of VAD.

[1] "A staple food is one that is eaten regularly and in such quantities as to constitute the dominant part of the diet and supply a major proportion of energy and nutrient needs" (FAO, 1995).

[2] HarvestPlus is a special or "challenge" program established by the Consultative Group for International Agricultural Research (CGIAR) to address the global problems of vitamin A, iron, and zinc malnutrition through biofortification of staple food crops. See www.harvestplus.org

[3] CIMMYT is a non-profit research for development institute, dedicated to sustainably increasing the productivity of wheat and maize systems to ensure global food security and alleviate poverty. See www.cimmyt.org

Following this introduction, Sects. "Breeding provitamin A biofortified maize" through "Overview of parallel and interdisciplinary efforts" describe the technical aspects leading to development of provitamin A biofortified maize varieties, Sect. "Creating and supplying demand for provitamin A maize" discusses the HarvestPlus strategies for creating and supplying demand for provitamin A biofortified maize varieties in Zambia, and Sect. "Achieving impact and conclusion" presents concluding thoughts, focusing on achieving sustainability of biofortification efforts after the HarvestPlus project concludes its activities in Zambia. A brief, general description of maize breeding methods is presented in Sect. "Annex: an introduction to plant breeding", and provides a quick reference for those unfamiliar with key terms that are used in Sect. "Overview of parallel and interdisciplinary efforts".

Breeding Provitamin A Biofortified Maize

The choice of strategy for a breeding program depends on the objectives and on the pertinent quality of both the starting material and the available sources of genetic variability for the trait(s) to improve. The main objective of the provitamin A-biofortified maize breeding project is to develop high-yielding, profitable varieties, with demonstrable effectiveness in reducing VAD, which are acceptable to consumers [7]. Following extensive discussion, a panel of nutritionists advising the HarvestPlus project initially determined that biofortified maize varieties should contain 15 μg/g of provitamin A carotenoids to have a high probability to reduce VAD; thus, 15 μg/g is the target value, and half of this became an intermediate target for the breeding program (see Sects. "Nutrition and bioavailability" and "Achieving impact and conclusion"). If maize had very little or no naturally occurring variation for provitamin A carotenoid concentrations, it would be impossible to improve the concentration of these carotenoids through conventional breeding approaches. Hence, the first step was to examine the carotenoid contents and profiles of hundreds of maize lines and varieties.

Genetic Variation for Provitamin A and Other Carotenoid Profiles

Several of the carotenoids present in maize have important roles in human health. Provitamin A carotenoids (e.g., β-cryptoxanthin, α- and β-carotene) are the precursors of vitamin A, which is essential in different systems in the human body and for the prevention of diet-related chronic diseases. Lutein and zeaxanthin, on the other hand, have been associated with lowering the risk of cataracts, age-related macular degeneration, and other degenerative diseases. Maize exhibits considerable natural variation in kernel carotenoids, with some genotypes accumulating as much as 80 μg total carotenoids/g dry weight (DW) (Table 17.1). The fraction of provitamin A carotenoids is typically only 10–20 %, whereas zeaxanthin and lutein each commonly represent 30–50 % of total carotenoids in maize [11].

A wide range of carotenoids are found in yellow temperate, tropical, and subtropical germplasm including landraces, inbred lines, and hybrids (Table 17.1). Most yellow maize grown and consumed throughout the world, however, has ≤2 μg provitamin A carotenoids/g DW. Significant progress in maize biofortification for provitamin A through conventional breeding has been achieved during the past 7 years. The genetic diversity found, not only for carotenoid content but also for haplotypes[4]

[4] Haplotypes are short DNA blocks or segments that are transmitted together from one generation to another and that exhibit variation among individuals. *Functional* haplotypes are often associated with differences in expression of a trait, such as content of provitamin A carotenoids in maize.

Table 17.1 Examples of ranges of carotenoid content in maize kernels

Germplasm adaptation	Lut	Zea	BCX	BC	AC	Total provitamin A	Total carotenoids	References
Temperate	0.0–27.5	0.01–7.7	0.07–2.4	0.07–7.6	0.0–0.7	0.1–8.8	0.15–33.1	[14]
	0.0–31.0	0.76–43.9	0.16–10.8	0.07–13.6	0.01–2.0	0.15–19.0	8.5–47.2	[12]
Tropical/ subtropical	1.3–32.3	0.3–34.8	0.0–6.13	0.7–5.8	0–2.31	0.7–8.8	2.42–81.3	[11]
	0.4–19	0.3–21.5	0.3–4.6	0.3–4.3	0.0–0.6	0.45–6.6	1.3–49.5	[15]

Data are expressed in μg/g DW
Lut lutein, *Zea* zeaxanthin, *BCX* β-cryptoxanthin, *BC* β-carotene, *AC* α-carotene

of genes encoding enzymes that affect the concentrations of provitamin A carotenoids in maize kernels, have significantly contributed to the advances in the breeding process (see Sects. "Molecular marker-assisted breeding for enhanced grain carotenoid content", "Development of the first provitamin A maize hybrids for Zambia" and "Development of the second and future generations of provitamin A maize hybrids").

In general, tropical maize contains more β-cryptoxanthin and less β-carotene than temperate maize, and because the emphasis was on enhancing β-carotene concentration, most of the initial breeding sources of high provitamin A germplasm were selected from temperate regions. Subsequently, genetic association mapping studies using three diverse maize germplasm panels, selected to encompass a wide range of carotenoid contents and ratios, have identified favorable alleles of genes encoding two key enzymes in the carotenoid biosynthetic pathway, i.e., lycopene epsilon cyclase (lycE) and β-carotene hydroxylase 1 (crtRB1), which substantially affect the accumulation of β-carotene in grain [12, 13]. Using molecular markers to select the favorable alleles for these two enzymes, the screening of germplasm has become faster and cheaper than selection based on high-performance liquid chromatography (HPLC) methodology to quantify carotenoids. Germplasm carrying the favorable crtRB1 allele in homozygous form has been identified with β-carotene concentrations up to 26 μg/g DW and total provitamin A as high as 30 μg/g DW. These newly identified sources of provitamin A are currently being used in breeding programs, leading to rapid gains in provitamin A carotenoid concentrations (Sect. "Molecular marker-assisted breeding for enhanced grain carotenoid content").

Breeding Provitamin A Biofortified Maize

In Sect. "Genetic variation for provitamin A and other carotenoid profiles" we noted that most yellow maize contains <2 μg/g while white maize has no provitamin A carotenoids. In contrast, after extensive search and characterization, a few maize types were found to have >15 μg provitamin A/g. The challenge to plant breeders is to develop new, provitamin A-rich, superior varieties by combining the excellent characteristics of already successful varieties, with the outstanding provitamin A concentration of source lines that come from distant and different environments and are thus often low-yielding and in several ways unsuitable for local use. Plant breeding is a science and an art, and is often referred to as a numbers game. Maize has more than 30,000 genes, and when a breeder crosses two very different maize plants, e.g., a local-favorite variety with a high-provitamin A maize from afar, the resulting progeny will contain 50 % genetic contribution from each of the parents. The plant breeder subsequently employs several of many diverse tools and strategies to examine hundreds to thousands of progeny over several years to select the best for use as new varieties. Nearly everything we eat is the result of centuries of effort by amateur and professional breeders.

Breeding biofortified crops requires combining knowledge and tools from nutritionists, biochemists, and food technologists to assure that the final varieties are not only high yielding and acceptable to farmers, but also contain superior quantities of provitamin A carotenoids, that these nutrients are bioavailable, and that the biofortified grains produce palatable foods.

Tools in Support of Breeding Efforts

Analytical Tools for Carotenoid Quantification in Maize

Analysis of carotenoids is inherently difficult due to: (1) the large number of naturally occurring carotenoids, which requires many tailor-made laboratory protocols to optimize the extraction and quantification for each; (2) their interactions with other molecules, which cause degradation or make complete extraction more difficult; (3) their wide range of concentrations; (4) their various isomers; (5) their rapid oxidation and degradation prior to and during analysis; and (6) the fact that only a few carotenoids have provitamin A activity [16]. Several basic precautions are recommended to maximize consistency of results when quantifying provitamin A carotenoids for maize, including analyzing kernels at similar physiological maturity and moisture content, minimizing sample storage time while ensuring low temperatures (−20 °C or preferably −80 °C), protecting samples from exposure to white light and oxygen, and minimizing time for extraction and analysis.

Several methods have been considered in search of a fast, accurate, and cheap assay to screen provitamin A content in maize kernels to support breeding programs. Candidate methods have included visual color scoring, the use of colorimetry, near infrared reflectance spectroscopy (NIRS), and liquid chromatography. However, given the characteristics and wide range of quantities of the carotenoids present in maize, visual color determination, colorimetric methods, and even NIRS have failed to provide consistent results that would endorse their use.

Non-significant phenotypic correlation coefficients have been reported between visual color score (shade of yellow) and β-cryptoxanthin ($r=0.21$) and β-carotene ($r=0.36$) contents in maize grain, respectively [12]. Color assessment scores using a HunterLab miniscan had a significant ($P<0.05$) correlation coefficient of $r=0.58$ with provitamin A concentration in maize flour [17]; however, this method has not proven reliable for a wide range of germplasm, perhaps due to confounding effects caused by the presence of other colored compounds (like polyphenolic compounds). Nevertheless, because deep-orange maize kernels are slightly more likely to have higher provitamin A content than pale yellow maize, breeders often select for deep-orange grain in the field and then conduct laboratory assays to quantify content for these.

NIRS is a rapid and inexpensive method that is widely used in plant breeding to measure numerous traits. Although the visible range (400–1,100 nm) is important for predicting carotenoid content in maize grain, calibration curves for estimating carotenoid concentrations have been successful for estimating the major carotenoids (lutein and zeaxanthin) and total carotenoid, but not for provitamin A carotenoids (18; Zum Felde, personal communication). Reverse-phase high-performance liquid chromatography (HPLC) coupled with a photodiode array detector is currently the most robust method available for provitamin A screening. However, the cost and time required for analysis make HPLC impractical when several thousand samples have to be analyzed in a short time. Ultra-performance liquid chromatography (UPLC) is a promising alternative to HPLC because its costs for reagents are lower, and throughput can be increased to more than six times that of HPLC.

In general, errors associated with chromatography are minor relative to those incurred during extraction procedures. To address this concern, several methods were compared in a HarvestPlus study to identify and recommend a standardized protocol for carotenoid extraction from maize [19].

The most widely accepted methods involve extraction of carotenoids with one or more organic solvents including hexanes, tetrahydrofuran, methanol, ethanol, or ethyl acetate. Many procedures require freeze-dried material, saponification to remove lipids, and the use of antioxidants like butylated hydroxytoluene (BHT) or pyrogallol. The most reproducible and therefore recommended method, based on coefficient of variation and extraction efficiency, is a modification of a method developed by Kurilich and Juvik [14]. A brief heat and saponification treatment is required, followed by the addition of an internal standard to account for mechanical losses. This modified method has been especially well-established for quantifying provitamin A carotenoids, and involves a relatively short extraction time [19]. Carotenoid analysis is complex and the use of internal standards, checks, and laboratory replicates are essential. Additionally, frequent inter-laboratory comparisons are recommended to help monitor data quality and accuracy.

Molecular Marker-Assisted Breeding for Enhanced Grain Carotenoid Content

Marker-assisted selection (MAS) in plant breeding involves selection of plants possessing genomic regions (DNA segments) that are involved in the expression of traits of interest by using DNA tags as signposts. Once associations between DNA markers and traits of interest are established and validated across diverse germplasm, MAS can save time and material resources in a breeding program. Importantly, unlike many traits that are affected by environmental conditions (e.g., drought affects yield), DNA markers are environment-neutral and can be used to select among plants grown anywhere, including in greenhouses or winter nurseries. In recent years, MAS has become a widely used tool in many breeding programs.

The carotenoid metabolic pathway has been well-researched in model species and key genes governing critical steps have been identified [20]. In maize, three important genes have been proposed to play crucial roles in the accumulation of provitamin A carotenoids. Phytoene synthase 1 (*Y1/Psy1*) catalyzes the first committed step in the pathway leading to formation of phytoene from geranylgeranyl diphosphate and is primarily responsible for the shift from white to yellow grain. Once the carotenoid pathway is activated, two other genes, lycopene epsilon cyclase (LcyE) and β-carotene hydroxylase 1 (crtRB1) regulate the accumulation of provitamin A-related compounds. LcyE converts lycopene into ζ-carotene and eventually to α-carotene through the action of other associated genes. Naturally existing, reduced-functionality, mutant alleles of LcyE result in increased apportioning of lycopene toward the β- (and less toward the α-) branch of the pathway, thereby enhancing the flux towards provitamin A-related compounds [12]. CrtRB1 is a hydroxylase gene that converts β-carotene into β-cryptoxanthin, whose theoretical provitamin A activity is only half that of β-carotene. Natural genetic variation for CrtRB1 that results in reduced functionality of this enzyme and increased retention of β-carotene in the maize endosperm has been discovered [13]. Molecular markers within the above-said three genes hold great potential for accelerating the development of high provitamin A carotenoid lines in a resource efficient manner. These molecular markers allow distinction between the wild-type and the desired mutant allele.

In 2008, the best experimental lines and hybrids had provitamin A concentrations from 5 to 8 μg/g, but lines developed recently using MAS have as much as 20 μg/g. Use of MAS, however, is not foolproof. Incorporating the favorable CrtRB1 allele into new lines results in a wide range of outcomes, and typically provitamin A level is increased by two- to ten-times. Thus, although using MAS is much cheaper than quantifying carotenoids by HPLC or UPLC, breeders still need to use these lab assays once or twice during the development of new lines to determine the outcome.

Breeding Progress

Development of the First Provitamin A Maize Hybrids for Zambia

A successful breeding program must integrate the knowledge from nutrition, social science, and plant genetics into new biofortified maize varieties that will be productive and desirable to farmers and consumers. Experienced breeders with a multidisciplinary background; analytical and molecular tools, such as HPLC and MAS; a little bit of "art" (intuition and skill); and a comprehensive strategy are necessary for success. Figure 17.1 summarizes the scheme used to develop biofortified maize at CIMMYT.

The first breeding crosses were made in 2004 and involved the best (elite) white-grained (i.e., 0 µg/g of provitamin A) inbred lines from the CIMMYT program in Harare, Zimbabwe, and temperate yellow lines with provitamin A concentrations ranging from 5 to 8 µg/g (received from T. Rocheford, University of Illinois, USA). Each F1 cross was back-crossed to its respective elite line prior to initiating new line development (Step 1, Fig. 17.1). Selection during the first two generations of inbreeding was primarily for deep yellow or orange grain color, as well as for resistances to lodging and plant and ear diseases (Step 2, Fig. 17.1). About 600–800 early generation (S2, most commonly) lines were then selected and crossed in isolation fields with one or two inbred line testers (Step 3, Fig. 17.1) to form hybrids for evaluation in Stage 1 trials at three locations in Mexico (Step 4, Fig. 17.1).

Yield and other agronomic data from Stage 1 trials were used to select approximately 20 % of the lines, which were further inbred and selected before crossing with three testers (Step 5, Fig. 17.1) for more extensive evaluation in Stage 2 trials (Step 6, Fig. 17.1). Stage 2 trials were grown at 5–6 locations, including key sites in Zambia and Zimbabwe. The best 10–20 % of lines evaluated in Stage 2 trials were selected to form hybrids with three single-cross testers (Step 7, Fig. 17.1), and these three-way-cross hybrids were evaluated in trials at 6–8 locations (Step 8, Fig. 17.1). The provitamin A hybrids were competitive at all sites except the highest yielding site, which is of minimal concern given that very few farmers in Zambia achieve yields above 10 tons/ha.

Although the provitamin A concentrations of the best experimental hybrids were only 6–9 µg/g, the Zambian HarvestPlus project steering committee endorsed submitting five of these hybrids to

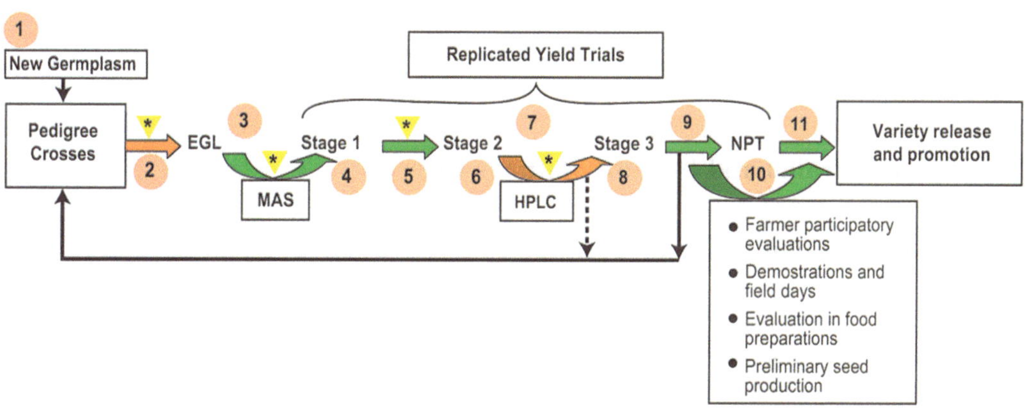

Fig. 17.1 Generalized plant breeding or biofortified product development scheme. *Circled numbers* refer to steps discussed in the text. *EGL* early generation line, *MAS* marker-assisted selection, *HPLC* high-performance liquid chromatography, *NPT* national performance trial (Zambia). *Asterisk* indicates major opportunities for agronomic selection, e.g., for disease resistance

National Performance Trials (NPT) during 2010–2011 (Step 10, Fig. 17.1). Two years of data from government-implemented NPTs are required to support applications for variety release and commercialization. During these 2 years, numerous parallel activities conducted to validate farmer and consumer acceptance of these promising hybrids (Step 10, Fig. 17.1) and to begin creating interest, demand, and supply for seed of the best hybrids for future commercialization and planting (Step 11, Fig. 17.1).

Development of the Second and Future Generations of Provitamin A Maize Hybrids

The breeding program is cyclic and continually reinitiates and executes the steps outlined above. Every year new crosses are made (Step 1, Fig. 17.1) and the entire process begins again. The "breeding pipeline" is always full and contains better products than currently ready for release and commercialization. There are at least two reasons for this: (1) better germplasm, including the best from previous years of work (see the downward and return arrows after Stage 2 and Stage 3 trials (Fig. 17.1)), the best from other breeding programs, and novel sources with higher provitamin A concentration, are used in making new crosses; and (2) faster, cheaper and more effective selection methods or tools become available, such as molecular markers for useful genes or improved methods for provitamin A analysis.

As described in Sect. "Molecular marker-assisted breeding for enhanced grain carotenoid content", the single most exciting advance in the past 3 years has been the discovery of useful allelic diversity for two genes in the carotenoid biosynthetic pathway, and development of molecular markers that we now use in selecting for these alleles in the breeding program (Step 3, Fig. 17.1). This identified source lines with >15 μg/g of provitamin A carotenoids, which are routinely used as parents for new crosses (Step 1, Fig. 17.1), and allows us to select lines with 40–250 % greater provitamin A carotenoid concentrations than lines without the favorable allele. A second important improvement in our breeding program was achieved by using UPLC in place of HPLC, which greatly increased the number of samples for which provitamin A can be evaluated, and allowed selection for this trait earlier in the breeding pipeline (Fig. 17.1).

The enormous challenge is to ensure that new biofortified varieties are competitive for all crucial traits, including seed production, grain yield, disease resistance, drought tolerance, food processing quality, taste, and other characteristics that determine acceptability to farmers and consumers (see Sect. "Creating and supplying demand for provitamin A maize").

Overview of Parallel and Interdisciplinary Efforts

Carotenoid Retention and Food Technology

Maize provides food for over 900 million people located mainly in sub-Saharan Africa, Mexico, and Central America [21]. It is consumed as whole kernels (boiled or roasted), or as flour produced by dry milling, wet milling, or lime cooking [2]. After harvest, maize is dried and stored in a variety of ways for differing time periods, depending on local uses and customs. Maize is commonly stored on the cob (with or without husks), as shelled grain (often in bags), or as flour. In some cultures, farmers remove the husks and hang the cobs, or place them under the sun to dry. Others shell the ears and dry the grain under the sun on a cement surface or in an open basket.

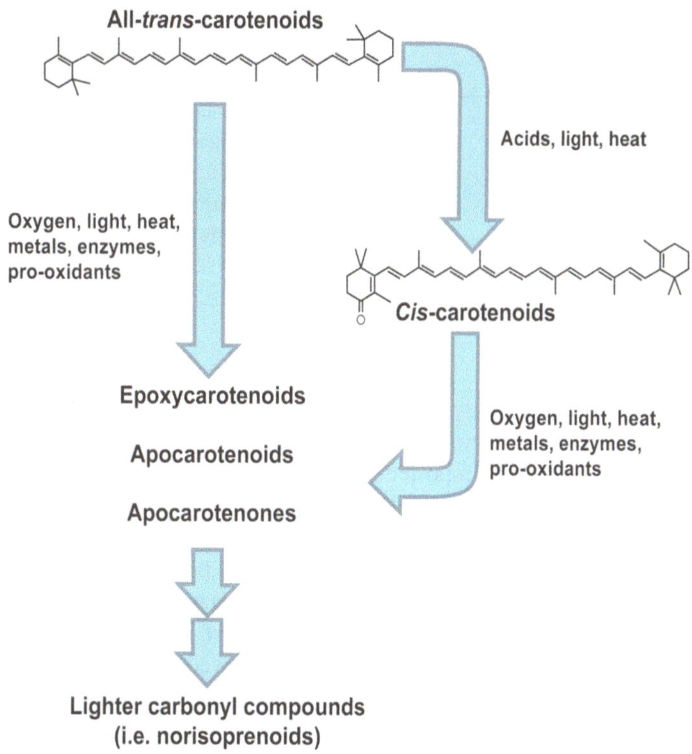

Fig. 17.2 Carotenoid losses scheme (modified from 23)

Carotenoid losses during grain or flour storage, food preparation, and industrial processing have been widely recognized and reported for various food products, and are important factors to consider when setting provitamin A target levels for biofortified maize [7]. Losses are due to physical removal of carotenoid-containing components during food preparation, catabolism (enzymatic oxidation), or degradation (nonenzymatic oxidation). Moisture and water activity affect the catabolism of carotenoids; nonenzymatic oxidation is also affected by water activity, thus higher degradation rates occur at low water activity due to decreased enzymatic activities, e.g., for peroxidases and dioxygenases. Provitamin A carotenoids are highly unsaturated compounds that are prone to isomerization and oxidation [22]. Carotenoid oxidation products include epoxides, apocarotenals, and apocarotenones (Fig. 17.2). Oxidative losses depend on the availability of oxygen and are enhanced by light, heat, presence of metals, and various enzymes [23]. Several studies have concluded that oxygen is a major factor determining carotenoid degradation during storage of foodstuffs [24, 25]. In addition to losses via oxidation, carotenoid isomerization can occur during food processing, leading to the formation of *cis*-isomers, loss of provitamin A activity, and altered bioavailability [26, 27].

Drying and storage temperature, oxygen availability, and light conditions are important in determining the stability of carotenoid compounds; however, these factors have only recently been tested for maize with increased levels of provitamin A carotenoids. As also reported for sweet potato [24], carotenoid losses during maize drying are small and independent of the form and method of drying (e.g., cobs, grain; sun, hot air) [28]. During maize storage, however, provitamin A losses can vary from 7 to 45 %, depending on the variety, and degradation is fastest during the first 2 months of storage (manuscript in preparation). Provitamin A losses are larger for finely milled flour stored in translucent permeable packaging than for grain or finely milled flour stored in vacuum sealed bags. These differences are mainly due to the destruction of the cellular structure during milling, and to increased exposure of the compounds to oxygen and pro-oxidant environments [23].

Table 17.2 Carotenoid retention studies in maize-derived products

Product	Processing	Cooking method	Provitamin A carotenoid losses	References
Sadza	Dry-milling	Boiling	37 %	[32]
Fermented Ogi	Wet-milling	Fermentation/boiling	27.5 %	[29]
Unfermented Ogi	Wet-milling	Boiling	25 %	[29]
Maize chips	Lime-cooking	Frying	36 %	[17]
Sweet tamal[a]	Lime-cooking	Steamed	40 %	Not published
Boiled maize cob	None	Boiling	17 %	Not published
Roasted maize cob	None	Roasting	0 %	Not published

[a]Traditional lime-cook maize dough

Degradation of carotenoids following dry-milling is dependent on the duration and conditions of storage. Li et al. [29] reported less than 10 % loss of provitamin A carotenoids after dry kernels were soaked and wet-milled. After processing, maize is boiled, steamed, fried, fermented, or cooked by many different methods. In Eastern and Southern Africa, maize is mainly consumed by adding maize flour to boiling water and stirring until a thick porridge is formed (e.g., *ugali, sadza*, or *nshima*). The traditional production of *ogi*, the fermented maize porridge consumed in West Africa, involves soaking dried whole maize kernels, milling, addition of water, and spontaneous fermentation. In Mexico and Central America, maize is lime-cooked, followed by steeping for 10–12 h, washing, and forming into dough, which is sheeted, cut, or extruded to make tortillas, tortilla chips, corn chips, and other products; provitamin A carotenoids are not significantly lost during these processes (unpublished data).

Carotenoid retention studies for common food products made with high-carotenoid maize are summarized in Table 17.2. In general, studies evaluating the retention of nutrients in cooked foods can be misinterpreted if raw and cooked samples differ in water content, texture, or other pertinent characteristics; if the extraction efficiency for the raw samples and cooked samples differ (see Sect. "Analytical tools for carotenoid quantification in maize"); if enzymatic oxidation occurs in the raw sample; and if calculation of retention is not corrected for weight loss or gain during cooking [30]. Several studies have found very large retention rates (some >100 %), perhaps due to the disruption of complex matrices during cooking, which may "release carotenoids" allowing more efficient or complete extraction and quantification [29, 31].

The original calculation of HarvestPlus target levels for development of provitamin A biofortified maize assumed 50 % loss of carotenoids during storage and processing [7]. Nevertheless, it is important to estimate carotenoid losses for foods prepared using promising provitamin A biofortified maize varieties before they are released, because genetic variation exists for the extent of provitamin A carotenoid losses and because of the complex nature of carotenoid retention during different food preparations.

Nutrition and Bioavailability

Biofortified crops are bred to improve the nutritional status of the consumer by increasing the micronutrient density in the edible portions of staple food crops; however, not all micronutrients present in food are available for human utilization. Release of nutrients from the food matrix during digestion, making them *bioaccessible*, is the first challenge towards the utilization of provitamin A carotenoids from maize [33]. Dietary fat is essential to *micellarization*, which is the process in which carotenoids are emulsified for absorption by the intestine's enterocytes making them *bioavailable*.

The fraction of carotenoids that are absorbed and remain in the lipid phase are then packaged into large lipoprotein particles (*chylomicrons*) and transported into the bloodstream, from where they are transferred to extrahepatic tissue before being cleared by the liver as chylomicron remnants [34].

In the intestine, provitamin A carotenoids can be converted to retinol (*bioconversion*) and stored as retinyl esters in the liver or recirculated back into the bloodstream to meet the needs of extrahepatic tissues [34]. If 100 % of provitamin A carotenoids were available, central cleavage would give a stoichiometric ratio of 1 μmole β-carotene to 2 μmole retinol, and 1 μmole of α-carotene or β-cryptoxanthin to 1 μmole retinol (*bioefficacy*). Based on human studies, and reflecting the average losses during all steps outlined above, the USA Institute of Medicine (IOM) has generalized the dietary conversion factors to be 12 μg β-carotene and 24 μg for the other provitamin A carotenoids to 1 μg retinol [35]. Variation of conversion factors in humans is influenced by species of carotenoids, dose size, food matrix, age, gender, health, and nutritional status of the host [36] (see Section I).

For children and women to meet the Estimated Average Requirement (EAR) for vitamin A, a preliminary target concentration of 15 μg provitamin A/g DW was set for biofortified maize in 2005 [7]. Assumptions made for provitamin A, based on the best available information, were an average of 50 % retention during processing and cooking, a 12:1 bioconversion ratio of β-carotene to retinol, 200 and 400 g daily maize consumption by children and women, respectively, and an EAR of 250 and 500 μg for children and women, respectively.

Recent evidence looking at bioefficacy and food retention of provitamin A maize suggests that this target value is adequate to meet the needs of the most vulnerable populations. Animal models provide a valuable tool for understanding and measuring carotenoid bioavailability, and Mongolian gerbils (*Meriones unguiculatus*) are a good model for evaluating bioefficacy of provitamin A carotenoids because they metabolize carotenoids similarly to humans [37]. A bioefficacy study using a vitamin A-depleted gerbil model with *ad libitum* feeding found the conversion factor for provitamin A maize to be 2.8 μg β-carotene: 1 μg retinol, which is much more efficient than predicted by the IOM (12:1) [38]. The authors hypothesized that the surprisingly efficient bioconversion rate was due to the presence of other provitamin A carotenoids and to the oil content in maize kernel (normally around 4 %). This study showed that carotenoids in provitamin A maize are as bioavailable as β-carotene supplements in a vitamin A-depleted gerbil model. Furthermore, bioconversion may be more dependent on vitamin A status than on the actual dietary intake of β-carotene from food or supplements.

Recent studies by Li et al. [39] and Muzhingi et al. [40] found that β-carotene in high provitamin A maize porridge was highly bioavailable when consumed by healthy adults. Conversion factors were reported to be 6.48 [39] or 3.2 [40] μg of β-carotene to 1 μg retinol. Li et al. [39] suggested that the starch matrix found in maize is an effective food matrix for biofortified foods, but there is currently no evidence to support this hypothesis. The difference in the bioconversion factors between the gerbil and the two human studies may be explained by the difference in vitamin A status as well as study design. Both the gerbils and the Muzhingi et al. [40] human subjects were vitamin A-depleted, which affects bioconversion of carotenoids from maize.

Davis et al. [41] studied the bioconversion of β-cryptoxanthin to retinol in gerbils and reported conversion factors of 2.74 μg β-cryptoxanthin in oil and 2.4 μg β-carotene equivalents in maize: 1 μg retinol. They hypothesized that the polar oxygenated structure of β-cryptoxanthin allows it to be more bioaccessible from the high provitamin A maize matrix, making it more than or equally as efficacious as β-carotene [41].

Food-based approaches for eliminating nutrient deficiencies may be considered more complete than single-nutrient fortification or supplementation approaches because nutrients often work together to enhance each other's absorption and utilization, and a deficiency in one nutrient may lead to an apparent deficiency in another. Vitamin A deficiency, for example, negatively affects iron metabolism leading to iron deficiency anemia, whereas iron deficiency may impair vitamin A mobilization from the liver [42]. Lutein, zeaxanthin, and β-carotene enhance iron absorption in humans on maize- or wheat-based diets; for example, adding 1.8 mg of lutein to a maize-based breakfast doubled iron absorption [43]. Changes in iron solubility are the proposed mechanism for this effect, but further research is needed to determine if the presence of carotenoids helps to solubilize the iron or if a carotenoid–iron complex is actually absorbed. The interaction between zinc deficiency and vitamin A status is less well-known, but evidence suggests that zinc has a role in the absorption, transport, and utilization of vitamin A [36]. Vitamin A deficiency may also negatively affect zinc absorption as well as metabolism by altering zinc mobilization from tissues and lowering plasma zinc levels [36]. Hence, breeding efforts to simultaneously increase both provitamin A concentration and zinc in maize may have a positive effect on provitamin A bioavailability.

Plant foods also contain anti-nutrients or inhibitors that negatively impact bioaccessibility of provitamin A carotenoids. The type and amount of fiber may negatively influence bioavailability, and interactions between fat and fiber during digestion may interfere with micellarization [33]. Furthermore, complications may arise when interpreting bioaccessibility results due to provitamin A carotenoid complexes with kernel proteins behaving differently during processing, extraction, digestion, and analysis [33]. Another anti-nutrient that may affect bioavailability of carotenoids is resistant starch, which acts as a dietary fiber in humans [36]. As with dietary fibers, resistant starches are not digested in the small intestine and may interfere with fat absorption. Typical maize contains 25 % amylose, whereas high-amylose varieties consist of as much as 70 % amylose [44]. Different methods and conditions of food processing and cooking may change the degree of solubility of fiber, micellarization of carotenoids, and release of carotenoids from proteins in maize. Cooking, chilling, and storage all affect the type and quantity of resistant starch in food [45]. It is therefore necessary to determine how popular food preparation methods affect carotenoid bioavailability and bioefficacy.

Determining bioavailability of provitamin A carotenoids in maize is currently complex, expensive, and very low throughput. However, as continued research generates more knowledge about the main factors influencing the bioavailability of provitamin A in maize, it may become possible to generate molecular markers for enhanced bioavailability for use in plant breeding programs.

For maize, the net outcome of all of these interacting, enhancing, and inhibiting factors is that provitamin A carotenoids are readily bioaccessible. Ultimately, however, only effectiveness trials in target populations can measure the likelihood of success of using biofortified maize as an intervention tool against malnutrition.

Creating and Supplying Demand for Provitamin A Maize

Farmer Participatory Evaluation and Demonstrations

Globally, about 50 % of maize farmers in nontemperate regions plant farm-saved seed of traditional (not "improved" or "modern") varieties, thus failing to meaningfully benefit from conventional maize breeding approaches [46]. Many new varieties have little or no impact because they are never adopted and thus remain "on the shelves" of research institutions. Even successful varieties are seldom adopted and used in the manner recommended or anticipated by the researcher. Farmers may plant in hills instead of rows, use more or less fertilizer, sow with intercrop instead of monoculture, use zero instead of conventional tillage, strip plant tops for fodder, sell produce in local instead of commercial markets, consume boiled instead of roasted, or otherwise modify or deviate from researcher-tested uses of the new varieties. Farmer-participatory evaluations enable researchers to identify and prioritize likely farmer modifications and to select varieties that are most likely to be desired and adopted for further promotion and commercialization. Pixley et al. [47] discuss challenges, merits, myths, and realities of participatory plant breeding and variety selection.

The maize provitamin A biofortification project in Zambia will use a farmer-participatory variety evaluation system that evaluates performance and acceptance of new varieties under farmers' conditions. The most promising biofortified maize varieties will be included in "mother/baby" trials [48] that are flexibly applied in different communities to suit local resources and conditions. The design consists of a "mother" trial, which is a complete, replicated trial, managed by a technician or trained partner, and several "baby" trials, which are incomplete replications grown by farmers on their own fields (within walking distance of the mother trial) and using their chosen crop management methods. Quantitative and qualitative traits from mother and baby trials are subjected to statistical analysis. Partners involved in conducting the trials include extension services, research stations, NGOs, rural development projects, farmer associations, and secondary schools. In addition to informing decisions about variety release and promotion, the trials facilitate a simple flow of information between breeders, extension staff, and farmers. Successful participatory evaluations [49] empower farmers to influence which varieties are promoted to variety release and commercialization. Participatory evaluations do raise expectations among participants and while it is difficult to gain the trust of partners, it is very easy to lose it. This fact was simply and clearly stated by a farmer during a field day at a "mother" trial in central Zimbabwe, when he said that many projects have come to his village seeking his participation, but very few ever came back.

Demonstration plots are a common marketing tool that are used when a very small number (often one to four) of exciting varieties are ready for widespread promotion. Seed companies generally display their current champion varieties alongside new releases, and farmers and general public are invited to field days where they can see the varieties and perhaps sample foods prepared from them. Demonstration plots are a showcase, and are usually "manicured" to look perfect and attractive, whereas participatory evaluations are conducted by farmers using their "real world" management practices. Both participatory variety evaluations and demonstration plots are important components of a demand-creation strategy, with participatory evaluations usually preceding demonstrations and including a preliminary selection of promising candidate varieties.

In addition to mother/baby trials and numerous demonstration plots, the Zambia maize biofortification project will distribute free samples of seed of the most promising two or three biofortified varieties to several hundred farmers. The sample packages will provide enough seed to plant a small plot and to harvest sufficient grain to enable testing its suitability for common household uses. This strategy of distributing small seed sample packs is a common demand-creation strategy among commercial seed companies.

Nutrition Education

Universally, parents care about the health and well-being of their children. Both demand for and intake of provitamin A biofortified crops can be increased by nutrition education campaigns that effectively empower caregivers with knowledge about the importance of vitamin A in health, and of dietary sources of provitamin A, including biofortified crops. Provitamin A-biofortified sweet potato projects in Kenya and Mozambique have documented the effectiveness of appropriate nutrition education, for example, through community theater, group demonstration sessions, and radio programs, in creating demand [50]. Tanumihardjo et al. [36] highlighted that nutrition education messages must go beyond encouraging healthy diets to also include teaching safe food storage techniques and preparation skills that conserve nutritional value. The provitamin A maize HarvestPlus project in Zambia is working closely with the Ministry of Health, the National Food and Nutrition Commission, the Ministry of Agriculture and Cooperatives (extension service), and others to develop nutrition education strategies to create lasting demand for provitamin A biofortified maize and other sources of vitamin A.

Consumer Acceptance

Several studies have examined consumer acceptance of yellow versus white maize, facilitated by the fact that both products are available in the market. Many of these studies tended to have an urban focus. Results from studies in Mozambique, Zimbabwe, and Kenya [51–53] paint a general picture that white is preferred over yellow maize, when the two are sold at equal prices. Only a price discount for yellow maize facilitated its preference, particularly by poor households. Yellow maize has typically not found acceptance in Zambia largely because such varieties were perceived as "drought food" (associated with bad times, since it was introduced as food aid), and are considered to have inferior taste (perhaps because food aid is not fresh, and may have endured harsh storage conditions during transport).

The literature comparing white with orange, rather than yellow maize, is limited. The study by Stevens and Winter-Nelson [54], which included white, yellow, and orange (imported from the USA) varieties of maize, suggests that orange maize meal is as preferred as white and that no price discounts are likely to be necessary to promote its consumption. This consumer acceptance study indicates that when nutrition information was provided regarding the importance and sources of vitamin A, families with young children and those that did not consume diets rich in animal products were more likely to accept orange maize. This conclusion is similar to those from biofortified sweet potato projects mentioned in Sect. "Nutrition education", where orange-fleshed have been widely accepted and demanded by consumers accustomed to white-fleshed sweet potatoes, following nutrition education campaigns [50].

A study of consumer acceptance of biofortified orange maize in Zambia was undertaken in 2009 [55]. The study elicited consumer willingness to pay by evaluating preference for orange maize relative to the already available white and yellow maize varieties in rural Zambia. It attempted to examine the impact of nutrition information delivered either as messages by simulated radio or by community leaders on consumer acceptance. It also assessed whether the opportunity to experience (cook and consume) the product in their own home setting influenced the magnitude of premiums or discounts required by consumers to accept orange maize. Both food and economic preferences were used to assess consumer acceptance, and both approaches led to the conclusions that: (1) orange maize is likely to be accepted by rural consumers in Zambia; (2) nutrition education campaigns translate into improved acceptance and willingness to pay for orange maize (other studies also indicated that nutrition information was the single most important factor in determining a household's decision to purchase nutritionally enhanced maize [31]); and (3) although both were effective, nutrition information received from community leaders was more effective than from the radio for influencing acceptance of orange maize [55].

The main message from these studies is that there are reasons to be confident that the negative connotations associated with yellow maize may not carryover to orange maize. In contrast to yellow maize, for which a price discount relative to white varieties is necessary for consumer acceptance, orange maize should require no price discount.

Seed Production

Seed has long been recognized as an efficient and sustainable mode for delivering agricultural technologies to farmers. According to Burke et al. [56], seed accounts for only 10 % of total maize production costs among small-scale farmers in Zambia; however, this estimate includes the effects of various subsidy programs. HarvestPlus plans to deliver technologies developed in breeding and nutritional research through seed of provitamin A biofortified maize varieties, beginning after the first release in 2012. Efficient, timely, and high quality seed production is a key component for success of the biofortification program.

Zambia has approximately 1.49 million small-scale farmers [57] who accounted for 90 % of the total maize production in the 2009/2010 cropping season. Use of improved seed in Zambia has increased from 23 % in 2001 to 73 % in 2007, and is currently estimated to cover 85 % of the maize area [58, 59]. These changes in adoption rates can be attributed to increased private sector participation and to private/public partnerships (through relief seed distribution). Increasing use of improved seed indicates that more farmers have access to the benefits of recent research efforts, and also suggests that reaching farmers with biofortified varieties will be possible through existing, growing channels.

Simfukwe [60] identified two parallel distribution networks for maize seed distribution in Zambia. The "commercial channel" operates through wholesale and the extensive distribution networks of seed companies (e.g., rural stockists), whereas the "noncommercial channel" operates through the Ministry of Agriculture and Cooperatives (MACO), relief agencies, and NGO farmer support programs. The noncommercial channel accounted for 50 % of total seed sales in the period 2002–2005, and the MACO input support program in the same period accounted for 35 % of sales by seed companies. The number of small-scale farmers targeted by this program has increased from 120,000 at inception in 2002 to 900,000 in the 2010/11 season. The input support program, therefore, now reaches about 60 % of the small-scale farmers with 9,000 tons of seed, and covers about 36 % of the total national seed requirements.

HarvestPlus will use and build upon the above-described, established seed production, certification and marketing systems in Zambia. Both commercial and noncommercial distribution channels will be important, but the noncommercial may be especially important in rural areas where Simfukwe [60] has noted that, despite the impressive urban network of seed distributors and stockists for seed companies, there is little permanent presence of commercial seed trade.

Market Development

The initial approach to market development that HarvestPlus will explore is creation of partnerships with organizations such as Concern Worldwide, World Vision International, and the World Food Program (WFP), whose missions are to support poor rural communities. Currently the Zambia HarvestPlus program is developing a joint action plan with the WFP's Purchase for Progress (P4P) project to encourage school governing boards to include provitamin A maize in their locally procured food baskets. The P4P project is supporting the government policy shift to Home-Grown School Meals project, a concept that links school feeding programs with local agricultural production and procurements of locally grown commodities (maize meal and pulses). This initiative will offer immense opportunities to local agricultural production and the resultant local market opportunities will stimulate adoption and consumption of provitamin A maize. Such arrangements will provide market outlets for rural households who achieve surplus production and for emergent commercial producers of provitamin A maize, while also achieving the HarvestPlus objective of providing poor rural communities with a micronutrient-dense food crop that addresses hidden hunger.

The major buyer of maize at the national level, which also reaches remote rural areas in Zambia where provitamin A maize is expected to be produced, is the government-owned Food Reserve Agency (FRA). The FRA also influences the price and distribution of maize by buying and selling a certain percentage of gross domestic maize at fixed prices. However, the FRA currently buys exclusively white maize, a policy that in itself creates barriers for provitamin A maize entering the mainstream maize markets. This means that until there is a change in this government policy, provitamin A maize will enter market channels operated only by private merchants and informal local traders. Another market channel for provitamin A maize is vertical integration with processors who may add value to the crop by processing it into products for sale to urban consumers.

Achieving Impact and Conclusion

Success, measured by significant contribution of provitamin A biofortified maize to the reduction of VAD in Zambia, will only follow sustained, long-term adoption and consumption of biofortified varieties. Excellent biofortified varieties are necessary and these will continue to become available (recall the cyclic nature of breeding projects, Sects. "Development of the first provitamin A maize hybrids for Zambia" and "Development of the second and future generations of provitamin A maize hybrids") if biofortification becomes institutionalized as part of a national strategy to combat malnutrition through productive and profitable agriculture.

Project Ownership

The critical step for long-term sustainability of the provitamin A maize biofortification effort in Zambia is for project ownership and the biofortification strategy to be fully embraced and assumed by Zambian partners. Continued success of biofortification in alleviating VAD in Zambia will also require that provitamin A maize become a widely demanded source of dietary provitamin A, and that biofortified varieties become a reliable source of crop income among small farmers and agribusiness firms in key agricultural production regions.

HarvestPlus has pursued two approaches towards achieving project ownership by its Zambian partners. First, it proposed and initiated the formation of a steering committee comprised of public and private sector members to guide and oversee the process of product development and delivery for provitamin A maize in Zambia. Through the steering committee, a negotiated agreement on how provitamin A maize will be introduced in Zambia was reached among Zambia's key stakeholders in agriculture, scientific research, food security, health, and nutrition. The members developed a product development and delivery plan to guide the implementation process. The Zambia Agricultural Research Institute (ZARI) chairs the committee in its capacity as the initiator and overseer of the product development process for provitamin A maize in Zambia. If this collaborative approach continues to grow, provitamin A maize production and consumption will be sustained beyond the existence of HarvestPlus.

Second, while several development and delivery activities are undertaken by Zambian stakeholders on the basis of a shared vision and mutual interests, HarvestPlus also promotes contractual relationships, and facilitates independent initiatives to create supply of and demand for biofortified maize. In contractual relationships, local Zambian institutions and community-based organizations are invited to tender offers and subsequently undertake provitamin A maize development and delivery activities. These activities include product development, seed multiplication and distribution, information dissemination, nutrition message formulation, and extension services. Independent public and private sector investments in the development of biofortified maize are facilitated through the establishment of a local carotenoid analysis service laboratory, a molecular-marker assisted breeding service, and collaborative biofortified maize breeding network. HarvestPlus envisages that these approaches will build local capabilities and will create demand for and promote production, distribution, and utilization of provitamin A maize.

Conclusion

Although simple in concept, reducing malnutrition through biofortification of maize is a complex undertaking which we have only superficially described. The complexity of the causes and consequences of VAD in Zambia, however, continue to defy solution, and biofortification contributes a novel approach that richly merits trying. During summer 2011–2012, more than 300 farmers grew trial plots of the experimental biofortified maize hybrids and more than 80 field days were organized at demonstration plots comparing these hybrids with currently successful commercial hybrids. The second year of National Performance Trials (NPTs) confirmed the agronomic competitiveness of these experimental biofortified hybrids, and in September 2012 three of the hybrids were approved for release and commercial production in Zambia. Although the eventual impact of the HarvestPlus project and biofortified varieties will take many years and perhaps a couple of generations to be fully achieved, immediate health benefits will be realized from nutrition education efforts at household, community, and national levels.

Annex: An Introduction to Plant Breeding

Plant breeding is the science and art of modifying plants to better serve our needs or preferences. All plant breeding begins with identifying or creating genetic variation for the trait(s) of interest, followed by selecting those variants that are most desirable. If variation is extensive, and the trait is highly *heritable*, a term that quantifies the degree to which offspring resemble their parents, or the reliability with which parents' characteristics can be expected to be reproduced in their offspring, then progress from plant breeding for that trait will likely be relatively fast and simple to achieve. Maize grain color varies and an ear may have kernels segregating for shades of yellow and orange. Deep yellow or orange kernels can be selected, planted, and expected to produce plants with ears that have kernels with deeper yellow or orange than the parental ear. This process would be largely an art, and would likely result over time in increasing the total concentration of carotenoids in the grain. Provitamin A carotenoids, however, cannot be visually distinguished, and selection for color, without relying on laboratory analysis is unlikely to result in maize biofortified with provitamin A.

The heritability of a trait is affected by several factors, including the number of genes involved in determining the expression of the trait, and the extent to which different growing environments alter the effect of each gene determining the trait. In general, the more genes involved, the less heritable the trait will be; simply put, the more complicated the trait, the less reliably we can predict its value based on that of its parents. Similarly, the more sensitive a trait's expression is to variation in environmental conditions, for example heat, drought or acidic soils, the lower its heritability tends to be. The carotenoid biosynthetic pathway has been well-characterized (see, for example, 20, 61–63) and involves more than a dozen crucial genes, each of which has multiple forms, variants or *alleles*, capable of acting singly or in combination with other genes within or outside the pathway, resulting in different final carotenoid profiles and concentrations in the maize kernels. The huge numbers of possible combinations of alleles among the genes of the carotenoid biosynthetic pathway represent opportunities for plant breeders to select combinations that increase individual carotenoid concentrations, or the total provitamin A concentration in grain.

Recurrent Selection

The simplest form of plant breeding is like an accelerated version of natural selection, which through hundreds of generations rids a population of unfit individuals and gradually exaggerates the fitness-enhancing traits of the ever-more-prevalent surviving types. In plant breeding, we might begin with a landrace or a popular variety of maize, and implement a cyclic process of evaluating the provitamin A concentration of a hundred or more individuals or families, selecting and inter-mating (or allowing them to intermate) only those with highest provitamin A concentration, again planting the new progeny generation, and repeating the process until we are satisfied with the average provitamin A concentration of the improved variety. This approach will only be successful if there was adequate variation for provitamin A concentration among the individuals of the original landrace or variety, and if provitamin A concentration is sufficiently heritable to allow progress from selection. Unfortunately, we have found that although provitamin A concentration is heritable, most yellow maize populations have insufficient variation for provitamin A concentration to allow us to reach nutritionally meaningful levels within an acceptable number of years.

Inbred Line and Hybrid Development

Most modern varieties of maize are hybrids, formed by crossing two parents to form a variety that has the best characteristics from each parent, and is therefore superior to both of them. Much of the effort in maize breeding is devoted to a painstaking process of identifying very unique pairs of parents that complement each other exceptionally well when producing offspring (the hybrid). Our primary interest is enhanced provitamin A concentration, but to be successful, a hybrid must also be high yielding, disease resistant, produce tasty grain, and have many more essential and desirable attributes. The effort is only useful if, once we create the outstanding hybrid, we are able to produce sufficient seed of it to plant many thousands of hectares year after year.

Maize is ideally suited for making hybrids because its female flowers (each maize kernel originates as a flower) are separate from its male flowers (contained in the tassel, at the top of the plant). By covering the young ear (with a small bag called a shoot bag) before any silks emerge from the tip of the ear leaves, breeders can pollinate the flowers of that ear with pollen collected from a tassel on the same plant or another plant. Pollinating an ear with pollen from the same plant, called *self-pollination*, results in a 50 % reduction in allelic variation, and repeated self-pollination for several generations results in an *inbred line*, which is genetically uniform, having for all genes only one, the same allele, on each chromosome. Inbred lines are pure breeding because self-pollinating them reproduces exactly the same line, which is a crucial feature for enabling hybrid varieties; once we develop pure lines and identify the specific combination of inbred lines that makes an excellent hybrid, we can produce the exact same hybrid over and over and over again, making seed available to many farmers for planting on large land areas during many years.

Several crucial activities are conducted during the process of self-pollinating maize plants to develop inbred lines for use in hybrid varieties. Highly heritable traits, such as resistance to many diseases, are evaluated for all lines, and only those with an acceptable level of resistance are self-pollinated, while all others—usually the vast majority—are discarded. Other traits, including grain yield in hybrid combination, are not highly heritable and breeders form experimental hybrids in parallel with the repeated self-pollination process. The hybrids are evaluated in multilocation trials and only the best hybrids, performing as well or better than commercial hybrid checks included in the trials, are selected. Breeders use the hybrid trial data to discard the vast majority of lines that are being self-pollinated in the parallel process of developing inbred lines. Plant breeding is thus a numbers game, and it is commonly said that only one of a million maize lines in a breeding program succeeds to be used in a commercial hybrid. Needless to say, a commercially successful inbred line is extremely valuable.

Commercial inbred lines, and *elite lines* that were nearly, but not quite good enough to become commercial lines, are used extensively as parents in crosses (usually with other elite or commercial lines) that are used to develop new inbred lines by repeating the long process of repeated self-pollination while selecting for all important traits. This process of elite or commercial line development, followed by their use in new breeding crosses to initiate new line development is indeed a variant of recurrent selection (described above).

Sometimes breeders wish to improve traits for which there is not sufficient or any useful variation among the elite and commercial lines. This has been the case for provitamin A carotenoid concentration, for which most commercial lines have <2 μg/g. Maize with 15 or 20 μg/g may only be found among landraces held in germplasm banks, or among lines from distant ecologies, and such sources of the desired trait (provitamin A in this case) must be used in breeding crosses despite their many defects which they will transmit to the offspring of these crosses. In such cases, the cross of elite line with source line is often *back-crossed* to the elite line one or more times in a process during which progeny with the desired trait are selected after each back-cross and prior to performing the additional back-cross. Back-cross breeding results in lines that are very similar to the elite parent, but have incorporated the desired trait(s) from the source parent. Back-cross breeding has been an important strategy in developing provitamin A biofortified maize.

Genetically Modified, or Transgenic Lines and Varieties

Transgenes are no different from any other genes, except that they originate from a different species. All the breeding methods described above rely on combining genes (or alleles of genes) from one parent with those of the other parent to achieve in the offspring the desired values for traits of interest, such as provitamin A concentration. Back-cross breeding is a less-preferred strategy, when the desired trait cannot be found in elite or commercial lines. For some traits, however, the desired values may not exist in the crop species of interest, and it may be possible to transgenically introduce these alleles or genes from another species. In making golden rice, for example, inserting a gene from maize (phytoene synthase) resulted in rice with 30 μg/g of β-carotene [64], whereas common rice varieties have no β-carotene. Transgenic strategies have not been used in developing provitamin A biofortified maize, because the natural genetic variation in maize is sufficient to achieve the target of 15 μg/g of provitamin A carotenoids.

Open-Pollinated Varieties

Not all improved and biofortified varieties will be hybrids. About 30 % of improved varieties, and about 50 % of all maize grown in sub-Saharan Africa are *open-pollinated varieties* (OPVs). An OPV differs in many ways from a commercial hybrid (see Pixley [65] for a discussion of advantages and disadvantages of hybrids relative to OPVs), but an OPV can be conceptualized as a hybrid with many parents, which may or may not be inbred lines. Some excellent OPVs have been created by intermating as few as five or six, or as many as 30 or more elite inbred lines. We are using this approach to develop and test OPVs that could be used as provitamin A biofortified varieties. As you might expect, it is easier to find two lines that make an excellent hybrid than to find 6–30 lines that form an equally good OPV (think that for every trait there will always be one or more "weak links" bringing down the overall performance of the OPV), so hybrids almost always out-perform OPVs. However, OPVs have the distinct advantage that farmers can save harvested grain for use as seed in several subsequent seasons, without much reduction in performance of the crop; by contrast, using harvested grain of hybrid varieties as seed generally results in important loss of performance, which is why farmers typically purchase new seed of hybrids each time they plant.

References

1. WHO. Global prevalence of vitamin A deficiency in populations at risk 1995–2005. WHO Global Database on Vitamin A Deficiency. World Health Organization, Geneva. http://www.who.int/nutrition/publications/micronutrients/vitamin_a_deficiency/9789241598019/en/. Accessed 4 Nov 2011.
2. Nuss ET, Tanumihardjo SA. Maize: a paramount staple crop in the context of global nutrition. Compr Rev Food Sci Food Saf. 2010;9:417–36.
3. Atlin GN, Palacios N, Babu R, Das B, Twumasi-Afriyie S, Friesen DK, DeGroote H, Vivek B, Pixley KV. Quality protein maize: progress and prospects. Plant Breed Rev. 2011;34:83–130.
4. Pfeiffer WH, McClafferty B. HarvestPlus: breeding crops for better nutrition. Crop Sci. 2007;47:S88–105.
5. Graham RD, Welch RM, Bouis HE. Addressing micronutrient malnutrition through enhancing the nutritional quality of staple foods: principles, perspectives and knowledge gaps. Adv Agron. 2001;70:77–142.
6. Hotz C, McClafferty B. From harvest to health: challenges for developing biofortified staple foods and determining their impacts on micronutrient status. Food Nutr Bull. 2007;28:S271–9.
7. Bouis HE, Welch RM. Biofortification—a sustainable agricultural strategy for reducing micronutrient malnutrition in the global South. Crop Sci. 2010;50:S20–32.
8. Qaim M, Stein AJ, Meenakshi JV. Economics of biofortification. Agric Econ. 2007;37(S1):119–33.
9. Copenhagen Consensus. 2008. www.copenhagenconsensus.com/Home.aspx. Accessed 5 Nov 2011.
10. Bhagwati J, Bourgignon F, Kydland FE, Mundell R, North DC, Schelling TC, Smith VL, Stokey NL. Expert panel ranking. In: Lomborg B, editor. Global crises, global solutions. 2nd ed. New York: Cambridge University Press; 2009. p. 605–8.
11. Ortiz-Monasterio JI, Palacios-Rojas N, Meng E, Pixley K, Trethowan R, Peña RJ. Enhancing the mineral and vitamin content of wheat and maize through plant breeding. J Cereal Sci. 2007;46:293–307.
12. Harjes C, Rocheford T, Bai L, Brutnell T, Bermudez-Kandiannis C, Sowinski S, Stapleton A, Vallabhaneni R, Williams M, Wurtzel E, Yan J, Buckler E. Natural genetic variation in lycopene epsilon cyclase tapped for maize biofortification. Science. 2008;319:330–3.
13. Yan J, Bermudez-Kandianis CB, Harjes CE, Bai L, Kim E, Yang X, Skinner D, Fu Z, Mitchell S, Li Q, Salas-Fernandez M, Zaharieva M, Babu R, Fu Y, Palacios N, Li J, DellaPenna D, Brutnell T, Buckler E, Warburton M, Rocheford T. Rare genetic variation at *Zea mays* crtRB1 increases β-carotene in maize grain. Nat Genet. 2010;42:322–7.
14. Kurilich A, Juvik J. Quantification of carotenoid and tocopherol antioxidants in *Zea mays*. J Agric Food Chem. 1999;47:1948–55.
15. Menkir A, Liu W, White W, Maziya-Dixon B, Rocheford T. Carotenoid diversity in tropical-adapted yellow maize inbred lines. Food Chem. 2008;109:521–9.
16. Kimura M, Rodriguez-Amaya DB. Sources of errors in the quantitative analysis of food carotenoids by HPLC. Arch Latinoam Nutr. 1999;49:58S–66.
17. Lozano-Alejo N, Vazquez-Carrillo G, Pixley K, Palacios-Rojas N. Effects of snack preparation by nixtamalization and frying on carotenoid profiles of Mexican maize landraces and hybrids. Innov Food Sci Emerg Technol. 2007;8:385–9.
18. Berardo N, Mazzinelli G, Valotti P, Lagianna P, Redaelli R. Characterization of maize germplasm for the chemical composition of the grain. J Agric Food Chem. 2009;57:2378–84.
19. Howe JA, Tanumihardjo SA. Carotenoid-biofortified maize maintains adequate vitamin A status in Mongolian gerbils. J Nutr. 2006;136:2562–7.
20. Giuliano G, Tavazza R, Diretto G, Beyer P, Taylor MA. Metabolic engineering of carotenoid biosynthesis in plants. Trends Biotechnol. 2008;26:139–45.
21. FAOSTAT. CountrySTAT. An integrated system for national food and agriculture statistics. http://www.countrystat.org. Accessed 3 May 2011.
22. Bechoff A, Dhuique-Mayer C, Dornier M, Tomlins K, Boulanger R, Dufour D, Westby A. Relationship between the kinetics of β-carotene degradation and formation of norisoprenoids in the storage of dried sweet potato chips. Food Chem. 2010;121:348–57.
23. Rodriguez-Amaya D, Nutti M, de Carvalho JL. Carotenoids of sweet potato, cassava and maize and their use in bread and flour fortification. In: Patel VB, Preedy VR, Watson RR, editors. Flour and breads and their fortification in health and disease prevention. London: Academic Press, Elsevier; 2011. p. 301–11.
24. Bechoff A, Westby A, Owori C, Menya G, Dhuique-Mayer C, Dofour D, Tomlins K. Effect of drying and storage on the degradation of total carotenoids in orange-fleshed sweet potato cultivars. J Sci Food Agric. 2010;90: 622–9.
25. Goldman M, Horev B, Saguy I. Decolorization of β-carotene in model systems simulating dehydrated foods. Mechanism and kinetic principles. J Food Sci. 1983;48:751–4.

26. Aman R, Schieber A, Carle R. Effects of heating and illumination on *trans-cis* isomerization and degradation of β-carotene and lutein in isolated spinach chloroplasts. J Agric Food Chem. 2005;53:9512–8.
27. Ilg A, Beyer P, Al-Babili S. Characterization of the rice carotenoid cleavage dioxygenase 1 reveals a novel route for geranial biosynthesis. FEBS J. 2009;276:736–47.
28. Burt A, Grainger C, Young C, Shelp B, Lee E. Impact of postharvest handling on carotenoid concentration and composition in high-carotenoid maize (*Zea mays* L.) kernels. J Agric Food Chem. 2010;58:8286–92.
29. Li S, Tayie F, Young M, Rocheford T, White W. Retention of provitamin A carotenoids in high β-carotene maize (*Zea mays*) during traditional African household processing. J Agric Food Chem. 2007;55:10744–50.
30. Rodriguez-Amaya DB. Carotenoids and food preparation: the retention of provitamin A carotenoids in prepared, processed, and stored foods. Arlington: Opportunities for Micronutrient Intervention (OMNI); 1997.
31. Muzhingi T, Langyintuo A, Malaba L, Banziger M. Consumer acceptability of yellow maize products in Zimbabwe. Food Policy. 2008;33:352–61.
32. Tayie FA, White WS. Effects of traditional African maize processing on the carotenoid contents of beta-carotene-rich yellow maize. Fam Consum Sci Res J. 2005;34:180–96.
33. Kean EG, Hamaker BR, Ferruzzi MG. Carotenoid bioaccesibility from whole grain and degermed maize meal products. J Agric Food Chem. 2008;56:9918–26.
34. Olson JA. Absorption, transport and metabolism of carotenoids in humans. Pure Appl Chem. 1994;66:1011–6.
35. Institute of Medicine. Dietary reference intakes for vitamin A, vitamin K, arsenic, boron, chromium, copper, iodine, iron, manganese, molybdenum, nickel, silicon, vanadium, and zinc. Washington, DC: National Academy Press; 2001. p. 65–126.
36. Tanumihardjo SA, Palacios N, Pixley KV. Provitamin A carotenoid bioavailability: what really matters? Int J Vitam Nutr Res. 2010;80:336–50.
37. Lee CM, Lederman JD, Hofmann NE, Erdman Jr JW. The Mongolian gerbil (*Meriones unguiculatus*) is an appropriate animal for evaluation of the conversion of carotene to vitamin A. J Nutr. 1998;128:280–6.
38. Howe JA, Tanumihardjo SA. Evaluation of analytical methods for carotenoid extraction from biofortified maize (*Zea mays* sp.). J Agric Food Chem. 2006;54:7992–7.
39. Li S, Nugroho A, Rocheford T, White WS. Vitamin A equivalence of the β-carotene in β-carotene biofortified maize porridge consumed by women. Am J Clin Nutr. 2010;92:1105–12.
40. Muzhingi T, Gadaga TH, Siwela AH, Grusak MA, Russell RM, Tang G. Yellow maize with high β-carotene is an effective source of vitamin A in healthy Zimbabwean men. Am J Clin Nutr. 2011;94:510–9.
41. Davis CR, Howe JA, Rocheford TR, Tanumihardjo SA. The xanthophyll composition of biofortified maize (*Zea mays* sp.) does not influence the bioefficacy of provitamin A carotenoids in Mongolian gerbils (*Meriones unguiculatus*). J Agric Food Chem. 2008;56:6745–50.
42. Munoz EC, Rosado JL, Lopez P, Furr HC, Allen LH. Iron and zinc supplementation improves indicators of vitamin A status of Mexican preschoolers. Am J Clin Nutr. 2000;71:789–94.
43. Garcia-Casal MN. Carotenoids increase iron absorption from cereal-based food in the human. Nutr Res. 2006;26:340–4.
44. Cauvain SP, Young LS. The ICC handbook of cereals, flour, dough and product testing. Lancaster, PA: DEStech Publications, Inc.; 2009.
45. Brown IL. High amylose starches-new development in human nutrition. Nutr Soc Aust. 1994;18:33–9.
46. Morris ML. Assessing the benefits of international maize breeding research: an overview of the global maize impacts study. In: Pingali PL, editor. CIMMYT 1999-2000 world maize facts and trends. Meeting world maize needs: technological opportunities and priorities for the public sector. Mexico, DF: CIMMYT; 2001. p. 25–34.
47. Pixley K, Fuentes M, Badstue L, Bergvinson D. Participatory plant breeding: science or dogma? Chapter 15. In: Chopra VL, Sharma RP, Bhat SR, Prasanna BM, editors. Search for new genes. New Delhi: Academic Foundation; 2007.
48. Snapp S. Mother and baby trials: a novel trial design being tried out in Malawi. In: TARGET, the Newsletter of the Soil Fertility Research Network for Maize-Based Cropping Systems in Malawi and Zimbabwe. 1999 Jan;17:8
49. Bänziger M, De Meyer J. Collaborative maize variety development for stress-prone environments in southern Africa. In: Cleveland DA, Soleri D, editors. Farmers, scientists and plant breeding. Wallingford, UK: CAB International; 2002. p. 269–96.
50. Low JW, Arimond M, Osman N, Cunguara B, Zano F, Tschirley D. Ensuring the supply of and creating demand for a biofortified crop with a visible trait: lessons learned from the introduction of orange-fleshed sweet potato in drought-prone areas of Mozambique. Food Nutr Bull. 2007;28:S258–70.
51. Tschirley DL, Santos AP. Who eats yellow maize? Preliminary results of a survey of consumer maize preferences in Maputo, Mozambique. In: International Development Working Paper 53. Michigan, USA: Michigan State University; 1995.
52. Rubey LR, Ward W, Tschirley D. Maize research priorities: the role of consumer preferences. In: Byerlee D, Eicher C, editors. Africa's Emerging maize revolution. Colorado: Lynne Eienner Publishers; 1997. p. 145–56.
53. De Groote H, Chege Kimenju S. Comparing consumer preferences for color and nutritional quality in maize: application of a semi-double-bound logistic model on urban consumers in Kenya. Food Policy. 2008;33:362–70.

54. Stevens R, Winter-Nelson A. Consumer acceptance of pro-vitamin A biofortified maize in Maputo, Mozambique. Food Policy. 2008;33:341–51.
55. Meenakshi JV, Banerji A, Manyong V, Tomlins K, Hamukwala P, Zulu R, Mungoma C. Consumer acceptance of provitamin A orange maize in rural Zambia. HarvestPlus Working Paper No. 4. 2010. http://www.dfid.gov.uk/r4d/PDF/Outputs/Misc_Crop/HarvestPlus_Working_paper_4.pdf. Accessed 4 Aug 2011.
56. Burke WJ, Hichaambwa M, Banda D, Jayne TS. The cost of maize production by small scale farmers in Zambia. Working Paper No. 50. http://www.aec.msu.edu/fs2/zambia/wp50.pdf. Accessed 31 Mar 2011.
57. Kuteya A, Kabwe S, Beaver M, Chapoto A, Burke B, Mason N, Weber M. Statistical report on categorization of rural cropping households in Zambia: Section III. Household-Level Demographics and Population Location. Working Paper No.51-3. Food Security Research Project Lusaka, Zambia Draft, Mar 2011. http://www.aec.msu.edu/fs2/zambia/wp51/wp51_Section_III.pdf. Accessed 4 Aug 2011.
58. Langyintuo AS, Mwangi W, Diallo AO, MacRobert J, Dixon J, Bänziger M. An analysis of the bottlenecks affecting the production and deployment of maize seed in eastern and southern Africa. 2008. http://ageconsearch.umn.edu/bitstream/51713/2/Seeds-paper-2009-uploaded.pdf. Accessed 4 Aug 2011.
59. La Rovere R, Kostandini G, Abdoulaye T, Dixon J, Mwangi W, Guo Z, Bänziger M. Potential impact of investments in drought tolerant maize in Africa. 2010. http://www.mtnforum.org/en/content/potential-impact-investments-drought-tolerant-maize-africa. Accessed 4 Aug 2011.
60. Simfukwe M. FANRPAN: relief seed trade study-Zambia. Mwalimu Simfukwe. 2006 Sep 1. Discussion Document. Food Agriculture, and Natural Resources Policy Analysis Network. http://www.fanrpan.org/documents/d00202/Zambia_Seed_Trade_Simfukwe_Sept2006.pdf. Accessed 4 Nov 2011.
61. DellaPenna D, Pogson B. Vitamin synthesis in plants: tocopherols and carotenoids. Annu Rev Plant Biol. 2006;57:711–38.
62. Hirschberg J, Cohen M, Harker M, Lotan T, Mann V, Pecker I. Molecular genetics of the carotenoid biosynthesis pathway in plants and algae. Pure Appl Chem. 1997;69:2151–8.
63. Just BJ, Santos CAF, Fonseca MEN, Boiteux LS, Oloizia BB, Simon PW. Carotenoid biosynthesis structural genes in carrot (*Daucus carota*): isolation, sequence-characterization, single nucleotide polymorphism (SNP) markers and genome mapping. Theor Appl Genet. 2007;114:693–704.
64. Paine JA, Shipton CA, Chaggar S, Howells RM, Kennedy MJ, Vernon G, Wright SY, Hinchliffe E, Adams JL, Silverstone AL, Drake R. Improving the nutritional value of golden rice through increased pro-vitamin A content. Nat Biotechnol. 2005;23:482–7.
65. Pixley KV. Hybrid and open-pollinated varieties in modern agriculture. Chapter 17. In: Lamkey KR, Lee M, editors. Plant breeding: the Arnel R. Hallauer international symposium. IA, USA: Blackwell Publishing Professional; 2006. p. 234–50.

Chapter 18
Horticultural Crops as a Source of Carotenoids

Philipp W. Simon, Megan J. Bowman, and Sherry A. Tanumihardjo

Key Points

- Horticultural crops are a rich and diverse source of carotenoids for consumers around the world.
- Crop production, storage, and delivery to market are often challenging but crop value can be high.
- A few international agencies and programs target horticultural crop improvement, and consequently play an important role in sustaining carotenoid availability to consumers in global regions with high incidence of vitamin A deficiency.
- Classical horticultural crop breeding as well as biotechnological approaches to increase carotenoid content and quality offer potential for developing more nutritious dietary sources of carotenoids.

Keywords Horticultural crops • Biotechnological approaches • Carotenoid sustainability • Vitamin A health

Introduction

Horticultural crops include several major food crops: vegetables, fruits, and nuts. These crops are usually grown on a relatively small scale compared to staple food crops, but they typically command a high value in the marketplace. Unlike cereal grains and dry legumes, many horticultural crops have a relatively short shelf-life, requiring ready access to cold storage to preserve market value. This limits their long-distance distribution, especially in less-developed regions of the world. Consequently,

P.W. Simon, Ph.D. (✉)
USDA-Agricultural Research Service, Vegetable Crops Research Unit, University of Wisconsin, 1575 Linden Drive, Madison, WI 53706, USA

Department of Horticulture, University of Wisconsin-Madison, 1575 Linden Drive, Madison, WI 53706, USA
e-mail: psimon@wisc.edu

M.J. Bowman, Ph.D.
Department of Horticulture, University of Wisconsin-Madison, 1575 Linden Drive, Madison, WI 53706, USA

S.A.Tanumihardjo, M.S., Ph.D.
Department of Nutritional Science, University of Wisconsin-Madison, 1415 Linden Drive, Madison, WI 53706, USA

S.A. Tanumihardjo (ed.), *Carotenoids and Human Health*, Nutrition and Health,
DOI 10.1007/978-1-62703-203-2_18,

numerous vegetable and fruit crops are extensively grown and used in small geographic regions but are not well known outside of local production areas, and many are regarded as indigenous. For widely grown horticultural crops, both the US Department of Agriculture (USDA) [1] and the Food and Agriculture Organization (FAO) [2] collect and summarize production statistics for 30–40 vegetable crops (including melons) and 30–40 fruit crops. The large number of horticultural crops combined with their often localized production make for a complex situation in determining the impact of horticultural crops, but both economic and nutritional values are considered to be high for vegetables and fruits.

Vegetables and fruits are a significant source of several dietary nutrients, and carotenoids are among the most important. In fact, horticultural crops are by far the most significant source of dietary carotenoids. A recent assessment of food and nutrient consumption in the US based upon the "What We Eat in America" component of the National Health and Nutrition Examination Survey (NHANES) [3] indicated that among food sources contributing at least 1.0% of a given carotenoid to the US diet, horticultural crops were the only sources of α- and β-carotene, lycopene, β-cryptoxanthin, and lutein + zeaxanthin, except for 1.5% of β-carotene coming from yellow margarine, 4.2% of lutein + zeaxanthin from eggs, and 1.2% of lutein + zeaxanthin from white taco corn [4]. Vegetables were predominant among carotenoid sources, with carrots, tomatoes, and spinach contributing more than 20% of the α- and β-carotene, lycopene, and lutein + zeaxanthin, respectively, but oranges were by far the major source of dietary β-cryptoxanthin. It is notable that while lutein + zeaxanthin came from 12 different horticultural crops, β-carotene from 9 crops, and β-cryptoxanthin from 5 crops, the predominant sources of α-carotene and lycopene were carrots and tomatoes, respectively.

While horticultural crops are clearly the largest source of dietary carotenoids in the USA, no comparable analysis based upon food intake has been performed for other countries or regions. Relevant information that has been reported from a global perspective includes Simpson [5] who noted that carotenoids in vegetables account for 68% of the world-wide dietary vitamin A and 82% in developing countries. FAO and the World Health Organization (WHO) estimated a similar value of >80% in developing countries in 2001 with 84% from "vegetable" (non-animal) sources in Africa, and 90% in SE Asia, as compared to 63% for Europe, 64% for the Americas, and 72% globally [6]. While details indicating documented specific food sources and their dietary intake were not provided for these global values, widely grown vegetables and fruits (e.g., spinach, amaranth, pumpkins, squash, carrots, mangoes, apricots, papayas) as well as red palm oil (a fruit crop) and indigenous fruits and leafy greens (annual vegetables and tree leaves) are noted as likely primary sources of provitamin A carotenoids. High carotenoid, cooler season vegetable crops, such as winter squash and carrots, are not as extensively grown in the developing world as in the USA. Fruit crops with high carotenoid content, such as mangoes and papayas, as well as orange-fleshed sweet potatoes, are more plentiful in markets of the developing world. Therefore, it may be surmised that these warm season crops provide more dietary carotenoids in the developing world than in the USA, but as in the USA, it can be concluded that horticultural crops are the primary sources of dietary carotenoids in the entire world.

Production and Delivery of Horticultural Crop Carotenoids to Consumers

Given this important status of horticultural crops in providing dietary carotenoids, and the crucial roles the intake of these compounds play in maintaining both vitamin A status and a broad range of other aspects of health, the prospects for sustaining and expanding the impacts of horticultural crops in global health warrant consideration. Several distinct, but not unrelated, issues arise in sustaining and ultimately increasing the delivery of dietary carotenoids to consumers from horticultural crops. These include sustaining and expanding crop production, improving post-harvest cold storage capacity, and crop improvement through plant breeding for higher carotenoid content or bioavailability (e.g., "biofortification"). Variation in horticultural crop production across years for a given production region tends to have relatively little influence on carotenoid content or composition (i.e., relative amounts of components), as long as relatively optimal production conditions are realized [7, 8]. Carotenoid content recorded in various nutrient composition tables from different regions of the world does vary widely for many horticultural crops [9]. For example, a recent evaluation of the carotenoid profile of 21 African indigenous leafy green vegetables from Cameroon revealed a broad range of provitamin A carotenoids with values ranging from ~1 to 40 mg β-carotene/100 g dry weight, which varied by processing method [10]. Therefore, quantification is important when making recommendations. Climatic variation likely accounts for some variation, but differences in predominant cultivars of a given crop grown in different geographic regions also account for much variation, as does lab methodology used to generate carotenoid content values. One aspect of horticultural crop production that does play a major role in delivering carotenoids to consumers is the fact that some crops like tree fruits are perennial and others like cassava are sometimes grown as perennials. Because of this, lead time to adjust production in anticipation of increased market demand is much greater than that required for rapidly growing annuals.

Long-term, post-harvest storage of most horticultural crops is not possible without a cold chain to deliver the crop to consumers, and carotenoid content can decrease, and composition can change, with sub-optimal cold storage. Cold chains are well-established in the developed world but often minimal and unreliable in regions where under-consumption of carotenoids raises the greatest health risks. The combined challenges of reliable horticultural crop production and post-harvest preservation in developing regions often reflects inadequate numbers of human capital such as trained horticulturists, and an under-developed infrastructure (e.g., transportation and communications) to ensure delivery of carotenoid-rich crops to consumers. As with other nutritional deficiencies in the developing world, poverty sustains sub-optimal production of horticultural crops.

Development of improved market profitability of horticultural crops can stimulate the development of local production expertise and post-harvest facilities with notable positive health consequences. For example, the development of local mango production industry driven by crop profitability was interpreted as the underlying basis for greater local consumption and consequent reduced incidence of vitamin A deficiency in Indonesian children [11]. However, if expanded horticultural crop production is focused on expanding export sales, local consumption may not be increased.

Genetic Improvement of Horticultural Crops as a Source of Carotenoids

Genetic improvement of horticultural crops can increase the delivery of dietary carotenoids to consumers in several ways. Genetic improvement to improve productivity and profitability for growers, for example, to incorporate genetic resistance to disease or extended shelf-life, can have an immediate effect on delivering more carotenoid-rich commodities to the local marketplace. In some situations, genetic improvement of a crop is not even necessary, but rather expanding the array of available cultivars for a given crop beyond local cultivars to include those bred for other regions can result in the discovery of commercially available but previously untested cultivars with superior productivity, post-harvest shelf-life, and/or carotenoid content. The World Vegetable Center, also known as the Asian Vegetable Research and Development Center (AVRDC), has established extensive innovative field testing for several vegetable crops. Trialing has been established for beans, sweet potatoes, and white potatoes by the International Center for Tropical Agriculture (CIAT) and the International Potato Center (CIP). Productivity, quality, and market value of many horticultural crops and global regions could be increased from expanded field testing of available crop cultivars to identify improved sources of dietary carotenoids.

Table 18.1 Sources of carotenoids in the US diet ranked by their relative contribution of total dietary intake, based on NHANES 2003–2004, all age groups 2 years and greater. All values % (modified from 4)

β-Carotene	α-Carotene	Lycopene	β-Cryptoxanthin	Lutein + zeaxanthin
Carrots 29.5	Carrots 66.8	Tomatoes 72.1	Oranges 60.6	Spinach 24.7
Spinach 8.2	Tomatoes 4.9	Other <1%—27.9	Carrots 5.7	Sweet corn 5.3
Sweet potatoes 7.7	Others <1%—28.3		Watermelons 3.3	Oranges 5.1
Tomatoes 6.8			Sweet corn 2.9	Collards 4.8
Lettuces 5.1			Persimmons 2.2	Lettuces 4.5
Melons 4.8			Others <1%—25.3	Eggs 4.2
Collards 2.2				Broccoli 3.6
Broccoli 1.6				Chicory 3.2
Margarine 1.5				Squashes 2.3
Watermelons 1.0				Kale 2.3
Other <1%—31.6				Beans 2.1
				Peas 1.6
				Tomatoes 1.5
				White corn 1.2
				Other <1%—33.6

For horticultural crops where plant breeding programs are established, there are often abundant opportunities to include breeding for higher carotenoid content or altered carotenoid profile as part of the breeding goals. A recent review comparing current content of the five carotenoids listed in Table 18.1, as well as total carotenoid content, revealed that for all crops surveyed, the upper range of genetic variation in carotenoid content was much higher, often several-fold, than the current average content of those carotenoids found in the US marketplace [4]. This indicates substantial room for genetic improvement of carotenoid content in horticultural crops. Given the fact that genetic variation for higher carotenoid content is usually discernable with the naked eye, visual evaluation and selection for darker orange, red, or yellow color among breeding stocks has been successful for crops like carrot, pepper, tomato, sweet potato, squash, melons, mangoes, and apricots. Consequently, breeding for higher carotenoid content is relatively straightforward. To get a sense of the impact breeding for high carotenoid would have in increasing the delivery of provitamin A carotenoids to consumers, Table 18.2 presents estimates of the number of adult males able to obtain their required dietary vitamin A from five vegetables and four fruits, based upon current carotenoid content for the US crop, the Institute of Medicine's conversion factor of 12 μg β-carotene equivalents to 1 μg retinol activity equivalents, and the recommended dietary allowance of 900 μg/day for an adult male [12]. While horticultural crops are already a significant source of vitamin A, breeding could increase their provitamin A carotenoid content by 1.5- to 10-fold [4].

It should be noted that breeding for higher carotenoid content in horticultural crops that typically contain carotenoids, like carrots, tomatoes, or mangoes, may result in nutritionally enriched cultivars that are not known to consumers to be any different than less nutritious cultivars. Breeding for higher carotenoid content in crops that are typically not known by consumers as containing carotenoids, like cauliflower or cucumbers, often requires some level of consumer education to assure them that the unusual color is safe and healthy. The issue of consumer acceptance has met with resistance or confusion in some cases where colorless or low-carotenoid containing forms of the crop are familiar and preferred in certain regions of the world (e.g., white vs. orange sweet potatoes). In other cases, breeding for different carotenoids than what consumers expect can also lead to reduced acceptance. For example, orange high β-carotene tomatoes and red high lycopene carrots. Similar consumer acceptance issues can, of course, also arise with high-carotene versions of staple crops like orange biofortified maize and "golden rice" (see Chap. 17).

Table 18.2 Productivity and potential provitamin A delivery of selected horticultural crops based on US cultivars to men based on the daily recommended intake of 900 μg retinol activity equivalents (RAE)

						Number of 900 μg RAE servings	
	Marketable yield of less-developed countries (FAO.stat) (total yield minus refuse)	Current crop content (per http://www.nal.usda.gov/fnic/foodcomp/search/)				Per kg crop	Per hectare crop (less-developed world yield)
Crop	(kg/ha)	β-carotene mg/kg	α-carotene mg/kg	β-cryptoxanthin mg/kg	μg RAE/kg		
Carrot	5,950	83	35	0	8,350	9.3	55,200
Tomato	8,680	4.5	1	0	420	0.5	4,050
Cantaloupe	7,600	20	0.16	0	1,690	1.9	14,300
Sweet potato	3,240	85	0.7	0	7,090	7.9	25,500
Spinach	3,900	56	0	0	4,690	5.2	20,300
Mango	3,370	6.4	0.1	0.1	540	0.6	2,020
Orange	5,320	0.9	0.1	1.2	120	0.13	709
Banana	3,830	0.26	0.25	0	30	0.03	128

On the topic of consumer acceptance, it is worth noting that even if consumers of horticultural crops with higher carotenoid content are willing to accept an unfamiliar color, they rarely will purchase and consume produce based upon nutritional value alone. Decisions to purchase and consume horticultural crops depend much more on price, size, shape, and especially flavor. While breeding for improved carotenoid content or profile is a worthy, and often achievable goal, growers rarely, if ever, appreciate any added value for enhanced nutritional value. All the other variables that growers and consumers take into consideration in making their decisions need to be as good or better than typical cultivars in local markets if nutritional improvements in the crop are to be realized as a healthier consumer.

Provitamin A Carotenoid Biofortification Research for Horticultural Crops

Research into the accumulation of provitamin A carotenoid pigments in horticultural crops has proven to be complex. The mechanism of carotenoid accumulation in a variety of plant tissues has been difficult to identify, as plant species accumulate these pigments in different organs, with a diverse array of methods for regulation. Much of the previously published research has focused on those plants that regulate the accumulation of carotenoids within the carotenoid biosynthetic pathway itself. For example, both the *y1* gene in corn (maize) [13] and *r* in tomato [14] are mutations in the gene phytoene synthase (PSY), the first determinant step in the carotenoid biosynthetic pathway. While the regulation of carotenoid accumulation may be found within the pathway for some horticultural crops, research has demonstrated that this may not always be the case.

Carotenoid pigments accumulate in chromoplasts, storage organelles differentiated from the plastid precursor proplastids. Found in flower petals, tomato fruits, and carrot storage roots, for example, these organelles serve as a sink for carotenoids to accumulate within the plant cell. If the regulation of carotenoid pigments is controlled at the level of chromoplast development, this sink can develop and provitamin A carotenoids can accumulate. Chromoplast-associated regulation of carotenoid accumulation has been demonstrated in cauliflower where the *Or* gene encodes a cysteine-rich domain containing protein that causes the accumulation of β-carotene in the curd tissue of this otherwise white plant organ, and also causes accumulation in the pith, leaf bases, and shoot meristems. This mutation does not impact carotenoid pigmentation of leaves, or cauliflower flower petals. The *Or* gene, and the discovery of the regulation of carotenoid accumulation not associated with the carotenoid biosynthesis pathway, has proven to be a useful resource in the biofortification of other horticultural crops [15–17].

Lessons learned from the study of the regulation and accumulation of carotenoid biosynthesis have provided information for increasing the amount of provitamin A carotenoids in a variety of plant species. The *Or* gene serves as an example of the complexity of this system, and the possibility that the regulation of carotenoid accumulation in other horticultural crops lies outside of the carotenoid biosynthetic pathway. Pinpointing the key regulatory steps of carotenoid pigment accumulation in other important horticultural crops such as carrot has proven to be difficult, but these new insights into the biology of carotenogenesis will be essential for furthering research into non-model plant species and the development of high carotene varieties.

Biofortification of Ketocarotenoids in Horticultural Crops

Ketocarotenoids are xanthophylls that are powerful antioxidants found in animals such as salmon, trout, krill, shrimp, and other crustaceans, and feathers in birds like the flamingo. While animals cannot produce ketocarotenoids endogenously, the consumption of these antioxidants in animal feed produces a pink pigmentation in these species. The production of ketocarotenoids in higher plants is rare, but has been found in the flower petals of species of the genus *Adonis* [18]. Because of the rarity of this carotenoid in horticultural crops, the development of food sources high in these carotenoids is of interest. While not a provitamin A carotenoid, astaxanthin is an important antioxidant and is used as a food supplement. Research into the regulation and manipulation of the carotenoid biosynthetic pathway has aided in the efforts to use biofortification in increasing the amounts of this important carotenoid in plants.

Ketocarotenoid biofortification of specific vegetable crops has been successful through transgenic means, as has been demonstrated in potato and carrot. For example, in the potato tuber, both the low carotenoid *Solanum tuberosum* cultivar "Desiree" and the *Solanum phureja* cultivar "Mayan Gold", which is a yellow-fleshed cultivar that already produces carotenoid pigments, were transformed with a β-carotene ketolase gene from algae. With the successful transformation of this gene into both of these cultivars, the amount of the ketocarotenoids astaxanthin and ketolutein was 14 μg/g dry weight in the transgenic *S. phureja* line, a significant increase in the total amount of ketocarotenoid accumulation [19]. In carrot, the successful transformation of the β-carotene ketolase gene to petiole explants of High Carotene Mass carrots, a USDA carrot inbred line with high levels of carotenes in the storage root, has been suggested as a possible candidate for the commercial production of ketocarotenoids. In the transgenic carrot lines, ketocarotenoids comprised approximately 70% of the total amount of carotenoids in the plant, representing an accumulation of up to 2,400 μg/g root dry weight [20]. The development of these transgenic horticultural crops could be important in increasing the amount of these ketocarotenoid pigments in the human diet, providing a new source for the healthful benefits found in the consumption of carotenoids.

International Biofortification Programs to Improve Provitamin A Carotenoids in Horticultural Crops

The provitamin A carotenoid content found in many of the previously discussed horticultural crops is high, and the availability of these food sources makes the prevalence of vitamin A micronutrient malnutrition much lower in the developed world. Research in production, post-harvest physiology, and increased carotenoid pigment content has certainly made gains in crops that have already been established as good sources of carotenoids. Alternatively, for many horticultural crops important to the developing world, significant efforts are needed and being implemented to increase provitamin A carotenoid content and/or crop productivity to reduce the likelihood of vitamin A deficiency [21]. Collaborative international research projects involving many agricultural scientists and nutritionists have focused their attention on the improvement of provitamin A carotenoid content in a variety of horticultural crops.

Cassava is a staple horticultural crop in many tropical and subtropical regions. According to the FAO in 2008 [22], this storage root is the third most important source of calories in the tropics. Unfortunately, the cassava root is void of many essential nutrients, including provitamin A carotenoids [23]. The enhancement of provitamin A carotenoids in cassava has been the focus of many research programs. BioCassava Plus [24] is an international research project addressing the issue of cassava root improvement for use in sub-Saharan Africa. Along with the Donald Danforth Plant Science Center in St. Louis, Missouri, this group is comprised of scientists from nine public research institutions. Partnering with researchers in Kenya and Nigeria, BioCassava Plus focuses on delivering biofortified cassava varieties that will serve the needs of people throughout Africa. Examples of the improvements made by this research consortium include varieties with significantly increased levels of protein and iron. Along with increasing the levels of these important nutritional components, the BioCassava Plus research group has successfully increased the amount of β-carotene in the cassava root by 30-fold, and this β-carotene is bioavailable according to nutritional studies [25]. Other areas of interest to this international research group are the food safety and environmental impacts these cassava varieties have in the African nations in which they are grown. BioCassava Plus has used biofortification techniques to increase several important nutritional compounds in cassava root [24].

HarvestPlus is another influential international research group working toward improving the provitamin A carotenoid content in horticultural crops throughout the world. An initiative of the Consultative Group for International Agricultural Research (CGIAR), HarvestPlus received the first funding for biofortification through the Bill and Melinda Gates Foundation. The project focuses on increasing the content of iron, zinc, and provitamin A in a variety of crops. These three nutrients were identified by the WHO as being the most limiting in the human diet for optimal health. This international group also partners with the International Center for Tropical Agriculture (CIAT) and the International Food Policy Research Institute (IFPRI).

Like BioCassava Plus, HarvestPlus has focused on breeding and development of cassava varieties with increased levels of provitamin A carotenoids. Setting the initial breeding goal of increasing carotenoid content to 15 μg/g fresh cassava root, HarvestPlus has used the variation already found in cassava germplasm toward breeding high carotenoid cassava roots, and uses modern breeding techniques such as molecular markers. Cassava varieties developed by HarvestPlus will be targeted for Democratic Republic of Congo and Nigeria, but more than a dozen countries in Africa may be receiving these biofortified provitamin A cassava varieties [26].

HarvestPlus has also focused on increasing the provitamin A carotenoid content of orange-fleshed sweet potato for regions throughout Africa. In collaboration with the International Food Policy Research Institute and the International Potato Center, HarvestPlus initially focused on releasing improved varieties in Uganda and Mozambique. An initial breeding goal in the development of sweet potato varieties was set at 32 μg provitamin A/g raw sweet potato. Already existing international sweet potato germplasm was found to be sufficient to meet this goal. Varieties with increased levels of carotenoid pigments were released in 2007, with a dozen countries receiving the improved varieties [27].

In addition to these projects improving the nutritional value of horticultural crops, USAID has initiated a Horticulture Collaborative Research Support Group to fund projects on post-harvest practices, seed systems, orange-fleshed sweet potatoes, and African indigenous vegetables that include evaluation of nutritional value as an objective. For example, nutritional studies that evaluate potential differences among similar vegetables, such as leafy greens, are important at both a basic science [10, 28] and applied community setting for dietary promotion [29].

Conclusions and Future Prospects

Horticultural crops have been the richest source of dietary carotenoids globally, and vitamin A, in the form of provitamin A carotenoids, in the developing world. New sources of provitamin A carotenoids are being developed in staple crops, but the prominent role of horticultural crops in maintaining vitamin A health will likely continue. Prospects for improving the carotenoid content and profile in horticultural crops are excellent, but improved nutritional value cannot be expected to bring added value to growers. Improved nutritional quality must be combined with improvements in crop productivity, post-harvest storability, and flavor if nutritional improvements are expected to be realized by consumers. To achieve this end, more horticultural crop production and marketing expertise must be available to farmers, especially in the developing world, given the challenges of growing horticultural crops and delivering them to market. Production trials for growers and basic nutrition education for consumers can improve the deployment of existing horticultural crops rich in carotenoids, and build a framework for more nutritious cultivars under development. The AVRDC, international agriculture research centers, and other programs are addressing some of the issues related to horticultural crop breeding, production, storage, marketing, and consumer education, but their resources are currently inadequate to include many crops that could provide provitamin A carotenoids in regions with vitamin A deficiency.

References

1. 2010 Agricultural statistics. http://nass.usda.gov/Publications/Ag_Statistics/. Accessed 28 July 2011.
2. FAOSTAT. http://faostat.fao.org/. Accessed 28 July 2011.
3. Raper N, Ingwersen L, Steinfeld L, Anand J. An overview of the USDA's Dietary Intake Data System. J Food Compost Anal. 2004;17:545–55.
4. Simon PW, Pollak LM, Clevidence BA, Holden JM, Haytowitz DB. Plant breeding for human nutrition. Plant Breed Rev. 2009;31:325–92.
5. Simpson KL. Relative value of the carotenoids as precursors of vitamin A. Proc Nutr Soc. 1983;42:7–17.
6. FAO-WHO. Human vitamin and mineral requirements. Report of a joint FAO/WHO expert consultation, FAO Rome. 2001.
7. Simon PW, Wolff XY. Carotenes in typical and dark orange carrots. J Agric Food Chem. 1987;35:1017–22.
8. Simon PW. Genetic improvement of vegetable carotene content. In: Bills DD, Kung S-D, editors. Biotechnology and nutrition. Proc. Third Internatl. Symposium Biotech and Nutrition. Boston, MA: Butterworth-Heinemann; 1992. p. 291–300.
9. Simon PW. Carrots and other horticultural crops as a source of provitamin A carotenes. Hortic Sci. 1990;25:1495–9.
10. Djuikwo VN, Ejoh RA, Gouado I, Mbofung CM, Tanumihardjo SA. Determination of major carotenoids in processed tropical leafy vegetables indigenous to Africa. Food Nutr Sci. 2011;2:793–802.
11. Tarwotjo IA, Sommer A, Soegihartjo T, Susanto D, Mulihal. Dietary practices and xerophthalmia among Indonesian children. Am J Clin Nutr. 1982;35:575–81.
12. Institute of Medicine. Dietary reference intakes for vitamin A, vitamin K, arsenic, boron, chromium, copper, iodine, iron, manganese, molybdenum, nickel, silicon, vanadium, and zinc. Washington, DC: National Academy Press; 2001. p. 65–126.
13. Buckner B, San Miguel P, Janick-Buckner D, Bennetzen JL. The *yl* gene of maize codes for phytoene synthase. Genetics. 1996;143:479–88.
14. Fray RJ, Grierson D. Identification and genetic analysis of normal and mutant phytoene synthase genes of tomato by sequencing, complementation and co-suppression. Plant Mol Biol. 1993;22:589–602.
15. Li L, Paolillo DJ, Parthasarathy MV, DiMuzio EM, Garvin DF. A novel gene mutation that confers abnormal patterns of beta-carotene accumulation in cauliflower (*Brassica oleracea* var. *botrytis*). Plant J. 2001;26:59–67.
16. Lu S, Van Eck J, Zhou X, Lopez AB, O'Halloran DM, Cosman KM, Conlin BJ, Paolillo DJ, Garvin DF, Vrebalov J, Kochian LV, Kupper H, Earle ED, Cao J, Li L. The cauliflower Or gene encodes a DnJ cysteine-rich domain containing protein that mediates high levels of beta carotene accumulation. Plant Cell. 2006;18:3594–605.

17. Li L, Van Eck J. Metabolic engineering of carotenoid accumulation by creating a metabolic sink. Transgenic Res. 2007;16:581–5.
18. Cunningham FX, Gantt E. A study in scarlet: enzymes of ketocarotenoid biosynthesis in the flowers of *Adonis aestivalis*. Plant J. 2005;41:478–92.
19. Morris WL, Ducreux LJM, Fraser PD, Millam S, Taylor MA. Engineering ketocarotenoid biosynthesis in potato roots. Metab Eng. 2006;8:253–63.
20. Jayaraj J, Devlin R, Punja Z. Metabolic engineering of novel ketocarotenoid production in carrot plants. Transgenic Res. 2008;17:489–501.
21. Tanumihardjo SA, Palacios N, Pixley KV. Provitamin A carotenoid bioavailability: what really matters? Int J Vitam Nutr Res. 2010;80:336–50.
22. FAO. Why cassava? 2008. http://www.fao.org/ag/agp/agpc/gcds/. Accessed 28 July 2011.
23. Montagnac JA, Davis CR, Tanumihardjo SA. The nutritional value of cassava for use as a staple food and recent advances for improvement. Compr Rev Food Sci Food Saf. 2009;8:181–94.
24. BioCassava Plus. http://www.danforthcenter.org/science/programs/INTERNATIONAL_PROGRAMS/BCP/default.as. Accessed 28 July 2011.
25. Howe JA, Maziya-Dixon B, Tanumihardjo SA. Cassava with enhanced β-carotene maintains adequate vitamin A status in Mongolian gerbils (*Meriones unguiculatus*) despite substantial *cis*-isomer content. Br J Nutr. 2009; 102:342–9.
26. Cassava. http://www.harvestplus.org/content/cassava. Accessed 28 July 2011.
27. Sweet potato. http://www.harvestplus.org/content/sweet-potato. Accessed 28 July 2011.
28. Ejoh RA, Dever JT, Mills JP, Tanumihardjo SA. Small quantities of carotenoid-rich tropical green leafy-vegetables indigenous to Africa maintain vitamin A status in Mongolian gerbils (*Meriones unguiculatus*). Br J Nutr. 2010;103:1594–601.
29. Tchum SK, Newton S, Tanumihardjo SA, Arthur FKN, Tetteh A, Owusu-Agyei S. Evaluation of a green leafy vegetable intervention in Ghanaian postpartum mothers. Afr J Food Agric Nutr Dev. 2009;9:1294–308.

Chapter 19
Orange Sweetpotato as a Staple or Complementary Food

Paul van Jaarsveld and Mieke Faber

Key Points

- Conventionally bred orange sweetpotato varieties with high β-carotene content accepted by consumers and small-scale rural African farmers are available.
- Efficacy and effectiveness studies proved that orange sweetpotato offers a complementary source of vitamin A to rural sweetpotato-producing communities to improve vitamin A intakes.
- A large variation in β-carotene content in sweetpotato varieties occurs and the amount needed to provide the dietary requirement of vitamin A varies substantially. For example, for South African varieties, between 25 and 265 g boiled yellow to orange sweetpotato will provide 100 % of the vitamin A dietary requirement for all age groups.
- Because considerable amounts of β-carotene are retained in boiled sweetpotato, the high β-carotene orange varieties can be eaten as a staple, vegetable, or in processed products.
- Orange sweetpotato processed products can make a significant contribution toward sustaining an increased vitamin A intake provided that high β-carotene varieties are used, orange sweetpotato comprise a considerable proportion as an ingredient, and optimal processing methods are used.
- Fat, salt, and sugar should be used sparingly in processed products to not exacerbate the increasing problem of chronic diseases.
- Vitamin A deficiency does not occur in isolation. Hence, the promotion of orange sweetpotato needs to be part of a more holistic dietary approach to address vitamin A deficiency and improve overall diet quality.

Keywords Orange sweetpotato • β-Carotene • Vitamin A status • β-Carotene retention • Processing

P. van Jaarsveld (✉) • M. Faber
Nutritional Intervention Research Unit, Medical Research Council of South Africa,
Francie van Zijl Drive, Parow Valley 7500, Cape Town, Western Cape Province, South Africa
email: paul.van.jaarsveld@mrc.ac.za; mieke.faber@mrc.ac.za

S.A. Tanumihardjo (ed.), *Carotenoids and Human Health*, Nutrition and Health,
DOI 10.1007/978-1-62703-203-2_19, © Springer Science+Business Media New York 2013

Background

Vitamin A Deficiency in Developing Countries

Globally 190 million (33.3 %) children under the age of 5 years are vitamin A deficient, with Southeast Asia and Africa having the highest prevalences at 49.9 % and 44.4 %, respectively [1]. Vitamin A is essential for maintaining eye health and normal functioning of the immune system as discussed in Chap. 16. Children who are vitamin A deficient have a lower resistance against common childhood infections such as respiratory and diarrhoeal diseases, measles, and malaria [2].

It is commonly believed that the major cause of the high rate of vitamin A deficiency in lower income countries is a chronic inadequate intake of vitamin A through the diet with poverty being the underlying factor for this inadequacy [1]. Healthier food choices are generally more expensive than the more commonly consumed foods [3]. Resource poor populations from the developing world usually consume monotonous diets that are predominantly based on starchy staples and often include little or no animal products and few vegetables and fruit. Foods of animal origin, the best dietary source of bioavailable preformed vitamin A, are often not within the financial reach of the poor. Yellow/orange-fleshed vegetables and fruit, as well as dark-green leafy vegetables, are inherently rich in provitamin A carotenoids (predominantly β-carotene), which achieve vitamin A activity when they are converted to retinol in the body. In South Africa, where vitamin A-rich vegetables and fruit are the least consumed foods [4], affordability and to a lesser extent availability have been identified as the major constraints for their consumption [5].

Strategies to Address Vitamin A Deficiency

There is no single strategy that will on its own eliminate vitamin A deficiency. An integrated approach, combining different complementary strategies supported by relevant public health measures for the prevention and control of infectious diseases should be used as discussed in Chap. 20. The orange sweetpotato is featured in both the biofortification and dietary diversification strategies (see Table 19.1).

Orange Sweetpotato

Potential Effect of Orange Sweetpotato to Address Vitamin A Deficiency

β-Carotene Content

Sweetpotato has a large genetic diversity of flesh color and β-carotene content. Whereas the white/cream-fleshed varieties that are generally grown and consumed in Africa contain virtually no β-carotene, the orange-fleshed varieties contain significant amounts of β-carotene. The intensity of the orange color generally reflects the amount of β-carotene in the sweetpotato [10, 11]. A joint biofortification program between several African countries introduced several conventionally bred, β-carotene-rich, orange-fleshed varieties since the late 1990s [12]. Biofortification, as discussed in Chap. 17, refers to the process of increasing the micronutrient content in staple foods through plant breeding. The mean β-carotene content in sweetpotato varieties varies from insignificant to large amounts, with a range of

Table 19.1 Strategies to address vitamin A deficiency [1, 6–9]

Supplementation	Periodic distribution of high-dose vitamin A supplements to: (1) All children of defined age (and other designated groups) within communities in specified regions according to a pre-established time schedule (blanket supplementation) (2) High-risk individuals through the existing health service infrastructure and/or community-based health programs (targeted supplementation)
Food fortification	Addition of vitamin A or β-carotene to accessible and affordable staple foods or condiments that are regularly consumed in constant amounts by a significant proportion of the target population
Biofortification	Breeding staple crops for increased provitamin A carotenoid content
Dietary diversification	(1) Increasing production, availability, and access to vitamin A-rich foods through horticultural approaches such as home-gardens (2) Increasing the consumption of vitamin A-rich foods through behavior change achieved through communications, social marketing, or nutrition education (3) Increasing the bioavailability of vitamin A in the diet through optimal preparation, preservation, and cooking methods to maximize the vitamin A and provitamin A carotenoid retention and utilization
Public health measures for the prevention and control of infectious diseases	Promoting breastfeeding Using oral rehydration therapy in the treatment of diarrhea Measles vaccination Hygiene and sanitation

10–28,100 μg/100 g fresh weight (FW) [11, 13–21]. When sweetpotato is used in food-based interventions to address vitamin A deficiency, a target breeding level of 7,500 μg β-carotene/100 g FW has been proposed for populations where sweetpotato is the sole source of β-carotene, and 3,700 μg β-carotene/100 g FW if a mixed diet is eaten [22].

Efficacy and Effectiveness

Orange sweetpotato naturally rich in β-carotene positively impacts vitamin A status. In adult Bangladeshi men, daily consumption of 160 g canned sweetpotato that was puréed and sautéed in corn oil, which provided 375 μg retinol activity equivalents (RAE)/day, had a positive effect on total body vitamin A stores. The vitamin A equivalency factor (μg β-carotene:μg retinol) was estimated as 13:1 [23], which is similar to 12:1 proposed by the Institute of Medicine for all-*trans*-β-carotene in mixed food eaten by healthy people in developed countries [24]. In a randomized controlled study, consumption of supplemental meals with β-carotene-rich red sweetpotato (prepared boiled, fried, or boiled and blended with wheat flour) providing 750 μg retinol equivalents (RE) (approximately 375 μg RAE), increased serum retinol concentrations at 21 days in 3–6 year old Indonesian children [25]. In a randomized controlled efficacy trial among 5–10 year old South African children, consumption of 125 g boiled and mashed orange sweetpotato providing 1,031 μg RAE/day for 53 days increased vitamin A liver stores [26].

A 2-year quasi-experimental effectiveness study that included an integrated package of agriculture, nutrition, and market interventions promoting orange sweetpotato in rural communities in Mozambique was successful at increasing consumption of orange sweetpotato among children (mean age 35 months at follow-up), which reduced the prevalence of low serum retinol. The median intake of 314 g orange sweetpotato/day by children as determined with dietary recall provided 90 % (approximately 380 μg RAE/day) of their vitamin A intake [27]. Between 2006 and 2009, Hotz et al. [21] conducted a randomized, controlled effectiveness study of an intervention in rural Mozambique to promote household-level orange sweetpotato production and consumption using integrated agricultural, demand creation/behavior change, and marketing components, comparing a low intensity (1 year; Model 1) and a high intensity (nearly 3 years; Model 2) training model. This large-scale intervention reached 10,800 direct beneficiaries from 12,000 farm households, compared to 1,094 direct beneficiaries in 53 farmer groups in the Low et al. [27] study. The primary nutrition outcomes were orange sweetpotato and vitamin A intakes by children 6–35 months and 3–5.5 years of age and women. Model 1 resulted in significant net increases in orange sweetpotato intakes of 46, 48, and 97 g/day (263, 254, and 492 μg RAE/day) among the younger children, older children, and women, respectively. Among the intervention children, orange sweetpotato provided 80 % of total vitamin A intakes. Dietary intakes of orange sweetpotato and vitamin A were similar for both models suggesting that group-level trainings in nutrition and agriculture could be limited to the first project year without compromising impact. These studies showed that the introduction of orange sweetpotato offers a complementary source of vitamin A to rural, sweetpotato-producing communities in Mozambique and other sweetpotato-producing communities in Africa. Overall, evidence shows that consumption of orange sweetpotato is an effective way to improve vitamin A intakes.

Fat in the Meal

Bioavailability and absorption of carotenoids in plant foods will improve if fat [25] or foods with fat content, e.g., avocado fruit [28], are added to the meal. Between 3 g [25] and 5 g [29] of fat per meal is required to ensure carotenoid absorption. Interventions promoting consumption of orange sweetpotato to improve vitamin A status of at-risk populations must therefore incorporate recommendations to add this minimum amount of fat to the meal containing orange sweetpotato.

Contribution of Sweetpotato to Dietary Vitamin A Requirements

The average portion sizes of boiled orange sweetpotato needed to provide the dietary requirements for different gender and age groups are given in Table 19.2. Three different portion sizes are given for boiled sweetpotato with dark-orange, orange, and pale-orange to yellow-orange flesh color. Based on South African sweetpotato varieties and the large variation in β-carotene content, the amount of cooked sweetpotato consumed needs to vary to provide the dietary requirement of vitamin A.

An additional benefit of orange sweetpotato is its high carbohydrate content making it a good source of energy [31]. Maternal and child undernutrition, including chronic energy deficiency, is highly prevalent in low- and middle-income countries [32]. The energy content of sweetpotato is thus highly beneficial in these at-risk populations. Considerable proportions of the rural population obtain much of their energy needs from staple foods; growing sweetpotato is therefore an important strategy for poor rural households that have limited access to fortified staple foods [12]. Also, the soft texture makes it suitable for infant feeding, as well as for the elderly and the ill.

Sensory Traits and Consumer Acceptance of Orange Sweetpotato

In areas where traditionally white/cream-fleshed sweetpotato is consumed, the success in reducing vitamin A deficiency by introducing orange varieties through food-based interventions will depend on consumer acceptance in terms of taste and other sensory characteristics. Studies in South Africa showed that cream and orange varieties differ in texture and flavor [20, 33, 34]. Cream varieties had a sweetpotato flavor and generally were lower in graininess. Orange varieties were sweeter, had higher

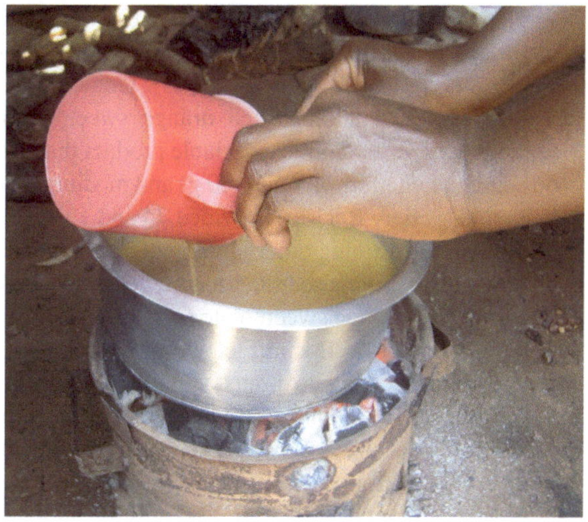

Fig. 19.1 Woman cooking orange sweetpotato-based porridge (photo with courtesy from Aurélie Bechoff)

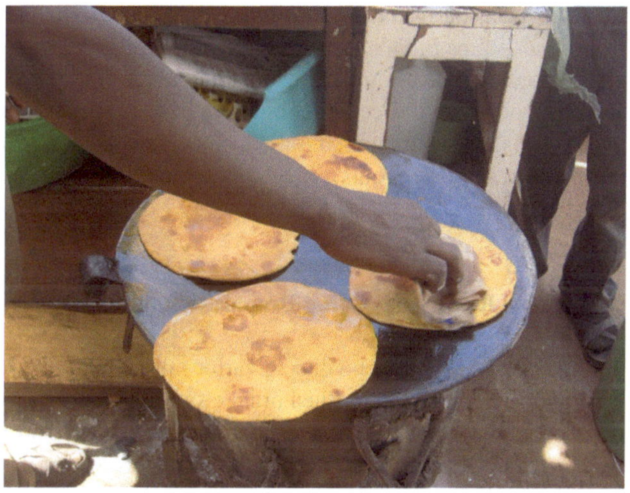

Fig. 19.2 Street vendor preparing orange sweetpotato-based chapattis (photo with courtesy from Aurélie Bechoff)

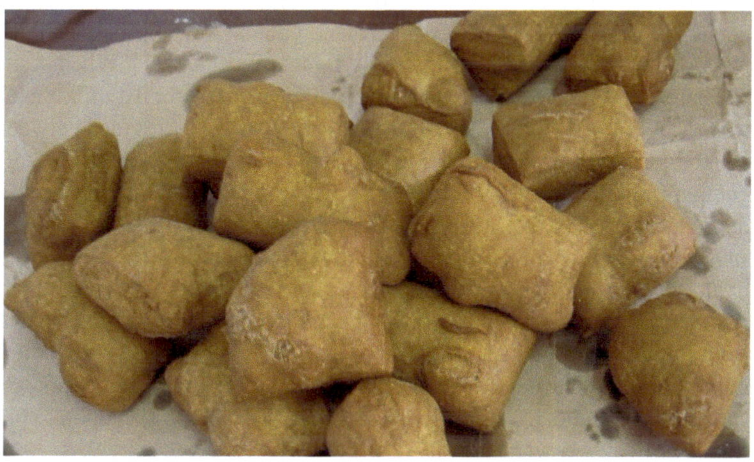

Fig. 19.3 Orange sweetpotato-based Mandazis (photo with courtesy from Aurélie Bechoff)

example, part of the wheat flour can be substituted with boiled and mashed orange sweetpotato, but it is important to use the β-carotene-rich dark-orange varieties to ensure that the baked bread provides adequate amounts of provitamin A [45]. Golden bread made by replacing 38 % of wheat flour by weight with boiled and mashed orange sweetpotato in recipes used by rural bakers in Central Mozambique is an economically viable product that has enough β-carotene content to be regarded as a good source of vitamin A. Small (60 g) and medium-sized (110 g) golden bread buns containing orange sweetpotato (variety Resisto) provided 74 and 136 μg RAE, respectively [45].

In Kenya, substituting other ingredients with orange sweetpotato in mandazis, chapattis, and bread buns dramatically increased the β-carotene content, and these products were popular among consumers. Substituting orange sweetpotato for wheat flour in mandazis made the product more profitable for market vendors [14]. Bechoff et al. [46] measured the all-*trans*-β-carotene content of chapatti (wheat:orange sweetpotato flours; 70:30; Fig. 19.2), mandazi (same ingredients as chapatti, deep-fried in oil; Fig. 19.3), and porridge (maize:soybean:orange sweetpotato flours; 30:35:35; Fig. 19.1) produced by local processors in Uganda using blended flours containing the Ejumula variety. The vitamin A values from these orange sweetpotato-based products were 232 μg RAE/300 g porridge, 273 μg RAE/100 g chapatti, and 290 μg RAE/90 g mandazis, making a considerable contribution to vitamin A intakes.

Sun-drying is a cheap and accessible method to preserve food and is used for storing sweetpotato roots. Products derived from sun-drying of roots in Uganda include *Atapa* (sweetpotato flour, derived from *Amukeke* or *Inginyo*, mixed with either millet or cassava flour, re-hydrated with boiling water and cooked over heat into a brown edible bread-like paste), *Amukeke* (roots are dried in the sun for 1–2 days, peeled and sliced into thin horizontal strips, and sun-dried), *Otere* (made from dried sweetpotato chips, which are boiled, salted, and either eaten in that form or mashed), *Inginyo* (chunks from crushed and sun-dried roots), *Kwon* (sweetpotato flour is mixed with millet/sorghum flour and added to boiling water), and flour [37].

β-Carotene Retention During Preparation and Processing

The retention of β-carotene during various processing methods has been reported. True retention of β-carotene in boiled and mashed orange sweetpotato (variety Resisto) using different cooking conditions ranged from 83 to 92 % for medium-sized roots and from 70 to 81 % when roots of different sizes were boiled together (all sweetpotatoes were from the same harvest batch). The best retention was obtained when the sweetpotato was boiled intact, covered with water using the pot lid, and cooked for the shortest possible time [19].

The effect of boiling, steaming, deep-frying, and drying on β-carotene retention in orange sweetpotato varieties (with all-*trans*-β-carotene content varying between 108 and 315 μg/g dry matter) released in Uganda was investigated by Bengtsson et al. [11]. When orange sweetpotato was boiled in water for 20 min, steamed for 30 min, and deep-fried for 10 min, the all-*trans*-β-carotene retention was 78 %, 77 %, and 78 %, respectively. These varieties provided between 243 and 627 μg RAE/100 g cooked portion. Oven-drying, solar-drying, and open-air sun-drying of 1–2 mm thick slices of the popular Ejumula orange sweetpotato variety (typically containing about 300 μg all-*trans*-β-carotene/g dry matter) resulted in all-*trans*-β-carotene retention of 88 %, 91 %, and 84 %, respectively, showing substantial amounts of β-carotene remaining in the dried slices. Bechoff et al. [47] confirmed the relatively low loss of all-*trans*-β-carotene using three different drying treatments for sweetpotato chips (i.e., hot air cross flow drying, 16 %; greenhouse solar-drying, 23 %; and open-air sun-drying, 34 %). Both Bengtsson et al. [11] and Bechoff et al. [47] reported favorable retention during rapid sun-drying under hot, dry, and windy weather conditions. Sun-dried crimped slices retained more all-*trans*-β-carotene than sun-dried chips, indicating that the shape of sweetpotato pieces affects carotenoid retention [47].

It is important to assess whether technologies that were evaluated under strictly controlled research conditions can be successfully transferred to on-farm situations where the farmers monitor the drying and storage of their crops. In Mozambique, on-farm evaluation using three locally built dryers (i.e., tunnel dryer, open-air sun dryer, and open-air shade dryer) and local storage conditions (traditional bags hung in a mud-house) on the total carotenoid content was assessed. Thin and thick chips and traditional slices of two orange sweetpotato varieties (i.e., MGCL01 with 35 % dry matter content and 236 μg carotenoids/g dry matter and Resisto with 27 % dry matter content and 434 μg carotenoids/g dry matter) were used [48]. The type of dryer, thickness of the chip/slice, and sweetpotato variety affected carotenoid loss. The open-air shade dryer resulted in the least amount of caroteniod loss (1.9 %) compared with the tunnel (13 %) and open-air sun dryers (10 %). The shade dryer worked well for thin chips, but hand-cut slices needed a longer drying time, which led to unacceptable off-odors. Thin chips and slices had similar carotenoid losses after drying, 11 % and 9 %, respectively, while drying thick chips resulted in a 15 % loss. On average, carotenoid loss after drying was higher in the Resisto variety (13.2 %) than the MGCL01 variety (5 %). During storage, further carotenoid losses in the dried sweetpotato chips/slices occurred over a 4-month period. After 1, 2, and 4 months of storage, the Resisto variety had total carotenoid losses of 27 %, 48 %, and 79 %, respectively, and the MGCL01 variety 39 %, 63 %, and 88 %, respectively. Although carotenoid loss during storage differed significantly between the two varieties, the loss of total carotenoids was similar for thin and thick chips and slices within a variety. Taking into account the quality of the product (particularly insect damage to Resisto chips) and nutritional value, Bechoff et al. [48] concluded that storage of dried chips should not exceed 3 months for Resisto and not more than 2 months for MGCL01.

The β-carotene content of products, such as mandazis, chapattis, and bread buns, can be increased by substituting other ingredients with orange sweetpotato. In two ready-to-eat products produced by local processors in Uganda using blended flours containing the Ejumula variety, e.g., chapatti (wheat:orange sweetpotato flours; 70:30) and porridge (maize:soybean:orange sweetpotato flours; 30:35:35) the average all-*trans*-β-carotene retention was 83 % (containing 3,010 μg/100 g chapatti) and 77 % (containing 698 μg/100 g porridge), respectively [46].

Year-Round Availability and Access of Orange Sweetpotato for Household Consumption

Production of orange sweetpotato is affected by climatic and seasonal patterns. In countries with two rainy seasons (e.g., Rwanda, Burundi, and Uganda), sweetpotato is available 11 months a year [12]. In most other sub-Saharan African countries, sweetpotato has one dominant growing season and is available for 4–8 months a year, depending on whether households can access lowland areas with sufficient moisture to sustain a dry season crop and on the maturity period of available varieties. Planting orange sweetpotato together with a variety of both warm-weather (e.g., butternut squash and pumpkin) and cool-weather β-carotene-rich food crops (e.g., carrot and spinach) will ensure year-round availability of β-carotene-rich vegetables for household consumption [49]. From an agronomic point of view, planting a variety of vegetables will help to maintain soil health, and protect against plant pests and diseases, especially soil-borne diseases [50], thereby reducing the risk of crop failure. Seasonal availability of orange sweetpotato can also be extended by manipulating agricultural practices such as using various planting and harvesting dates, plant spacing, and soil storage [51]. Staggered planting at different time points during the season prevents the roots from maturing at the same time prolonging sweetpotato availability [12].

Freshly harvested orange sweetpotato of the Resisto variety can be stored at room temperature for a maximum of approximately 12 weeks [52]. After maturity, roots are often stored in-ground, and farmers harvest just enough roots for a single meal (piece-meal harvesting) [12]. The β-carotene content of Resisto sweetpotato is substantial after 22 weeks of in-ground storage [52]. The roots can also be stored in a simple pit structure for 12 weeks without any effect on sensory traits or consumer acceptance [36]. In-ground storage may, however, present a challenge for later consumption because of weevil attacks to the roots, especially when the soil is dry and cracked [12]. On the other hand, early maturing orange sweetpotato varieties have low in-ground storability making them particularly vulnerable to rotting and pest damage [37]. Drying fresh sweetpotato roots will further extend their use for consumption during the dry season [12, 37].

Low et al. [27] recommended market development that enables farmers to earn income from orange sweetpotato sales and for maintaining an increased demand and intake of provitamin A carotenoids. Marketing can, however, be hampered by the perishable and bulky nature of fresh sweetpotato, which limits storage and transportation [12, 53]. Using a variety of economically viable post-harvest products could enhance demand, sustainability of local production, and market possibilities [45].

Challenges

Uncured fresh sweetpotato roots are bulky and perishable with a maximum shelf-life of 12 weeks [52]. Infrastructures, such as roads, transport, and facilities, are needed for market access, to reduce transaction costs, and to provide adequate storage to minimize losses enabling households to sell surplus [54]. Bovell-Benjamin [53] argued that inadequate storage, processing, and post-harvest technologies, along with insubstantial estimates of the market demand for value-added sweetpotato-based products must be overcome for the orange sweetpotato to reach its full potential in sub-Saharan Africa. Optimal technologies should be easily accessible, culturally acceptable, affordable, and cause minimum loss of carotenoid content with no unfavorable effect on sensory characteristics of the product.

Creating a demand for orange sweetpotato-based, post-harvest products has become part of the overall strategy to combat vitamin A deficiency. Sweetpotato products that are high in fat, salt, and/or sugar should be avoided because of the escalating prevalence of overweight and obesity (a risk factor for noncommunicable diseases such as cardiovascular disease, diabetes, osteoarthritis, and certain cancers) and the co-existence of childhood undernutrition and maternal obesity within households in low- and middle-income countries [55].

The biofortification program for orange sweetpotato to alleviate vitamin A deficiency is based on the replacement of white sweetpotato (devoid of β-carotene), or at least part, with β-carotene-rich orange sweetpotato. In order for wide-spread farmer adoption, orange sweetpotato varieties should compare favorably with white/cream sweetpotato varieties in terms of agronomic (e.g., yield), consumer (e.g., taste), and economic characteristics. In addition, a significant degree of behavior change is needed to adopt new sweetpotato varieties that have a distinct visible trait (i.e., flesh with an orange color). An intensive nutrition education and promotion program is needed. Nevertheless, the orange color of the sweetpotato is not a barrier, but a very strong marketing tool for vitamin A nutrition education [27].

Strategies including orange sweetpotato to address vitamin A deficiency focus primarily on local production. Challenges experienced with gardening projects in South Africa, which are similar in other African countries, include a shortage of water for irrigation; lack of fencing, resulting in wild and domestic livestock destroying the crops; lack of funds to procure agricultural supplies; insects and plant diseases; and the lack of access to orange sweetpotato vine cuttings [56]. For the success and sustainability of initiatives promoting the production and consumption of orange sweetpotato, an improved sweetpotato vine reproduction system and easy access to a regular supply of virus-free plant cuttings at an affordable price are critical [27, 56]. These initiatives therefore often include community-based field nurseries [57], but sustainability of these nurseries remains a challenge.

Conclusions

Conventionally bred orange sweetpotato varieties with high β-carotene content are available. Efficacy and effectiveness to improve vitamin A intake and reduce vitamin A deficiency have been shown. Consumer acceptance in terms of taste and other sensory characteristics is important for consumers to adopt orange varieties. Orange sweetpotato can be eaten as a staple, vegetable, or used in processed products. Considerable amounts of β-carotene are retained in boiled sweetpotato. In processed products, retention of β-carotene depends on the method of preparation and processing. Orange sweetpotato-based post-harvest products can make a significant contribution toward sustaining an increased vitamin A intake provided that high β-carotene varieties are used, orange sweetpotato comprises a considerable proportion as an ingredient, and optimal processing methods are used. Seasonal availability of orange sweetpotato can be prolonged through manipulating agricultural practices and storage. Orange sweetpotato needs to be promoted as part of a holistic dietary approach to address vitamin A deficiency.

Future Directions

One of the remaining challenges is to strengthen the evidence base to give orange sweetpotato the visibility it deserves. Large-scale access and promoting production and consumption of orange sweetpotato to address vitamin A deficiency integrated with existing health, agricultural, and development programs will enhance sustainability and cost-effectiveness to result in national implementation.

References

1. WHO. Global prevalence of vitamin A deficiency in populations at risk 1995–2005. WHO Global Database on Vitamin A Deficiency. Geneva: World Health Organization; 2009. http://whqlibdoc.who.int/publications/2009/9789241598019_eng.pdf. Accessed 12 Dec 2011.
2. Rice AL, West Jr KP, Black RE. Vitamin A deficiency. In: Ezzati M, Lopez AD, Rodgers A, Murray CJL, editors. Comparative quantification of health risks. Global and regional burden of disease attributable to selected major risk factors. Geneva: World Health Organization; 2004.
3. Temple NJ, Steyn NP, Fourie J, De Villiers A. Price and availability of healthy food: a study in rural South Africa. Nutrition. 2011;27:55–8.
4. Labadarios D, Steyn NP, Nel J. How diverse is the diet of adult South Africans? Nutr J. 2011;10:33. doi:10.1186/1475-2891-10-33.
5. Love P, Maunder E, Green M, Ross F, Smale-Lovely J, Charlton K. South African food-based dietary guidelines. Testing of the preliminary guidelines among women in KwaZulu-Natal and the Western Cape. S Afr J Clin Nutr. 2001;14:9–19.
6. Dary O, Mora JO. Food fortification to reduce vitamin A deficiency: International Vitamin A Consultative Group recommendations. J Nutr. 2002;132:2927S–33S.
7. Bouis HE, Graham RD, Welch RM. The Consultative Group on International Agricultural Research (CGIAR) micronutrients project: justification and objectives. Food Nutr Bull. 2000;21:374–81.
8. Ruel MT. Can food-based strategies help reduce vitamin A and iron deficiencies? A review of recent evidence. Washington, DC: International Food Policy Research Institute; 2001.
9. Gillespie S, Mason J. Controlling vitamin A deficiency. ACC/SCN state-of-the-art series. ACC/SCN, Geneva; 1994. Nutrition policy discussion paper, No. 14.
10. Takahata Y, Noda T, Nagata T. HPLC determination of β-carotene content of sweet potato cultivars and its relationship with color values. Jpn J Breed. 1993;43:421–7.
11. Bengtsson A, Namutebi A, Larsson Alminger M, Svanberg U. Effects of various traditional processing methods on the all-*trans*-β-carotene content of orange-fleshed sweet potato. J Food Comp Anal. 2008;21:134–43.

12. Low J, Lynam J, Lemaga B, et al. Sweetpotato in sub-Saharan Africa. In: Lobenstein G, Thottappilly G, editors. The sweetpotato. Heidelberg, Germany: Springer Science and Business Media; 2009. p. 359–90.
13. Almeida-Muradian LB, Penteado MVC. Carotenoids and provitamin A value of some Brazilian sweet potato cultivars (*Ipomoea batatas* Lam.). Rev Farm Bioquím Univ São Paulo. 1992;28:145–54.
14. Hagenimana V, Carey EE, Gichuki ST, Oyunga MA, Imungi JK. Carotenoid contents in fresh, dried and processed sweet potato products. Ecol Food Nutr. 1999;37:455–73.
15. Huang AS, Tanudjaja L, Lum D. Content of alpha-, beta-carotene, and dietary fiber in 18 sweetpotato varieties grown in Hawaii. J Food Comp Anal. 1999;12:147–51.
16. K'osambo LM, Carey EE, Misra AK, Wilkes J, Hagenimana V. Influence of age, farming site, and boiling on provitamin A content in sweet potato (*Ipomoea batatas* (L.) Lam.) storage roots. J Food Comp Anal. 1998;11:305–21.
17. Takahata Y, Noda T, Nagata T. Varietal differences in chemical composition of the sweet potato storage root. Acta Hort. 1993;343:77–80.
18. Failla ML, Thakkar SK, Kim JY. In vitro bioaccessibility of beta-carotene in orange-fleshed sweet potato (*Ipomoea batatas*, Lam.). J Agric Food Chem. 2009;57:10922–7.
19. Van Jaarsveld PJ, Marais DeW, Harmse E, Nestel P, Rodriguez-Amaya DB. Retention of β-carotene in boiled, mashed orange-fleshed sweet potato. J Food Comp Anal. 2006;19:321–9.
20. Laurie SM. Agronomic performance, consumer acceptability and nutrient content of new sweet potato varieties in South Africa. University of the Free State, South Africa; 2010. PhD Thesis.
21. Hotz C, Loechl C, de Brauw A, et al. A large-scale intervention to introduce orange sweet potato in rural Mozambique increases vitamin A intakes among children and women. Br J Nutr. 2012;108(1):163–76.
22. Nestel P, Bouis HE, Meenakshi JV, Pfeiffer W. Biofortification of staple food crops. J Nutr. 2006;136:1064–7.
23. Haskell MJ, Jamil KM, Hassan F, et al. Daily consumption of Indian spinach (*Basella alba*) or sweet potatoes has a positive effect on total-body vitamin A stores in Bangladeshi men. Am J Clin Nutr. 2004;80:705–14.
24. Otten JJ, Hellwig JP, Meyers LD, editors. Dietary reference intakes. The essential guide to nutrient requirements. Washington, DC: The National Academic Press; 2006.
25. Jalal F, Nesheim MC, Agus Z, Sanjur D, Habicht JP. Serum retinol concentrations in children are affected by food sources of β-carotene, fat intake, and anthelmintic drug treatment. Am J Clin Nutr. 1998;68:623–9.
26. Van Jaarsveld PJ, Faber M, Tanumihardjo SA, Nestel P, Lombard CJ, Benadé AJS. β-Carotene-rich orange-fleshed sweet potato improves the vitamin A status of primary school children assessed with the modified-relative-dose-response test. Am J Clin Nutr. 2005;1:1080–7.
27. Low JW, Arimond M, Osman N, Cunguara B, Zano F, Tschirley D. Ensuring supply and creating demand for a biofortified crop with a visible trait: Lessons learned from the introduction of orange-fleshed sweet potato in drought-prone areas of Mozambique. Food Nutr Bull. 2007;28:S258–70.
28. Unlu NZ, Bohn T, Clinton SK, Schwartz SJ. Carotenoid absorption from salad and salsa by humans is enhanced by the addition of avocado or avocado oil. J Nutr. 2005;135:431–6.
29. Jayarajan P, Reddy V, Mohanram M. Effect of dietary fat on absorption of β-carotene from green leafy vegetables in children. Indian J Med Res. 1980;71:53–66.
30. Faber M, Laurie S, van Jaarsveld P. Nutrient content and consumer acceptability for different cultivars of orange-fleshed sweetpotato. Report to the South African Sugar Association; 2008. Project no 202.
31. Woolfe JA. Sweet potato—past and present. In: Sweet potato: an untapped food resource. Cambridge, United Kingdom: Cambridge University Press; 1992. p. 15–40.
32. Black RE, Allen LH, Bhutta ZA, et al. Maternal and child undernutrition: global and regional exposures and health consequences. Lancet. 2008;371:243–60.
33. Leighton CS. Nutrient and sensory quality of orange-fleshed sweetpotato. University of Pretoria, Pretoria, South Africa; 2007. MSc Thesis.
34. Leighton CS, Schönfeldt HC, Kruger R. Quantitative descriptive sensory analysis of five different cultivars of sweet potato to determine sensory and textural profiles. J Sensory Studies. 2010;25:2–18.
35. Kays SJ, Wang Y. Thermally induced flavor compounds. HortSci. 2000;35:1002–12.
36. Tomlins K, Ndunguru G, Stambul K, et al. Sensory evaluation and consumer acceptability of pale-fleshed and orange-fleshed sweetpotato by school children and mothers of preschool children. J Sci Food Agric. 2007;87:2436–46.
37. Yanggen D, Nagujja S. The use of orange-fleshed sweet potato to combat vitamin A deficiency in Uganda. A study of varietal preferences, extension strategies and post-harvest utilization. Lima, Peru: International Potato Center (CIP); 2006. p. 80.
38. Tomlins K, Rwiza E, Nyangon A, et al. The use of sensory evaluation and consumer preference for the selection of sweetpotato cultivars in East Africa. J Sci Food Agric. 2004;84:791–9.
39. Masumba E, Kapinga R, Tollan SM, Mary O, Yongolo, Kitundu CD. Adaptability and acceptability of new orange-fleshed sweetpotato varieties in selected areas of Eastern and Central zones of Tanzania. Proceedings of the 13th

ISTRC Symposium; 2007:737-745. http://www.istrc.org/Symposiums/Tanzania_03/vitaa_masumba.pdf. Accessed 12 Dec 2011.

40. Low J, Walker T, Hijmans R. The potential impact of orange-fleshed sweet potatoes on vitamin A intake in Sub-Saharan Africa. The VITAA Project, Vitamin A and orange-fleshed sweetpotatoes in sub-Saharan Africa, Nairobi, Kenya, 2001. http://www.cipotato.org/publications/pdf/002221.pdf. Accessed 12 Dec 2011
41. Rodriguez-Amaya DB. Some considerations in generating carotenoid data for food composition tables. J Food Comp Anal. 2000;13:641–7.
42. Laurie SM. Sweetpotato in perspective. In: Niederwieser JG, editor. Guide to sweet potato production in South Africa. Pretoria: Agricultural Research Council; 2004. p. 1–6.
43. Department of Agriculture, Forestry and Fisheries (DAFF). A profile of the South African sweet potato market value chain 2010. DAFF, Pretoria, South Africa. http://www.daff.gov.za/docs/AMCP/SweetPotatoVCP2010-11.pdf. Accessed 12 Dec 2011.
44. Ukpabi UJ, Ekeledo EN. Feasibility of using orange-fleshed sweet potato as an alternative to carrot in Nigerian salad preparations. Agric J. 2009;4:216–20.
45. Low JW, van Jaarsveld PJ. The potential contribution of bread buns fortified with β-carotene-rich sweet potato in Central Mozambique. Food Nutr Bull. 2008;29:98–107.
46. Bechoff A, Poulaert M, Tomlins KI, et al. Retention and bioaccessibility of β-carotene in blended foods containing orange-fleshed sweet potato flour. J Agric Food Chem. 2011;59:10373–80.
47. Bechoff A, Dufour D, Dhuique-Mayer C, Marouzé C, Reynes M, Westby A. Effect of hot air, solar and sun drying treatments on provitamin A retention in orange-fleshed sweetpotato. J Food Eng. 2009;92:164–71.
48. Bechoff A, Tomlins K, Dhuique-Mayer C, Dove R, Westby A. On-farm evaluation of the impact of drying and storage on the carotenoid content of orange-fleshed sweet potato (*Ipomea batata* Lam.). Int J Food Sci Technol. 2011;46:52–60.
49. Faber M, Laubscher R. Seasonal availability and dietary intake of β-carotene-rich vegetables and fruit of 2-year-old to 5-year-old children in a rural South African setting growing these crops at household level. Int J Food Sci Nutr. 2008;59:46–60.
50. Agrios GN. Plant pathology, 5th ed. Elsevier Academic Press; 2005. p. 300–301.
51. Du Plooy CP, van den Berg AA, Laurie SM. Production systems for orange-flesh sweetpotato. In: Faber M, Laurie S, van Jaarsveld P, editors. Proceedings orange-fleshed sweetpotato symposium. Pretoria, 3 Oct 2007. Cape Town, South African Medical Research Council; 2008. p. 25–8.
52. Van Jaarsveld P. Retention of β-carotene in boiled orange-fleshed sweetpotato and during storage: Importance of nutrient content for nutritional impact. In: Faber M, Laurie S, van Jaarsveld P, editors. Proceedings orange-fleshed sweetpotato symposium. Pretoria, 3 Oct 2007. Cape Town, South African Medical Research Council; 2008. p. 63–8.
53. Bovell-Benjamin AC. Sweet potato: a review of its past, present, and future role in human nutrition. Adv Food Nutr Res. 2007;52:1–59.
54. Hendriks SL. The potential for nutritional benefits from increased agricultural production in rural KwaZulu-Natal. S Afr J Agric Ext. 2003;32:28–44.
55. Prentice AM. The emerging epidemic of obesity in developing countries. Int J Epidemiol. 2006;35:93–9.
56. Faber M, Laurie SM. A home-gardening approach developed in South Africa to address vitamin A deficiency. In: Thompson B, Amoroso L, editors. Combating micronutrient deficiencies: Food-based approaches. CABI and FAO; 2011. p. 163–82.
57. Laurie S, Faber M. Integrated community-based growth monitoring and vegetable gardens focusing on crops rich in β-carotene: Project evaluation in a rural community in the Eastern Cape, South Africa. J Sci Food Agric. 2008;88:2093–101.

Chapter 20
International Efforts to Eradicate Vitamin A Deficiency

Sherry A. Tanumihardjo and Harold C. Furr

Key Points

- Achieving food security of macronutrients and micronutrients is of paramount concern, both for humanitarian and security reasons.
- Although its biology and chemistry are unique, vitamin A serves as a paradigm for micronutrient public health interventions. Alleviation of vitamin A deficiency can be achieved by administration of preformed vitamin A through supplementation and food fortification. However, long-term solutions should involve increased intake of provitamin A carotenoids (i.e., β-carotene, α-carotene, and β-cryptoxanthin) from foods.
- Dietary diversification includes increased consumption of naturally occurring rich sources of β-carotene such as red palm oil, orange and yellow fruits and vegetables, and green leafy vegetables.
- Both traditional plant breeding techniques and molecular biology can be used to increase provitamin A carotenoid content of these foods.
- A number of international organizations, including the Consultative Group for International Agricultural Research, the Global Alliance for Improved Nutrition, Heller Keller International, Sight and Life, the United Nations Children's Fund, the World Health Organization, and the World Vegetable Center, are involved in alleviating vitamin A deficiency with different combinations of the approaches outlined here.
- A multipronged approach is needed to eradicate vitamin A deficiency in the world.

Keywords Dietary diversification • Fortification • International organizations • Supplementation • Vitamin A

S.A. Tanumihardjo, M.S., Ph.D. (✉) • H.C. Furr, M.N.S., Ph.D.
Department of Nutritional Sciences, University of Wisconsin-Madison, 1415 Linden Dr, Madison, WI 53706, USA
e-mail: sherry@nutrisci.wisc.edu

S.A. Tanumihardjo (ed.), *Carotenoids and Human Health*, Nutrition and Health,
DOI 10.1007/978-1-62703-203-2_20, © Springer Science+Business Media New York 2013

Introduction

Individual and household food security must be a basic right for all, but achieving this goal continues to challenge us. Hunger, malnutrition, and associated poor health afflict as many as 2 billion people today [1], and may affect greater numbers as the world's population grows to 9 billion by 2050, further challenging availability and access to sufficient nutritious food. Achieving universal food security involves much more than ensuring a sufficient supply of food to feed the world's population; food security "exists when all people, at all times, have physical and economic access to sufficient, safe, and nutritious food to meet their dietary needs and food preferences for an active and healthy life" [2]. There is no simple or single solution to such a complex challenge for any nutrient, including the vitamin A needs of the world.

No single approach will be adequate for alleviation of vitamin A deficiency in all settings. Each situation of apparent vitamin A inadequacy must be evaluated to determine the subgroup(s) of the population most at risk, the extent of the problem, and appropriate approaches to meet vitamin A needs. Methods to alleviate vitamin A deficiency have included supplementation programs, food fortification, and promotion of vitamin A-rich (or provitamin A carotenoid-rich) foods [3]. Supplementation programs, whether using tablets or orally administered oil solutions, are usually more expensive when one considers the resources needed to implement them [4], the fact that the intervention needs to be frequently repeated, and supplements may not provide adequate coverage in all settings. However, vitamin A supplements to preschool children have proven to reduce childhood mortality [5] and programs should continue until other more sustainable interventions are in place. Food fortification has proven to be effective in some environments, but requires identification of a suitable vehicle for fortification that reaches the target audience. Dietary diversification supported by nutrition education, use of home gardens, and plant breeding for higher provitamin A carotenoids will most likely provide long-term, sustainable results, but is slowest to implement. Supplementation and/or food fortification are efficacious as short-term interventions until long-term solutions are universally available. Table 20.1 outlines the relative costs of various intervention strategies used to alleviate vitamin A deficiency.

Eradication of vitamin A deficiency is indeed a global effort to improve human health and prevent mortality. The Vitamin A Global Initiative partners currently include the United Nations Children's Fund (UNICEF), the World Health Organization (WHO), the Canadian International Development Agency (CIDA), the United Kingdom's Department for International Development (DfID), the United States Agency for International Development (USAID), and the Micronutrient Initiative (MI) [6]. This chapter reviews current efforts to eradicate vitamin A deficiency including those which involve provitamin A carotenoids and discusses some of the organizations dedicated to the cause.

Supplementation

The WHO gives advice to member states on vitamin A supplementation regimens as discussed in Chaps. 15 and 16. All vitamin A supplements in public health programs are provided as retinyl ester, although β-carotene supplements have been used in research settings to women [7, 8]. Meta-analyses of vitamin A supplementation trials have found that supplementation is effective in reducing all-cause mortality by about 24 % compared with no treatment and further placebo-controlled trials in children between 6 months and 5 years of age are not needed [5]. Thus, WHO continues to recommend supplementation to this age group of children to reduce mortality risk [9]. Although vitamin A supplements have been successfully implemented by many developing countries, more sustainable, long-term solutions are recommended by experts. Thus, promoting provitamin A sources alongside of supplementation efforts is desirable in achieving the goal of eradicating vitamin A deficiency [10].

Table 20.1 Economic costs of alternative interventions

Criteria	Fortification	Tablets	Injections	Nutrition education	Home gardens	Plant breeding
Costs						
Initial capital investments	Moderate	Low	Low	Low	Low	High
Continuing personnel	Low	High	High	High	Low	High
Continuing materials	Low	Low	Moderate	Low	Moderate	High
Personnel requirements						
Skill level	Moderate	Moderate	High	Low	Moderate	High
Numbers	Low	High	High	Moderate	High	Low
Administrative requirements						
Supervision	Moderate	High	High	Moderate	Moderate	High
Health system organization	Low	High	High	Moderate	Low	Low
Technical feasibility						
Technological dependability	High	High	Moderate	Moderate	High	Moderate
Side effects risk	Low	Moderate	High	Low	Low	Moderate
Beneficiary role						
Acceptability	High	Moderate	Moderate	Moderate	Moderate	Moderate
Community involvement	Low	Moderate	Moderate	High	High	Low
Impact						
Population coverage	High	Moderate	Moderate	Moderate	Moderate	Moderate
Time needed to show benefit	Moderate	Low	Low	Moderate	Low	High
Permanency of benefit	High	Low	Low	Moderate	High	High

Adapted from [27]

Food Fortification and Biofortification

Fortification of staple foods with preformed vitamin A has been used to alleviate vitamin A deficiency in countries with appropriate infrastructure. Carrier vehicles (foods) have been chosen to effectively deliver vitamin A to specific target groups, including milk, cooking oil, margarine, wheat and maize flours, sugar, and monosodium glutamate. The acetate and palmitate esters of vitamin A (retinyl acetate and palmitate) have been the usual forms of vitamin A chosen because they are highly bioavailable, relatively stable chemically, and are readily incorporated into oil matrices. Programs using these fortified foods are successful in some settings, especially sugar fortification [11, 12]. But conventional food fortification requires development and implementation of appropriate technology (an expense which must be covered by either local or international governmental support), may require appropriate storage of the fortified food or fortificant before mixing, and also requires distribution of the fortified food to the target population.

Although fortification with preformed vitamin A is successful at eradicating vitamin A deficiency, there is always the risk of toxicity with preformed sources of vitamin A [3]. Fears of excessive intakes have inhibited or prevented implementation of some fortification programs. Fortification of foods with provitamin A carotenoids is proposed as the safest means of increasing vitamin A intake of a population, because there is little or no known danger of over-intake of carotenoids and also because conversion of provitamin A carotenoids to vitamin A is highly regulated as discussed in Chap. 3. The major disadvantages of fortifying foods with provitamin A carotenoids are that these compounds are highly pigmented and chemically unstable when exposed to light and oxygen. Nonetheless, hypervitaminosis A from dietary intake of provitamin A carotenoids has never been demonstrated as discussed in Chaps. 14 and 15. This is a clear advantage of biofortification approaches as discussed extensively in Section III of this book. However, as shown in Section I of this book, the extent of conversion of carotenoids to vitamin A depends on a number of factors, and varies widely from one individual to another. Factors that positively affect the efficiency of bioavailability and bioconversion include co-consumption of fat and cooking [10], but those that negatively affect conversion are still being elucidated and may include individual genetic polymorphisms as discussed in Chap. 7. Lack of knowledge will not prevent successful implementation of biofortification programs, but increased knowledge of these factors will promote more efficient implementation.

Dietary Diversification

UNICEF suggests that wherever possible, including meat, eggs, fruit, red palm-oil, green leafy vegetables, and carrots in the diet will further ensure adequate vitamin A consumption [6]. Red palm oil is naturally high in β-carotene and has been promoted as an efficacious source of vitamin A especially in tropical regions [13]. Promoting vegetable consumption in general is always considered part of a healthy diet because of the associated benefits.

Biofortification is a form of dietary diversification and for vitamin A refers to breeding a staple crop, vegetable, or fruit with enhanced concentrations of provitamin A carotenoids. As this book has demonstrated, particularly in Chap. 17, a wide variety of scientific disciplines must interact in order to establish an effective biofortification program: biology (plant biochemistry, molecular biology), plant physiology, plant breeding and agronomy, seed technology, food technology, analytical chemistry, nutrition, socioeconomics, extension and communication, education, and medicine (Table 20.2; [10]).

In principle, any food which naturally contains provitamin A carotenoids (β-carotene, α-carotene, or β-cryptoxanthin) can potentially be bred to have enhanced dietary vitamin A value. Thus, orange-yellow fruits and vegetables (e.g., carrots, mango, papaya, orange, and tangerine) and leafy green vegetables (e.g., kale, spinach, brussels sprouts, and ivy gourd leaf) have been studied. In addition to

Table 20.2 Some of the disciplines involved in establishing a biofortified crop from seeds to bowls

Disciplines	Tasks
Biology (plant biochemistry, molecular biology)	Knowledge and cutting-edge technologies for rapid breeding of biofortified varieties
Plant breeding and agronomy	Development and testing of the agricultural suitability of biofortified varieties
Plant physiology	Knowledge of metabolic pathways to enhance efficiency of breeding and foresight of selection effects (biofortification of seed) on plant function
Analytical chemistry	Method development to analyze nutrients in crops, screen crops for nutrient concentrations
Food technology	Food product development, optional markets, retention studies
Nutrition	Test food products in animal and human models, nutrition education
Socioeconomics	Market, impact, acceptability
Extension	Farmer-participatory variety evaluation, validation, and demand-creation
Education	Behavior change
Medicine	Morbidity studies, health status of target populations
Communication	Product dissemination, nutrition education, public and private sector awareness, and engagement
Seed technology	Maintenance and production of high-quality, affordable seed parent stocks, and commercial seed

From reference [10], Int J Vitamin Nutr Res. 2010;80:336–350 (c)

traditional breeding, genetic techniques allow incorporation of carotenoid-producing genes into foods which traditionally have not contained carotenoids, such as rice [14].

Plant-based dietary sources of provitamin A, e.g., red palm oil, green vegetables, or biofortified staple crops, are the desirable approach to meeting vitamin A needs [10]. Indigenous leafy green vegetables can make a difference in vitamin A status [15], and horticultural development as discussed in Chap. 18 could help ensure their availability and consumption in appropriate amounts to make a difference in vitamin A status [16, 17].

Organizations and Institutions Dedicated to Eradicating Vitamin A Deficiency

Consultative Group for International Agricultural Research

The Consultative Group for International Agricultural Research (CGIAR), briefly mentioned in Chaps. 17 and 18, is a global partnership that unites international and regional organizations and funders engaged in research for sustainable development including governments and foundations. The Consortium of International Agricultural Research Centers has 15 members in close collaboration with hundreds of partner organizations, including national and regional research institutes, civil society organizations, academia, and the private sector [18]. The CGIAR centers not only support global food security but also the need for agricultural development to support nutritional security and human health [19]. Part of the mission is to support biofortification of staple foods (e.g., maize, sweet potato, cassava, rice) with provitamin A carotenoids to improve vitamin A status in developing countries.

Global Alliance for Improved Nutrition

Global Alliance for Improved Nutrition (GAIN) is an international alliance headquartered in Geneva, Switzerland whose vision is to have a world without malnutrition. It was created in 2002 and supports public–private partnerships to increase access to missing nutrients in poor quality diets. GAIN has scaled-up its operations by working with more than 600 companies in more than 25 countries [20]. Although they are currently reaching about 400 million people with nutritionally enhanced foods, their goal is to reach >1 billion people with fortified foods that are sustainable. One of the targeted nutrients for GAIN is vitamin A. Examples of products that GAIN has supported include vitamin A-fortified cooking oil, rice, and "sprinkles," which are small sachets of micronutrients that can be mixed into weaning foods. All of these products contain preformed retinyl palmitate.

Helen Keller International

Helen Keller International (HKI) is among the oldest nongovernmental organizations (founded in 1915) which is devoted to preventing blindness and reducing malnutrition [21]. They work in 22 countries, which include 13 in Africa, 8 in Asia, and the USA. HKI designs, implements, and monitors programs that ensure delivery of vitamin A supplements to vulnerable populations. These programs help to save the sight and lives of thousands of children. The promotion of orange-fleshed sweetpotato high in β-carotene in West Africa is among HKI's agendas [22], and its benefits are discussed extensively in Chap. 19.

Sight and Life

Sight and Life, which was founded in 1986, is a nonprofit humanitarian initiative originally organized by the DSM company. It participates in the global fight to prevent micronutrient deficiencies through sharing funds, knowledge, policy, and technology [23]. In 2012, DSM decided to channel Sight and Life activities through the charitable organization called Vitamin Angels. Sight and Life provides vitamin A, mostly in the form of capsules, to children's and women's supplementation projects to support those who are most at risk of vitamin A deficiency in developing countries. To ensure that the supplements are provided according to international guidelines and recommendations, they also provide technical assistance.

United Nations Children's Fund

United Nations Children's Fund (UNICEF) works in about 190 countries and territories with the purpose of advancing children's rights. UNICEF has been involved in the progress made to eliminate vitamin A deficiency and desires that this progress be sustainable and in reach to all children in need [6]. Currently, many vitamin A supplementation programs are linked to polio immunization campaigns, but as the world nears its goal of eradicating polio, another delivery mechanism must be found.

UNICEF understands the importance of educating governments, health professionals, policymakers, and the public about the benefits of vitamin A and they support three strategies to eliminate vitamin A deficiency: vitamin A supplements during health interventions especially to children 6–59 months, fortifying staples such as sugar in Central America, and diversifying foods. UNICEF further supports logistical planning, provides supplements, and assists in monitoring and evaluation. Today the majority of children in more than 40 countries are receiving at least one vitamin A supplement yearly. UNICEF estimates that as many as 300,000 child deaths are prevented each year due to vitamin A supplementation [6].

World Health Organization

One of WHO's core functions is to provide evidence-based recommendations on global guidelines to improve human health [24]. WHO's guidelines for nutrition include vitamin A supplementation programs [25]. As discussed briefly in Chaps. 15 and 16, at the present time high-dose vitamin A supplementation is only recommended for children 6–59 months of age and may be the single most cost-effective child survival intervention [6]. Recommended doses are 100,000 IU for infants 6–11 months of age and 200,000 IU for children 12–59 months of age, which provides adequate protection from clinical deficiency in most populations for 4–6 months [9]. Evidence to reduce maternal and infant mortality by supplementing other vulnerable groups is currently lacking.

World Vegetable Center (AVRDC)

The AVRDC, briefly covered in Chap. 18, is a nonprofit research and development institution whose mission is to alleviate poverty and malnutrition in the developing world through the increased production and consumption of nutritious and health-promoting vegetables [26]. Some of their programs include vegetable seed kits for sub-Saharan Africa and South Asia for use in home gardening. The kits contain approximately 20 different kinds of high yielding and nutritious vegetables, with enough seeds to plant a home garden to provide a family with a healthy diet for a year. The vegetable crops are selected to meet local environmental conditions and dietary preferences and can supply vitamin A requirements as provitamin A carotenoids.

Conclusions

Achieving universal food security, including alleviating the chronic malnutrition problems that afflict nearly one-third of the world's population, will require multidisciplinary partnerships across agriculture, nutrition, health, education, and other fields. The catalytic role of agricultural development in contributing to poverty alleviation is well-recognized, but the intermediate outcomes of improved nutrition and health are often overlooked. Multidisciplinary teamwork along a research and outreach continuum from field to bowl is needed to truly improve human health through the adoption of biofortified foods or diversification of diets. Key steps to alleviating vitamin A deficiency include developing the foods, validating the nutritional effects, and promoting foods with provitamin A carotenoids. Scaling up nutritional interventions, such as those associated with improving vitamin A status through higher consumption of provitamin A carotenoids, needs to be coupled with scaling up agriculture to sustainably improve global health.

References

1. Barrett CB. Measuring food insecurity. Science. 2010;327:825–8.
2. FAO. Rome declaration on world food security and world food summit plan of action. FAO corporate document repository. 1996. http://www.fao.org/docrep/003/w3613e/w3613e00.HTM.
3. Tanumihardjo SA. Food-based approaches for ensuring adequate vitamin A nutrition. Compr Rev Food Sci Food Saf. 2008;7:373–81.
4. Neidecker-Gonzales O, Nestel P, Bouis H. Estimating the global costs of vitamin A capsule supplementation: a review of the literature. Food Nutr Bull. 2007;28(3):307–16.
5. Imdad A, Herzer K, Mayo-Wilson E, Yakoob MY, Bhutta ZA. Vitamin A supplementation for preventing morbidity and mortality in children from 6 months to 5 years of age. Cochrane Database Syst Rev. 2010;12:CD008524.
6. UNICEF. Micronutrients—iodine, iron and vitamin A. http://www.unicef.org/nutrition/index_iodine.html. Accessed Dec 2011.
7. West Jr KP, Christian P, Labrique AB, Rashid M, Shamim AA, Klemm RD, Massie AB, Mehra S, Schulze KJ, Ali H, Ullah B, Wu LS, Katz J, Banu H, Akhter HH, Sommer A. Effects of vitamin A or beta-carotene supplementation on pregnancy-related mortality and infant mortality in rural Bangladesh: a cluster randomized trial. JAMA. 2011;305(19):1986–95.
8. Rice AL, Stoltzfus RJ, de Francisco A, Chakraborty J, Kjolhede CL, Wahed MA. Maternal vitamin A or beta-carotene supplementation in lactating Bangladeshi women benefits mothers and infants but does not prevent sub-clinical deficiency. J Nutr. 1999;129(2):356–65.
9. World Health Organization. Guideline: vitamin A supplementation for infants and children 6-59 months of age. Geneva: World Health Organization; 2011.
10. Tanumihardjo SA, Palacios N, Pixley KV. Provitamin A carotenoid bioavailability: what really matters? Int J Vitam Nutr Res. 2010;80:336–50.
11. Dary O, Mora JO. Food fortification to reduce vitamin A deficiency: International Vitamin A Consultative Group Recommendations. J Nutr. 2002;132:2927S–33.
12. Ribaya-Mercado JD, Solomons NW, Medrano Y, Bulux J, Dolnikowski GG, Russell RM, Wallace CB. Use of the deuterated-retinol-dilution technique to monitor the vitamin A status of Nicaraguan schoolchildren 1 y after initiation of the Nicaraguan national program of sugar fortification with vitamin A. Am J Clin Nutr. 2004;80:1291–8.
13. Rice AL, Burns JB. Moving from efficacy to effectiveness: red palm oil's role in preventing vitamin A deficiency. J Am Coll Nutr. 2010;29(3 Suppl):302S–13.

14. Paine JA, Shipton CA, Chaggar S, Howells RM, Kennedy MJ, Vernon G, Wright SY, Hinchliffe E, Adams JL, Silverstone AL, Drake R. Improving the nutritional value of golden rice through increased pro-vitamin A content. Nat Biotechnol. 2005;23:482–7.
15. Ejoh RA, Dever JT, Mills JP, Tanumihardjo SA. Small quantities of carotenoid-rich tropical green leafy-vegetables indigenous to Africa maintain vitamin A status in Mongolian gerbils (*Meriones unguiculatus*). Br J Nutr. 2010;103:1594–601.
16. De Pee S, West CE, Muhilal, Karyadi D, Hautvast JG. Lack of improvement in vitamin A status with increased consumption of dark-green leafy vegetables. Lancet. 1995;346:75–81.
17. Tanumihardjo SA. Can lack of improvement in vitamin A status indicators be explained by little or no overall change in vitamin A status of humans? J Nutr. 2001;131:3316–8.
18. Consultative Group for International Agricultural Research CGIAR. www.cgiar.org. Accessed Dec 2011.
19. CGIAR Fund Office. The CGIAR at 40 and Beyond: Impacts that Matter for the Poor and the Planet. June 2011.
20. GAIN (Global Alliance for Improved Nutrition). http://www.gainhealth.org. Accessed Dec 2011.
21. Helen Keller International. http://www.hki.org/. Accessed Dec 2011.
22. Biofortification. http://www.hki.org/reducing-malnutrition/biofortification/. Accessed Dec 2011.
23. Sight and Life. http://www.sightandlife.org/. Accessed Dec 2011.
24. World Health Organization. http://www.who.int/publications/guidelines/en/index.html. Accessed Dec 2011.
25. World Health Organization. http://www.who.int/publications/guidelines/nutrition/en/index.html. Accessed Dec 2011.
26. AVRDC - The World Vegetable Center. http://www.avrdc.org/. Accessed Dec 2011.
27. Bauernfeind JC. Nutrification of foods. In: Shils ME, Olson JA, Shike M, editors. Modern nutrition in health and disease. Philadelphia: Lea & Febiger; 1994. p. 1579–92.

Index

S.A. Tanumihardjo (ed.), *Carotenoids and Human Health*, Nutrition and Health,
DOI 10.1007/978-1-62703-203-2, © Springer Science+Business Media New York 2013

MIX
Papier aus verantwortungsvollen Quellen
Paper from responsible sources
FSC® C105338

If you have any concerns about our products,
you can contact us on
ProductSafety@springernature.com

In case Publisher is established outside the EU,
the EU authorized representative is:
Springer Nature Customer Service Center GmbH
Europaplatz 3, 69115 Heidelberg, Germany

Printed by Libri Plureos GmbH
in Hamburg, Germany